HIV/AIDS

HIV/AIDS

A Guide to Nursing Care

THIRD EDITION

Jacquelyn Haak Flaskerud, PhD, RN, FAAN
Professor, School of Nursing
University of California, Los Angeles
Los Angeles, California

Peter J. Ungvarski, MS, RN, FAAN
Clinical Nurse Specialist, HIV Infection
VNS Home Care
Visiting Nurse Service of New York
New York, New York

W.B. SAUNDERS COMPANY

A Division of Harcourt Brace & Company
Philadelphia   London   Toronto   Montreal   Sydney   Tokyo

W.B. SAUNDERS COMPANY
A Division of Harcourt Brace & Company

The Curtis Center
Independence Square West
Philadelphia, PA 19106

Library of Congress Cataloging-in-Publication Data
HIV/AIDS : a guide to nursing care / [edited by] Jacquelyn Haak Flaskerud, Peter J. Ungvarski.—3rd ed.
p.   cm.
Includes bibliographical references and index.
ISBN 0-7216-5239-5
1. AIDS (Disease)—Nursing.   I. Flaskerud, Jacquelyn Haak.
II. Ungvarski, Peter J.
[DNLM: 1. Acquired Immunodeficiency Syndrome—nursing.
2. HIV Infections—nursing.   WY   150   H676   1995]
RC607.A26A3473   1995
610.73'699—dc20
DNLM/DLC
94-32150

HIV/AIDS: A GUIDE TO NURSING CARE   ISBN   0-7216-5239-5

Printed in United States of America

Last digit is the print number: 9 8 7 6 5 4 3 2

To Tom
For his courage, commitment, and intelligence
and to
John and Jimie
For their faith and love

Contributors

MARY G. BOLAND, MSN, RN, CPNP

Associate in Pediatrics, University of Medicine and Dentistry of New Jersey, New Jersey Medical School; Director, Children's Hospital AIDS Program and National Pediatric HIV Resource Center, United Hospital Medical Center, Newark, New Jersey

Nursing Care of the Child

PENNY S. BROOKE, JD, MS, RN

Assistant Dean and Associate Professor, University of Utah College of Nursing; Trustee, Intermountain Health Care; Board of Governors, Salt Lake Valley Hospitals, Salt Lake City, Utah

Legal Issues Related to the Care of Persons With HIV

KATHLEEN McMAHON CASEY, MEd, MA, RN, OCN

Associate, Columbia University School of Nursing, New York, New York; National Director, Clinical Program Development, Caremark Healthcare Services Division, Caremark, Northbrook, Illinois

Pathophysiology of HIV-1, Clinical Course, and Treatment

MAUREEN CONNOLLY, BSN

Director, High Tech Program, Visiting Nurse Association of Staten Island, Staten Island, New York

Personal Perspectives on Nursing Care

LYNN CZARNIECKI, MSN, RN

Clinical Nurse Specialist, Children's Hospital AIDS Program, Children's Hospital of New Jersey, Newark, New Jersey

Nursing Care of the Child

THOMAS E. EMANUELE, RN, C, MsT

Nurse Consultant, HIV Early Intervention Program, HIV/AIDS/STD Bureau, Public Health Division, New Mexico Department of Health, Albuquerque, New Mexico

Personal Perspectives on Nursing Care

CHRISTINE FEGAN, BSN, RN

Nursing Director, AIDS Clinical Trials Group, University of California at San Diego, San Diego, California

Personal Perspectives on Nursing Care

JACQUELYN HAAK FLASKERUD, PhD, RN, FAAN

Professor and Associate Dean for Academic Affairs, University of California at Los Angeles, Los Angeles, California

Overview of HIV Disease and Nursing
Health Promotion and Disease Prevention
Psychosocial and Psychiatric Aspects
Culture and Ethnicity

KATHRYN J. FOLEY, MS, RN

Public Health Nurse, TB Control, Department of Health and Hospitals, Boston, Massachusetts

Personal Perspectives on Nursing Care

MARTHA W. MOON, MS, RN

Family Nurse Practitioner; Doctoral Student, University of California at San Francisco School of Nursing, San Francisco, California

Nursing Care of the Adolescent

KATHLEEN M. NOKES, PhD, RN, FAAN

Associate Professor and Project Director, Nursing of Persons with HIV/AIDS Subspecialty; HIV Nurse Clinician, Wordhull Medical and Mental Health Center, Brooklyn, New York

Nursing Care of Women

NANCY B. PARRIS, MPH, RN, CIC

Assistant Clinical Professor, University of California at Los Angeles School of Nursing; Infection Control and Epidemiology Consultant, Santa Marta Hospital and Clinical Science Laboratory, Los Angeles, California

Infection Control

JUDITH M. SAUNDERS, DNSc, FAAN

Clinical Associate Professor, Department of Nursing, University of Southern California, Los Angeles; Assistant Research Scientist, Department of Nursing Research, City of Hope National Medical Center, Duarte, California

Ethical Issues Related to the Care of Persons With HIV

JOAN SCHMIDT, MS, MPH, RN

Clinical Instructor, AIDS Services, Visiting Nurse Service of New York, New York, New York

Nursing Management of the Adult Client
Community-Based and Long-Term Care

JO ANNE STAATS, MSN, RN, ANP

Adult Nurse Practitioner, St. Vincent's Hospital and Medical Center, AIDS Center, New York, New York

Clinical Manifestations of AIDS in Adults
Nursing Care of Chemically Dependent Clients

PETER J. UNGVARSKI, MS, RN, FAAN

Clinical Associate, City University of New York, Hunter College–Bellevue School of Nursing; Clinical Nurse Specialist, HIV Infection, Visiting Nurse Service of New York, New York, New York

Clinical Manifestations of AIDS in Adults
Nursing Management of the Adult Client
Community-Based and Long-Term Care

DEBORAH L. WOLEN, RN, CMS

Nurse Practitioner, HIV Primary Care Center, Cook County Hospital, Chicago, Illinois

Personal Perspectives on Nursing Care

Preface

HIV disease is an individual and public health problem in which nurses and nursing care play a vital and comprehensive role. This text grew out of a need among nurses for information about AIDS and HIV infection. The content of the first two editions of the book was based on surveys of nurses in which they identified their needs for information about HIV/AIDS. These nurses made valuable suggestions for defining the scope of the book. Since the second edition was published, nurses have made major contributions to public awareness, scientific advances, and state-of-the-art clinical practice in HIV disease. Two important events were the reports of the National Commission on AIDS (1993) and the Early HIV Infection Clinical Practice Guidelines published by the Agency for Health Care Policy and Research (1994), both of which included noteworthy contributions by nurses. These documents are incorporated into this text and reflect the significant work of nurses in advancing and defining clinical practice in HIV nursing. Notably a nurse, Kristine Gebbie, was elevated to national prominence when she was appointed by President Clinton as the Coordinator of AIDS Programs in the United States. Although she has since stepped down, these events plus changes in the science of HIV, consequent changes in practice, and the changing knowledge needs of nurses have influenced the content of this third edition.

The third edition constitutes a greatly expanded and detailed guide to nursing, human service, and medical care, including the care of women, adolescents, children, and intravenous drug users. As in the first two editions, the focus of the text remains on clinical practice. The book provides a comprehensive view of the spectrum of HIV disease to assist the nurse in clinical practice, whether that practice be in primary, secondary, or tertiary prevention of HIV. It serves, as well, as an in-depth text for students learning the practice of nursing or specializing in a nursing clinical area. A special section provides nursing faculty with guidelines for incorporating HIV into the curriculum. All health and human service workers who use a case management approach to HIV care will find the book invaluable.

There are several noteworthy new features in the third edition. Each chapter summarizes the nursing research in its content area and makes recommendations for research needed in nursing. This nursing text is unique in that respect. The research needed takes its general direction from the nursing research priorities set by the National Institute of Nursing Research. Also new, the nursing care of adolescents is addressed in depth in its own chapter. Additionally, the book includes a section on issues in HIV nursing that have an impact on practice. These issues include the legal and ethical concerns related to the care of persons with HIV (PWHIV). For the first time, the text includes a chapter on the cultural issues involved in the care of the PWHIV. This chapter is another unique feature of the book; it offers both a conceptual and practical view of environment, social structures, beliefs, and practices.

The introductory chapter provides a context into which the HIV epidemic and the consequent demands on nursing care can be placed:

- An overview of the history of the epidemic; the changing sociodemographic distribution of AIDS in the United States; nurses' knowledge and attitudes, and strategies for changing these; and a model for a developing HIV curriculum with reference to content areas in this text.

Nursing care of persons infected with HIV are addressed in Chapters 2 through 12. These chapters provide guidelines for nursing care that can be applied in the hospital or in the community.

- Health promotion and disease prevention with a detailed section on HIV testing and counseling; a focus on cofactors of transmission and disease expression; and a review of successful primary prevention programs.
- A description of the characteristics of HIV and how it affects the immune system; the pathophysiologic effects of HIV on organ systems; an overview of therapies.
- A comprehensive delineation of common infections and neoplasms associated with AIDS in adults and their medical treatment; a summary of common drugs in use and their side effects.
- An in-depth nursing care plan for managing the adult client with HIV disease through primary, secondary, and tertiary prevention measures; the plan is based on symptom assessment and organized by nursing diagnosis.
- A multifaceted look at the nursing care of children with HIV/AIDS; current treatments available, home care and the changing needs of children and their families.
- Epidemiology of HIV in teenagers; pertinent growth and development issues; educational strategies; providing care for disenfranchised youth; monitoring the course of HIV in adolescents.
- The special problems of women with HIV/AIDS: prevention, transmission, presenting diagnoses, treatment, pregnancy.
- Issues and nursing care specific to persons with chemical dependencies: substance abuse, transmission and treatments available.
- Infection control guidelines applicable to the hospital, the home, and community facilities; information on risk to health care workers (HCWs) and household contacts; transmission of HIV from HCWs to their patients.
- The psychosocial and spiritual needs of persons with HIV disease, their families, lovers, spouses, and friends, and the nurses caring for them; common psychiatric and neuropsychiatric disorders of PWHIV and their nursing and medical treatment.

Additional information that will assist nurses in counseling, education, referrals, and community care is provided in Chapter 12.

- The various community activities that occur surrounding HIV disease: education, counseling, referrals, home care and hospice care organized from a case management perspective.

Several issues involved in the care of persons with HIV influence their nursing care and are addressed in Chapters 13 through 15.

- Principles of ethical care with examples for decision making in treatment, testing, assisted suicide; nursing's caring perspective and how that influences ethical dilemmas.
- Legal guidelines, regulations and laws governing HIV testing, malicious intent, liability of HCWs, assisted suicide.

• Cultural and social diversity issues related to beliefs, practices, models of illness and care, prevention, and nursing practice.

Finally, bringing together and giving meaning to much of the information presented in other chapters, several nurses involved in HIV care share their personal experiences of providing such care on a daily basis (Chapter 16).

Readers of this text should be aware of two phenomena associated with the burgeoning literature on HIV/AIDS. First, information on HIV disease is constantly developing. For instance, knowledge of infection and the markers of disease progression, of early intervention, and of effective treatment may change on a day-to-day basis. This information will affect the care and teaching that nurses provide. Nurses should be cognizant of this constant change and keep themselves up-to-date through continuing education courses and by reading the voluminous literature on HIV/AIDS.

Second, because of the vast amount of literature available, there is a diversity of opinion on risk of infection, transmission, disease expression, and preferred treatment. This diversity is common to all areas of knowledge that are developing and constantly changing but is exaggerated in the case of HIV because of the high rate of mortality associated with the disease, because of the social stigma and moral disapproval associated with the largest transmission groups, and because of the intense competition in the scientific community to discover effective treatment and vaccines. There are currently many unknowns regarding HIV/AIDS. This is partially due to the constant and consistent change in information and partially to the differences in human nature. Opinion on what current information means can reflect attempts to exploit public fear for personal or political gain, competition in the scientific community, public policy and political expediency, professional vs. lay opinion, individual pessimism vs. optimism, and the focus of one discipline as opposed to another. It is important that nurses stay well-informed and abreast of information on HIV disease so that they can sift through the diversity of opinion, give informed care to their clients, and allay their own fears and those of the public. It is in this spirit and with confidence in the intelligence, sensitivity, intentions, and motivation of nurses that the book was written.

Several persons and organizations made important contributions to the development of this third edition. The survey of nurses' information needs and staff support for the project was funded for the two initial editions by the National Institute of Allergy and Infectious Diseases. Special appreciation goes to John Fahey, Director of the Center for Interdisciplinary Research in Immunology and Diseases (CIRID) at UCLA for his belief in and support of the value of the project and his constant encouragement, interest, and ideas. Karen Taka and Diana Shin provided valuable library, editing, and computer assistance and support. The contributing authors were spirited, cooperative, and inspiring, an intelligent and knowledgeable group with whom it was an honor to work. Our editor, Thomas Eoyang, facilitated this project through his constant belief in it and his unflagging attention, assistance, and editorial advice. Thanks to our friends and family for encouragement, valued critiques, and suggestions. And finally a special thank you once more to our best friends, John Flaskerud and Jimie Rottner, for their good cheer, love, and dedication to the detail, excellence, and completion of this project.

Contents

Overview of HIV Disease and Nursing

Jacquelyn Haak Flaskerud

At this writing, more than 340,000 cases of acquired immunodeficiency syndrome (AIDS) have been documented in the United States and 1,167,000 people are estimated to be infected by the virus (Centers for Disease Control and Prevention [CDC], October 1993; Mann et al., 1992). Using mortality data for the most recent year available, the CDC projected human immunodeficiency virus (HIV) infection in 1994 as the fifth leading cause of years of potential life lost before age 65 years. This represents a 12.7% increase from 1989 and the largest increase in any of the leading causes of death in the United States during the period (CDC, April 9, 1993). The CDC projects that by the end of 1994 the cumulative number of AIDS cases in the United States will total more than 400,000, with more than 300,000 deaths (*HIV/AIDS Prevention*, May 1993). To date, no cure or vaccine has been found for HIV infection, and predictions are that AIDS will be with us well into the twenty-first century.

WHAT IS HIV DISEASE?

To speak knowledgeably and to understand the disease known as AIDS, one must define the problem in all its complexity. The term *AIDS* is used to indicate only the most severe diseases or clinical conditions (i.e., infections, neoplasms) observed in the continuum of illness related to infection with the retrovirus human immunodeficiency virus type 1 (HIV-1). *Infection with HIV* and *AIDS* are not synonymous terms. Studies of the natural history of HIV infection have documented a wide spectrum of disease conditions ranging from asymptomatic infection to life-threatening conditions characterized by severe immunodeficiency, serious opportunistic infections, and cancers (CDC, Dec. 18, 1992). This range of disease conditions has a strong association with the levels of CD4$^+$ T-lymphocytes per microliter of blood (CDC, 1992b). In the past, published classification schemes for HIV infection stratified various HIV-related illnesses into separate syndromes such as AIDS-related complex and lymphadenopathy syndrome. AIDS itself was classified according to various clinical conditions known as AIDS indicator conditions (CDC, 1986). These different presentations of HIV disease are now considered a continuum of host response to HIV infection and not separate syndromes (Abrams, 1990; Najera et al., 1987; Osmond, 1990). Today in the United States, HIV disease is classified according to CD4$^+$ T-lymphocyte count and clinical conditions associated with HIV infection (CDC, Dec. 18, 1992). The World Health Organization (WHO) has proposed a somewhat different classification scheme based on *stages* of clinical condition and CD4$^+$ T-lymphocyte count. The WHO system incorporates a performance scale and total lymphocyte count in lieu of CD4$^+$ determinations to be used in countries where these are not available (*Global AIDS News*, 1993). These two classification schemes are presented in Table 1–1 for comparison purposes.

Asymptomatic Stage

For purposes of description here, the CDC and WHO classifications are combined. The asymptomatic stage of HIV disease includes an acute primary HIV infection, an asymptomatic condition, and/or persistent generalized lymphadenopathy (PGL) (CDC, Dec. 18, 1992). In the acute infection phase, there is an initial depression of T cells as a result of

Table 1–1. Comparison: 1993 Revised Classification System for HIV Infection (CDC) and WHO Proposed Staging System for HIV Infection and Disease, 1993

CD4+ T-CELL CATEGORIES CDC: 1, 2, 3 WHO: A, B, C	CLINICAL CATEGORIES (CDC): A, B, C CLINICAL STAGING CATEGORIES (WHO): 1, 2, 3, 4					
	(A) ASYMPTOMATIC, HIV, PGL (1) ASYMPTOMATIC		(B) SYMPTOMATIC (2) EARLY (3) INTERMEDIATE		(C) AIDS-INDICATOR (3) INTERMEDIATE (4) LATE	
	CDC	WHO	CDC	WHO	CDC	WHO
1 or A CD4+ ≥500	A1	1A	B1	2A & 3A	C1	3A & 4A
2 or B CD4+ 200–499	A2	1B	B2	2B & 3B	C2	3B & 4B
3 or C CD4+ <200	A3	1C	B3	2C & 3C	C3	3C & 4C

a buildup in p24 antigen levels. A majority of infected people—as many as 90%—have symptoms that resemble a severe flu. These symptoms occur 1 to 3 weeks after infection. Signs and symptoms may include fever, rigors, sore throat, headache, malaise, arthralgias, and myalgias lasting 1 to 2 weeks. A widespread rash, abdominal cramps, and diarrhea may also occur. About 75% of the time a diffuse lymphadenopathy also occurs. Immunologic abnormalities during primary illness may include mild leukopenia, lymphopenia, thrombocytopenia, elevated erythrocyte sedimentation rate, and relative monocytosis (Tindall & Cooper, 1991). During this phase the result of the common test for HIV antibody is usually not positive.

During the asymptomatic phase most people have no significant symptoms. Early in this phase (2 to 18 weeks after infection), the HIV antibody test result will become positive. Commonly used tests are the enzyme-linked immunosorbent assay (ELISA) and the enzyme immunoassay (EIA); the Western blot assay and the immunofluorescence assay (IFA) are used to confirm positive results. Performed correctly and repeatedly, these tests together can identify previous exposure to the virus and avoid false-positive results. In some situations an error might occur, but in general these tests are more than 99% accurate (Menitove, 1990). A test for the p24 part of HIV antigen may detect HIV infection when results of tests for the HIV antibody are negative. However, the practical utility of the test might not match its theoretic importance

given the accuracy of repeated antibody tests (Menitove, 1990). In addition, it has been shown recently that p24 antigenemia is present during only a fraction of the seronegative "window" period (de Saussure et al., 1993).

As noted above, about 75% of persons have a diffuse lymphadenopathy. This swelling of lymph nodes persists in about a third of cases. PGL describes a phase of HIV infection that is characterized by lymph nodes that are located in at least two extrainguinal sites and that are swollen to more than 1 cm for 3 months or longer. In addition to the swollen, sometimes painful nodes, symptoms include fever, night sweats, weight loss, and an enlarged spleen. Prospective studies of persons with clinical signs and symptoms of PGL report rates of progression to AIDS similar to those of symptom-free HIV-seropositive persons (Osmond, 1990).

The asymptomatic stage of infection is matched by the latent phase of virus replication shown in low levels of p24 antigen. Based on estimates and prospective studies, the current median incubation period from infection with HIV until the emergence of symptoms is 9 to 10 years (Osmond, 1990). Nevertheless, there is a steady decrease in CD4+ T-cell levels during this stage—about 40 to 80 cells per microliter for each year of infection (CDC, 1992b).

Early Symptomatic Stage

The early symptomatic stage develops when CD4+ T-cell counts drop to around 500 cells per microliter. Constitutional symptoms such as fever, drenching night sweats, weight loss, fatigue, and lymphadenopathy characterize this stage. Examples of clinical conditions in this stage include candidiasis (oropharyngeal and vulvovaginal), cervical dysplasia, herpes zoster, pelvic inflammatory disease, listeriosis, and peripheral neuropathy (CDC, Dec. 18, 1992).

Late Symptomatic Stage

The late symptomatic stage begins when the $CD4^+$ T-cell count drops to less than 200 cells per microliter. Severe symptoms along with life-threatening infections and cancers characterize this stage. At this stage, infections and cancers are generally treatable. Furthermore, at this stage the infection has reached a level where it meets the CDC criteria for AIDS (CDC, Dec. 18, 1992). In addition to the 1986 and 1987 clinical conditions (Kaposi's sarcoma, *Pneumocystis carinii* pneumonia, other opportunistic infections, HIV encephalopathy, HIV wasting syndrome), the CDC has added pulmonary tuberculosis, recurrent bacterial pneumonia, and invasive cervical cancer to the list of AIDS indicator illnesses. These conditions are covered in depth in Chapter 4.

Advanced HIV Disease Stage

When the $CD4^+$ cell count drops to less than 50 cells per microliter, the immune system is so impaired that there is an increasing chance of treatment failure. In this stage, severe opportunistic infections and malignancies occur. Death becomes likely, usually within 1 year (Fahey et al., 1990; Lange et al., 1989).

HISTORY OF AIDS

The history of the AIDS epidemic in the United States is very recent. In June 1981 the first description of what would soon be referred to as AIDS appeared in the CDC's *Morbidity and Mortality Weekly Report* of June 5, 1981. The report described the occurrence of *Pneumocystic carinii* pneumonia (PCP) in five previously healthy, sexually active, young homosexual men from Los Angeles. This report was quickly followed by case reports of an unusual and extremely rare tumor, Kaposi's sarcoma (KS) in a male homosexual population in New York City. Both conditions occur infrequently and had previously been seen only in severely immunosuppressed individuals.

Between June 1981 and May 1982, similar cases were reported to the CDC in increasing numbers. Initially the number of cases was doubling every 6 months. In addition to PCP and KS, other unusual viral, fungal, and parasitic infections were being diagnosed in young homosexual men. Again, these diseases had previously been seen only in severely immunosuppressed individuals. Laboratory studies of patients with these opportunistic infections and cancers revealed that all of them had severe immunodeficiencies; clinically their condition deteriorated and they died of these unusual infections quickly (CDC, 1982a).

At first only homosexual and bisexual men were thought to be affected, and some aspect of the gay lifestyle was hypothesized to be the probable cause of the immunodeficiency. The disease was named gay-related immunodeficiency at that time. However, as the complex of diseases became more widely recognized, other cases reported to the CDC made it obvious that this was not a disease limited to homosexuals. The same infections and tumors were reported in heterosexual injection drug users (IDUs); Haitian immigrants; persons with hemophilia; spouses, sexual partners, and children of persons with the disease; and recipients of blood or blood components from infected persons (CDC, 1982b, 1982c). In September 1982 the CDC designated the disease as AIDS and defined its characteristics. With the exception of Haitian immigrants, in whom infections were found to be related to the other modes of transmission, the originally identified groups became and currently remain those most frequently exposed to the virus. It soon became apparent that AIDS was transmitted through an exchange of body fluids, principally blood and semen.

Persons at increased risk of contracting HIV infection are those who have unprotected sex with multiple partners; share needles; receive blood, blood products, or tissue from HIV-infected individuals; have hemophilia or a coagulation disorder; or are the sexual partners or children of these persons. Transmission occurs through sexual contact between men and men and between men and women, but currently the largest transmission group in the United States remains men who have sex with men (55%); the next largest group is IDUs (24%), both male and female. These two groups and a combination of the two groups account for 85% of persons 13 years of age and older with AIDS nationwide; 88% of adolescent and adult persons with AIDS are male (CDC, October 1993). The World Health Organization (WHO) has designated this pattern of transmission as pattern 1. However, the proportion of IDUs among those with newly diagnosed infection is increasing, especially along the Eastern Seaboard (Selik et al., 1993). The proportion of cases related to each exposure category varies significantly among the geographic regions of the United States. These differences are addressed later in this chapter.

While the number of cases was mounting in the United States, AIDS started appearing in Europe, where an interesting phenomenon was observed. Although in many European countries transmission patterns were similar to those in the United States (pattern 1 transmission), a sizable number of cases were occurring in immigrants from central Africa or in Europeans who had traveled the major trade routes in sub-Saharan Africa. When investigators turned their attention to Africa, they discovered an epidemic that could be traced through serologic studies to 1959 (von Reyn & Mann, 1987). A different aspect of the epidemic in Africa was that it affected men and women equally and was widespread in the heterosexual population (WHO designation, pattern 2). The disease has been reported in all but seven countries in Africa and has been transmitted principally through heterosexual contact between multiple partners, including commercial sex workers (Mann et al., 1992; Quinn, 1990; Sandman, 1992). In Africa, in addition to HIV-1, retroviruses designated HIV-2 and HTLV-IV were isolated in 1985

(Mann et al., 1992; Quinn, 1990). The highest rates of HIV-2 infection have been reported in West Africa. HIV-2 infection also exists in Angola and Mozambique and sporadic cases have been reported in the Americas, India, and Europe. HIV-2 infection has transmission patterns, clinical features, and public health interventions similar to those of HIV-1 (Mann et al., 1992; Quinn, 1990).

HIV-1 was identified and named in stages. Not until early 1983 was there any indication that a virus first discovered in France in 1980, human T-cell leukemia/lymphotropic virus, might be the causative agent of AIDS (Barre-Sinoussi et al., 1983). Luc Montagnier and scientists at the Institut Pasteur in France named the virus lymphadenopathy-associated virus (LAV). In the United States in May 1984, Robert Gallo and other investigators at the National Institutes of Health reported the isolation of a group of cytopathic retroviruses and antibodies against those viruses in persons with AIDS. They termed their discovery human T-lymphotropic virus type III (HTLV-III) (Popovic et al., 1984). At the same time, West Coast scientists at the University of California San Francisco who were studying the virus named it the AIDS-associated retrovirus (ARV) (Levy et al., 1984). In the summer of 1986, the International Society on the Taxonomy of Viruses arbitrated, changing the name to human immunodeficiency virus type 1 (HIV-1). Through legal arbitration, Montagnier and Gallo have been recognized as codiscoverers of the virus. For the sake of standardization and communication, the virus is now known worldwide as HIV-1.

Identification of the virus led to development of a test for HIV antibody in the blood. This test made it possible to determine which persons carried HIV antibody and therefore had been infected by HIV; it also permitted the screening of blood and blood products to prevent transmission by blood transfusion (Abrams, 1986; Najera et al., 1987).

Since 1981 the AIDS pandemic has assumed major proportions. It has been characterized as a global epidemic out of control (Mann et al., 1992). The Global AIDS Policy Coalition (GAPC), made up of ranking scientists, educators, and health workers around the world, has described the epidemic as volatile, dynamic, unstable, and with its major impact yet to come (Mann et al., 1992). WHO officials estimate that 12 million people around the world carry the virus and that as many as 100 million will become infected by the year 2000 (*Global AIDS News,* 1993). The GAPC estimates that by 1995 an additional 6.9 million people will become infected and that by the year 2000 a possible 110 million might be infected (Mann et al., 1992). They project a changing epidemiology by the year 2000, with the largest proportion of HIV infections in Asia and Oceania (42%), compared with 31% in sub-Saharan Africa and 14% in Latin America and the Caribbean (Mann et al., 1992). Currently there are 7.5 million infected people in sub-Saharan Africa, 2 million infected in the Americas, 1.5 million in South and Southeast Asia, 500,000 in Western Europe, 75,000 in North Africa and the Middle East, 50,000 in Eastern Europe and Central Asia, 25,000 in East Asia and the Pacific, and 25,000 in Australia (*Global AIDS News,* 1993). Worldwide about 75% of HIV infections are transmitted sexually, with four cases transmitted by male-female contact to each one case transmitted by male-male sexual contact. The remainder of infections are about equally divided between the exposure routes of injectable drug use, perinatal transmission, and transfusion transmission. From these data it is obvious that the picture of the epidemic worldwide is very different from that in the United States.

After careful study of the global epidemic, the GAPC characterized the epidemic and its lessons:

1. No community or country in the world already affected by AIDS has been able to stop the spread of HIV.
2. HIV is spreading rapidly to new communities and countries around the world, and HIV will reach most, if not all, human communities. Geography may delay the spread but will not protect against it.
3. The global epidemic becomes more complex as it matures and is composed of thousands of smaller, complicated epidemics as HIV exploits every potential avenue for spread.

4. HIV has demonstrated repeatedly its ability to cross all borders—social, economic, cultural, political, and geographic—and the conditions that foster HIV spread are complex and changing.
5. A plateau of the efforts against HIV dominates the global picture while at the same time the pandemic is expanding at a dynamic pace (Mann et al., 1992, pp. 2, 3, 8).

Current Issues

The picture of HIV infection today is pessimistic and realistic. Yet it is necessary to focus on the knowledge, commitment, and action that can make a difference. When the first edition of this text was published in 1989, the progress made against the disease from 1981 to that time was summarized: the probable causative agent of AIDS had been discovered, the virus had been cloned, a blood screening program had been implemented, work on the development of a vaccine had begun, and therapies that extend life had been identified. In the second edition, many major changes had occurred in the progression and epidemiology of the disease, treatment and nursing care, and the delivery of care. These changes included increased survival time after diagnosis, a decline in Kaposi's sarcoma as a presenting diagnosis, testing of several vaccines, changes in biologic and behavioral cofactors to infection and disease progression, expanded use of zidovudine (AZT; azidothymidine) and prophylactic antibiotics, a shift in treatment and care from acute care centers to the community, changes in the cost of care, and changes in the efficacy and ethics of HIV antibody testing (Becker & Joseph, 1988; Brandt, 1988; Gail et al., 1990; Jason et al., 1989; Lemp et al., 1990; Lifson et al., 1990; Nanda & Minkoff, 1989; Osmond & Moss, 1989; Scitovsky, 1989).

Again, since the second edition was published, several changes have occurred in the epidemiology of HIV infection, disease expression, treatment, costs of care, and the political climate. Each change is noteworthy, caught the public's attention, and/or is essential to nursing care. Some of the changes are highlighted here. Those essential to current nursing care are addressed in depth in following chapters.

A major change that occurred as the previous edition went to press was the revised classification system for HIV infection and an expansion of the AIDS surveillance case definition. The CDC added three clinical conditions and a laboratory marker of immunodeficiency to the case definition. The revised system was described earlier in this chapter. It has resulted in a national increase of reported cases in 1993 of approximately 75% (CDC, April 30, 1993). In the first 3 months of 1993, the number of reported AIDS cases increased 204% over the first quarter of 1992. The first quarter increase was inflated over that expected for the rest of the year because of the reporting of persons with previously diagnosed conditions added to the surveillance definition in 1993 that could not be reported as persons with AIDS before January 1. The new definition will not lead to earlier identification of people with HIV antibodies, but it will allow earlier classification of people in the AIDS category (CDC, Oct. 1, 1993). The majority of additional cases will come from those people who have HIV antibodies and a T-cell count less than 200. The effect will be that people will now live longer, on average, after a diagnosis of AIDS than they would have under the old definition of AIDS.

Some cities and clinical settings have already assessed the impact of the revised definition on the prevalence of AIDS. Chaisson and colleagues (1993), at Johns Hopkins in Baltimore, found that the new case definition doubled the number of prevalent AIDS cases, with significant increases in the proportion of patients who were female, IDUs, or without symptoms. Survival of patients was also significantly longer. Investigators in San Francisco estimated a 100% to 250% increase in prevalent AIDS cases (Katz et al., 1993; Sheppard et al., 1993).

The change in case definition was not without controversy within the United States and in the world. Sheppard and colleagues (1993) warned that a case definition using a specific T-cell subset value will be compromised by the inherent variability of these measures and the substantial overlap in the results for those with and without clinical manifestations of HIV disease.

Differences in the CDC and WHO classifications also generated controversy. The CDC proposed that their revised classification system would provide a framework for categorizing HIV-related morbidity and immunosuppression. Additionally it would assist efforts to track the epidemic, make accurate clinical assessments, provide prophylactic and therapeutic interventions, and provide a greater access to treatment for those Americans who are insured (CDC, Dec. 18, 1992). The WHO noted that the CDC definition could be applied in countries where $CD4^+$ counts are widely used for the clinical management of HIV-infected people. However, it also noted that the new definition will make trend analysis and international comparisons difficult; it requires sophisticated diagnostic technology; it labels some symptom-free people as having AIDS just because their $CD4^+$ count is less than 200; and the number of reported cases will depend in part on how many seropositive people have their $CD4^+$ counts monitored (*Global AIDS News,* 1993). This controversy regarding case definitions has not been resolved and may await arbitration, as did naming the virus and establishing the discoverers of the virus.

A second major change since the previous edition of this text occurred in HIV disease expression with the resurgence of a pulmonary tuberculosis (TB) epidemic exacerbated by HIV. After three decades of steadily decreasing TB morbidity, from 1985 to 1991, TB increased 18% in males and 20% in females (CDC, Aug. 13, 1993; U.S. CDC, *TB Weekly,* April 5, 1993). By ethnicity, the largest rise was among Latinos (72.4%), followed by Asians (32.3%) and African Americans (25.6%). In 1991, 71% of new cases occurred in ethnic people of color. A strong epidemiologic link exists between HIV infection and the development of pulmonary TB (Agency for Health Care Policy and Research [AHCPR], January 1994; De Cock et al., 1992). TB morbidity parallels HIV morbidity in geographic areas and demographic groups (CDC, 1991c). However, not all TB cases are HIV related: the poor are disproportionately affected; immigrants from countries with high TB prevalence are contributing to the increase; and living in congregate living facilities (nursing homes, prisons, homeless shelters) has increased the rate of infection by two to four times over noncongregate living (U.S. CDC, *TB Weekly*, April 5, 1993). A similar trend has been observed in Western Europe (CDC, Aug. 20, 1993; van Deutekom et al., 1993). There is also a strong immunologic association between pulmonary TB and HIV infection as affected by the $CD4^+$ T-lymphocyte count (De Cock et al., 1992). Lowered T-cell counts in persons with HIV increase the risk of active TB and reactivation of disease (Allen & Ownby, 1991). Each disease exacerbates the expression of the other. On the basis of epidemiologic and immunologic evidence, pulmonary TB was added to AIDS surveillance criteria in 1993.

Greatly complicating the resurging TB epidemic has been the emergence of multidrug-resistant (MDR) TB (TB isolate resistant to at least isoniazid and rifampin). MDR-TB most often develops in patients who do not complete an appropriate course of therapy. Homeless persons, alcoholics, and IDUs frequently do not complete therapy (Allen & Ownby, 1991; Bayer et al., 1993; U.S. CDC, *TB Weekly*, April 5, 1993). Other persons with an increased risk of MDR-TB are foreign-born persons from Asia, Africa, and Latin America; persons with a history of previous treatment for TB; and contacts of persons with drug-resistant cases through geographic or personal proximity (CDC, 1991c).

Since 1990, CDC has investigated large outbreaks of MDR-TB in hospitals and correctional facilities in Florida, New York, and New Jersey. The outbreaks have been characterized by association with HIV infection, high fatality rates (70% to 80%), a brief interval between TB diagnosis and death (4 to 16 weeks), and evidence of nosocomial infection (CDC, June 11, 1993; U.S. CDC, *TB Weekly*, April 5, 1993). Nationwide, more than 100 health care workers (HCWs) have been infected with MDR-TB, presumably because

their exposure was to others with MDR-TB (U.S. CDC, *TB Weekly*, April 5, 1993).

Another change—a treatment issue that has received major attention in the past year—is the efficacy of early retroviral therapy with AZT. The Concorde trial, reported in a letter to *Lancet*, was at the center of the controversy (Aboulker & Swart, 1993). The Concorde trial was a multicenter, randomized, double-blind, placebo-controlled trial of 1749 patients in Europe. It was designed to determine whether HIV-infected adults benefit from starting AZT therapy while still free of symptoms, rather than waiting until symptoms develop. At the Ninth International Conference on AIDS, in Berlin (June 7 to 11, 1993), a full presentation of the Concorde trial was given (Cotton, 1993). The investigators concluded after 3 years of study that the use of prophylactic AZT in symptom-free patients neither prolongs life nor delays AIDS onset (Cotton & Friedland, 1993). Other AIDS clinical trial group studies reported in Berlin suggested confusing and inconsistent results of monotherapy with AZT, didanosine or dideoxyinosine (ddI), dideoxycytidine (ddC), and stavudine (D4T), and of comparisons of their effectiveness in the treatment of advanced HIV disease. One general conclusion was that monotherapy with these drugs is relatively ineffective in persons with advanced disease (Cotton, 1993; Kozal et al., 1993). Since the Berlin conference and the Concorde trial, other investigators have reported better outcomes (probability of disease progression and decline in $CD4^+$ counts to less than 350) for patients with $CD4^+$ cell counts more than 400 who receive monotherapy with AZT than for those receiving placebos (Bartlett, 1993; Cooper et al., 1993). These investigators concluded that the benefit of early antiretroviral therapy might be greatest if it is begun when $CD4^+$ cell counts are more than 300 to 400 per cubic millimeter. Guidelines for the initiation of antiretroviral therapy were published by the AHCPR, U.S. Public Health Service, in January 1994. These guidelines are included in Appendix I, Managing Early HIV Infection (AHCPR, January 1994).

Drug resistance to AZT has resulted in

switching to therapy with ddI or ddC if CD4$^+$ cell counts decrease, opportunistic infections occur, or weight loss or constitutional symptoms occur. However, at the Berlin conference the validity of the CD4$^+$ marker for determining the efficacy of such drugs was called into serious question. Changes in the CD4$^+$ cell count did not predict outcome in several clinical trials (Choi et al., 1993; Lin et al., 1993). CD4$^+$ response did not entirely explain the benefits or failures of antiretroviral therapy (Cotton, 1993; Henry, 1993). At the conference, interest in combination therapies was high and many large clinical trials currently are addressing its efficacy. There was also a great deal of interest in gene therapy (Goldsmith, 1993) and gene inoculation (Wang et al., 1993). However, the use of CD4$^+$ as a surrogate marker will continue to be a problem in evaluations of antiretroviral drugs, but it is currently the most practical marker available (Fischl et al., 1993).

AZT has been used prophylactically in health care workers (HCWs) after an occupational exposure to HIV (Gerberding, 1993; Tokars et al., 1993). The seroconversion rate from occupational exposure is still extremely low (0.36%), but workers using AZT after exposure had increased by 31% from 1988 to 1993. One HCW became infected with a strain of HIV sensitive to AZT after a full course of treatment with it. Other treatment failures have also been reported (American Health Consultants, *AIDS Alert,* 1992). Because of side effects, many HCWs did not complete planned courses of AZT therapy. Both the prospective surveillance of exposed HCWs and the results of clinical trials make it clear that patients should be fully informed of the value and limits of early antiretroviral therapy.

A continuing issue in the epidemic is the cost of health care for persons with HIV disease (Andrulis et al., 1992). Costs brought to attention the shifts in the settings of health care, the threats to health care facilities, and evaluation of health care delivery models (Aiken et al., 1993). Costs of treating persons with HIV/AIDS are staggering to inner city hospitals and may result in limitation of the number of persons served by these hospitals (Andrulis et al., 1992). One possible solution for reducing hospital costs is a case-managed model of care that may result in reduced hospital charges (Sowell et al., 1992). Another proposed solution is a community nursing center for person(s) with HIV disease (PWHIV), with both cost-effectiveness and quality of care as demonstrated outcomes (Schroeder, 1993). Nevertheless, the setting for care appears to continue to shift from inpatient to outpatient settings, and a significant portion of costs are incurred by patients in whom AIDS has not yet developed (Johnson et al., 1993; Rietmeijer et al., 1993). A probable contributor to high costs of care in symptom-free PWHIV may be the early prophylactic use of AZT. An entire national treatment program of early intervention has been built around the use of AZT monotherapy, resulting in a dramatic increase in HIV antibody testing, monitoring of disease progression through CD4$^+$ cell testing, and aggressive use of immunizations and PCP prophylaxis. All these interventions greatly increased costs. The recent confusing and sometimes disappointing assessment of early monotherapy with the current antiretroviral agents calls for a reevaluation of present treatment plans in view of their costs.

Finally, a major issue on the sociopolitical front during the past 2 years, the Florida dentist case (Dr. David Acer and patient Kimberly Bergalis), directed public attention and often hysteria to HIV transmission from HCWs to patients (CDC, 1990). Much controversy over epidemiologic evidence and viral sequencing evidence, together with calls for mandatory testing of HCWs and restriction of the practice of HCWs, kept this story at the forefront of public and professional consciousness for the past 2 years. Media attention resulted in CDC recommendations (two versions) for prevention of transmission of HIV and hepatitis B virus to patients during exposure-prone invasive procedures, infection control practices for dentists, legislative efforts to impose mandatory testing on HCWs, and several investigations of potential HIV transmission to patients by infected HCWs (CDC, 1991a and

1991b, May 7, 1993, May 28, 1993; Dickinson et al., 1993; Rogers et al., 1993; Saah, 1993; von Reyn et al., 1993). Still, HIV transmission from HCWs to patients remains a very unimportant means of HIV transmission. The public, governmental, and scientific furor over the case may be partly attributed to the tendency to avoid talking about sex and drug use, the real forces behind the epidemic (Saah, 1993). A possible positive result of this controversy may have been that health professionals of all disciplines came together and stood together in their opposition to mandatory testing and the original set of CDC guidelines for invasive procedures.

The epidemiology of AIDS and nurses' knowledge, attitudes, and practices related to the disease have also changed in the past 2 years. The epidemiology of AIDS for special populations is discussed in Chapters 6 through 9. An overview of epidemiologic changes is given here. The issue of risks to nurses and other health care workers, as well as nurses' practices in relation to universal precautions, are addressed in Chapter 10. An overview of nurses' knowledge, attitudes, and practices is provided later in this chapter.

CHANGES IN EPIDEMIOLOGY OF HIV INFECTION

The sociodemographic characteristics of persons with HIV disease differ with geographic regions in the United States. These differences have become more pronounced during the past 2 years and have come to characterize the population with AIDS in each region. The national statistics often do not adequately reflect the sex, ethnicity, or route of transmission of PWHIV in a particular city or region. To mount effective prevention and treatment programs, nurses must be aware of the sociodemographic characteristics of PWHIV in their own region. The demographics of the 10 metropolitan statistical areas (MSAs) and the 10 states or commonwealths with the most AIDS cases are presented in Table 1–2. As may be noted in the table, the geographic distribution of AIDS has changed in the past 2 years. The percentage of the total number of AIDS cases represented in the 10 leading MSAs has decreased, representing a spread of AIDS to smaller cities and rural areas of the United States. The Miami MSA has moved to fourth in the percentage of total cases, and San Juan, Puerto Rico, is now

Table 1–2. Demographics of Total AIDS Cases

TEN LEADING MSAs*	% OF TOTAL U.S. CASES		TEN LEADING STATES OR COMMONWEALTHS	% OF TOTAL U.S. CASES	
	1993	1991		1993	1991
New York City (1)	16.6	19.0	New York (1)	19.2	22.0
Los Angeles (2)	6.4	7.0	California (2)	18.3	19.0
San Francisco (3)	5.0	6.0	Florida (3)	9.8	8.0
Miami (8)	2.86	2.4	Texas (4)	7.0	7.0
Chicago (7)	2.79	2.4	New Jersey (5)	5.7	6.5
Washington, D.C. (5)	2.77	2.8	Puerto Rico (7)	3.22	2.9
Houston (4)	2.73	3.0	Illinois (6)	3.18	3.0
Newark (6)	2.2	2.7	Georgia (9)	2.75	2.6
Philadelphia (9)	2.1	2.0	Pennsylvania (8)	2.68	2.8
San Juan, P.R.	2.05	—	Massachusetts (10)	2.13	2.0
Atlanta (10)	2.03	2.0	Combined % of total	73.96	75.8
Combined % of total	45.05	49.3			

Statistics from Centers for Disease Control and Prevention (October 1993): *HIV/AIDS Surveillance Report.* United States AIDS Program, Atlanta, Ga.
*MSA, Metropolitan Statistical Area.
(1) Position in 1991.

among the leading 10 MSAs. Other U.S. cities with close to 2% of the total cases were Boston and Dallas. The 10 leading states have decreased slightly their percentage of total cases. However, looking at individual states, Florida and Puerto Rico have noticeably increased their percentage of the total. Michigan also has increased and now has more than 2% of total cases.

The statistics for route of exposure, gender, and ethnicity in the Eastern Seaboard states and MSAs differ from the national statistics and those in the Midwest and West. Infection of IDUs, women, and ethnic subgroups is greater in the East. Infection of IDUs, according to 1993 surveillance statistics and 92 seroprevalence studies of this group in the United States, is highest in the Northeast (10% to 65%) and Puerto Rico (45% to 59%); lower in the South Atlantic states (7% to 29%) and in the metropolitan areas of Atlanta (10%), Detroit (7% to 13%), and San Francisco (7% to 13%); and 5% or less in other areas of the West, Midwest, and South (Hahn et al., 1989). See Table 1–3 for additional comparative data on injection drug use.

The number of infections in women, according to seroprevalence data from reproductive health clinics and delivery room settings (parturient women), is highest in the urban areas of New Jersey (290 per million female population), New York (270 per mil-

Table 1–3. Geographic Distribution of AIDS Cases (in Percent)

	UNITED STATES	NEW YORK STATE	NEW YORK CITY	NEW JERSEY
Exposure Category				
Male-male sexual contact	55	39	40	11
Injection drug use (IDU)	24	44	43	47
Male-male sexual contact/IDU	6	4	3	3
Hemophilia/coagulation disorder	1	0	0	0
Male-female sexual contact	7	6	6	20
Transfusion with blood/products	2	1	1	1
Undetermined	5	7	7	19
Age and Gender				
*Adult**	98.5	98	98	98
Male	88	83	83	77
Female	12	17	17	23
Children†	1.5	2	2	2
Age and Race or Ethnic Group				
Adults				
White	52	34	31	32
Black	31	37	38	54
Hispanic	16	27	29	14
Other‡	1	1	2	0
Children				
White	20	11	10	17
Black	55	53	53	63
Hispanic	24	35	37	20
Other†	1	1	0	1

Statistics based on surveillance data provided by the Centers for Disease Control and Prevention and the states and cities listed as of summer 1993.
*Includes all patients 13 years of age and older.
†Includes all patients less than 13 years of age.
‡Includes Asian/Pacific Islander and American Indian/Alaska Native.
Note: Totals may not equal 100% because of rounding.

lion), the District of Columbia (216 per million), and Florida (138 per million). States or commonwealths with 40 or more cases of AIDS per million female population include those just listed plus Rhode Island, Delaware, Connecticut, Massachusetts, Maryland, and Puerto Rico. States with 20 to 39 cases per million female population include Pennsylvania, Virginia, South Carolina, Georgia, Mississippi, Louisiana, Colorado, Arizona, Nevada, California, Alaska, and Hawaii (Shapiro et al., 1989). Table 1–3 provides additional comparative data on gender.

Data on HIV seroprevalence in women seeking an abortion have been reported in Atlanta, Georgia, New York City, and Washington, D.C. The seroprevalence of HIV-1

was reported as similar to that of parturient women in Atlanta and New York City and lower than that of parturients in Washington, D.C. (Araneta et al., 1992; Lindsay et al., 1990; Rosenberg et al., 1993). Investigators in the Washington, D.C., area suggested that the lower rates in women having an abortion was related to the higher social class of these women (Rosenberg et al., 1993). In October 1987 the District of Columbia stopped funding public abortions, and abortions are now available only to those who can afford them. Researchers in the New York City study warned that if access to abortion services were curtailed for low-income women, the rate of HIV-1 infection by perinatal transmission could potentially increase by 400 cases an-

DADE CO. (MIAMI), FL	SAN JUAN, P.R.	CHICAGO	HOUSTON	DALLAS	LOS ANGELES	SAN FRANCISCO
45	18	64	71	82	80	84
23	55	20	8	4	6	5
4	8	5	9	9	7	9
0	0	1	0	0	1	0
20	14	6	3	1	1	1
1	3	2	1	1	2	1
6	3	2	7	3	3	1
97	98	99	99	99	99	99
82	81	90	95	96	96	98
18	19	10	5	4	4	2
3	2	1	1	1	1	1
23	0	41	67	74	58	79
46	0	44	21	17	18	9
31	99	14	12	8	23	9
0	0	1	0	0	2	2
3	0	9	66	42	23	49
88	0	64	22	42	30	37
9	100	26	12	11	43	11
0	0	0	0	5	3	3

nually (Araneta et al., 1992). In Atlanta, the majority of HIV-infected women were infected through heterosexual transmission (Lindsay et al., 1990). The other two studies did not report exposure categories.

Infection rates of African Americans and Latinos are also higher along the Eastern Seaboard than in other parts of the country. For example, the racial breakdown of cases in New York City is 31% white, 38% African American, 29% Latino, and less than 1% others. This compares with a New York City population distribution of 52% white, 24% African American, 20% Latino, and 4% other. The ethnic distribution of the AIDS epidemic is related to the proportion of infected drug users and the proportion of infected women (CDC, October 1993). Ethnicity, gender, and injection drug use are interrelated and are associated with the proportion of infected individuals in a specific geographic region. Table 1–3 presents the exposure category, gender, age, and ethnic distribution of AIDS patients in selected geographic regions and compares them with the national distribution of patients in these categories for June 1993. Compared with 2 years ago, general trends can be observed in all tabled states and metropolitan areas. There has been a steady and sometimes dramatic increase in injection drug use and heterosexual exposure to HIV, in the proportion of women infected, and in the proportion of African Americans and Latinos infected. There has been a corresponding decrease in exposure through male-male sexual contact and in white persons.

As can be noted from Table 1–3, routes of exposure differ widely between the East Coast and both the Midwest and West, with higher percentages of injection drug use among the total cases in the East and South. The number of new cases of AIDS among IDUs has been increasing yearly, with Eastern Seaboard states reporting an increase of 43% between 1988 and 1989. The number of new cases of AIDS in sexual partners of IDUs increased 58% during this same period in the East. In geographic areas where IDUs make up a greater percentage of the total number of AIDS patients, the numbers of African Americans and Latinos also make up a greater

percentage. The ranges in the distribution of cases by exposure category and the ethnic makeup of these groups call for new knowledge, prevention, and treatment approaches among nurses. Chapters 2, 6 through 9, and 15 deal with these topics.

Gender of HIV-infected persons also differs regionally and is closely related to cases of AIDS in children. Because a greater proportion of women make up the total number of persons with AIDS, predictably the proportion of infected children also rises. The proportion of AIDS cases among women and children who are African American or Latino is particularly striking. The proportion of ethnic women of color who have AIDS closely parallels the percentages among children with AIDS (percentages among children are depicted in Table 1–3). For example, in Dade County, Florida, of women with AIDS, 84% are African American, 9% white, 7% Hispanic/Latina, and 1% other. In New York City, women with AIDS are 52% African American, 33% Latina, and 14% white. In contrast, women with AIDS in San Francisco are 43% white, 38% African American, 12% Latina, and 7% other. Despite these differences between the East and West coasts, the proportion of cases of AIDS among people of color has been increasing steadily on both coasts. For instance, in Los Angeles County the proportion of new adult cases of AIDS has decreased among whites from 60% in 1988 to 55% in 1990 to 47% in 1992. During this same period the percentage of new adult cases in African Americans has increased from 18% in 1988 to 21% in 1992, and in Latinos from 19.5% in 1988 to 29.4% in 1992. The danger of the spread of AIDS in the African American and Latino communities cannot be overstated. This is especially true among women and children. Chapters 6 and 8 deal with HIV infection in children and women, respectively.

The relation of age to infection with HIV has also become a concern, especially among adolescents who might be at risk. In a national survey, disadvantaged and out-of-school youth (aged 16 to 21 years) who received Job Corps training from 1988 to 1992 were screened for HIV seropositivity (Conway et al., 1993). Seroprevalence decreased for young men from 3.6 per 1000 in 1988 to 2.2 per 1000 in 1992 but increased for young women from 2.1 per 1000 to 4.2 per 1000. The decreasing and increasing trends were due to changes in seroprevalence in African American trainees. In African American women the greatest increase was in those from the South who reported heterosexual exposure to HIV. Higher HIV seroprevalence among young women than young men has been reported in other surveys of adolescents (D'Angelo et al., 1991; Wendell et al., 1991). The only other national survey among adolescents and young adults is the HIV screening of military applicants. A decline in seroprevalence among male applicants was noted for the same period (U.S. Department of Defense, 1992). Declines in seropositivity for men in both the Job Corps and military surveys may be due to self-deferral from either of these programs by young men who realize the risk of male-to-male sexual contact, whereas young women may not recognize the risk of male-to-female sexual contact and may not be self-deferring from these programs.

A second cause for concern in the relation of age to HIV infection is that AIDS has become the leading cause of death among young adults (25 to 44 years old) in several U.S. cities with a population of 100,000 or more (Selik et al., 1993). Infection with HIV was the leading determinant of death in 1990 among young men in five states, causing 29% of their deaths in New York, 28% in New Jersey, 24% in California and Florida, and 16% in Massachusetts. Furthermore, HIV infection was the second leading cause of death of young men in eight other states. In U.S. cities with a population of 100,000 or more, HIV was the leading cause of death among young men in 64 cities, ranging from 16% in Bridgeport, Connecticut, to 61% in San Francisco (see Fig. 1–1).

Among young women, HIV was the leading cause of death in nine cities, ranging from 15% in Baltimore to 43% in Newark, New Jersey (see Fig. 1–2). Clearly the HIV epidemic is making major inroads into young populations, threatening premature death, with consequent disruption to the labor force,

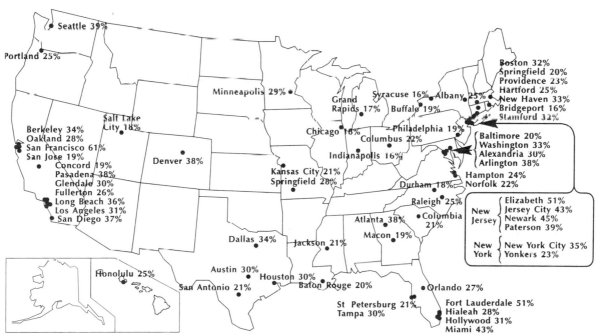

Figure 1–1. The proportion of deaths caused by HIV infection among deaths in 1990 in young men (aged 25 to 44 years) in U.S. cities of at least 100,000 population in which HIV infection was the leading cause of death in young men and the denominator was at least 25 deaths from all causes. (From Selik, R.M., Chu, S.Y., Buehler, J.W. (1993). HIV infection as leading cause of death among young adults in U.S. cities and states. *Journal of the American Medical Association*, 269(23), 2993.)

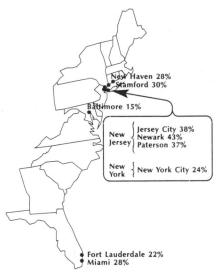

New Haven 28%
Stamford 30%
Baltimore 15%

New Jersey { Jersey City 38%
Newark 43%
Paterson 37%

New York { New York City 24%

Fort Lauderdale 22%
Miami 28%

Figure 1–2. The proportion of deaths caused by HIV infection among deaths in 1990 in young women (aged 25 to 44 years) in U.S. cities of at least 100,000 population in which HIV infection was the leading cause of death in young women and the denominator was at least 25 deaths from all causes. (From Selik, R.M., Chu, S.Y., Buehler, J.W. (1993). HIV infection as leading cause of death among young adults in U.S. cities and states. *Journal of the American Medical Association,* 269(23), 2994.)

and depriving young children of their parents.

The threat of HIV infection in special populations has become a growing concern. Studies of the homeless who are mentally ill have found seroprevalence rates ranging from 6.4% to 19.4%; HIV seropositivity was related to younger age and injection drug use (Empfield et al., 1993; Susser et al., 1993). Even among long-stay patients in a state psychiatric hospital, a 4% seroprevalence rate was found (Meyer et al., 1993). Among mentally ill persons who do not use injection drugs, unprotected sexual activity with multiple partners is frequent. Partners are chosen casually from persons met on the street, in parks, or in other public places (Kelly et al., 1992). This is a population in which education is difficult and the risk factors for infection are numerous. Other populations needing special consideration are incarcerated populations.

The AIDS epidemic in the United States has taken on many faces: in the last 2 years greater concern regarding adolescents, homeless persons, women, children, and ethnic people of color has arisen. As of this writing, it is clear that AIDS is spreading inexorably to the smaller cities and rural areas of the United States. The epidemiology of AIDS makes it clear that providing health care services in the United States is virtually impossible without knowledge of AIDS and the multiple epidemics it spawns in the various regions and human groups that it affects.

The explosion of knowledge about AIDS has been phenomenal. Nurses and other health care workers need in-depth and up-to-date knowledge of AIDS to practice. Nurses have close and constant contact with PWHIV in a variety of settings, and nursing is one of the principal professions involved in AIDS education and prevention.

NURSES' NEEDS FOR KNOWLEDGE ABOUT AIDS AND HIV INFECTION

With few exceptions, the management of AIDS and the care of PWHIV become the responsibility of nurses in secondary and tertiary care centers. In acute care hospitals, nurses provide constant, direct care to patients with HIV infection and to those with AIDS who have had exacerbations of their disease. To do so, they need knowledge regarding nursing management of the alterations in health status caused by the disease and regarding precautions to prevent transmission in the workplace.

In home health care settings, as well as in intermediate- and long-term care settings, nurses are often the only professionals involved daily with patients in the remission or chronic phase of the disease. Knowledge regarding prevention, precautions, infection control in the home, nutrition, transmission among household contacts, and safer sexual practices is necessary.

Schoolchildren, their parents, and teachers, to allay their fears of having a child with HIV/AIDS in the classroom, sometimes request information from nurses on how HIV infection is spread. In addition, teenagers need information on safer sexual practices and the dangers of drug use to reduce the likelihood of transmission.

In primary care settings, nurses are in positions to screen and counsel populations at risk of having HIV infection and AIDS and to assist in the identification of cases. Nurses need knowledge of sexual and drug use practices to assess these practices in their clients. They also need knowledge of sexual and drug use counseling. Nurses have contact with HIV-infected persons and their families in a variety of occupational and outpatient settings and may assume one or more roles in the prevention or treatment of HIV infection. Nurses working in occupational health settings or as independent practitioners need assessment skills to determine whether referral for HIV testing is needed.

Nurses in acute care and mental health settings must be familiar with the psychosocial and neuropsychiatric aspects of HIV disease, because they may have to deal with the depression and anxiety that accompany a diagnosis of HIV infection or AIDS, with comorbidity of HIV and psychiatric disorders, and with the dementia associated with AIDS. Knowledge of HIV disease is necessary for counseling persons in any stage of infection, as well as the "worried well." Mental health nurses, hospital nurses, community health nurses, and nurses working in hospices need knowledge of supportive therapies to deal with death and dying.

Community health nurses need information on prevention, transmission, risk assessment and case finding, HIV antibody testing, and psychosocial support to be of service to their clients. In addition, they must know the sexual and lifestyle practices of various subcultures in the United States to work effectively and to educate. Nurses are commonly the source of referrals for PWHIV and their families and friends in dealing with many of the problems associated with AIDS. They provide information about AIDS to the general public.

Nurses need knowledge about HIV infection, AIDS, and management of the disease because they have a greater range of contact with PWHIV and their families than does any other health care professional group. Nurses

are also frequently consulted about AIDS by laypersons and community groups. Finally, to give safe and sensitive care to PWHIV, nurses must understand the disease, its effects on patients, transmission, precautions for avoiding infection, and the supportive care of persons with HIV infection. Questions have been raised about whether nurses have adequate knowledge of HIV disease and the care of infected persons and whether their attitudes interfere with sensitive, supportive, and safe care.

NURSES' KNOWLEDGE AND ATTITUDES AND THEIR EFFECT ON PRACTICE

Often knowledge and attitudes are interrelated in the care of PWHIV. Anxiety, fear, discomfort, embarrassment, and negative social attitudes may decrease as knowledge of the disease and its transmission increases. Fear of the disease and its transmissibility has been an overriding concern of nurses and physicians. As a result of this fear, some nurses have left their jobs, refused to care for PWHIV, or given only minimal care to these patients. Nurses have sometimes used inappropriate precautions and isolation techniques with patients who have AIDS.

Early studies of nurses' knowledge of AIDS and attitudes toward PWHIV showed that knowledge was inadequate and attitudes were sometimes negative. In February 1986 the American Nurses' Association released a survey of state nurses' associations: 14 states reported instances in which registered nurses refused to care for AIDS patients, and in nine states employees were permitted to request reassignment to avoid caring for persons with AIDS. In most cases, nurses backed down on threats to resign when told that refusal to care for persons with AIDS would result in termination of employment. At the time of the survey, hospitals and health care facilities were just beginning to adopt specific guidelines for care of PWHIV and for employee protection from exposure.

During these early days it was apparent that knowledge of AIDS was inaccurate and inadequate. In large surveys of hospital employees, beliefs were still widespread that AIDS could be spread through casual contact or through coughing and sneezing. The majority could not identify the symptoms of AIDS or take a sexual history (Macks, 1986; van Servellen et al., 1988). A large percentage said that they absolutely would not care for patients with AIDS, that nurses should be allowed to refuse to care for patients having or suspected of having HIV infection, and that they spent less time with AIDS patients than with others. Nurses who had recently cared for patients with AIDS and for those at risk, and who had attended lectures and education forums on AIDS, were more likely to know AIDS symptoms, groups at risk, and necessary precautions. They were also more willing to give care to PWHIV. Early in the AIDS epidemic the nursing community believed that knowledge would increase and attitudes would improve with adequate education.

During the period from 1988 to 1991, many more studies were conducted of nurses' knowledge and attitudes about AIDS and the effect of these on the nurses' practice. From these studies, reported in the previous edition of this text, it was apparent that although AIDS knowledge had increased appreciably there had not been a concomitant change in attitudes. Nurses generally had correct knowledge about AIDS and its transmission but harbored irrational fears about casual transmission and held negative views of homosexuals. They believed they should have the right to refuse to care for a PWHIV (Damrosch et al., 1990; D'Augelli, 1989; Scherer et al., 1989).

On the other hand, some of the early studies had opposite results, showing that accurate knowledge about AIDS was significantly correlated with lower anxiety, willingness to work with PWHIV, and appropriate professional behavior toward PWHIV (Christ & Wiener, 1985; Lawrence & Lawrence, 1989; Malik-Nitto & Plantemoli, 1986). In general, accurate and regular in-service education on transmission and infection control, clear and consistent institutional policies on precautions for HCWs, and clear and consistent institutional guidelines on the obligation to treat had decreased the fears and inappropriate behaviors

of nurses working with HIV-infected persons (Malik-Nitto & Plantemoli, 1986).

Several early studies reported the effects of continuing education conferences or workshops and experience working with PWHIV on nurses' knowledge and attitudes. The findings were generally positive. The essential aspects of psychoeducational interventions for changing nurses' knowledge and attitudes were identified: accurate information on precautions and infection control guidelines; experience in sexual history taking and counseling; psychosocial support; and involvement in the establishment of institutional policies (All, 1989; Damrosh et al., 1990; Flaskerud et al., 1989; Wiley et al., 1990; Young, 1988; Young et al., 1989).

Three preliminary studies of nursing students offered evidence of the positive effects of direct experience with care of PWHIV on knowledge and attitudes (Cassels & Redman, 1989; Klisch, 1990; Matocha, 1990). Students progressed from fear and ambivalence to readily providing direct care for a person with HIV disease and taking appropriate precautions.

Studies of nurses' AIDS knowledge, attitudes, and practices are still being conducted to the present. Few differences during the past 7 years have been observed (Alexander & Fitzpatrick, 1991; Bell, 1993; Bond et al., 1990; Breault & Polifroni, 1992; Campbell et al., 1991; Curry et al., 1990; Dow & Knox, 1991; Downes, 1991; Huerta & Oddi, 1992; Kemppainen et al., 1992; Martindale & Barnett, 1992; Passannante et al., 1993; Strasser & Damrosch, 1992; Tesch et al., 1990). Subjects in these studies have been staff nurses, students, and nursing faculty from across the United States and several settings in Europe. In the great majority of studies, knowledge of pathogenesis and modes of transmission were high (Plant & Foster, 1993). However, much uncertainty was expressed about risk to HCWs from occupational exposure. Fear of contagion was a primary concern in nurses' and other health care workers' belief that they should be able to refuse to care for PWHIV, in their selection of clinical specialties, and in their decision of where to work (or in some cases to leave nursing) (van Wissen & Siebers, 1993). Negative attitudes in these studies were apparent in homophobia, discomfort with IDUs and homosexuals, and discomfort with death and dying. The level of AIDS knowledge was generally not related to these variables (Martindale & Barnett, 1992; Robbins et al., 1992; Scherer et al., 1991). In one particularly alarming study, the investigators found that nurses who provided sustained AIDS patient care had more negative attitudes than those who worked in hospitals with a lower prevalence of AIDS (Kemppainen et al., 1992). This finding was attributed to the fatigue, stress, and dissonance that occur with sustained care. Another study reported an increase in nurses' negative attitudes since the AIDS crisis began (Alexander & Fitzpatrick, 1991). This finding supports earlier studies with similar results (Scherer et al., 1989; Wallack, 1989; Young et al., 1989).

OCCUPATIONAL EXPOSURE, FEARS, AND PRACTICES

Fear of occupational exposure to HIV surfaced in most studies and may be one cause of negative attitudes toward caring for PWHIV. For some time now, evidence has indicated that the risk to HCWs is small and that the precautions recommended for them are adequate (Gerberding, 1989; Marcus et al., 1993). Recent studies support the findings of continued low risk of occupational HIV infection in HCWs (Ippolito et al., 1993). However, fears of occupational exposure remain and are often irrational (Gallop et al., 1992a; Taerk et al., 1993). Some nurses and physicians continue to believe that the government, their hospital, researchers, or the CDC is withholding information on the transmission of AIDS (Currey et al., 1990; Wallack, 1989). This attitude is more prevalent among minority physicians and nurses, many of whom are foreign born.

Recent studies have documented health care providers' doubts about whether universal precautions are effective and their distrust of information about their safety provided by national experts (Campbell et al., 1991; Elford et al., 1991b). Ficarrotto and colleagues (1991) found that graduate-level nursing students had exaggerated fears of occupational HIV contagion, believing that they were at risk from casual contacts such as holding a patient, shaking hands with a patient, or entering a room without a mask and gown. In a study of staff nurses, Campbell and associates (1991) reported a moderate to high level of anxiety over occupational HIV infection even though one third of their respondents had never cared for a PWHIV and 45% had cared for only one to four AIDS patients. Exaggerated perceptions of risk in these studies and in others were associated with negative attitudes toward PWHIV (Breault & Polifroni, 1992; Dow & Knox, 1991; Huerta & Oddi, 1992). Many studies report evidence of bias against gays or homophobia (Campbell et al., 1991; Damrosch et al., 1990; Scherer et al., 1991; Strasser & Damrosch, 1992; Wallack, 1989). It is difficult to determine whether fear of exposure or negative attitudes is behind nurses' continued reluctance to provide care to PWHIV (Campbell et al., 1991; Currey et al., 1990; Martindale & Barnett, 1992).

Paradoxically, several recent studies have found that despite the widespread fear of occupational HIV infection, nurses fail to implement universal precautions in actual practice. In a study by Gruber and colleagues (1989), nurses' knowledge of HIV transmission was high, and yet few nurses were wearing a gown when changing the linen of incontinent patients or wearing goggles and a mask when suctioning the airway of patients with a tracheostomy. More recent studies also have found a high level of knowledge of universal precautions and a perception of high occupational risk accompanied by failure to observe universal precautions (Abiteboul et al., 1991; Gershon et al., 1991). Only 50% of nurses treated all body fluids as potentially infected with HIV in a study by van Wissen and Siebers (1993), and the same number did not wear gloves when handling a variety of body fluids or tissues. In a study that included 1,520 nurses, Colombotos and associates (1991) found that a significant number failed to follow universal precautions and used barrier procedures only when HIV status was known. A review of research of nurses' knowledge, attitudes, and practices identified gaps in knowledge about transmission of HIV, infection control, and occupational exposure (Swanson et al., 1990).

Clearly there is ample room for improvement in nurses' HIV-related attitudes and work practices. In most cases, knowledge of HIV and AIDS appears to be adequate, but fears, negative attitudes, and unsafe practices persist.

NURSE-IDENTIFIED AIDS INFORMATIONAL NEEDS

As the AIDS epidemic spreads and takes form across the United States, all nurses need information about HIV disease to provide optimal care for their clients and to protect themselves. The content of the first edition of this book was based on an assessment of nurses' needs for AIDS information. A national survey of 832 nurses was conducted to identify nurses' AIDS informational needs, the groups of clients to whom they were providing care, and their preferred educational resources for information about HIV. For the second edition, a random sample of 200 nurses from the original survey was selected. These nurses received a copy of the book and a questionnaire to use in evaluating the text; 162 of the sample (81%) completed and returned the evaluation. Respondents were asked to indicate in which areas they needed more information about AIDS. The following areas were identified:

1. Current treatment   60%
2. Drugs in use   65%
3. Symptom assessment   70%
4. Precautions for health care
   workers   68%
5. Transmission in the workplace   66%
6. Sexual history taking   60%
7. Sexual counseling   70%
8. Prevention   65%
9. Psychosocial aspects   73%
10. Ethical issues   75%

The respondents also expressed an interest in information on special topics: 95% were interested in epidemiologic trends in the United States; 89% desired information on IDUs; about three fourths wanted information on the differences in HIV disease among women (75%) and children (79%); 97% were interested in changes in treatment of HIV disease; and 85% wanted to learn about changes in the virus and virus strains. Change in general was of particular interest to the nurses. They recognized that the HIV/AIDS arena changes rapidly and that their information on the subject requires constant updating. The content of this current edition was planned also to address the changes in HIV epidemiology, disease, medical treatment, nursing care, and the needs of special populations. In the development of the content areas, nurses' needs for AIDS information were inferred also from the studies of nurses' knowledge, attitudes, and practices reviewed in this chapter. Several implications for nursing educational efforts may be drawn from these sources of data as well as from recent trends in nursing research.

PLANNING HIV EDUCATION INTERVENTIONS

In planning educational intervention programs for peers or nursing students, nurses may be guided by a relatively new trend in the research on AIDS knowledge, attitudes, and practices. Several recent studies have used various theories of behavior and learning to explain changes in attitudes, beliefs, practices, and knowledge (Gallop et al., 1992b; Goldenberg & Laschinger, 1991; L.S. Jemmott et al., 1992; Pederson, 1993; Siminoff et al., 1991). In a review of studies of knowledge, attitudes, and practices, Swanson and colleagues (1990) pointed out that the majority were atheoretical, descriptive surveys. They recommended areas for improvement in research designs and research questions. Furthermore, the CDC has recently been disseminating information and data on the use of a conceptual framework for behavioral change based on a stages-of-change model (CDC, 1992c; Prochaska et al., 1992). The CDC supports use of such a model to evaluate change in specific behaviors.

To date, many of these models have been applied in only an exploratory fashion. The theory of reasoned action has been used to identify significant predictors of intentions to care for AIDS patients (Goldenberg & Laschinger, 1991; J.B. Jemmott et al., 1992; L.S. Jemmott et al., 1992). This theory has not been tested for the relationship between stated intentions to care for patients and actual caregiving behavior among nurses. Other investigators have recommended the use of concepts such as stigma or constructs from theories of decision making, psychoanalysis, and cognitive psychology to design programs that will resolve fears and modify behavior (Gallop et al., 1992b; Siminoff et al., 1991). Kemppainen and colleagues (1992) suggested the theory of cognitive dissonance as a plausible explanation for the inconsistencies found between behavior and attitudes.

Some conceptual teaching models have been applied. Pederson (1993) tested the use of structured controversy versus lecture to change nursing students' beliefs and attitudes about providing care for PWHIV. Structured controversy resulted in more positive changes; however, once again intentions were measured rather than actual changes. Models of adult learning were used by one state professional organization to educate care providers about the risk of HIV in women (California Nurses' Association, 1992). Significant changes were made in learners' knowledge, cultural beliefs and practices, and clinical skills. The use of theories of behavior and learning is a significant step forward in the effort to change nurses' attitudes and practices.

Staff Development

Nurses planning educational programs for their peers or for graduate nursing students may be guided also by researchers' findings in addressing nurses' knowledge and attitudes. In general, investigators have found that nurses' knowledge of AIDS is high. Therefore continuing education should now be directed at changes in information rather than at basic AIDS information. Nurses are interested in changes in the virus and new virus strains; in treatment and experimental uses of zidovudine; in nursing assessment of symptoms and effective nursing care (skin care, mouth care, nutrition planning, treatment of diarrhea, and so forth); and in antibiotic and antiviral drugs and their effectiveness against the various opportunistic infections and neoplasms. They are interested also in areas that were not explored in depth in the past: the components of a neuropsychiatric examination, the care of IDUs, differences in HIV disease in women, and current prognosis of the disease and treatment of children. Changes in the epidemiology of the disease are of interest also because of differences in the exposure categories in the various parts of the United States. These changes help identify the groups to whom nurses will be providing increased care—for instance, heterosexual adolescents and people of color.

Many areas of patient education are of interest to nurses: What is the latest information on early intervention? What are the roles of cofactors? How can persons with HIV infection enroll in research protocols? What alternative therapies are available and what is their effectiveness? How is partner notification handled? What community resources are available to PWHIV? What resources are available for long-term care and home care?

Continuing education courses that provide information and an opportunity to practice clinical skills may be sufficient to address these deficits in knowledge and skills. However, equally important are educational experiences that address fears, anxieties, and attitudes. Courses that focus on knowledge only are unlikely to affect attitudes (Robbins et al., 1992). Flaskerud (1991) has proposed a three-tiered psychoeducational model to address knowledge, clinical skills, and attitudes and fears. The first tier addresses knowledge and clinical skills that are not emotion laden. Content areas and teaching-learning strategies for these areas are listed in Table 1–4.

There are several areas of knowledge and clinical skills, however, that are laden with emotion and are related to feelings of anxiety and insecurity among nurses. The second tier of the model addresses these areas. Foremost among them are occupational exposure to

Table 1–4. Content and Strategies for Increasing Knowledge and Clinical Skills

CONTENT	STRATEGIES
Immunology, viral strains	Provide information
Treatment, uses of zidovudine or AZT	
Specific antibiotic and antiviral therapies for specific opportunistic infections and neoplasms	
Regional epidemiology	
HIV in injection drug users	
HIV in women	
HIV in adolescents	
HIV in children	
Nursing assessment of symptoms	Provide information
Neuropsychiatric assessment	Provide practice for skill attainment
Effective nursing care: mouth care, skin care, nutrition, diarrhea, providing a safe environment	Provide demonstration
Client education	Provide information
Information on early intervention	Include service providers as sponsors and resources
Role of cofactors	
Enrolling in research protocols	
Alternative therapies	
Partner notification	
Community resources	

HIV, transmission in the workplace, and precautions for HCWs. For nurses' fears to be allayed, they must frequently be given up-to-date information on risks to nurses and on infection control procedures.

As noted in the review of research on nurses' knowledge and attitudes, nurses are skeptical of information on transmission in the workplace given to them by national experts. Some believe that new strains of the virus have developed and require new precautions. Repeated information on the documented risk to HCWs and the effectiveness of universal precautions may calm nurses' fears in this regard. However, a second area of concern is nurses' apparent failure to use universal precautions even when these are well known and a matter of hospital policy. Educational efforts with an affective component (opportunity for dialogue, expression of feelings in a nonthreatening atmosphere) may help motivate nurses to change behaviors and thereby reduce their risk (Irvine et al., 1993) (Table 1–5).

Group discussions of institutional policies with a knowledgeable leader may be an effective means of educating nurses about univer-

sal precautions and other areas of AIDS care. Group discussions give nurses practice and information for involvement in institutional policy making. A comprehensive institutional policy should include direction on reporting HIV exposure, information on the care and treatment of HCWs who are exposed, clear and relatively stable information on universal precautions, a commitment to provide adequate equipment for implementing precautions, psychosocial support services for health care personnel working with HIV-infected persons, and legal and ethical support services for HCWs (Taerk et al., 1993).

Feelings of anxiety, insecurity, and discomfort among nurses also arise in response to a lack of knowledge about sexual practices, sexual history taking, and sexual counseling. Information in these areas, followed by practice in the form of role playing, may provide education and allay anxieties, insecurities, and discomfort with topics of sexuality. Providing information about HIV infection and actual practice in developing skills in areas in which nurses are less knowledgeable and comfortable (e.g., sexual history taking and counseling) may also affect their attitudes. Role play-

Table 1–5. Content and Strategies for Increasing Knowledge, Clinical Skills, and Attitudes

CONTENT	STRATEGIES
Occupational exposure	Provide information
Transmission in the workplace	Group discussions with knowledgeable leaders (e.g., in-
Precautions for health care workers	fection control nurses)
Failure to use universal precautions	
Hospital and institutional HIV policies	Provide practice in designing comprehensive policy
Sexual practices, history taking, and counselings	Provide information
Drug use practices, history taking, counseling,	Provide practice through role playing
and referral	Include service providers as sponsors/resources

ing and practice tend to normalize behavior that at first might be considered strange. The same is true of drug use behavior. Most nurses know little about assessing drug use behavior, counseling about drug use, and resources in the community for treating and rehabilitating drug users. Again, a combination of educational and behavioral strategies such as role playing may reduce anxiety and discomfort with this topic.

Changing nurses' attitudes requires more than just providing more information or education about AIDS. As noted previously, attitudes are influenced by fears of infection and anxiety associated with a lack of information and skills in some areas such as sexual behavior and drug use. However, attitudes are also formed by deeply held negative social and moral judgments about homosexuals and homosexuality, injection drug use, and involvement with multiple sexual partners. Nurses share these attitudes with other HCWs and the public.

The third tier of the psychoeducational model addresses attitudes alone (Table 1–6). The studies reviewed in this chapter indicate that nurses' attitudes have not changed substantially in the past 2 years and that education alone does not motivate attitude change. The most effective educational strategies for influencing attitudes have a strong affective component in which feelings can be expressed openly and in a nonthreatening atmosphere. This includes negative feelings about homosexuals and IDUs, about various sexual practices, and about hospitals' forcing nurses to care for PWHIV against their wishes. It also includes identifying what angers or frightens nurses about homosexuality, drug use, or caring for a PWHIV.

However, expression of negative feelings and identification of fears and hostilities cannot be the only components of an affective educational program. Researchers have reported that nurses with positive attitudes share a number of characteristics: they have a homosexual friend or family member; they have cared for a person with AIDS; they have more knowledge about AIDS, sexuality, and drug use; they are younger; they are better educated; they are United States born and white; and they have no religion or belong to

Table 1–6. Content and Strategies for Attitude Change

CONTENT	STRATEGIES
Homosexuality	Provide information
Drug use	Exploration of feelings in small group format
Multiple sexual partners	Provide knowledgeable group leaders who share participants' social, cultural background (include culturally diverse nurses)
	Include gay men, IDUs, PWHIV in discussion groups
	Include clergy, religious representatives, ethicists, and attorneys in discussion groups

a religious group that does not condemn homosexuality.

Educational program planners can take these participant-learner characteristics into account. Whenever possible, educators can compensate by providing supplemental information when feasible and designing specific interventions for nurses based on their social and cultural differences. For example, involving gay men, PWHIV, and injection and recreational drug users in educational programs gives participants in these programs a chance to meet and engage in a dialogue with people whom they may not have known previously. A positive group experience with PWHIV, drug users, and gay men assists respondents in knowing and understanding them a little better (Gallop et al., 1992b).

Programs with different emphases might have to be developed for nurses who are, for instance, from various cultural backgrounds. Distrust of government (e.g., CDC) statements on transmission, unfounded fears of risks from casual contact, and moral disapproval and denial of homosexuality and drug use by some cultural groups might be issues that would require specific educational programs for nurses in some communities. Programs or group discussions led by a knowledgeable nurse with a social and cultural background similar to that of the participants may significantly reduce feelings of distrust and skepticism. On the other hand, the group's makeup does not have to be homogeneous. The value of discussion with persons who hold differing social and moral positions should not be minimized in its role of producing individual growth and understanding. Educational programs that bring nurses together to discuss their various views can facilitate their acceptance and understanding of their patients and each other.

The part that religion plays in condemning homosexuals, drug users, and sexually promiscuous persons should not be underestimated in its influence on nurses' attitudes toward PWHIV. However, most religions have at their core a commitment to charity and goodwill that can be cited to persuade nurses of the worth of PWHIV and other stigmatized groups. In fact, in some religions the highest good can be achieved by service to those who are considered by society to have the "least worth." Many dedicated clergy and representatives of all the major religions have been involved in providing care to PWHIV. Whenever possible, including such religious leaders in program and group discussions should be considered. These persons can serve as role models to nurses who share the same religious affiliation. Furthermore, frank group discussions of religious beliefs may remind nurses of the commitments to charity and compassion that characterize most major religions. In addition, the inclusion of ethicists and attorneys in group discussions may further nurses' understanding and acceptance of their obligations to patient care.

Nurses employing this model for educational program planning are urged to consider two aspects of model development and use. The first is assessment. The audience for any educational program must be assessed for levels of knowledge, skill attainment, and attitudes. It is possible that any given audience will benefit from only one tier of the model, whereas others might need all three. To evaluate the model appropriately, one must know the audience and its needs. Second, the model is as yet untested. It is based on previous research and experience. It is highly recommended that educators attempting to use the model employ evaluative strategies in implementing the model.

Undergraduate Teaching

Duffy (1993) proposed a model for the integration of HIV/AIDS content into baccalaureate nursing curricula. A three-stage model of curriculum development allows faculty to introduce HIV content gradually, taking into account the process and practicality of curriculum change and the level of faculty expertise. However, faculty could begin the introduction of HIV content at any of the three proposed stages and not progress through all three stages, depending on the specific situation. Each of the stages is described here. Relevant content from this textbook related to each stage is described in Appendix II.

The three-stage model begins with Stage I, entitled "The Guest Speaker," in which the school recognizes the need for HIV content but faculty members do not have the expertise to deliver this content. Duffy (1993) describes this stage as introductory, delivered by guest lecturer(s), and consisting of a one-shot AIDS program, lecture, or workshop for the school. Stage II, entitled "Mainstreaming HIV Content," involves the inclusion of HIV content in appropriate places in the traditional curriculum but relies heavily on expert guest faculty. For instance, mainstreaming would include the presentation of HIV content along with discussion of other blood-borne pathogens in the fundamental skills course or incorporation of content regarding PCP into a medical-surgical nursing course or of content on psychosocial care into a psychiatric nursing course. Stage III, entitled "Integration," is characterized by the recognition that the clinical challenges of HIV care illuminate important learning needs, not limited to HIV care, in core nursing curricula. At this stage, core nursing faculty provide HIV content; clinical experiences with PWHIV are part of student skills learning; and HIV intervention research exemplifies nursing prevention and intervention research. New areas of content and clinical skills that have not received attention in traditional undergraduate curricula are identified and integrated on the basis of the clinical challenges of HIV care.

Many of the strategies for learning discussed in the preceding section on staff development may be used in any of the three stages of the model proposed for undergraduate curriculum development. In addition, specific suggestions for learning at each stage are included in Appendix II.

RESEARCH IN HIV NURSING

Several reviews of nursing research and HIV/AIDS have been published recently (Gaskins et al., 1991; Larson, 1988, Larson & Ropka, 1991; Ragsdale, 1993; Swanson et al., 1990; Zeller et al., 1993). These reviews have summarized the research to date, recommended areas for further study, discussed methodologic and ethical issues, and proposed collaborative efforts between clinicians and researchers. In addition, the National Center for Nursing Research (NCNR) (now the National Institute for Nursing Research [NINR]) in 1988 and again in 1993 set the national research agenda for nursing.

From 1988 through 1994 the priorities of NCNR were low birth weight, HIV infection, long-term care, symptom management, nursing informatics, health promotion, and technology dependency. In the area of HIV nursing research, the NCNR identified five areas for study (1993): physiologic nursing care, psychosocial nursing care, delivery of nursing care, prevention of transmission, and applied ethics. Larson and Ropka (1991) reviewed nursing research published to that date and categorized published reports according to the HIV nursing priorities of the NCNR. They identified a continued need for research in all areas but a particular need in the areas of physiologic nursing care and applied ethics. They also noted the need for research with vulnerable populations: adolescents, injection drug users, pregnant women and newborn infants, homeless people, and people of color. Finally, they identified a need for research on high-quality, efficient, and cost-effective care for persons with HIV disease and their caregivers.

A somewhat different interpretation of HIV research needs was made as the result of a review of all HIV/AIDS entries indexed by MEDLINE between 1981 and 1990 (Elford et al., 1991a). After reviewing the topics of more than 30,000 papers on HIV/AIDS, these reviewers recommended that priority be given to research on prevention and control, the psychological aspects of HIV/AIDS, and the further development of drug therapies.

In this edition of the textbook, a section on HIV nursing research has been added to each chapter. The topic of HIV nursing research will be addressed from two perspectives in each chapter. The first will be a summary review of nursing research to date on the chapter topic. The second will be an identification of nursing research needs in the topic area. Special attention will be given to the new (1994–1999) research agenda of the NINR and the possibilities for its application to HIV nursing research (*NCNR Outreach*, 1993).

The new priorities—one to be emphasized each year from 1995 through 1999—are identified below, with examples of HIV nursing research that might be considered in each category.

1. *Developing and testing community-based nursing models.* The care of persons with HIV disease is given increasingly in the community. The range of care and services needed by persons with HIV disease and their families makes this population particularly appropriate to the development and testing of community-based nursing models. Every aspect of nursing care from health promotion to treatment and palliation, from physiologic to psychosocial, from acute to long term, and from cost-effective home care to referral for care could be studied in a community-based nursing care system for persons with HIV. Results of these studies might be generalized to the community care and service needs of other populations as well. A summary of research in this area and recommendations for future research are addressed in more depth in Chapter 12.

2. *Assessing the effectiveness of nursing interventions in HIV/AIDS.* Both physiologic nursing care interventions and psychosocial interventions could be identified and tested with the use of experimental designs. Research in the area of physiologic care, especially, is needed to test nursing interventions into human responses to HIV: fatigue, nausea, weight loss, dry skin, diarrhea, shortness of breath, cough, fever, pain, and so forth. Zeller and colleagues (1993) suggested some of these same areas for research, identifying them as symptom management. Interventions specific to adults and children, men and women, and various cultural groups should be identified and tested. Studies on interventions into human responses to illness might be generalizable to other illness conditions as well. A summary of research specific to these areas and recommendations for HIV nursing research are addressed particularly in Chapter 5 but also in the chapters on women, adolescents, and children.

3. *Developing and testing approaches to re-mediating cognitive impairment.* For persons with HIV disease, cognitive dysfunction occurs because of HIV dementia and because of various other fungal, parasitic, and viral infections. In addition to treatment with drugs, persons with cognitive dysfunction can be retrained in memory and concentration and in self-care skills (activities of daily living). Interventions could be designed and tested to determine the outcomes for the person with HIV in self-care skills and the reduction of stress in caregivers. Results might be generalizable to other cognitively impaired persons, such as those with Alzheimer's disease, and their caregivers. A summary of research specific to this area and recommendations for future research are addressed in more depth in Chapters 5 and 11.

4. *Testing interventions for coping with chronic illness.* Increasingly, HIV disease is considered a chronic illness. From the early infection stage to advanced HIV disease, PWHIV need a range of coping skills, supportive services, and nursing therapeutics. All of them can be identified and tested with a population of PWHIV. Study results may be generalized to persons with other chronic, life-threatening diseases such as cancer. A research summary and recommendations in this area are addressed in greater depth in Chapter 12.

5. *Identifying biologic-behavioral factors and testing interventions to promote immunocompetence.* The effects of nutrition, exercise, rest, stress reduction, changes in lifestyle factors such as smoking and the use of recreational drugs, preventive and therapeutic health care, and so forth, all suggest interventions that may enhance immunocompetence. Programs instituting these biobehavioral factors need to be designed and tested with PWHIV. Study results may be generalizable to persons with other immunodeficiency diseases as well. Research to date and research needed in this area are addressed in more depth in Chapter 2.

Finally, some investigators have encouraged collaborative research between clinicians and researchers (Ragsdale, 1993). The benefits of such research are obvious in terms of applicability to nursing practice. Such research would also be more likely to take the direction suggested by the new NINR priorities for research.

SUMMARY

Many changes in HIV disease and the AIDS epidemic have occurred in the past 2 years. This chapter provides an overview of those changes and refers the reader to subsequent chapters in which current information is presented in depth. Two areas of change not addressed elsewhere are covered here: the changing regional epidemiology of HIV infection and changes in nurses' knowledge, attitudes, and practices. Suggestions are given for planning nursing education workshops and conferences to improve nurses' knowledge, skills, and attitudes in the care of persons with HIV disease. Finally, suggestions are made for HIV nursing research using the new NINR priorities for 1995 through 1999.

Information about HIV disease is changing so rapidly that it is impossible to publish anything that is completely up-to-date. For this reason, it is especially important for nurses to remain aware of new developments and changes in information about HIV. Close attention to AIDS- and HIV-related research, conferences, and information in the professional and popular media can help nurses keep up with issues and information about HIV disease and the AIDS epidemic.

REFERENCES

Abiteboul, D., Fourrier, A., Anoulay, S., et al. (1991). Occupational exposure to blood: A descriptive survey of risk management in public assistance hospital of Paris. Paper presented to the 7th International Conference on AIDS, Florence, Italy.

Abrams, D.I. (1986). AIDS: Battling a retroviral enemy. *California Nursing Review, 8*(6), 36–37, 44.

Abrams, D.I. (1990). Definition of ARC. In P.T. Cohen, M.A. Sande, & P.A. Volberding (Eds.), *The AIDS knowledge base* (pp. 1-4.1.13 to 3-4.1.3). Waltham, MA: Medical Publishing Group.

Aboulker, J.P., Swart, A.M. (1993). Preliminary analysis of the Concorde trial. *Lancet, 341,* 889–890.

Agency for Health Care Policy and Research (AHCPR), Public Health Service, USDHHS (January 1994). Evaluation and management of early HIV infection. Clinical Practice Guideline, No. 7 (AHCPR publication No. 94-0572). Rockville, MD: The Agency.

Aiken, L.H., Semaan, S., Lehman, H.P., et al. (1993). Nurse practitioner managed care for persons with HIV infection. *IMAGE: Journal of Nursing Scholarship, 25* (3), 172–177.

Alexander, R., Fitzpatrick, J. (1991). Variables influencing nurses' attitudes toward AIDS and AIDS patients. *AIDS Patient Care, 5*(6), 315–320.

All, A. (1989). Health care workers' anxieties and fears concerning AIDS: A literature review. *The Journal of Continuing Education in Nursing, 20*(4), 162–165.

Allen, M.A., Ownby, K.K. (1991). Tuberculosis: The other epidemic. *Journal of the Association of Nurses in AIDS Care, 2*(4), 9–14.

American Health Consultants (1992). Failures renew doubts about zidovudine prophylaxis. *AIDS Alert, 7*(2), 177–180.

Andrulis, D.P., Weslowski, V.B., Hintz, E., et al. (1992). Comparisons of hospital care for patients with AIDS and other HIV-related conditions. *Journal of the American Medical Association, 267,* 2482–2486.

Araneta, M.R.G., Weisfuse, I.B., Greenberg, B., et al. (1992). Abortions and HIV-1 infection in New York City, 1987–1989. *AIDS, 6*(10), 1195–1201.

Barre-Sinoussi, F., Chermann, J.C., Rey, F., et al. (1983). Isolation of a T-lymphotropic retrovirus from a patient at risk for acquired immune deficiency syndrome (AIDS). *Science, 220*(4599), 868–871.

Bartlett, J.G. (1993). Zidovudine now or later? *New England Journal of Medicine, 329*(5), 351–352.

Bayer, R., Dubler, N.N., Landesman, S. (1993). The dual epidemics of tuberculosis and AIDS: Ethical and policy issues in screening and treatment. *American Journal of Public Health, 83*(5), 649–654.

Becker, M.H., Joseph, J.G. (1988). AIDS and behavioral change to reduce risk: A review. *The American Journal of Public Health, 78*(4), 394–410.

Bell, D.M. (1993). Information gap: HIV and the health worker. *Harvard Medical Alumni Bulletin, 67,* 15–22.

Bond, S., Rhodes, T., Philips, P., et al. (1990). HIV infection and AIDS in England: The experience, knowledge and intentions of community nursing staff, *Journal of Advanced Nursing, 15,* 249–255.

Brandt, A.M. (1988). AIDS in historical perspective: Four lessons from the history of sexually transmitted diseases. *The American Journal of Public Health. 78*(4), 367–371.

Breault, A.J., Polifroni, E.C. (1992). Caring for people with AIDS: Nurses' attitudes and feelings. *Journal of Advanced Nursing, 17,* 21–27.

California Nurses' Association (1992). Women at risk: AIDS/HIV training for care providers. Funded by the Department of Health Services of the State of California, developed by California Nurses' Association (CNA), AIDS Education and Training. San Francisco, CA.

Campbell, S., Maki, M., Willenbring, K., et al. (1991). AIDS-related knowledge, attitudes, and behaviors among 629 registered nurses at a Minnesota hospital: A descriptive study. *Journal of the Association of Nurses in AIDS Care, 2*(1), 15–23.

Cassels, J.M., Redman, B.K. (1989). New baccalaureate graduates in care of AIDS patients: Perceptions of preparedness and information accessibility. *The Journal of Continuing Education in Nursing, 20*(4), 156–161.

Centers for Disease Control (1981). *Pneumocystis* pneumonia—Los Angeles. *Morbidity and Mortality Weekly Report, 30*(21), 250–252.

Centers for Disease Control (1982a). Update on acquired immune deficiency syndrome (AIDS)—United States. *Morbidity and Mortality Weekly Report, 31*(37), 507–514.

Centers for Disease Control (1982b). Opportunistic infections and Kaposi's sarcoma among Haitians in the

United States. *Morbidity and Mortality Weekly Report, 31*(26), 353–354, 360–361.

Centers for Disease Control (1982c). *Pneumocystis carinii* pneumonia among persons with hemophilia A. *Morbidity and Mortality Weekly Report, 31*(27), 365–367.

Centers for Disease Control (1986). Classification system for human T-lymphotropic virus III/lymphadenopathy–associated virus infection. *Morbidity and Mortality Weekly Report, 35,* 335.

Centers for Disease Control (1990). Possible transmission of human immunodeficiency virus to a patient during an invasive dental procedure. *Morbidity and Mortality Weekly Report, 39*(29), 489–493.

Centers for Disease Control (1991a). Update: Transmission of HIV infection during an invasive dental procedure—Florida. *Morbidity and Mortality Weekly Report, 40*(2), 21–27.

Centers for Disease Control (1991b). Recommendations for preventing transmission of human immunodeficiency virus and hepatitis B virus to patients during invasive procedures. *Morbidity and Mortality Weekly Report, 40*(RR-8), 1–7.

Centers for Disease Control and Prevention (1991c). Epidemiology of tuberculosis in the United States. *Core Curriculum on Tuberculosis,* 19–20.

Centers for Disease Control and Prevention (Dec. 18, 1992). 1993 revised classification system for HIV infection and expanded surveillance case definition for AIDS among adolescents and adults. *Morbidity and Mortality Weekly Report, 41*(RR-17), 1–19.

Centers for Disease Control and Prevention (1992b). Guidelines for the performance of CD4+ T-cell determinations in persons with human immunodeficiency virus infections. *Morbidity and Mortality Weekly Report, 41*(RR-8), 1–12.

Centers for Disease Control and Prevention (1992c). A conceptual framework for evaluating behavior change. *CDC HIV/AIDS Prevention, 3*(4), 2–3.

Centers for Disease Control and Prevention (April 9, 1993). Years of potential life lost before age 65. *Morbidity and Mortality Weekly Report, 42*(13), 251–253.

Centers for Disease Control and Prevention (April 30, 1993). Impact of the expanded AIDS surveillance case definition on AIDS case reporting. *Morbidity and Mortality Weekly Report, 42*(16), 308–314.

Centers for Disease Control and Prevention (May 7, 1993). Update: Investigations of persons treated by HIV-infected health-care workers—United States. *Morbidity and Mortality Weekly Report, 42*(17), 329–337.

Centers for Disease Control and Prevention (May 28, 1993). Recommended infection-control practices for dentistry, 1993. *Morbidity and Mortality Weekly Report, 42*(RR-8), 1–11.

Centers for Disease Control and Prevention (May 1993). Summaries of Reports and Recommendations. Projections of the number of persons diagnosed with AIDS and the number of immunosuppressed HIV-infected persons—United States, 1992–1994 (December 25). *HIV/AIDS Prevention, 4*(1), 10.

Centers for Disease Control and Prevention (June 11, 1993). Outbreak of multidrug-resistant tuberculosis at a hospital—New York City, 1991. *Morbidity and Mortality Weekly Report, 42*(22), 427–437.

Centers for Disease Control and Prevention (Aug. 13, 1993). Tuberculosis among pregnant women—New York City 1985–1992. *Morbidity and Mortality Weekly Report, 42*(31), 605–612.

Centers for Disease Control and Prevention (Aug. 20, 1993). Tuberculosis—Western Europe, 1974–1991. *Morbidity and Mortality Weekly Report, 42*(32), 628–631.

Centers for Disease Control and Prevention (October 1993). *HIV/AIDS Surveillance Report* (Third Quarter Edition), *5*(3).

Centers for Disease Control and Prevention (Oct. 1, 1993). Assessment of laboratory reporting to supplement active AIDS surveillance—Colorado. *Morbidity and Mortality Weekly Report, 42*(38), 749–752.

Chaisson, R.E., Stanton, D.L., Gallant, J.E., et al. (1993). Impact of the 1993 revision of the AIDS case definition on the prevalence of AIDS in a clinical setting. *AIDS, 7*(6), 857–862.

Choi, S., Lagakos, S.W., Schooley, R.T., et al. (1993). CD4+ lymphocytes are an incomplete surrogate marker for clinical progression in persons with asymptomatic HIV infection taking zidovudine. *Annals of Internal Medicine, 118*(9), 674–680.

Christ, G.H., Wiener, L.S. (1985). Psychosocial issues in AIDS. In V.T. DeVita, Jr. (Ed.), *AIDS etiology, diagnosis, treatment and prevention* (pp. 275–297). Philadelphia: J.B. Lippincott.

Colombotos, J., Messeri, P., Burgunder, M., et al. (1991). Physicians, nurses and AIDS: Preliminary findings from a national study. *Agency for Health Care Policy and Research Program Note,* (AHCPR Pub. No. 0024). Rockville, MD, U.S. Department of Health and Human Services.

Conway, G.A., Epstein, M.R., Hayman, C.R., et al. (1993). Trends in HIV prevalence among disadvantaged youth: Survey results from a national job training program, 1988 through 1992. *Journal of the American Medical Association, 269*(22), 2887–2889.

Cooper, D.A., Gatell, J.M., Kroon, S., et al. (1993). Zidovudine in persons with asymptomatic HIV infection and CD4+ cell counts greater than 400 per cubic millimeter. *New England Journal of Medicine, 329*(5), 297–303.

Cotton, D.J. (1993). Reports from Berlin. *AIDS Clinical Care, 5*(7), 51.

Cotton, D.J., Friedland, G.H. (1993). The Concorde study: The long-term benefit of early vs. delayed AZT remains uncertain. *AIDS Clinical Care, 5*(5), 38.

Currey, C.J., Johnson, M., Ogden, B. (1990). Willingness of health-professions students to treat patients with AIDS. *Academic Medicine, 65,* 472–474.

Damrosch, S., Abbey, S., Warner, A., et al. (1990). Critical care nurses' attitudes toward, concerns about, and knowledge of, the acquired immunodeficiency syndrome. *Heart and Lung, 19,* 395–400.

D'Angelo, L., Getson, P.R., Luban, N.L.C., et al. (1991). HIV infection in urban adolescents: Can we predict who is at risk? *Pediatrics, 88,* 982–986.

D'Augelli, A.R. (1989). AIDS fears and homophobia among rural nursing personnel. *AIDS Education and Prevention, 1*(4), 277–284.

De Cock, K.M., Soro, B., Coulibaly, I.M., et al. (1992). Tuberculosis and HIV infection in sub-Saharan Africa. *Journal of the American Medical Association, 268,* 1581–1587.

de Saussure, P., Yerly, S., Tullen, E., et al. (1993). Human immunodeficiency virus type 1 nucleic acids detected before p24 antigenemia in a blood donor. *Transfusion, 3*(2), 164–167.

Dickinson, G.M., Morhart, R.E., Klimas, N.G., et al. (1993). Absence of HIV transmission from an infected dentist to his patients. *Journal of the American Medical Association, 269,* 1802–1806.

Dow. M.G., Knox, M.D. (1991). Mental health and substance abuse staff: HIV/AIDS knowledge and attitudes. *AIDS Care, 3*(1), 75–87.

Downes, J. (1991). Acquired immunodeficiency syndrome: The nurse's legal duty to serve. *Journal of Professional Nursing, 7*(6), 333–340.

Duffy, P.R. (1993). A model for the integration of HIV/AIDS content into baccalaureate nursing curricula. *Journal of Nursing Education, 32*(8), 347–351.

Elford, J., Bor, R., Summers, R. (1991a). Research into HIV and AIDS between 1981 and 1990: The epidemic curve. *AIDS, 5,* 1515–1519.

Elford, J., Bor, R., Cockroft, A. (1991b). Teaching medical students to examine their own preconceptions about HIV/AIDS. Paper presented at the 7th International Conference on AIDS. Florence, Italy.

Empfield, M., McKinnon, K., Cournos, F., et al. (1993). HIV seroprevalence among homeless patients admitted to a psychiatric inpatient unit. *American Journal of Psychiatry, 150,* 47–52.

Fahey, J.L., Taylor, J.M.G., Detels, R., et al. (1990). The prognostic value of cellular and serologic markers in infection with human immunodeficiency virus type 1. *New England Journal of Medicine, 332,* 166–172.

Ficarrotto, T.J., Grade, M., Zegans, L.S. (1991). Occupational and personal risk estimates for HIV contagion among incoming graduate nursing students. *Journal of the Association of Nurses in AIDS Care, 2*(1), 5–11.

Fischl, M.A., Olson, R.M., Follansbee, S.F., et al. (1993). Zalcitabine compared with zidovudine in patients with advanced HIV-1 infection who received previous zidovudine therapy. *Annals of Internal Medicine, 118,* 762–769.

Flaskerud, J.H. (1991). A psychoeducational model for changing nurses' AIDS knowledge, attitudes, and practices. *The Journal of Continuing Education in Nursing, 22*(6), 237–244.

Flaskerud, J.H., Lewis, M.A., Shin, D. (1989). Changing nurses' AIDS-related knowledge and attitudes through continuing education. *The Journal of Continuing Education in Nursing, 20*(4), 148–154.

Gail, M.H., Rosenberg, P.S., Goedert, J.J. (1990). Therapy may explain recent deficits in AIDS incidence. *Journal of Acquired Immune Deficiency Syndromes, 3*(1), 296–306.

Gallop, R.M., Lancee, W.J., Taerk, G., et al. (1992a). Fear of contagion and AIDS: Nurses' perception of risk. *AIDS Care, 4*(1), 103–109.

Gallop, R.M., Taerk, G., Lancee, W.J. (1992b). A randomized trial of group interventions for hospital staff caring for persons with AIDS. *AIDS Care, 4*(2), 177–185.

Gaskins, S., Sowell, R., Gueldner, S. (1991). Overcoming methodological barriers to HIV/AIDS nursing research. *Journal of the Association of Nurses in AIDS Care, 2*(4), 33–37.

Gerberding, J.L. (1989). Risks to health care workers from occupational exposure to hepatitis B virus, human immunodeficiency virus, and cytomegalovirus. *Infectious Disease Clinics of North America, 3*(3), 735–743.

Gerberding, J. (1993). Is antiretroviral treatment after percutaneous HIV exposure justified? *Annals of Internal Medicine, 118*(12), 979–980.

Gershon, R., Curbow, B., Vlahov, D., et al. (June 1991). Low compliance with universal precautions among hospital employees despite high perceived risk. Paper presented at the 7th International AIDS Conference, Florence, Italy.

Global AIDS News (1993). New CDC definition will cause surge in reported U.S. AIDS cases. *Global AIDS News, 1,* 4.

Goldenberg, D., Laschinger, H. (1991). Attitudes and normative beliefs of nursing students as predictors of intended care behaviors with AIDS patients: A test of the Ajzen-Fishbein theory of reasoned action. *Journal of Nursing Education, 30*(3), 119–126.

Goldsmith, M.F. (1993). For AIDS treatment, vaccines, now think genes. *Journal of the American Medical Association, 269*(17), 2189–2190.

Gruber, M., Beavers, F.E., Johnson, B., et al. (1989). The relationship between knowledge about acquired immunodeficiency syndrome and the implementation of universal precautions by registered nurses. *Clinical Nurse Specialist, 3*(4), 182–185.

Hahn, R.A., Onorato, I.M., Jones, T.S. (1989). Prevalence of HIV infection among intravenous drug users in the United States. *Journal of the American Medical Association, 261*(18), 2677–2684.

Henry, K. (1993). Switching and combining antiretroviral therapies. *AIDS Clinical Care, 5*(5), 33.

Huerta, S.R., Oddi, L.F. (1992). Refusal to care for patients with human immunodeficiency virus/acquired immunodeficiency syndrome: Issues and responses. *Journal of Professional Nursing, 8*(4), 221–230.

Ippolito, G., Puro, V., De Carli, G. (1993). The risk of occupational human immunodeficiency virus infection in health care workers. *Archives of Internal Medicine, 153*(12), 1451–1458.

Irvine, S., Penny, R., Anns, M. (1993). Developing quality primary care services in HIV/AIDS care: The education imperative. *Journal of Acquired Immune Deficiency Syndromes, 6*(Suppl. 1): S72–S76.

Jason, J., Lui, K., Ragni, M.V., et al. (1989). Risk of developing AIDS in HIV-infected cohorts of hemophilic and homosexual men. *Journal of the American Medical Association, 26*(5), 725–727.

Jemmott III, J.B., Freleicher, J., Jemmott, L.S. (1992). Perceived risk of infection and attitudes toward risk groups: Determinants of nurses' behavioral intentions regarding AIDS patients. *Research in Nursing and Health, 15,* 295–301.

Jemmott, L.S., Jemmott III, J.B., Cruz-Collins, M. (1992). Predicting AIDS patient care intentions among nursing students. *Nursing Research, 41*(3), 172–177.

Johnson, A.M., Shergold, C., Hawkins, A., et al. (1993). Patterns of hospital care for patients with HIV infection and AIDS. *Journal of Epidemiology and Community Health, 47*(3), 232–237.

Katz, M.H., Hessol, N.A., Buchbinder, S.P., et al. (1993). Use of Bayes theorem to estimate the impact of the proposed CD4-based expansion of the AIDS case definition. *Journal of Acquired Immune Deficiency Syndromes, 6*(3), 295–297.

Kelly, J.A., Murphy, D.A., Bahr, G.R., et al. (1992). AIDS/HIV risk behavior among the chronic mentally ill. *American Journal of Psychiatry, 149*(7), 886–889.

Kemppainen, J., St. Lawrence, J.S., Irizarry, A., et al. (1992). Nurses' willingness to perform AIDS patient care. *Journal of Continuing Education in Nursing, 23*(3), 110–117.

Klisch, M.L. (1990). Caring for persons with AIDS: Student reactions. *Nursing Educator, 15*(4), 16–20.

Kozal, M.J., Shafer, M.A., Winters, D.A., et al. (1993). A mutation in human immunodeficiency virus reverse transcriptase and decline in CD4 lymphocyte numbers in long-term zidovudine recipients. *Journal of Infectious Disease, 167*(3), 526–532.

Lange, M.A., de Wolf, F., Goudsmit, J. (1989). Markers for progression of HIV infection. *AIDS, 3*(Suppl. 1), s153–160.

Larson, E. (1988). Nursing research and AIDS. *Nursing Research, 37*(1), 60–62.

Larson, E., Ropka, M. (1991). An update on nursing research and HIV infection. *Image, 23*(1), 4–12.

Lawrence, S., Lawrence, R. (1989). Knowledge and attitudes about aquired immunodeficiency syndrome in nursing and non-nursing groups. *Journal of Professional Nursing, 5,* 92–101.

Lemp, G.F., Payne, S.F., Neal, D., et al. (1990). Survival trends for patients with AIDS. *Journal of the American Medical Association, 263*(3), 402–406.

Levy, J.A., Hoffman, A.D., Kramer, S.M., et al. (1984). Isolation of lymphocytopathic retroviruses from San Francisco patients with AIDS. *Science, 225*(4664), 840–842.

Lifson, A.R., Darrow, W.W., Hessol, N.A., et al. (1990). Kaposi's sarcoma in a cohort of homosexual and bisexual men. *American Journal of Epidemiology, 131*(2), 221–231.

Lin, D.Y., Fischl, M.A., Schoenfeld, D.A. (1993). Evaluating the role of CD4-lymphocyte counts as surrogate endpoints in human immunodeficiency virus clinical trials. *Statistics in Medicine, 12*(9), 834–865.

Lindsay, M.K., Peterson, H.B., Taylor, E.B., et al. (1990). Routine human immunodeficiency virus infection screening of women requesting induced first-trimester abortion in an inner-city population. *Obstetrics & Gynecology, 76*(3), 347–350.

Macks, J. (1986). The Paris AIDS conference: Psychosocial research. *Focus, 1*(10), 1–2.

Malik-Nitto, S., Plantemoli, L. (1986). A strategic plan for the management of patients with AIDS. *Nursing Management, 17*(6), 46–48.

Mann, J., Tarantola, D.J.M., Netter, T. (Eds.), (1992). *AIDS in the world: A global report,* Cambridge, MA: Harvard University Press.

Marcus, R., Srivastava, P.U., Zalenski, R.J., et al. (1993). Risk of human immunodeficiency virus infection among emergency department workers. *The American Journal of Medicine, 94,* 363–370.

Martindale, L., Barnett, C. (1992). Nursing faculty's knowledge and attitudes toward persons with AIDS. *Journal of the Association of Nurses in AIDS Care, 3*(2), 9–13.

Matocha, L.K. (1990). Student clinical experience with persons who are HIV-positive or have ARC/AIDS: A model of success. *Journal of Nursing Education, 29*(2), 90–92.

Menitove, J.E. (1990). Current risk of transfusion-associated human immunodeficiency virus infection. *Archives of Pathology and Laboratory Medicine, 114,* 330–334.

Meyer, I.K., McKinnon, F., Cournos, M., et al. (1993). Seroprevalence among long-stay patients in a state psychiatric hospital. *Hospital and Community Psychiatry, 44*(3), 282–284.

Najera, R., Herrera, M.I., de Andres, R. (1987). Human immunodeficiency virus and related retroviruses. *Western Journal of Medicine, 147,* 694–701.

Nanda, D., Minkoff, H.L. (1989). HIV in pregnancy: transmission and immune effects. *Clinical Obstetrics and Gynecology, 32*(3), 456–466.

NCNR Outreach (Spring 1993) (p. 1). National Center for Nursing Research, National Institutes of Health, Bethesda, MD.

Osmond, D. (1990). Progression to AIDS in persons testing seropositive for antibody to HIV. In P.T. Cohen, M.A. Sande, & P.A. Volberding (Eds.). *The AIDS knowledge base* (pp. 1-1.1.6 to 8-1.1.6). Waltham, MA: Medical Publishing Group.

Osmond, D.H., Moss, A.R. (1989). The prevalence of HIV infection in the United States: A reappraisal of the public health service estimate. In P. Volberding & M.A. Jacobson (Eds.), *AIDS clinical review 1989* (pp. 1–17). New York: Marcel Dekker.

Passannante, M.R., French, J.D.B., Louria, B. (1993). How much do health care providers know about AIDS? *American Journal of Preventive Medicine, 9*(1), 6–14.

Pederson, C. (1993). Structured controversy versus lecture on nursing students' beliefs about and attitude toward providing care for persons with AIDS. *The Journal of Continuing Education in Nursing, 24*(2), 74–81.

Plant, M.L., Foster, J. (1993). AIDS-related experience, knowledge, attitudes and beliefs amongst nurses in an area with a high rate of HIV infection. *Journal of Advanced Nursing, 18,* 80–88.

Popovic, M., Sarngodharan, M.G., Read, E., et al. (1984). Detection, isolation, and continuous production of cytopathic retrovirus (HTLV-III) from patients with AIDS and pre-AIDS. *Science, 224*(4648), 497–500.

Prochaska, J.O., DiClemente, C.C., Norcorss, J.C. (1992). In search of how people change. *American Psychologist, 47*(9), 1102–1114.

Quinn, T.C., (Aug. 9, 1990). The global epidemiology of the human immunodeficiency virus. Paper presented at the Clinical Care and Management of the HIV-Infected Patient Conference, Medical College of Ohio, Toledo, OH.

Ragsdale, D. (1993). A call for help: Collaborative nursing research. *Journal of the Association of Nurses in AIDS Care, 4*(2), 48–52.

Rietmeijer, C.A., Davidson, A.J., Foster, C.T., et al. (1993). Cost of care for patients with human immunodeficiency virus infection: Patterns of utilization and charges in a public health care system. *Archives of Internal Medicine, 153*(2), 219–225.

Robbins, I., Cooper, A., Bender, M.P. (1992). The relationship between knowledge, attitudes and degree of contact with AIDS and HIV. *Journal of Advanced Nursing, 17,* 198–203.

Rogers, A.S., Froggatt III, J.W., Townsend, T., et al. (1993). Investigation of potential HIV transmission to the patients of an HIV-infected surgeon. *Journal of the American Medical Association, 269,* 1795–1801.

Rosenberg, P.S., Gail, M.H., Biggar, R.J., et al. (1993). HIV prevalence among Washington, D.C. residents having abortions. *Journal of the American Medical Association, 269*(4), 472–473.

Saah, A.J. (1993). The Florida dentist case revisited. *AIDS Targeted Information, 7*(4), 1.

Sandman, J. (1992). AIDS, the world health organization, and Central Africa. *Journal of the Association of Nurses in AIDS Care, 3*(4), 33–41.

Scherer, Y.K., Haughey, B.P., Wu, Y.B. (1989). AIDS: What are nurses' concerns? *Clinical Nurse Specialist, 3*(1), 48–54.

Scherer, Y., Wu, Y., Haughey, B. (1991). AIDS and homophobia among nurses. *Journal of Homosexuality, 21*(4), 85–101.

Schroeder, C. (1993). Nursing's response to the crisis of access, costs, and quality in health care. *Advance Nursing Science, 16*(1), 1–20.

Scitovsky, A.A. (1989). The cost of AIDS: An agenda for research. *Health Policy, 11,* 197–208.

Selik, R.M., Chu, S.Y., Buehler, J.W. (1993). HIV infection as leading cause of death among young adults in U.S. cities and states. *Journal of the American Medical Association, 269*(23), 2991.

Shapiro, C.N., Schulz, S.L., Lee, N.C., et al. (1989). Review of human immunodeficiency virus infection in women in the United States. *Obstetrics and Gynecology, 74*(5), 800–808.

Sheppard, H.W., Ascher, M.S., Winkelstein, Jr., E., et al. (1993). Use of T-lymphocyte subset analysis in the case definition for AIDS. *Journal of Acquired Immune Deficiency Syndromes, 6*(3), 287–294.

Siminoff, L.A., Erlen, J.A., Lidz, C.W. (1991). Stigma, AIDS and quality of nursing care: State of the science. *Journal of Advanced Nursing, 16,* 262–269.

Sowell, R.L., Gueldner, S.H., Killeen, M.R., et al. (1992). Impact of case management on hospital charges of PWAs in Georgia. *Journal of the Association of Nurses in AIDS Care, 3*(2), 24–31.

Strasser, J., Damrosch, S. (1992). Graduate nursing students' attitudes toward gay and hemophiliac men with AIDS. *Evaluation and the Health Professions, 15*(4), 115–127.

Susser, E., Valencia, E., Conover, S. (1993). Prevalence of HIV infection among psychiatric patients in a New York City men's shelter. *American Journal of Public Health, 83*(4), 568–570.

Swanson, J.M., Chenitz, C., Zalar, M., et al. (1990). A critical review of human immunodeficiency virus infection and acquired immunodeficiency syndrome–related research: The knowledge, attitudes, and practice of nurses. *Journal of Professional Nursing, 6*(6), 341–355.

Taerk, G.R.M., Gallop, W.J., Lancee, R.A., et al. (1993). Recurrent themes of concern in groups of health care professionals. *AIDS Care, 5*(2), 215–222.

Tesch, B.J., Simpson, D.E., Kirby, B.D. (1990). Medical and nursing students' attitudes about AIDS issues. *Academic Medicine, 65*(7), 467–469.

Tindall, B., Cooper, D.A. (1991). Primary HIV infection: Host responses and intervention strategies. *AIDS, 5,* 1–14.

Tokars, J.I., Marcus, R., Culter, D.H., et al. (1993). Surveillance of HIV infection and zidovudine use among health care workers after occupational exposure to HIV-infected blood. *Annals of Internal Medicine, 118*(12), 913–919.

U.S. Centers for Disease Control and Prevention (April 5, 1993). Director testifies before Congressional subcommittee on TB. *TB Weekly,* 9–12.

U.S. Department of Defense (1992). Prevalence of HIV-1 antibody in civilian applicants for military service. October 1985–March 1992, Washington, D.C.

van Deutekom, H., Warris-Versteegen, A.A., Krijnen, P., et al. (1993). The HIV epidemic and its effect on the tuberculosis situation in the Netherlands. *Tubercle Lung Disease, 74*(3), 159–162.

van Servellen, G.M., Lewis, C.E., Leake, B. (1988). Nurses' responses to the AIDS crisis: Implications for continuing education programs. *The Journal of Continuing Education in Nursing, 19,* 4–8.

van Wissen, K.A., Siebers, R.W.L. (1993). Nurses' attitudes and concerns pertaining to HIV and AIDS. *Journal of Advanced Nursing, 18,* 912–917.

von Reyn, C.F., Gilbert, T.T., Shaw, F.W., et al. (1993). Absence of HIV transmission from an infected orthopedic surgeon: A 13-year look back. *Journal of the American Medical Association, 269*(4), 1807–1811.

von Reyn, C.F., Mann, J.M. (1987). AIDS—a global perspective: Global epidemiology. *Western Journal of Medicine, 147*(6), 694–701.

Wallack, J.J. (1989). AIDS anxiety among health care professionals. *Hospital and Community Psychiatry, 40*(5), 507–510.

Wang, B.K., Ugen, E., Srikantan, M.G., et al. (1993). Gene inoculation generates immune responses against human immunodeficiency virus type 1. *Proceedings of the National Academy of Science, 90*(9), 4156–4160.

Wendell, D., Onorato, I.M., McCray, E., et al. (1991). Youth at risk: Sex, drugs, and human immunodeficiency virus. *American Journal of Diseases in Children, 146*(1), 76–81.

Wiley, K., Heath, L., Acklin, M., et al. (1990). Care of HIV-infected patients: Nurses' concerns, opinions, and precautions. *Applied Nursing Research, 3*(1), 27–33.

Young, E.W. (1988). Nurses' attitudes toward homosexuality: Analysis of change in AIDS workshops. *Journal of Continuing Education in Nursing, 19*(1), 9–12.

Young, E.W., Koch, P.B., Preston, D.B. (1989) AIDS and homosexuality: A longitudinal study of knowledge and attitude change among rural nurses. *Public Health Nursing, 6*(4), 189–196.

Zeller, J.M., Swanson, B., Cohen, F.L. (1993). Suggestions for clinical nursing research: Symptom management in AIDS patients. *Journal of the Association of Nurses in AIDS Care, 4*(3), 13–17.

2 Health Promotion and Disease Prevention

Jacquelyn Haak Flaskerud

Health promotion in the case of HIV disease means promoting a lifestyle and behaviors that will prevent infection with HIV as well as promoting a healthy lifestyle and behaviors in people who are already infected. Similarly, disease prevention means not only preventing the behaviors that cause initial infection with the virus but also preventing behaviors and conditions that foster disease expression, prolonging the asymptomatic stage of HIV infection, and postponing the occurrence of AIDS-indicator diseases. Finally, disease prevention in AIDS means prophylactic and therapeutic treatment of the AIDS-indicator conditions, rehabilitation, and palliation. From this perspective, the public health nursing model of primary prevention, early intervention, and rehabilitative and palliative efforts is exceptionally applicable to the spectrum of HIV disease. From a community perspective also, the health promotion framework is uniquely suited to HIV prevention work (Wardrop, 1993). Ever since HIV/AIDS was first recognized, it has been apparent that the rate at which persons become immunodeficient or contract complicating diseases when infected with HIV varies considerably. Within groups of infected individuals, it is still uncertain in whom and when AIDS will develop. This variable expression of pathogenic properties is true of all but a few microorganisms infecting humans (Osborn, 1986; Siegel, 1986).

The proportion of people who are exposed to HIV and become infected or who are infected and will develop AIDS cannot be absolutely determined on the basis of observed data. However, more and more frequently the cofactors to infection and disease progression are being identified for persons in all exposure categories. The knowledge of these cofactors makes targeted health promotion and disease prevention a more practical reality.

Several recent developments have encouraged health care workers to implement health-promoting behaviors and lifestyles even in persons who are infected. Clinical and research findings have provided nurses with knowledge to give concrete direction and advice to their clients in specific situations. Several reports of long-term survivors of HIV disease have prompted investigators to study healthy persons to learn about resistance to HIV. The National Institutes of Health (NIH), in February 1992, identified three groups of resistant "rule breakers": (1) those exposed to HIV but not infected, (2) those who are infected but do not show immunologic progression (CD4$^+$ T-cell counts stabilize at above 200), and (3) those who show progression (CD4$^+$ T-cell counts fall to less than 200) but do not develop advanced HIV disease (Rowe, 1993). In San Francisco, Buchbinder and colleagues (1992) are studying gay men, some of whom have remained healthy and AIDS free for as long as 14 years. There are 135 men who have survived for 10 years or longer and who are in either group 2 or 3 of the rule breakers categorized above. Some of them have not taken any antiretroviral drugs. In another study of long-term survivors in New South Wales, Australia, six persons who acquired HIV infection through a common donor have been followed up for 10 or more years. These subjects have maintained normal CD4$^+$ T-lymphocyte counts and have persistently negative results on tests for p24 antigenemia. The blood donor who infected them also has not developed signs or symptoms (Learmont et al., 1992).

Long-term survivors have several immunologic characteristics in common. They maintain strong cytotoxic lymphocyte activity many years after HIV infection. They maintain strong suppressor T-cell activity, and they have higher levels of antibodies directed against several HIV proteins and subregions of proteins (Sheppard et al., 1993). Various reasons for the delay in the progression to AIDS have been postulated, such as infection with a less pathogenic strain of HIV, and genetic protection through a stronger human leukocyte antigen (HLA) type (Levy, 1993). Conversely, other cofactors might increase the rate of progression: older age, exposure through transfusion, and reexposure to HIV or to pathogens that cause other sexually transmitted diseases (STDs).

An intensive psychoimmunologic study of long-term survivors who are alive and well after an AIDS diagnosis was begun in 1987 by investigators in California (Solomon et al., 1987). They are studying psychosocial and immunologic variables associated with survival. These variables will include hardiness, the use of problem-solving help, altered lifestyle, hopeful psychological mood, an emotionally expressive personality type, a "fighting spirit," and several immunologic markers. Until the results of studies such as these are available, clinicians and researchers recommend healthy lifestyle practices and safer sexual practices to prevent reexposure to additional strains of HIV or to pathogens that cause other STDs.

There is new and consistent evidence also of "rule breakers" in NIH group 1: those exposed to HIV and not infected. This evidence comes from several exposure categories: perinatal, male-male sexual contact, and male-female sexual contact. In all these cases, the rate of HIV transmission was related to the immunologic status of the infected person. Infected sexual partners and pregnant women with low CD4$^+$ cell counts (<400) or percentages (<0.50) and detectable p24 antigen had high rates of transmission to partners and the fetus in comparison with those who had higher counts and no antigenemia (Saracco et al., 1993; Seage et al., 1993b; St. Louis et al., 1993; Tibaldi et al., 1993). In pregnant women the risk of infection to the fetus in-

creased tenfold with decreased immunologic status of the mother (St. Louis et al., 1993; Tibaldi et al., 1993). In the study of heterosexual exposure, the risk of infection to the female partner increased fivefold with lower immunologic status of the male partner (Saracco et al., 1993).

Currently, HIV disease is understood as a chronic disease with a recognizable course. Several prospective studies and estimates have shown that the asymptomatic incubation period of HIV disease is long (median of 9+ years) (Levy, 1993; Osmond, 1990). Without treatment, 33% of infected persons will progress to AIDS after 7 years, and 50% will develop AIDS within 9.2 years (Hendriks et al., 1993). These figures are averages and a way of looking at all persons with AIDS. It is possible from clinical and immunologic findings to look at smaller groups as well and to make a more specific prognosis about the rate of progression to AIDS. Individuals who are at high risk of having a rapid progression to AIDS can be recognized by the clinical presentation of symptomatic primary HIV infection with fever and skin rash, the presence of HIV p24 antigenemia, and the absence of a serologic response to HIV core protein (Keet et al., 1993). It may be assumed that for persons without these clinical and laboratory findings, the prognosis would be for a longer asymptomatic incubation period and perhaps for long-term survival. Survival is enhanced also by the use of prophylactic treatment of conditions such as *Pneumocystis carinii* pneumonia (Munoz et al., 1993).

The trend in increased survival time also varies considerably on the basis of geographic region, race or ethnicity, gender, and exposure category (Seage et al., 1993a). For example, in Massachusetts, increased survival time did not occur in Latinos/Hispanics, in men who have sex with men (MWSM) and are also injection drug users (IDUs), in residents of Boston, or in persons with Kaposi's sarcoma (Seage et al., 1993a). Some of these characteristics are not modifiable, whereas others may be amenable to change if the client concurs. For instance, a study of IDUs showed that concurrent infection with an STD, current injection drug use, abscess at the injection site, and multiple sexual partners predicted the transmission rate. All these behaviors are potentially modifiable. Such findings raise three important questions: Why do some people not become infected? Why do some who are infected not become immunodeficient or contract disease? And what is there about some persons that makes them susceptible to infection and disease progression? Something in addition to HIV exposure seems to be required both to acquire the virus and to become ill from it. One or more cofactors must exist. Knowledge of these cofactors and the various human groups most affected by them will assist nurses in developing health promotion and disease prevention programs.

COFACTORS AND HIV

Several cofactors appear to be involved in determining the pathogenesis of HIV disease (Levy, 1993). These cofactors might be viewed as occurring in two categories: exposure cofactors and trigger cofactors (Table 2–1) (Flaskerud, 1992). Exposure cofactors are those which might affect acquisition of HIV infection. Trigger cofactors are those which either increase a person's likelihood of being infected during exposure to HIV or contribute to HIV disease progression in those who have been infected.

Exposure Cofactors

Numerous studies in the United States and Europe have documented the relationship between specific sexual and lifestyle practices and exposure to HIV infection (Evans et al., 1993; Fennema et al., 1993; Koziol et al., 1993; Levy, 1993; Seage et al., 1993b; Winkelstein et al., 1993). Receptive anal intercourse, multiple anonymous sexual partners, douching or having rectal enemas before receptive anal intercourse, the presence of genital ulcers, and not being circumcised are all cofactors associated with the acquisition of HIV infection. These cofactors expose a person to HIV by increasing the probability of sexual contact with an infectious partner, providing a route for transmission, causing

Table 2–1. Cofactors for HIV Infection

Exposure Cofactors
Anal receptive sex
Rectal douching
Multiple sexual partners
Presence of genital ulcers
Needle and syringe sharing
Use of "shooting galleries"
Frequency of injection
Use of recreational drugs
Receipt of factor VIII concentrate
Receipt of blood, blood products, tissue
Needlestick
In utero and intrapartal exposure

Trigger Cofactors
Noninfectious
Malnutrition
Use of injection drugs
Use of recreational substances
Allergic conditions
Genetics
Emotional stress
Age
Pregnancy
Gender
Infectious
Antigenic overload from multiple infectious diseases (e.g., sexually transmitted diseases, soft tissue infections, bacterial endocarditis, tubercular infections)
Coincident viral infection and immune suppression (e.g., cytomegalovirus, hepatitis B virus, Epstein-Barr virus, herpesviruses)

trauma to the local mucosa, exposing a larger mucosal surface, and/or producing membrane disruption that permits access of the viral agent to the bloodstream. It should be noted that evidence suggests that the virus probably can pass through an intact mucous membrane as well (Levy, 1993; Rietmeijer et al., 1989; van der Graaf & Diepersloot, 1989).

Other cofactors for acquisition of HIV infection have been associated with various aspects of drug and alcohol use (Bagasra et al., 1993; Finelli et al., 1993; Kelly et al., 1993; McCoy & Inciardi, 1993; Rosenblum et al., 1993). The disinhibiting effects on behavior caused by alcohol and other drugs such as crack cocaine are well known and possibly allow more frequent and/or anonymous sexual exposure to the virus. Some drugs also blunt the sensation of pain, permitting or extending sexual practices that might not ordinarily be tolerated. The most obvious association of drugs and HIV infection is the direct transmission of the virus through the sharing of hypodermic needles, syringes, and other paraphernalia among IDUs. The risk of seropositivity increases with increasing numbers of persons with whom needles are regularly shared and with more frequent injections. In addition, a consistent relationship has been shown between the use of "shooting galleries" and seropositivity (Friedman et al., 1990; Ickovics & Rodin, 1992; Mann et al., 1992, p. 412; Metzger et al., 1993). These cofactors produce exposure by increasing the probability of contact with the virus.

Other exposure factors exist for persons with hemophilia and for recipients of blood, blood products, and tissue (Levy, 1993; Petersen et al., 1993). The risk of seropositivity associated with hemophilia increases as the number of exposures to factor VIII concentrate, pooled blood components, and multiple strains of HIV increases. Similarly, among recipients of blood and blood products, the exposure to plasma-rich pooled blood components and multiple strains of HIV and the volume of blood received are significant risk factors for HIV seropositivity (Balfour, 1993; Levy, 1993; Mann et al., 1992, p. 427). Transfusion of HIV-infected blood is the most efficient mode of HIV transmission and is associated with a 95% or higher probability of becoming infected.

The probability of being infected through *in utero* or intrapartal exposure has been estimated downward (Levy, 1993) and varies geographically from 14% in Europe, to 31% in New York City and San Francisco, to 45% in Kenya (Wara, 1993). Poor clinical health, depressed immunologic status of the mother, and the method of delivery (vaginal vs cesarean section) are exposure cofactors related to an increased risk of perinatal transmission (Hague et al., 1993; Nair et al., 1993; St. Louis et al., 1993; Wara, 1993). There is also a possibility of infant infection through breast milk.

Trigger Cofactors

Trigger cofactors exert an effect on the expression of disease that is independent of any role in producing exposure to HIV. These cofactors augment or accelerate immunodeficiency. They increase the likelihood of being infected during exposure or contribute to the expression of active disease in those with HIV positivity. Trigger cofactors may have additive, deterministic, synergistic, or facilitative roles in the cytopathic effects of HIV on the immune system. Trigger cofactors are postulated to contribute to T-cell immunodeficiency and immunologic abnormality through a variety of mechanisms.

Noninfectious Cofactors. Both noninfectious and infectious cofactors are involved in the cause of and susceptibility to HIV infection and symptomatic AIDS. Noninfectious cofactors include dietary factors; use of injection, recreational, or prescribed drugs; genetic predisposition; allergic disorders; stress; age; gender; and pregnancy. The most common cause of T-cell immunodeficiency worldwide is protein-calorie malnutrition. Malnutrition reduces the total number of T-lymphocytes and helper and suppressor cells, impairs cell-mediated immunity and secretory immunity, reduces complement secretion, alters phagocytic function, and decreases natural killer cell activity (Chandra, 1993). In addition, malnourishment leads to significant mineral, trace element, and vitamin deficiencies that affect overall immune function (Hickey & Weaver, 1988). Hypocholesterolemia has also been associated with immune dysfunction (Guillou, 1993; Shor-Posner et al., 1993). Malnutrition may be related to a lack of food supplies, to nonnutritional food choices, to the use of drugs to control appetite, and to loss of appetite related to injection and/or recreational drug use. Moore and colleagues (1993) have suggested that weight loss might be causally related to susceptibility to HIV infection.

Alcohol, nitrites (poppers), amphetamines, marijuana, tobacco (cigarettes), and injection drugs (heroin, cocaine, and morphine) have all been suggested as possible factors in immunosuppression (Bagasra et al., 1993; Messiah et al., 1993; Nieman et al., 1993; Park et al., 1993; Siddiqui et al., 1993). Cohort studies of persons with HIV infection (PWHIV) have sometimes supported the association of substance use and decreased immune function and other times have not (Ascher et al., 1993; Lifson et al., 1988; Park et al., 1993). However, smoking tobacco or marijuana and nitrite inhalation might predispose the lungs to opportunistic infection, especially PCP (Nieman et al., 1993).

Exposure to allogeneic semen and sperm has been suggested as a possible cofactor in HIV disease (Hoff & Peterson, 1989). Immunosuppression could result from exposure to allogeneic cells in passive partners during anogenital sex if sperm and semen can reach the lymphatic and vascular systems. This could occur by way of rectal or lower bowel lesions resulting from trauma caused by sexual practices or from viral infections.

A relationship between emotional stress and decreased immune function has been proposed frequently (Ickovics & Rodin, 1992). In the case of HIV disease this relationship has been hypothesized to be related to disease progression and to decline in lymphocyte function. Findings have been mixed. Kessler and colleagues (1989) found an association among stressor events, distressed mood, and illness onset. Researchers at San Francisco General Hospital found that depression was related to declines in CD4$^+$ cell count among HIV-infected gay and bisexual men and proposed that depression may accelerate disease progression (Burack et al., 1993). However, other investigators studying a larger sample in several geographic areas did not find a relationship between depression and a decline in CD4$^+$ cell count, AIDS-related symptoms over time, and time to death (Lyketsos et al., 1993). Depression may affect the immune system, or it may affect behavior, causing people to take poorer care of themselves and engage in unhealthy behaviors. A case in point is one study of HIV-infected men which demonstrated that a stress reduction program significantly lowered the number of sexual partners but did not affect lymphocyte numbers or function (Coates et al., 1989b). A

further clarification of this relationship came from a study of immune function and psychologic distress associated with the reaction to news of HIV seropositivity; the study showed no association between psychologic and immunologic phenomena (Ironson et al., 1990). These investigators concluded that the viral contribution to immune functioning overrides any influence of environmental stimuli.

Age is related to immunologic status. Infants have undeveloped natural resistance systems, which makes them susceptible to multiple infections including HIV infection. Younger infants (<6 months of age) with HIV infection also have the poorest prognosis (Turner et al., 1993). Additionally, the more premature that infants are, the more immunologically abnormal they are and the more likely to be infected with HIV (Ward et al., 1993). Older adults have an age-related loss of natural resistance, which might make them more susceptible to HIV and other infections (Buchbinder et al., 1992; Tichy & Talashek, 1992). Among heterosexual men, seropositivity is associated with older age (Chiasson et al., 1990). Among persons with hemophilia and other recipients of blood transfusions, older age is strongly related to disease progression (Phillips et al., 1991; Sutin et al., 1993). In two large cohorts (New York City, N = 5833; San Francisco, N = 4323) that included both homosexual and heterosexual PWHIV, survival was significantly related to age: increasing age reduced survival (Lemp et al., 1990; Rothenberg et al., 1987).

Pregnancy is another cofactor that contributes to immunosuppression. Gestational immunosuppression occurs naturally in the second and third trimesters and can be measured by depressed lymphocyte numbers and functions, which return to normal 1 month post partum (Hoff & Peterson, 1989; Nanda & Minkoff, 1989). A relationship between pregnancy and disease progression in seropositive women has been hypothesized. Current evidence suggests that pregnancy may exert an influence on the course of HIV disease (Ellerbrock & Rogers, 1990). Trends toward earlier manifestation of HIV-related symptoms in pregnant women and toward a higher maternal mortality rate in seropositive than seronegative women have been found, but these trends did not reach statistical significance (Deschamps et al., 1993; Mmiro et al., 1993).

Gender differences in response to HIV infection have been noted among persons with PCP in New York City (Bastian et al., 1993). Women had higher mortality rates from PCP. Comparing median survival times in men and women in San Francisco, researchers found that men had a median survival of 14.6 months after an AIDS diagnosis and women 11.1 months (Staff, *AIDS Alert,* 1992). This difference was attributed to different exposure cofactors and access to health care. Hormonal differences may also play a role in HIV disease progression (Ickovics & Rodin, 1992). In a review of U.S. adult AIDS cases diagnosed between January 1988 and June 1991, the prevalence of certain AIDS-defining conditions were reported significantly more frequently in women than men: infection with herpes simplex virus (HSV), infection with cytomegalovirus (CMV), and esophageal candidiasis (Fleming et al., 1993). These conditions commonly are associated with CD4[+] cell counts in a more advanced stage of disease progression.

Genetics may also play a role in HIV disease progression and the likelihood that specific disease manifestations will develop. In studies of persons with hemophilia and homosexual men, HLA type has been associated with clinical disease progression (Lifson et al., 1988; Meropol et al., 1989). HLA type may also protect HIV-infected persons from disease progression (Buchbinder et al., 1992).

Finally, of the possible noninfectious cofactors to HIV, allogeneic blood and blood products, especially plasma-rich blood components such as fresh frozen plasma, whole blood, and platelets, may be immunosuppressive. The transfer of allogeneic blood and blood products might compromise the immune system of recipients (Vamvakas & Kaplan, 1993). In persons with hemophilia, immunosuppression may result from infusion of factor VIII as replacement therapy (Blumberg & Heal, 1989). The tranfusion of stored anticoagulated plasma has been suggested as

one factor that may affect host immune defenses and facilitate expression of clinical HIV disease.

Infectious Cofactors. Infectious cofactors are involved also in the cause of and susceptibility to AIDS. In an immunosuppressed person, infection that leads to antigenic overload and stimulation can contribute to the progression to AIDS. If the immune system is continually overstimulated by a high antigenic load in association with various chronic infections, this overstimulation may interfere with the host's capacity to eliminate infectious agents. A history of multiple infectious diseases, among them syphilis, giardiasis, gonorrhea, chancroid, and parasitic diseases, has been suggested as a cofactor in the acquisition of HIV infection (Elifson et al., 1993; Laga et al., 1993, Schoenbach et al., 1993; Solomon et al., 1993). Soft tissue infections, such as injection site abscesses, as well as infections such as viral hepatitis and bacterial endocarditis, may result from the injection of drugs dissolved in nonsterile water, mixed with contaminated diluents and impure narcotics, and self-administered through needles and syringes contaminated by blood and dirt (Alcabes et al., 1993; Chiasson et al., 1990; Solomon et al., 1993). These infections are thought to produce sufficient insult to the immune system to enhance the pathologic effects of HIV on the host.

Another infectious cofactor that might be operative in the progression from asymptomatic infection to overt disease is coincident immunosuppression caused by viruses other than HIV. Chief among those suggested as playing an additive or synergistic role in potentiating the cytopathic effects of HIV are chronic infections with CMV, Epstein-Barr virus (EBV), hepatitis B and C viruses (HBV and HCV), herpesviruses, and human papillomavirus (HPV) (Elifson et al., 1993; Leach et al., 1993; Newton-Nash et al., 1993; Sabin et al., 1993; Spitzer et al., 1993; Staff, *AIDS Alert,* 1992; Swanson, 1992; Twu et al., 1993). These viruses significantly impair the immune system and may facilitate the progression of HIV infection. The effect of infection with other viruses might be simply immunosuppressive, providing opportunities for reactivation of HIV, or the viruses may activate cells that carry HIV, resulting in the full expression of cytopathologic effects (Leach et al., 1993).

Finally, reinfection with HIV, stage of HIV infectivity, and type of HIV strain may be interacting cofactors in the acquisition of HIV infection and in progression to clinical disease (Buchbinder et al., 1992; Learmont et al., 1992). The stage of infectivity determines the amounts of circulating virus and antibody. Transmission of the virus to others may vary depending on the amount of circulating virus or stage of infection in an HIV-infected individual (Saracco et al., 1993; Seage et al., 1993b; St. Louis et al., 1993). Furthermore, several investigators working with HIV-infected cohorts of blood recipients and homosexual men have hypothesized that HIV strain type may differ between persons and between populations (Buchbinder et al., 1992; Learmont et al., 1992; Zhang et al., 1993). If strains of HIV vary in their virulence, strain type may be related to primary HIV infection, disease course, and clinical outcome. If HIV strain types differ, a more virulent strain of HIV may infect a person who has thus far avoided infection even though exposed and may alter the course of disease progression in a person who has remained free of symptoms.

The various cofactors discussed here play a role in exposure to the virus, transmission of the virus, immunosuppression of the host, and activation or facilitation of the virus. Depending on their virulence and combination, they can increase or decrease the risk of HIV infection and the risk of expression of HIV disease.

PERSONAL AND SOCIAL GROUP EFFORTS

A comprehensive approach to cause, prevention, and cure is needed to control the spread of HIV infection. A comprehensive approach to combating disease considers changes in the host, the agent, and the environment. Host-related changes are behaviors that individuals, partners, and families can engage in or modify to prevent exposure to HIV or progression to disease expression. Agent-related efforts include identifying the virus, finding antiviral treatments, and developing a vaccine against the virus. Environmental efforts involve HIV infection control in the community. This section begins with health promotion and disease prevention changes needed in host behavior. A later section in this chapter addresses environmental (community) efforts to promote health and prevent disease.

Health Promotion

Knowledge of the exposure and trigger cofactors of HIV disease can assist nurses in planning health care activities that individuals and their partners, families, and friends can implement on their own behalf or with the assistance of health care workers. These take the form of health promotion and disease prevention activities.

Health promotion behaviors and activities are applicable to all persons regardless of HIV status. Behaviors and activities discussed here are those related to a healthy lifestyle and those believed to enhance immunocompetence. These behaviors apply also to persons who are infected with HIV and to those in all stages of HIV disease.

Diet. As noted earlier, malnutrition is the major cause of immunosuppression worldwide. The impact of specific nutrients on immune status has been documented: deficiencies in calorie-protein intake have consistent and profound effects on cell-mediated immunity, lymphocyte subsets, complement secretion, phagocyte function, secretory antibody response, and antibody affinity (Chandra, 1993; Keithley et al., 1992). T-lymphocytes are the primary target of HIV.

Currently, a health-promoting diet and one that promotes optimal immune functioning consists of a variety of foods from each of seven food groups and is composed of 50% to 55% calories from carbohydrates, 15% to 20% calories from protein, and 30% or less calories from fat (Wong, 1993). Two or three servings of food from each of the protein and dairy groups are recommended for each day, 7 to 12 servings from the starch-grain group, two servings of vitamin C–rich fruits and vegetables, one serving of vitamin A–rich fruits and vegetables, and three servings of other fruits and vegetables.

Micronutrients. Vitamins and minerals are essential for optimal immune functioning (Chandra, 1993; Hickey & Weaver, 1988; Task Force on Nutrition Support in AIDS, 1989). A diet rich in micronutrients should supply the vitamins and minerals essential for immune functioning. The addition of a multivitamin-mineral supplement to the diet provides sufficient essential nutrients (Wong, 1993). Recent reports have suggested that enhanced immune response may be related to adequate amounts of vitamins A and E, beta-carotene, zinc, and selenium (Chandra, 1993; Ward et al., 1993). Researchers at Johns Hopkins Medical Center have been studying the use of vitamins A, B_1, C, and niacin in doses larger than the recommended amount with 28 HIV positive men for up to 6–8 years. In an interim report these investigators found that micronutrient intake for at least 2 years, started early in the course of HIV infection, seemed to slow the onset of AIDS (*HIV Frontline Update*, 1994). According to the researchers, these results need to be confirmed by additional studies. It should be noted carefully that megadoses of vitamins and minerals may be dangerous. Megadoses can create nutrient-nutrient or nutrient-medication competitive environments, cause toxic effects and neurologic damage, and result in a weakening of the immune system (Wong, 1993).

Information on nutrition and meal planning is an important aspect of health promotion education for all groups. Special attention may be required for some groups. Some homosexual men and heterosexual women may have eating disorders or may diet excessively in an effort to be exceptionally thin to enhance their physical attractiveness. Information on the dangers of this kind of dieting and on what constitutes adequate nutrition may be needed (Karan, 1989).

Another group that may need nutrition information is the urban poor. Even when diets are adequate in calories in this group, they are often deficient in protein, vitamins, vegetables, and fruit, and high in fat. Among the urban poor are the IDUs and other substance abusers, who often are poorly nourished because of the appetite-suppressant effects of drugs, toxic effects of alcohol on the gastrointestinal tract, and inadequate assimilation of vitamins and amino acids as a result of damaged liver cells (Karan, 1989; Mondanaro, 1990).

Regular Exercise. Physical exercise is recommended as a health-promoting activity because it increases lung capacity, muscle-to-fat ratio, endurance, energy, and flexibility, and improves circulation (Centers for Disease Control and Prevention [CDC], Sept. 10, 1993). It also improves sleeping, appetite, and regular bowel activity and decreases stress (Wong, 1993). Solomon (1991) has proposed a relationship between psychosocial factors, exercise, and immunity based on studies of athletes, elderly persons, and PWHIV. Currently an exercise program of 30 to 45 minutes 4 or more days per week is recommended. Exercise should use muscle groups in both the arms and legs, should be fitted to personal endurance, and should not be painful or boring.

Acceptable and feasible exercise programs must be designed specifically for individual interests, physical capabilities, financial restrictions, and other personal characteristics. Walking is an exercise available to all that is not overly taxing and may be done in the company of children and/or other adults. The benefits of exercise are not readily apparent to some people who may believe that it is too expensive and will make them more tired and pressured for time, such as mothers with young children.

Balancing the need for regular exercise is the need for adequate, regular rest and sleep. For some persons, sleep programs must be designed that will allow them to fall asleep and stay asleep. Others need education on the negative effects of sleep deprivation.

Stress and Emotions. Reducing and controlling stress is the goal of stress management programs. Stress is often associated with immunosuppression and may increase an individual's vulnerability to disease (Ickovics & Rodin, 1992). Adequate sleep and rest and regular exercise are important stress-reduction activities (Solomon, 1991; Solomon et al., 1987). Mental exercises such as meditation, visualization, and biofeedback are all types of relaxation techniques that may reduce stress.

An adequate coping response may also moderate stress. Active or involved coping is believed to have beneficial health effects (Folkman et al., 1993; Solomon et al., 1987). Active coping includes problem-solving activity, increased expression of emotions, seeking advice and information, altering one's lifestyle, taking control of one's health and well-being, and having a sense of purpose and commitment to life (Ickovics & Rodin, 1992; Nyamathi & Lewis, 1991; Nyamathi et al., 1993b; Solomon et al., 1987). To date, the relationship of most of these behaviors, attitudes, and values are in a hypothetical stage of research.

Other stress reduction techniques involve social group relationships. These include being involved in altruistic ways with other individuals and groups, providing and receiving social support, taking part in recreational activities and play, taking breaks at work and vacations, and being involved in committed relationships (Ickovics & Rodin, 1992; Solomon et al., 1987; van Servellen et al., 1993). Avoiding stress-producing situations has also been recommended. However, it should be noted that avoiding stress is almost impossible in today's world, and using it as a health promotion strategy may be guilt producing.

Special attention should be given to the benefit of emotional expression (Linn et al., 1993). In several studies, strong sympathetic nervous system reactivity to the expression of basic emotions (fear, anger, surprise, disgust, happiness, and sadness) was related to more natural killer cell activity and enhanced mental and physical health (Dienstbier, 1989; Solomon et al., 1987; Temoshok et al., 1990). Some people may believe mistakenly that suppression of emotion is one method of stress reduction and that by suppressing emotions they will reduce stress and promote immune function. The studies cited above found the opposite. There were complex interactions among emotional expression, strong autonomic reactivity, and increased immune response. Helping individuals find avenues for emotional expression through family, friends, partners, social groups, and professional counseling may enhance both physical and mental health (Burack et al., 1993).

Recommending stress reduction programs as a health promotion activity on the basis of current evidence may seem premature, but there are probably at least three reasons for doing so. These programs pose few risks, they may have a positive effect on well-being, and they increase participation of people in their own health care (Jewett & Hecht, 1993). Such programs also provide more general information about health promotion, stress, and immune function that may be applicable to HIV disease as well. Finally, if the possibility exists that health promotion and stress reduction may affect immune status and, consequently, HIV disease status, it would be unthinkable not to offer these programs, especially since they involve no adverse side effects and have a psychologic benefit.

Recreational Drug Use. The overuse of chemical stimulants, alcohol, and recreational drugs such as tobacco, marijuana, and "speed" may have an immunosuppressant effect. These substances are associated with a variety of physical and mental health problems. Avoiding or limiting their use should be part of health promotion activities. Several self-help programs as well as professional programs exist to assist individuals who wish to modify their substance use behaviors. These substances, in addition to their possible immunosuppressant characteristics, limit or interfere with the health promotion activities and behaviors described earlier in this section. These substances suppress appetite, irritate the gastrointestinal tract, lead to impaired absorption of food, and damage liver cells. All these consequences reduce the health-promoting benefits of nutrition. They also interfere with regular exercise, sleep, and rest and may therefore exacerbate stress indirectly; direct exacerbation of stress may come from their effect on personal and social relationships.

Prevention of Primary Infection with HIV

The cofactors for exposure to HIV are most frequently behaviors that might lead to the transfer of blood, semen, or vaginal fluid from an infected person into the bloodstream of someone who is not infected. This happens through unprotected anal and vaginal intercourse, the sharing of injection drug equipment, *in utero* and intrapartal infection, and blood, blood product, and tissue transfusions and transplants. Transmission can occur also in health care settings through needle stick injuries and exposures to cuts or mucous membranes. This form of transmission is discussed in depth in Chapter 10. Each of these forms of exposure can be prevented.

Sexual Exposure. No risk of sexual transmission exists for those who practice sexual abstinence. Likewise, there is no risk of infection if neither partner is infected. This would be true of couples who have been mutually monogamous since the introduction of HIV in the United States (mid-1970s) and of mutually monogamous couples who have been shown to have HIV antibody negativity in serologic testing.

For persons outside these situations, the risk can be decreased by limiting the number of sexual partners and practicing protective sex. Protective sex is sexual activity in which no semen, vaginal secretions, or blood is exchanged between partners. Such practices involve kissing, hugging, caressing, and genital manipulation (all in the absence of an open lesion). Risks can be reduced in vaginal and anal intercourse provided a condom is worn (CDC, Aug. 6, 1993; Rosenberg & Holmes, 1993). It is *important to note* here that the use of spermicides with condom use was recommended in the past. It is now thought that spermicides may increase transmission through irritation of rectal mucosa or vaginal lining cells (Levy 1993). The relative risk of sexual transmission in various practices is provided in Table 2–2.

The risk of infection can be reduced by avoiding specific sexual behaviors and practices. These include anal receptive intercourse, rectal douching, and multiple sexual partners. In combination, these behaviors and practices produce the highest risk of HIV infection in the United States, probably because they involve tears in the fragile rectal mucosa that permit entry of the virus into the bloodstream (Messiah et al., 1993). Genital sores also increase the risk of infection. Avoidance of unprotected anal intercourse is the principal focus of efforts to reduce risk in male-to-male sexual contact (Elifson et al., 1993; Levy, 1993; Peterson et al., 1992).

Vaginal intercourse has lower risks than anal but has become a more frequent route of exposure (Ickovics & Rodin, 1992). Women are infected at a higher rate than men through this means of exposure. The risk of transmission is higher if there are preexisting sores in the genital area, such as herpes lesions (Stall, *AIDS Alert*, 1992; Levy, 1993).

For those engaging in vaginal intercourse, reducing the number of sexual partners and

Table 2–2. Risk of Exposure to HIV Related to Behaviors and Practices

RISK/LEVELS OF SAFETY	SEXUAL CONTACT	INJECTION DRUG USE	PERINATAL EXPOSURE
Absolutely safe	Abstinence Mutually monogamous with noninfected persons	Not using injection drugs	Abstinence Sterilization
Very safe	Noninsertive sexual practices	Using sterilized injection paraphernalia	Birth control measures and abortion
Probably safe	Insertive sexual practices with use of condoms	Cleaning injection paraphernalia with full-strength bleach	Use of condoms
Risky	Everything else	All other activities	Pregnancy Breast-feeding

practicing protective sex at all times can reduce the risk of infection. In an effort to assist its health care workers in an area that many find difficult and uncomfortable, Kaiser Permanente has been teaching its health care workers to use a 60-second sexual history interview. This interview is presented in Table 2–3.

Oral sex may play a role in transmission through exposure of the oral mucosa to semen or vaginal fluid. Sores around or in the mouth could theoretically provide an exposure route. Condoms can also help reduce risk in oral sex. Deep kissing with an exchange of saliva has theoretical but no practical risk (Richman & Rickman, 1993; Yeung et al., 1993).

There are also cofactors to exposure that may modify sexual behaviors. By reducing inhibitions and affecting judgment, the use of alcohol may lead to risky sexual activities. The use of crack cocaine has been consistently implicated in these behaviors (Bagasra et al., 1993; Diaz & Chu, 1993; McCoy & Inciardi, 1993; Temple et al., 1993; Weatherburn et al., 1993).

Injection Drug Use. The risk of HIV infection from injection drug use differs by geographic region, social setting of injection (e.g., shooting galleries), and frequency of injection (Vlahov et al., 1990). A history of STDs, pyogenic bacterial infections, and soft tissue infection at the injection site increases the risk of infection for IDUs (Alcabes et al., 1993; Nelson et al., 1993; Solomon et al., 1993). IDUs can eliminate their chance of exposure to HIV infection by stopping the use of injection drugs. For this to occur, addicted persons need referrals to rehabilitation programs. Currently, the number of rehabilitation programs available is inadequate to meet

---

Table 2–3. A 60-Second Sexual History Screening Interview

---

1. "Are you sexually active?" ("Do you have sex on a regular basis?")
    a. If YES: "Are you . . . " (GO TO QUESTION 2.)
    b. If NO: "How long since you've been sexually active?"
    c. If >10 years: STOP
    d. If <10 years:
        (1) "How long has it been since you had sexual relations on a regular basis?"
        (2) "When you were sexually active, were you . . . ?" (GO TO QUESTION 2.)
2. ". . . sexually active with men, women, or both?"
    a. If response indicates only one partner (man or woman), ask: "How long have you had just one partner?"
    b. If >10 years: (GO TO QUESTION 4.)
    c. If <10 years: "And before that?" (GO TO QUESTION 3.)
3. "How many partners do you [did you] have during the last 2 years [of activity]?" If more than one:
    a. "How many men?"
       "How many women?"
    b. "How long have you been or were you active with each?"
4. "How likely is it that your partner(s) had sexual contacts with an intravenous drug user?" "Several other persons?"
    a. If monogamous, partner is not bisexual and has no-risk contacts. (GO TO QUESTION 5.)
    b. If multiple partners, regardless of sex, ask:
        (1) "How often do you have sex with each?"
        (2) "What kind of sexual practices do you engage in, that is, oral, anal, or vaginal sex?"
        (3) If anal, ask: "Receptive or insertive?"
5. "Do you have any problems with sexual functioning that you would like to talk about?" Give examples depending on gender of patient.
6. If relevant, on the basis of answers to questions 1 through 4: "Have you ever had a sexually transmitted disease, such as gonorrhea or syphilis?"
7. If relevent (multiple partners/partner at risk), ask: "Do you use condoms?"

From Southern California Kaiser Permanente Medical Group, Physicians AIDS Symposium, February 1992.

the need if the goal is to stop drug use or if all drug users wish to enroll in such a program. A massive infusion of government and public support is necessary for a major rehabilitation effort (Mann et al., 1992, p. 406). Because epidemiologic evidence suggests that HIV infection affects African American and Latino IDUs disproportionately, much of this effort and money will have to be concentrated in communities of color.

If injection drug use cannot be stopped, exposure to HIV infection can be prevented by ending the sharing of unsterilized injection paraphernalia. Risk to female IDUs may be greater than to male IDUs because some investigators have found that females are more likely to share equipment, especially with partners (Wayment et al., 1993). At a minimum, persons who use injection drugs should clean their equipment with bleach. Recently the CDC (June 4, 1993) recommended the use of full-strength bleach to clean disposable needles and syringes because they are not intended for reuse and are very difficult to clean. Another possibility is to provide sterile needles and syringes for IDUs (Ginzburg, 1993; Schwartz, 1993). Needle exchange programs have been effective in decreasing the spread of HIV and have not encouraged drug use in the process (Guydish et al., 1993). To decrease their risk of seropositivity through parenteral and injection drug use, drug users should also stop using shooting galleries for injection and decrease the frequency of injection (see Table 2–2) (Metzger et al., 1993).

Outside the addicted population there are a substantial number of persons who experiment with drugs. Educational programs for teenagers, for communities in which drug use is high, and for the staff of drug clinics must emphasize the danger of sharing needles and equipment. The use of drugs in conjunction with sexual practices dramatically increases the risk of exposure to HIV.

Perinatal Exposure. Perinatal transmission of HIV can be avoided if infected women do not become pregnant. Pregnancy is associated with a moderate risk of infection to infants and may accelerate the development of AIDS in HIV-infected mothers (Des-

champs et al., 1993). The risk of perinatal transmission of HIV is higher in women with clinical symptoms of AIDS, with viremia and viral replication, with p24 antigenemia, and with $CD4^+$ cell counts less than 400 (Feng et al., 1992; Wara, 1993). Women at greater risk of exposure (IDUs, prostitutes, and women with multiple sexual partners, with STDs, or with sexual partners at high risk of exposure) should be encouraged to undergo testing for HIV infection. Those who are infected may be encouraged to postpone pregnancy until more is known about the risks to themselves and their infants. Infected women should be counseled about the risk of transmission based on their immunologic and clinical status and their risk behaviors (Nair et al., 1993). Women should be counseled about the advantages of AZT therapy perinatally and of enrolling in clinical trials of AZT. The most recent evidence of the perinatal use of AZT demonstrated a 67.5% reduction in the risk of vertical HIV transmission in 364 women participating in on-going clinical trials (CDC, April 29, 1994). AZT is given to the mother during pregnancy and delivery and to the newborn for the first 6 weeks of life. Women who are infected with HIV and become pregnant also should be given family planning and abortion counseling in the first trimester (Shayne & Kaplan, 1991; Stein, 1990). Women who decide to have their babies should be told not to breast feed because the infant may be exposed to HIV through this route as well.

Blood and Blood Product Transfusion and Tissue Transplantation. Infection through the use of donated blood, blood products, and tissue can be prevented by donor exclusion, serologic testing for HIV antibodies, and heat inactivation of products such as factor VIII concentrate (Levy, 1993; Petersen et al., 1993). Because processing semen from HIV-infected persons has not been shown to prevent transmission of HIV, semen implantation should be avoided (Edlin & Holmberg, 1993). Donor exclusion can be facilitated by education of donors, interviews at blood banks, and confidential postdonation self-exclusion (Asselmeier et al., 1993; Menitove, 1990; Patijn et al., 1993). Serologic testing of donors for HIV antibody uses both the enzyme-linked immunosorbent assay (ELISA) or enzyme immunoassay (EIA) technique and the confirmatory Western blot assay. Recently the indirect immunofluorescence assay (IFA) has provided an external standard against which ELISA performance can be judged (Pappaioanou et al., 1993). Early hopes that the testing for p24 antigen could "close the window" of false-negative results have not been met because p24 antigenemia is present during only a portion of the window period (de Saussure et al., 1993).

The recent addition of HBV antibody core testing of blood donors might further eliminate donors at risk of acquiring HIV infection, because a substantial proportion of those at risk of acquiring HIV infection are also at risk of acquiring HBV infection (Hart et al., 1993, Mann et al., 1992, p. 428). Heat inactivation of factor VIII concentrate suggests that this approach can protect persons with hemophilia who receive factor VIII from acquiring HIV infection. Another recommendation is the use of cryoprecipitate instead of concentrated products, because a product from only one individual should be safer than pooled blood products. These precautions in combination would virtually eliminate the risk of HIV infection from transfusion of blood and blood products. Worst scenario estimates indicate that 1 of 36,000 to 1 of 300,000 components may be collected from donors who have false-negative test results (Menitove, 1990). Currently in the United States the risk of acquiring HIV from screened blood is estimated at 1 in 225,000 units (Levy, 1993).

Several practices can further reduce the risk of exposure through blood and blood products. One of these is participation in autologous blood donation programs for persons who are seronegative. Autologous blood programs are also important for persons who are seropositive, to prevent reinfection with other HIV strains and to prevent transfusion-related lowering of CD4$^+$ cell counts (Mintz, 1993; Vamvakas & Kaplan, 1993). Another practice that will reduce transfusion transmission is the institution of appropriate transfusion protocols (Craighead & Knowles, 1993; Mann et al., 1992, p. 422). Single-unit trans-

fusions and transfusions of blood as a prophylactic measure are almost never necessary (Mann et al., 1992). In 1984 the World Health Organization estimated that 20% to 25% of blood transfusions and 90% of albumin transfusions were not necessary. In industrialized countries such as the United States, excessive and inappropriate use of transfusions may be common because they are available and affordable.

Asymptomatic HIV Disease: Health Education and Maintenance

Primary health education begins at the time of HIV antibody testing and counseling. A program of HIV testing and counseling must be concerned with complex social and psychologic issues. Testing has both benefits and harms, and pretest and posttest counseling guidelines must be followed to ensure a safe and beneficial program (Agency for Health Care Policy and Research [AHCPR], January 1994; CDC, Jan. 15, 1993a; Killian, 1990; McMahon, 1988). Hospitals and clinics, drug treatment centers, mental health facilities, and independent practitioners should consider the provision of voluntary HIV counseling for their clients. These settings can offer ready access, appropriate client referral, evaluation, and therapy (Janssen et al., 1992). Knowledge of HIV status allows individuals and their partners to seek treatment and prolong their lives, and to change high-risk behaviors and prevent transmission. Routine, voluntary HIV testing services can result not only in benefits to clients but in societal and economic benefits as well (Holgrave et al., 1993; Janssen et al., 1992). Despite these benefits, before embarking on an HIV testing and counseling program, health care facilities and professionals should consider carefully the social issues involved and the wide-ranging responsibilities engendered by such a service.

Issues in HIV Testing. The assurance of confidentiality is of the highest importance among the issues associated with testing. Disclosure of confidential information can result in discrimination in health care, insurance, employment, and housing. In addition, the impact on interpersonal relationships can be devastating. To protect themselves and their clients, agencies must have clearly written and enforced policies regarding disclosure of test results and maintenance of confidentiality throughout the system. Chapters 13 and 14 provide detailed information related to HIV testing and legal and ethical issues.

A second concern is the presence of a comprehensive standard of care or teaching program within which HIV antibody testing is conducted. Severe psychologic trauma to individuals being tested has occurred because of the way in which seropositive test results were revealed to them. This trauma is compounded by lack of counseling, failure to make referrals, disclosure of inaccurate test results, or institution of inappropriate procedures (e.g., isolation) based on test results. The standard of care for HIV testing and counseling is mandated by law in some states and is recommended in guidelines by the CDC and the U.S. Public Health Service AHCPR (AHCPR, January 1994, pp. 15-21; CDC, Jan. 15, 1993a). The AHCPR Clinical Practice Guidelines for Managing Early HIV Infection may be found in Appendix I and includes guidelines for communicating HIV serostatus.

The standard of care involves pretest and posttest counseling and may be characterized by emphasis on completeness and consistency. A personalized client risk assessment is the foundation of pretest counseling. Chapter 5 contains detailed information on taking a comprehensive health history. All relevant information must be provided to persons considering testing. The information provided must be consistent from one person to the next and in accord with standards of practice (CDC guidelines) and the current understanding of HIV disease. Problems arise when clients are provided with more or less information or with conflicting information. For this reason the CDC recommends adequate training for HIV counselors with ongoing periodic observation, and monitoring of counseling sessions and subsequent feedback for quality assurance. Finally, as part of any comprehensive standard of care, appropriate referral sources for continued counseling, education, medical care, and psychiatric emer-

gencies must be in place before HIV testing begins. HIV counseling should result in a personalized risk reduction, health promotion, and health maintenance plan negotiated with the client.

A final issue is the predictive value of HIV antibody testing. Like all laboratory tests, HIV antibody tests are imperfect. Both false-positive and false-negative results can occur. Because false-positive results may have tragic psychologic and legal consequences, additional testing of a second specimen by means of the Western blot test should be required before test results are communicated. In persons with no high-risk behaviors, positive results should be repeated on two new serum specimens in a reference laboratory. For instance, false-positive results have been reported among blood donors after influenza vaccination (CDC, March 12, 1993). False-negative antibody results also may occur. After infection, a window period takes place in which antibody cannot be detected. A negative result may be misleading and falsely reassuring to a tested person. Seroconversion may take up to 3 months or in rare cases longer. Continued high-risk behaviors may lead to infection of the person and of his or her sexual or needle-sharing partners. Before HIV testing is conducted, persons considering testing must be carefully instructed about the occurrence of false-positive and false-negative test results. They must also be informed in detail about what an HIV antibody test result does and does not mean.

Benefits and Risks of Testing. More than most clinical laboratory tests, HIV antibody testing has benefits, risks, and responsibilities that must be weighed before health facilities and professionals offer a program of testing and before an individual decides on whether to be tested (Holgrave et al., 1993; Janssen et al., 1992; McMahon, 1988). The benefits to individuals and society follow. For persons with seronegative test results, the benefits include the following:

- Reassurance and reduction of anxiety
- Motivation for behavior change to prevent infection

- Information on which to base decisions about marriage, sexual relationships, childbearing, breast-feeding, and immunizations for infants
- Support for an alternative medical diagnosis for unexplained symptoms when HIV disease is under consideration

Symptom-free persons with seropositive test results may receive these benefits:

- Closer medical follow-up
- Laboratory measurement of disease prognostic markers
- Opportunity for involvement in experimental protocols, early intervention programs, and alternative therapies
- Treatment or prophylaxis for other infectious diseases
- Protection of sexual partners
- Information as a basis for decisions about marriage, sexual relationships, childbearing, breast-feeding, and immunizations for infants
- Information for use in future plans for employment, insurance, housing, legal affairs, and so forth

Society receives these benefits from testing:

- Prevention of new HIV infections through sexual exposure, injection drug use, the blood supply and organ donations, and perinatal exposure
- Assistance to scientists and researchers through enrollment in experimental protocols, through tracking of the natural history of HIV infection and disease, and through establishment of the incidence and prevalence of infection
- Assistance to health providers and planners in designing programs to meet the HIV-related needs of the community and to provide treatment and services
- Decrease of the economic costs to society of HIV disease

There are also risks and harm associated with HIV antibody testing programs. Persons with seronegative test results may have had a false-negative result, resuling in a false sense of security, high-risk behaviors, and infection of others (Otten et al., 1993). Symptom-free persons with seropositive test results may have these problems:

- Possibility of false-positive test results accompanied by psychologic trauma
- Discrimination and ostracism by health care professionals, resulting in medically inappropriate procedures
- Severe psychologic reactions, including anxiety, depression, sleep disturbances, and suicidal behavior
- Disrupted interpersonal relationships
- Sexual dysfunction
- Preoccupation with physical symptoms
- Stigmatization and ostracism by society
- Discrimination in housing and employment
- Loss of insurance
- Exposure to hatred and violence

The potential harm of HIV testing far exceeds that of any other laboratory clinical test. Therefore in any HIV antibody testing program every effort must be made to maximize the benefits and minimize the harm to persons tested. These goals can be achieved best through a comprehensive pretest and posttest counseling program.

Pretest Counseling. A comprehensive pretest counseling program that meets standards of care in both completeness and consistency has several essential elements (AHCPR, January 1994; CDC, Jan. 15, 1993a; Killian, 1990; McMahon, 1988). The pretest counseling program should be extremely comprehensive both to maximize its benefits and because posttest counseling often occurs in a situation of such relief or anxiety that concentration is compromised. HIV counseling should be culturally competent, sensitive to issues of sexual identity, developmentally appropriate, and linguistically relevant (CDC, Jan. 15, 1993a; Valdiserri et al., 1993). The essential elements of a comprehensive pretest counseling program include the following:

- A personalized client risk assessment
- Analysis of reasons for seeking testing and assessment of risk behaviors
- Review of test procedures
- Review of what both positive and nega-

tive test results mean and do not mean
- Review of possibility of false-negative and false-positive results
- Review of agency's policy for protecting confidentiality
- General information on the virus and AIDS
- A personalized risk-reduction plan that will include the following as necessary:
  - Advice on safer sexual practices, abstinence, and safer drug use
  - Information on drug treatment programs
  - Provision of condoms and bleach
  - Information on pregnancy, breast-feeding, and immunizations for infants
  - General health information on diet, rest, exercise, alcohol and tobacco use, and avoidance of infections (e.g., STDs and soft tissue infections)
  - Review of potential psychologic and emotional reactions to test results
  - Review of potential interpersonal and societal reactions to test results
  - Information on alternative testing sites for partners
  - Information on medical, social, and psychiatric resources and follow-up counseling
  - Review of the risks and benefits of testing

When the pretest counseling session is completed, the counselor should obtain a written informed consent for testing.

Posttest Counseling. As noted earlier, often when the HIV antibody test results are disclosed, the person may be distracted by feelings of relief or anxiety. Therefore a comprehensive approach should be taken during pretest counseling. However, some elements of posttest counseling are essential. These should be both discussed with the person and given in a written format so that he or she can review them later. For persons with seronegative test results, posttest counseling includes the following:

- Interpretation of the test results
- Advice on HIV retesting after 3 months if the person engages in high-risk behaviors
- Information on safer sex and drug use practices
- Provision of condoms and bleach if desired
- Information on needle exchange programs where available
- Information on how to maintain a negative status
- General information on healthy lifestyle practices
- Information on alternative test sites for partners
- Referral for psychologic, social, medical, and psychiatric services and drug rehabilitation programs as needed
- Follow-up for retesting of persons engaging in high-risk behaviors
- An assessment of whether further posttest counseling is needed

For symptom-free persons with seropositive test results, posttest counseling includes the following:

- Reconfirmation of test results on a second serum specimen in a reference laboratory
- Interpretation of the results (including the information that the person does not have AIDS)
- Evaluation for suicide potential
- Crisis intervention counseling as needed
- Information on alternative test sites for partners
- Discussion of follow-up for partners and children
- Referral to a partner notification program if needed
- Information on transmission, safer sex and drug use practices, and reinfection
- Information on pregnancy and perinatal transmission
- Information on symptoms associated with the spectrum of HIV disease
- Referral to an early intervention program that includes attention to lifestyle practices that may suppress the immune system and activate the disease
- Referral to the appropriate support group(s)

- Referral for medical follow-up
- Referral to drug rehabilitation program(s)
- Information on entering experimental protocols
- Referral for psychologic, social, and psychiatric services as needed
- Discussion of potential discrimination and effects on housing, employment, insurance, and so forth
- Assessment of whether further posttest counseling is needed

Symptom-free infected persons will benefit from a full range of health and human services during the course of their HIV disease. At the time of immediate posttest counseling, they may be extremely anxious and unable to absorb the information presented. They should be given written information as well and encouraged to return for additional counseling. Such persons need continual reassurance and support and access to consistent health care. That health care should promote clients' concern for their condition and encourage monitoring and prevention, but it should avoid an excessive approach that can lead to undue anxiety. One of the most useful forms of support is an ongoing involvement with groups or individuals who share the person's situation and concerns. The overall goals of a comprehensive program for HIV-infected persons with no symptoms are to assist them to (1) cope with psychologic reactions, (2) manage information and resources, and (3) develop a personal health and medical care plan.

The same guidelines and procedures may be used for pretest and posttest counseling for HIV-2 and human T-lymphotropic viruses I and II (CDC, June 25, 1993; Mann et al., 1992). Transmission is similar although perhaps not as efficient. Health maintenance and monitoring guidelines are likewise very similar.

Health Education and Maintenance

Primary health maintenance involves taking a comprehensive health history and making a physical and psychosocial assessment. Taking a health history and physical assessment are covered in depth in Chapter 5 and Appendix IV. Psychosocial, psychiatric, and neuropsychologic assessment are discussed in Chapter 11.

Secondary health education and maintenance begins when HIV seropositivity has been established and the client enters the longest period of HIV disease, known as the asymptomatic stage. This stage may last for 9 or more years and is thought to be enhanced and possibly extended by health promotion activities and behaviors that increase immunocompetence. Persons who have HIV antibody and are free of symptoms can engage in a number of activities that may slow or prevent progression to clinical disease. These activities center on minimizing or eliminating the effects of both infectious and noninfectious cofactors and may be broadly categorized as health education and health maintenance activities.

Health Education. All persons who are infected with HIV need information on the meaning of infection. Secondary health education should include the person's sexual partner and family whenever possible. Persons with HIV infection should not assume that they will or will not develop clinical disease and should take all precautions possible to extend life. However, they should be informed that they are probably infected for life and probably contagious for life. This information means that they should not engage in unsafe sexual practices or needle sharing, nor should they donate blood, plasma, body organs, or other tissue. Additionally they should be told that anything that may be contaminated by their blood, semen, or vaginal fluid may constitute a risk of infection. For example, toothbrushes and razors should not be shared. Tampons and other blood-contaminated articles should be double bagged in plastic bags and marked as contaminated, and any needles or sharp objects used in treatment should be disposed of in a rigid container. Persons with HIV can thus help to prevent the spread of HIV to noninfected individuals. On the other hand, sharing food and toilet facilities, sneezing and coughing, and expressing affection in a casual manner will not transmit HIV.

It is important that persons with HIV not engage in unsafe sexual practices or share needles with other seropositive persons. Repeated exposures to the virus may involve more virulent strains and may increase the likelihood of progression to AIDS (Levy, 1993). Unsafe (unprotected) anal sexual practices also expose the person to allogeneic sperm and semen. Repeated exposure to sperm and semen through the rectum can have immunosuppressant effects that HIV-infected persons need to avoid.

Health education must be directed also at prevention of infections other than HIV. Many of the infectious cofactors of HIV infection can be prevented by the same changes in sexual practices that could prevent HIV infection: avoiding anal intercourse and multiple sexual partners. These practices are associated not only with HIV infection but also with other STDs that present a health threat: HBV, CMV, and HSV infections, amebiasis, syphilis, and gonorrhea. Whether through the ability of immunosuppression to provide opportunity for activation of HIV, or through actual activation of cells carrying HIV, coincident chronic infections have significant effects on the immune system and on the progression of HIV infection. Avoiding concurrent STDs should be a principal focus of any health education program. Short of abstinence, condoms should be used, at a minimum, for all insertive sexual practices, to reduce the risk of infection.

Injection drug users can eliminate or significantly reduce the risks of infectious cofactors by stopping the use of intravenous drugs, using disinfected needles and syringes, stopping needle and equipment sharing, decreasing the number of injections, and avoiding the use of shooting galleries for injection. All of these practices, uncorrected, result not only in HIV infection but also in other infections among IDUs. Chief among these infections are frequent and chronic soft tissue infections (cellulitis, abscesses), bacterial endocarditis, and the viral hepatitides. In addition, injection drug users may be infected with all the STDs described previously. These chronic multiple infections can play a role as cofactors in the progression of disease in HIV-infected individuals. The focus of health education for drug users should be on stopping the use of drugs, stopping the sharing of dirty needles and syringes, and encouraging safer sex (use of condoms, cessation of anal receptive intercourse, and reduction in number of sexual partners).

Other strategies for infection prevention revolve around controlling exposure to pathogens that naturally exist in such things as soil, pets, other humans, and food. Food safety may be maintained by keeping foods at the proper temperature (cold or hot); cooking them properly; washing foods, food preparation areas, and utensils thoroughly; and avoiding contamination of foods with one another. Finally, good hygiene practices and maintaining skin integrity are barriers to infection. These strategies are addressed also in Chapter 5.

Health Maintenance. Lovejoy and colleagues (1991) considered a health maintenance program to involve symptom surveillance, therapy, hygiene, nutrition, stress reduction, and involvement in supportive interpersonal relationships. Through lifestyle changes, persons with HIV infection can also minimize or eliminate immunosuppressive factors and emphasize factors that promote immune function. First, regular medical and psychiatric evaluations and follow-up are advised for HIV-infected persons (monitoring of health status requires an initial evaluation to establish baseline findings). Secondary health maintenance involves prophylaxis and treatments to prevent disease progression (these are addressed in depth in Chapter 5). Finally, health maintenance efforts include proper nutrition, elimination of recreational drug and alcohol use, stress management, and prevention of pregnancy, all of which may be influential in slowing the rate of disease progression. Secondary health maintenance should be directed at lifestyle changes in these areas.

Nutrition was discussed earlier in this chapter in the section on health promotion. In addition to the health-promoting activities described there, persons in the asymptomatic stage of HIV disease should focus on maintaining their weight and increasing calorie and protein intake as necessary. High-calorie, high-protein foods are from the protein, dairy, starch and grain, and fat food groups. Using food supplements and eating between meals are strategies for increasing intake. Evidence that nutrition plays a role in enhancing immunocompetence in persons with HIV comes from a prospective study of dietary intake in HIV seropositive homosexual men (Abrams et al., 1993). In this study, dietary intake affected CD4$^+$ cell count and HIV symptom variables. Furthermore, the use of micronutrients (vitamin A, B$_1$, C, and niacin) may slow the onset of AIDS (*HIV Frontline Update*, 1994).

Assisting persons with HIV to limit or give up the use of alcohol, recreational drugs, and tobacco is also part of secondary health maintenance. These substances reduce immunocompetence. Limiting or removing their use may slow or prevent disease progression in HIV-infected individuals. Programs such as Alcoholics Anonymous, smoking cessation, and drug rehabilitation may be indicated.

Women who are infected with HIV must be informed of the effects of pregnancy on the progression of disease. Pregnancy itself has an immunosuppressant effect; it is possible that pregnancy accelerates the pace of disease expression. Evidence on this point is conflicting. However, seropositive women should be cautioned against pregnancy; they should use a reliable method of birth control (Shayne & Kaplan, 1991). Other information that women need to know about pregnancy and AIDS is that more than 80% of pediatric AIDS is attributed to maternal transmission, that they do not need to be sick to pass HIV to the fetus, that there is no way to prevent the fetus from becoming infected if the mother is infected, and that the virus may be contracted through breast milk. Women also need information on the use of AZT during pregnancy. Counseling on birth control, pregnancy, enrolling in clinical trials, abortion, and breast-feeding should be part of any health maintenance program for women.

Stress reduction programs may also be useful in secondary health maintenance. They contribute to quality of life and may also contribute to immunocompetence. Information on stress reduction was given in the section on health promotion, above. In addition to regular exercise, rest, and sleep, personal use of relaxation techniques may be of help to some persons. Providing avenues for expression of emotion can be obtained through friends and family, social support groups, and professional counseling. Treatment of depression is recommended both to enhance quality of life and perhaps to enhance immunocompetence (Burack et al., 1993). All these measures are discussed in depth in Chapter 11.

Symptomatic HIV Disease

During the symptomatic stage of HIV disease, the person has various kinds of opportunistic infections and malignancies. They may also have weakness, fatigue, pain, weight loss, and wasting. Chronic diarrhea may be a particular problem, causing a deterioration in social activity, work, daily living, energy, and cognition (Lubeck et al., 1993). Clinical manifestations of AIDS are discussed comprehensively in Chapter 4. The nursing management of the symptomatic stage of HIV disease is discussed in Chapter 5 and focuses on symptoms and human responses to HIV illness. At this stage, infections generally respond to medical treatment. Symptom control is a major goal of nursing care.

Secondary health maintenance behaviors and activities discussed in the previous section are also applicable here. Enhancing immunocompetence to prevent infections is still the focus of care for the person with HIV, whether provided by self and family or by health care providers. In addition to the information provided above, further information on nutrition is given here. Common problems related to nutrition in symptomatic-stage HIV infection may be lack of appetite; mouth soreness and problems in swallowing; taste changes; bloating, fullness, and heartburn; nausea and diarrhea; and weight loss.

The latter course of HIV disease is most

frequently influenced by malnutrition (Mascioli, 1993; Task Force on Nutrition Support in AIDS, 1989). In particular, protein-calorie malnutrition significantly affects the immune system and the ability to deal with infection (Chandra, 1993). Therapies to reverse or alter the progressive weight loss associated with AIDS may be critical. Assessment of nutritional status is a necessary first step in supporting HIV-infected individuals, particularly in a syndrome whose treatment has yet to be established. Assessment and follow-up should include anthropometric measures and evaluation of visceral proteins (serum albumin, total iron-binding capacity, a complete blood cell count, and serum potassium level). Blood urea nitrogen, creatinine, and liver function tests should be performed as indicated. Weight should be assessed at least weekly, and frequent assessment of appetite is recommended.

Special high-calorie, high-protein, low-fat, lactose-free oral diets in combination with a full-strength food supplement are recommended as the first line of nutritional therapy (Hickey & Weaver, 1988). These diets are associated with few complications, require limited nursing management and pretherapy education, and do not restrict daily activities. A detailed nutritional plan is important to provide guidance in meal preparation (Hickey & Weaver, 1988; Mascioli, 1993).

When diarrhea is a problem, replacement therapy, antidiarrheal agents, diet modification, or bowel rest may be indicated. If oral intake is limited, tube feeding may provide nutrients if the gastrointestinal system is functioning. If the person has severely compromised bowel function and if oral or gastrointestinal tube feedings are inadequate or contraindicated, a short course of either peripheral parenteral nutrition or total parenteral nutrition should be considered (Hickey & Weaver, 1988). When the person returns to an oral diet, it should be high in protein and calories to maintain and nourish the existing functioning immune system.

Chapters 5, 6, 7, and 8 address in detail the nursing care needs of persons with HIV disease. These chapters include information on the care of various subgroups of patients in all stages of disease.

Late HIV Disease

In the late stage of HIV disease, immune functioning is severely compromised and pharmacologic treatments have little effect. Palliation and quality of life become the major goals of care. Management of pain, skin care, mouth care, provision of fluids and oxygen, and positioning take precedence in making clients comfortable (Butters et al., 1993). Spiritual care and psychosocial care are important for clients, partners, and family. These aspects of care are addressed in Chapters 5 and 11 in depth. They are considered the final stage of a health promotion and disease prevention approach on an individual and family level.

COMMUNITY EFFORTS

Health promotion and disease prevention also occur at the community level. Community interventions are discussed next with an emphasis on cofactors to HIV disease, various human groups, strategies for successful community programs, and existing community resources.

Cofactors to HIV tend to cluster in different human groups, producing social groups more or less at risk of acquiring infection by the virus through various exposure routes. It is important to note that behaviors and circumstances put people at risk, not the groups with whom they are associated. However, these behaviors and circumstances occur more or less frequently in some groups than others, and therefore the terms "populations at risk" and "vulnerable populations" have emerged. Identification of vulnerable at-risk populations has the possible negative result of stigmatizing these groups. A possible positive effect is the opportunity to design health education programs specific to the lifestyle, practices, and circumstances of specific population groups. Each of the exposure categories identified by the CDC suggests targeted community interventions for high-risk behaviors. These are discussed here under the categories of sexual practices, injection drug use, and blood product safety.

Changes in Sexual Practices

Nearly a decade has passed in which the public media and community groups have tried to educate the population about HIV disease and how to prevent its transmission. Epidemiologic reports from various geographic areas in the United States and Europe provide evidence of the effectiveness of these efforts. Changes in sexual practices appear to be greatest in men who have sex with men (MWSM) and self-identify as homosexuals. MWSM who do not identify as homosexual have not had the same changes. Less change in sexual behavior is observed in adolescents and women. Finally, among ethnic groups, African Americans and Latinos have experienced less change (CDC, Aug. 13, 1993).

Certain behaviors often are assessed to determine change in sexual behavior. In San Francisco, use of condoms and a sharp decline in the percentage of self-identified homosexual men who perform anogenital intercourse have been reported (Catania et al., 1992; Coates, 1990; Coates et al., 1989a and 1989b; van Griensvan et al., 1993). Similar findings have been reported in Australia, France, and England (Hart et al., 1993; Kippax et al., 1993; Messiah et al., 1993). However, in these studies several remaining behavioral problems emerged: safer practices did not extend to young homosexual men; some risky sexual practices were still being practiced; and safer sex practices were not consistent (Offir et al., 1993). Risky practices that continued were use of extraneous lubricants with condoms and anorectal douching after intercourse (Messiah et al., 1993). It was considered possible that these practices were misunderstood as safer sex or that these practices were not considered a true risk by those engaged in them (Messiah et al., 1993; Offir et al., 1993).

Despite the substantial increase in knowledge of HIV, including modes of transmission and the recognition of sexual transmission, risk behaviors in teenage and young adult MWSM have not changed substantially (CDC,

May 1993; Coates et al., 1989b; DeWit et al., 1993; Hart et al., 1993; Silvestre et al., 1993). The high number of newly infected homosexual and bisexual men has led investigators to call for additional intervention initiatives (Melbye & Smith, 1993). Among MWSM who do not self-identify as homosexual or who do not disclose their homosexuality or bisexuality, unprotected anal intercourse continues at high rates and the use of condoms is infrequent and inconsistent (CDC, Jan. 15, 1993b; Doll et al., 1992; Peterson et al., 1992). Ethnic identity is related both to failure to disclose or identify as homosexual and to a greater risk of HIV infection (Doll et al., 1992; Ostrow et al., 1991; Peterson et al., 1992; Schwartz et al., 1993).

Changes in sexual practices among heterosexuals have not been observed. Most sexually active heterosexuals are not using condoms (Catania et al., 1992). Even among heterosexual couples who were aware of a partner's seropositive status, use of condoms was not consistent (Saracco et al., 1993). Sexual risk behaviors continued in female partners of HIV-infected men with hemophilia (Dublin et al., 1992). The lack of safer sexual practices is particularly notable in young and adolescent heterosexuals, among whom sexual activity has been steadily increasing since the 1970s (Anon, 1993; CDC, 1991; CDC, Aug. 13, 1993; Hein, 1993; Pleck et al., 1993; Sonenstein et al., 1989). Among heterosexuals, women are more likely than men to continue unsafe sexual practices (Eversley et al., 1993a, 1993b; Kost & Forrest, 1992). Personal perception of risk, involvement with multiple sexual partners, and infection with an STD did not motivate women to adopt low-risk behaviors (Eversley et al., 1993a, 1993b; Finelli et al., 1993; Kost & Forrest, 1992). Unsafe sexual practices were greater among ethnic women of color than among white women (Eversley et al., 1993a, 1993b; Finelli et al., 1993).

Among persons who identified multiple sexual partners as a major risk factor, men, regardless of sexual orientation, were more likely to use condoms than women (CDC, May 28, 1993). Furthermore, among persons whose sexual contacts were both paying and nonpaying partners, the use of condoms was more frequent with paying partners (Elifson et al., 1993). Although there have been some positive changes overall in sexual behavior, it is apparent that for many groups risk practices have not decreased in response to public health campaigns and programs.

Changes in Injection Drug Use Practices

For IDUs also there has been a barrage of information on prevention, the use of bleach, distribution of condoms, and in some cases free needle and syringe exchanges. Despite these efforts there has been a continued rise in the number of HIV seroprevalent persons whose risk behavior is injection drug use (CDC, July 23, 1993). Similar findings have been reported in Europe (Worm & Gottschau, 1993). Sharing needles and using shooting galleries have been reported as high-risk behaviors for HIV exposure (Ickovics & Rodin, 1992; Metzger et al., 1993). Some studies have found that IDUs have modified their needle use (Guydish et al., 1990; van den Hoek et al., 1990; Wayment et al., 1993). However, sharing needles has been reported as more prevalent among women than men (Wayment et al., 1993). Women inject drugs more frequently with a partner than do men, and sharing tends to go on in this situation and role relationship.

Complicating injection drug use practices are the sexual behaviors of IDUs. It is frequently impossible to know whether exposure to HIV is occurring because of injection drug use or because of sexual practices (Ickovics & Rodin, 1992). For example, the severity of heroin dependence was found to be related to unprotected sexual activity with multiple partners, often for money or drugs (Gossop et al., 1993). Crack cocaine use also has been related to high-risk sexual activities (Finelli et al., 1993). Finally, intravenous drug use was significantly associated with sexual risk taking, with women more likely than men to have an IDU as a sexual partner (Kim et al., 1993). It becomes apparent from these reports that it is extremely difficult to separate the risks of exposure because of drug use from those of drug-related sex practices.

Needle exchange programs and needle disinfection programs have been supported and implemented to decrease the risk of transmission among IDUs. It is not clear that these programs have caused a change in needle use behavior. It is also far from certain that changing needle use will decrease transmission of HIV in IDUs. Changes in sexual behavior may be a more overriding concern.

Components of Successful Community Intervention

Several intervention models and strategies for change in sexual and drug use behavior have been implemented and evaluated. Some of these have been successful and have identified common and unique characteristics that may provide guidelines for future community prevention efforts. The CDC has recommended HIV-prevention case management to prevent transmission of HIV when one partner is infected (CDC, June 18, 1993). On the basis of the experiences of community health centers in Miami, New York City, and Newark, New Jersey, the CDC reported changes in risk behaviors related to case managed care. The essential features of this care were (1) a one-on-one client service, (2) associated with ongoing medical preventive care, and (3) for an extended period. Case managed care was designed around HIV testing and counseling, risk reduction counseling, and a care plan for medical and psychosocial services. Although the study employed no comparison group, the participants reported reduced sexual risk behaviors (CDC, June 18, 1993).

A successful strategy of couple counseling and providing social support was reported by Padian and colleagues (1993) in San Francisco. Heterosexual couples recruited from public health facilities and private providers were counseled on safer sexual practices and the use of condoms, and were given the opportunity to develop skills and participate in role playing. Counseling was ongoing every 6 months for an average of 1½ years. The study was limited by the absence of a control group but did find significant sexual behavior change and no HIV seroconversion during the follow-up period.

Intervention for HIV prevention with inner-city adolescent and young adult women in Boston compared a peer educator–delivered intervention with a provider-delivered intervention (Quirk et al., 1993). The study took place in a community family health center. Both interventions significantly affected knowledge, attitudes, and sexual behaviors (reduced vaginal intercourse, increased skills in discussing sexual behavior with a partner). Peer education achieved greater knowledge of injection drug use, and provider education achieved greater knowledge of sexual risks.

An already existing community agency to which women were attracted for food coupons was used to deliver an HIV prevention intervention for low income Latina (Mexican and Central American) women in Los Angeles (Flaskerud, personal communication, 1994). Women attending the Public Health Foundation's Nutrition Program for Women, Infants, and Children (WIC) in an inner-city neighborhood were given free HIV antibody testing and counseling and 1 year of follow-up care. The program consisted of counseling before and after HIV testing, counseling in risk reduction and health promotion, skill development in condom use and in negotiating with a partner, free condoms as often as desired, and referral and advocacy for medical, psychosocial, financial, legal, and social services. The intervention was based on a conceptual model of illness, prevention, and treatment that was specific to the cultural beliefs of the subjects (Flaskerud & Calvillo, 1991a). A one-on-one intervention was delivered by peer educators who shared the ethnicity, language, and gender of the participants. Snacks and child care were provided during visits. Three visits during the 1-year period were required. Additional visits for condoms and additional counseling were encouraged. The program employed a study group and a comparison group who did not receive the intervention. Significant changes occurred in knowledge of HIV transmission, in sexual behavior, and in condom use. These

changes did not occur in the comparison group. No HIV seroconversions occurred during the follow-up period. Eighty-five percent of the women came for more than the required three visits to obtain additional condoms and medical and human services referral and advocacy.

Coates (1990) described the essential features of the San Francisco model for changing high-risk sexual behavior among gay and bisexual men. Dramatic changes in behavior in this population have been attributed to the design and implementation of this multifaceted community program (Catania et al., 1992; van Griensven et al., 1993). The program was built on the same principles of community-level intervention derived from cardiovascular disease risk-reduction programs, smoking cessation programs, and family planning interventions to reduce adolescent pregnancy. These programs incorporated information, motivation, skills training, existing community structures and social networks, attention to normative behaviors, and methods of diffusing information. These programs used peer educators; they were approached as long-term efforts with multiple and repeated strategies to initiate and sustain ongoing change; they incorporated a comprehensive range of services (medical, psychosocial, and so forth); and they used a field experimental design to evaluate their effectiveness.

In a call for action for effective AIDS education for adolescents, Hein (1993) emphasized some of these same principles: peer education, realistic behavior change expectations, normative and explicit risk reduction messages, joining of HIV prevention with HIV services, and joining of HIV programs with existing community agencies serving youth. The CDC (1992a) noted that HIV prevention programs will be translated into prevention *practices* if the personal relevance of information is made clear, that is, if the client recognizes "what I do" to facilitate exposure. The cultural norms or beliefs that shape an individual's understanding of specific behaviors must frame the message. Finally, motivation through role models and examples of others like the participants who have been successful will encourage belief in personal capability.

The International Counterpart Forum, held during the Eighth International Conference on AIDS in Amsterdam, The Netherlands, issued a report summarizing HIV/AIDS prevention and treatment strategies for community educators (International Counterpart Forum, 1992). The Forum considered community programs and strategies for gay men, women, IDUs, children and adolescents, rural populations, and low-literacy populations. Common prevention strategies recommended for all these groups included one-on-one peer education, involvement of the community to be served, use of existing social networks and community agencies, ability to speak the language of the community served and use of images common to its culture, provision of HIV prevention within a comprehensive program of primary and public health care, provision of long-term ongoing services with follow-up repetitions of the intervention, and use of the mass media to reinforce messages and create behavioral norms. Several unique strategies also were identified: using beauty operators and bartenders to provide education and condoms, using pharmacists who exchange needles and syringes to provide education, including food in HIV/AIDS prevention activities, and using mobile care units in neighborhoods with a range of services or access to services. All successful intervention programs reviewed in this section have incorporated many and sometimes most of the common principles and components identified by these various groups and organizations and considered essential to behavior change and maintenance strategies.

Community Settings for HIV Prevention

Several existing community resources lend themselves to the prevention of HIV. Their relationship to known exposure to HIV, trigger cofactors for HIV infection, and human groups most at risk of having these cofactors recommends them for special consideration in community efforts to control the disease (Kalichman et al., 1992). Targeted interventions in conjunction with these existing resources may make a major difference where some others have so far failed. In designing community intervention programs in these settings, public health educators may take direction from the success of programs described in the preceding section.

Sexually Transmitted Disease Clinics. The relationship between HIV and other STDs is highly dynamic and synergistic (AHCPR, January 1994; Mann et al., 1992, pp. 165-193). Persons who have a history of STD are at increased risk of acquiring HIV, and HIV-infected persons have an increased susceptibility to infection with other STDs. Persons with HIV who are coinfected with other STDs usually have severe and protracted courses of these infections. In addition, the STD may facilitate disease expression (AIDS) in persons with HIV. Transmission is similar, and issues for STD prevention and control are applicable to the full range of infections, including HIV.

Locating education programs for HIV prevention in STD (or STI, sexually transmitted infection) clinics makes use of the concept of *core groups* for preventive interventions. Core groups are defined as segments of the population who are (in this case) more likely than others to transmit infections sexually. The public health importance of this concept rests in its potential to permit targeting of limited resources to groups that are most susceptible to transmission. The concept of the core group suggests a focus for behavioral interventions in persons with risky sexual practices (Richert et al., 1993). Comprehensive and well-integrated preventive services that address both HIV infection and other STDs may have a greater chance of success than separate programs. STD programs have a long history of control measures, treatment, follow-up and partner notification, and professional experience and expertise. The programs are an existing community resource, and they are used by sexually active persons who are engaged in risky sexual practices (Finelli et al., 1993). For many persons, such sexual practices are inextricably intermixed with drug use practices.

Family Planning and Perinatal Clinics. There is a dynamic interaction between HIV and various activities related to reproduction. Women of reproductive age and their infants may constitute another core group for HIV infection prevention programs. Reproductive clinics provide opportunities to educate women about sexual transmission, *in utero* and intrapartal transmission, and breast-feeding. Furthermore, pregnancy itself may enhance disease expression (AIDS) in women who are infected with HIV. In addition to contraceptive services, prenatal and postnatal care, and infant care, family planning and perinatal clinics also might offer voluntary HIV testing and counseling, prevention education, health promotion teaching, and follow-up (AHCPR, January 1994; Kass et al., 1992; Lindsay, 1993). These clinics constitute an existing community resource. The established history of such clinics, the professional experience and expertise which they embody, and their frequent use by women of reproductive age all recommend them for well-integrated preventive services that address both HIV infection and pregnancy. Family planning clinics also treat substantial numbers of women who are infected with STDs (Eversley et al., 1993a, 1993b). Another possible setting for reaching women of reproductive age is abortion clinics.

Prevention interventions for women differ substantially from those for men (Ickovics & Rodin, 1992). Locating these interventions in clinics associated with reproduction will ensure that these programs are specific to women and teach prevention methods unique to women (Gollub & Stein, 1993). Because reproductive clinics are often community based, it would be possible to design programs specific to the unique concerns of the population(s) served, such as teenagers and ethnic and cultural groups. As with the core groups who use STD clinics, women who use reproductive health clinics might be susceptible not only to sexual exposure but also to drug-use exposure or drug-related sexual exposure.

Programs Related to Drug (and Needle Use). Injection drug use and HIV infection have an obvious link because the injection provides a parenteral route for infection. The interaction between HIV infection and the use of noninjectable drugs may also have an effect on sexual transmission. Combining HIV prevention and education in conjunction with various programs related to drug use may provide another opportunity for reaching a core group of susceptible persons. Drug rehabilitation programs provide one such existing community resource that may be utilized for HIV prevention. Once again, professional experience and expertise and a history of working with drug users on a continuous, long-term basis recommend these programs for combination preventive strategies. Methadone programs provide the potential for reaching heroin IDUs. Oral opiate substitution programs can also be effective in reducing the risk of acquiring HIV infection (Mann et al., 1992). Needle and syringe exchange centers or pharmacies also offer the opportunity for education on HIV prevention and transmission. In all these existing community facilities, the risk of transmission through sexual practices needs equal emphasis with the risk of transmission through injection, or the parenteral route.

Despite the potential represented by these existing community resources, a tremendous amount of information must still be learned about addiction itself, needle-sharing practices, gender-specific risks, and sexual behavior of drug users. With this gap in understanding, prevention efforts currently focus on reduction of risk and reduction of harm (i.e., through the use of clean needles). Harm reduction messages have had success, but more must be done about the social roots of drug use to stop the spread of HIV in drug users through injection or sexual exposure.

In-School Programs. Children and adolescents who attend school can be targeted for health education and disease prevention programs that include prevention of HIV infection. To meet the needs of students and their communities, HIV prevention programs in schools should be integrated into a comprehensive health promotion approach that begins in elementary school (CDC, 1992b). The CDC has initiated youth risk behavior surveys to help monitor and evaluate changes in behavior related to comprehensive school health programs. Among children and adolescents, health promotion and counseling must focus on the prevalence and threat of intentional and unintentional injuries, tobacco use, alcohol and other drug use, unsafe sexual behaviors, poor dietary habits, and the lack of physical fitness (CDC, 1992c).

For students who are engaged already in unsafe behaviors, schools may plan and implement HIV prevention programs that meet local standards. These programs are usually designed to help students stop risky behaviors or teach them methods to reduce risk. In some instances, local areas have permitted the distribution of condoms and bleach. According to one leading clinician-researcher-educator who works with adolescents, HIV education in schools must be joined with on-site condom availability (Hein, 1993). A national survey by the CDC in 1990 showed that 54% of U.S. teenagers engaged in sexual intercourse, many with multiple partners. Of these, only 41% used condoms (CDC, 1992b). An alarming report issued by the CDC (Aug. 13, 1993) noted that during the period from 1981 through 1991, 24% to 30% of the reported morbidity from gonorrhea and 10% to 12% of the reported morbidity from syphilis in the United States were in adolescent age groups. Prevalence was higher in the South and in African American youth.

Other aspects of in-school programs related to HIV specifically and to healthy attitudes and behaviors in general are coordination of in-school programs with a variety of community health services and health professionals. In-school programs should also help teachers, parents, and students understand HIV disease and deal compassionately with students who are infected.

Other Community Settings. Selecting community settings for HIV education, prevention, and treatment that are in existence already and are providing health and human services makes sense for several reasons. These settings are known to the community and are being used by community members. Recruitment of core groups is not a problem.

Professionals working in these settings have experience and expertise in specific areas that involve the behaviors of their core group. The structure for administering and delivering services is in place. If these existing agencies would incorporate the new strategies gained in field experiments of community HIV prevention programs, they would offer advantages over other settings in the battle to prevent HIV infection.

Several in-place community settings come to mind other than those described here: WIC programs, Job Corps programs, and college campuses, to name a few. Community health nurses are aware of many others that would be similarly well suited.

HIV NURSING RESEARCH IN HEALTH PROMOTION AND DISEASE PREVENTION

Summary of Research

For our purposes here, research on health promotion and disease prevention is considered behavioral in that it focuses on behaviors of people and communities that promote health, prevent disease, and enhance immunocompetence. Although biologic research may also include health promotion through the discovery of the roles of chemicals, micronutrients, and genetics and their effects on immune function, the area of research emphasized here focuses on behaviors involved with biologic processes, such as drinking, smoking, eating, and reproducing. Nurses have been engaged in several important dimensions of research in this area. For example, nursing research related to cofactors of HIV disease has explored the role of nutrition in the immunocompetence of persons with HIV, the role of stress management in the quality of life of PWHIV and correlates of stress in HIV disease, and the coping responses used by persons at risk of acquiring HIV infection (Keithley et al., 1992; McCain, 1993; Nyamathi & Lewis, 1991; Nyamathi et al., 1993b; van Servellen et al., 1993). These areas of research lend themselves to nursing questions and interventions and are being pursued all over the country. Several studies of health promotion and disease prevention have direct applicability to HIV: predicting the health-promoting behaviors of gay men; changing codependent and health-promoting behaviors in families of substance abusers; reducing sexual transmission of STD; and identifying condom-use control variables for women and their partners (Haram, 1993; Jemmott, 1993; Marion, 1993; Saunders, 1991–1995; Swanson, 1992, 1993; Waller, 1993).

Nursing research has focused also on health promotion and health maintenance activities by and for persons with HIV infection, such as accessibility of health care, utilization of health care services, and involvement in self-care activities (Ballantyne, 1993; Butz et al., 1993; Lovejoy et al., 1991). Especially in the AIDS epicenters in the United States, these areas of research are of interest to nurses because of their direct effects on and applicability to nursing practice. Furthermore, HIV nursing research has been involved with designing and testing the effects of community-based AIDS prevention programs on changes in knowledge and behaviors (Flaskerud & Nyamathi, 1988, 1989a, 1990) and with evaluating community-based nurse case management of symptoms in PWHIV (Wright et al., 1993). The nursing research provided as examples here has involved a wide range of subjects—homosexual and bisexual men, women, children and adolescents, ethnic people of color, homeless persons, low income persons, elderly persons, and state employees—to exemplify a range of study participants (Butz et al., 1993; Flaskerud & colleagues, 1988, 1989b, 1990, 1991a, 1991b, 1993; Lovejoy et al., 1991; Nyamathi, 1992; Nyamathi & colleagues 1989, 1991, 1993a, 1993b; Tichy & Talashek, 1992; van Servellen et al., 1993). The results of this research have made meaningful contributions to a science of health promotion and disease prevention for nursing and other health-related disciplines.

Research Needed

Health promotion and disease prevention are fruitful areas of research for nursing because of the long-standing interest and support among nurses for preventive nursing practice. Research that continues to be needed may be divided into four categories: (1) behavioral cofactors to prevent exposure, (2) behavioral cofactors to promote health, (3) behavioral cofactors to maintain health, and (4) community-based interventions to change knowledge and behaviors. Each of these areas may be further subdivided on the basis of the population(s) served.

1. Research that describes, explains, and predicts behavioral cofactors to exposure:

   - Preventing or limiting risky sexual practices
   - Preventing or decreasing risky drug use practices
   - Preventing behaviors resulting from an interaction of drug use and sexual practices
   - Preventing or limiting pregnancy, intrapartal infection, and transmission through breast-feeding
   - Preventing inappropriate use of transfusions, tissue transplants, and unsafe donations

2. Research that describes, explains, and predicts cofactors to health promotion:

   - Effects of nutrition
   - Effects of physical exercise, rest, and sleep
   - Effects of stress management

3. Research that describes, explains, and predicts cofactors to health maintenance in HIV-infected persons:

   - Prevention of infections
   - Effects of health promotion behaviors (listed above)
   - Effects of treatment: physiologic, psychosocial, and neuropsychiatric
   - Effects of comfort measures
   - Effects of palliation
   - Accessibility, availability, and responsiveness of health care services
   - Promotion and maintenance of self-care activities

4. Research that describes, explains, and predicts successful community-level interventions:

- Essential elements of successful programs
- Strategies of successful programs with a wide variety of populations
- Effect of the use of in-place community settings for HIV prevention programs
- Field experiments testing the effectiveness of specific community programs with specific populations

Nurses have a special interest in all these areas of research. They also are uniquely qualified because of their practice to conduct research in these areas. Finally, research in these areas will help develop a science of nursing that reflects nursing expertise.

SUMMARY

Cofactors play a major role not only in exposure to HIV infection but also in disease expression and progression. Identifying these cofactors and making them a focus of public health education programs are crucial. Health promotion, health education, and health maintenance programs can be designed to take into account cofactors related to immunocompetence and immunosuppression. Changes in behaviors related to known cofactors have been demonstrated to improve health for everyone and at all stages of HIV infection.

Community health promotion and prevention programs have identified the essential components of successful intervention programs. However, these need further testing and evaluation. When validated, these components can be incorporated into the design of future programs. Placing these programs in community settings that are already providing services for similar behaviors may enhance their effect and appeal. Nursing research in all areas of health promotion and disease prevention should inform nursing practice and develop the base for nursing interventions.

REFERENCES

Abrams, B., Duncan, D., Hert-Picciotto, I. (1993). A prospective study of dietary intake and acquired immune deficiency syndrome in HIV-seropositive homosexual men. *Journal of Acquired Immune Deficiency Syndromes, 6*(8), 949–958.

Agency for Health Care Policy and Research (AHCPR), Public Health Service, USDHHS (January 1994). Evaluation and management of early HIV infection. Clinical Practice Guideline, No. 7. AHCPR publication No. 94-0572, Rockville, MD.

Alcabes, P., Schoenbaum, E.E., Klein, R.S. (1993). Correlates of the rate of decline of CD4$^+$ lymphocytes among injection drug users infected with the human immunodeficiency virus. *American Journal of Epidemiology, 137*(9), 989–1000.

Anon. (1993). Heterosexual AIDS: Pessimism, pandemics, and plain hard facts. *Lancet, 341*(8849), 863–864.

Ascher, M.S., Sheppard, H.W., Winkelstein, W., Jr., et al. (1993). Does drug use cause AIDS? *Nature, 361*(6416), 103–104.

Asselmeier, M.A., Caspari, R.B., Bottenfield, S. (1993). A review of allograft processing and sterilization techniques and their role in transmission of the human immunodeficiency virus. *American Journal of Sports Medicine, 21*(2), 170–175.

Bagasra, O., Kajdacsy-Balla, A., Lischner, H.W., et al. (1993). Alcohol intake increases human immunodeficiency virus type 1 replication in human peripheral blood mononuclear cells. *The Journal of Infectious Diseases, 167*, 789–797.

Balfour, H.H., Jr. (1993). Transfusion and the human immunodeficiency virus. *Transfusion, 33*(2), 101–102.

Ballantyne, J.E. (Nov. 12-15, 1993). Experiences of HIV-infected men with rural health care. Paper presented at the 1993 scientific sessions of the ANA Council of Nurse Researchers, Washington, D.C.

Bastian, L., Bennett, C.L., Adams, J., et al. (1993). Differences between men and women with HIV-related *Pneumocystis carinii* pneumonia: Experiences from 3,070 cases in New York City in 1987. *Journal of Acquired Immune Deficiency Syndromes, 6*(6), 617–623.

Blumberg, N., Heal, J.M. (1989). Transfusion and recipient immune function. *Archives of Pathology and Laboratory Medicine, 113*, 246–253.

Buchbinder, S.P., Katz, M., Hessol, N., et al. (1992, July). Healthy long-term positives: Men infected with HIV for more than 10 years with CD4 counts of 500 cells. Presented at the Eighth International Conference on AIDS, Amsterdam, The Netherlands.

Burack, J.H., Barrett, D.C., Stall, R.D., et al. (1993). Depressive symptoms and CD4 lymphocyte decline among HIV-infected men. *Journal of the American Medical Association, 270*, 2568–2573.

Butters, E., Higginson, I., George, R., et al. (1993). Palliative care for people with HIV/AIDS: Views of patients, carers and providers. *AIDS Care, 5*(1), 105–116.

Butz, A.M., Hutton, N., Joyner, M., et al. (1993). HIV-infected women and infants: Social and health factors impeding utilization of health care. *Journal of Nurse-Midwifery, 38*(2), 103–109.

Catania, J.A., Coates, T.J., Kegeles, S., et al. (1992). Condom use in multi-ethnic neighborhoods of San Francisco: The population-based AMEN (AIDS in Multi-Ethnic Neighborhoods) Study. *American Journal of Public Health, 82*, 284–287.

Centers for Disease Control (1991). Premarital sexual experience among adolescent women—United States, 1970–1988. *Morbidity and Mortality Weekly Report, 39,* 929–932.

Centers for Disease Control (1992a, August). Improving public understanding of the HIV epidemic. *HIV/AIDS Prevention, 3*(2), 1–2.

Centers for Disease Control (1992b, October). Preventing risk behaviors among students. *HIV/AIDS Prevention, 3*(3), 1.

Centers for Disease Control (1992c, October). YRBSS helps monitor student health behavior. *HIV/AIDS Prevention, 3*(3), 5–6.

Centers for Disease Control and Prevention (Jan. 15, 1993a). Recommendations for HIV testing services for inpatients and outpatients in acute-care hospital settings and technical guidance on HIV counseling. *Morbidity and Mortality Weekly Report, 42*(RR-2), 1–5, 11–16.

Centers for Disease Control and Prevention (Jan. 15, 1993b). Condom use and sexual identity among men who have sex with men—Dallas, 1991. *Morbidity and Mortality Weekly Report, 42*(1), 7.

Centers for Disease Control and Prevention (March 12, 1993). False-positive serologic tests for human T-cell lymphotropic virus type among blood donors following influenza vaccination, 1992. *Morbidity and Mortality Weekly Report, 42*(9).

Centers for Disease Control and Prevention (1993, May). Condoms and HIV/STD prevention: Clarifying the message. *HIV/AIDS Prevention, 4*(1), 2–4.

Centers for Disease Control and Prevention (May 28, 1993). Sexual behavior and condom use—District of Columbia, January-February, 1992. *Morbidity and Mortality Weekly Report, 42*(20), 390–398.

Centers for Disease Control and Prevention (June 4, 1993). Use of bleach for disinfection of drug injection equipment. *Morbidity and Mortality Weekly Report, 42*(2), 418–419.

Centers for Disease Control and Prevention (June 18, 1993). HIV prevention through case management for HIV-infected persons: Selected sites. *Morbidity and Mortality Weekly Report, 42*(23), 448–456.

Centers for Disease Control and Prevention (June 25, 1993). Recommendations for counseling persons infected with human T-lymphotrophic virus, types I and II. *Morbidity and Mortality Weekly Report, 42,* No. RR-9, 1–13.

Centers for Disease Control and Prevention (July 23, 1993). Update: Acquired immunodeficiency syndrome—United States, 1992. *Morbidity and Mortality Weekly Report, 42*(28), 547–557.

Centers for Disease Control and Prevention (Aug. 6, 1993). Update: Barrier protection against HIV infection and other sexually transmitted diseases. *Morbidity and Mortality Weekly Report, 42*(30), 589–597.

Centers for Disease Control and Prevention (Aug. 13, 1993). Special focus: Surveillance for sexually transmitted diseases. *Morbidity and Mortality Weekly Report, 42,* (No. SS-3), 1–39.

Centers for Disease Control and Prevention (Sept. 10, 1993). Physical activity and the prevention of coronary heart disease. *Morbidity and Mortality Weekly Report, 42*(35), 669–672.

Centers for Disease Control and Prevention (April 29, 1994). Zidovudine for the prevention of HIV transmission from mother to infant. *Morbidity and Mortality Weekly Report, 43*(16), 285–287.

Chandra, R.K. (1993). Symposium on nutrition and im-

munity in serious illness. *Proceedings of the Nutrition Society, 52,* 77–84.

Chiasson, M.A., Stoneburner, R.L., Lifson, A.R., et al. (1990). Risk factors for human immunodeficiency virus type 1 (HIV-1) infection in patients at a sexually transmitted disease clinic in New York City. *American Journal of Epidemiology, 131*(2), 208–220.

Coates, T.J. (1990). Strategies for modifying sexual behavior for primary and secondary prevention of HIV disease. *Journal of Consulting and Clinical Pathology, 58*(1), 57–69.

Coates, T.J., Ekstrand, M., Kegeles, S.M., et al. (1989a, June). HIV antibody status and behavior change in two cohorts of gay men in San Francisco: The San Francisco Men's Health Study (SFMHS) and the AIDS Behavioral Research Project (ABRP). Presented at the 5th International Conference on AIDS: The Scientific and Social Challenge, Montreal, Quebec, Canada.

Coats, T.J., McKusick, L., Kuno, R., et al. (1989b). Stress reduction training changed number of sexual partners but not immune function in men with HIV. *American Journal of Public Health, 79*(7), 885–887.

Craighead, I.B., Knowles, J.K. (1993). Prevention of transfusion-associated HIV transmission with the use of a transfusion protocol for under-5s. *Tropical Doctor, 23*(2), 59–61.

de Saussure, P., Yerly, S., Tullen, E., et al. (1993). Human immunodeficiency virus type 1 nucleic acids detected before p24 antigenemia in a blood donor. *Transfusion, 33*(2), 164–167.

Deschamps, M., Pape, M.J.W., Desvarieux, M., et al. (1993). A prospective study of HIV-seropositive asymptomatic women of childbearing age in a developing country. *Journal of Acquired Immune Deficiency Syndromes, 6*(5), 446–451.

DeWit, J.B.F., van Griensven, G.J.P., Kok, G., et al. (1993). Why do homosexual men relapse into unsafe sex? Predictors of resumption of unprotected anogenital intercourse with casual partners. *AIDS, 7*(8), 1113–1118.

Diaz, T., Chu, S.Y. (1993). Crack cocaine use and sexual behavior among people with AIDS. *Journal of the American Medical Association, 269*(22), 2845–2846.

Dienstbier, R.A. (1989). Arousal and physiological toughness: Implications for mental and physical health. *Psychological Review, 96,* 84–100.

Doll, L.S., Petersen, L.R., White, C.R., et al. (1992). Homosexually and nonsexually identified men who have sex with men: A behavioral comparison. *Journal of Sex Research, 29,* 1–14.

Dublin, S., Rosenberg, P.S., Goedert, J.J. (1992). Patterns and predictors of high-risk sexual behavior in female partners of HIV-infected men with hemophilia. *AIDS, 6,* 475–482.

Edlin, B.R., Holmberg, S.D. (1993). Insemination of HIV-negative women with processed semen of HIV-positive partners. *Lancet, 341*(8844), 570–571.

Elifson, K.W., Boles, J., Sweat, M. (1993). Risk factors associated with HIV infection among male prostitutes. *American Journal of Public Health, 83*(1), 79–83.

Ellerbrock, T.V., Rogers, M.F. (1990). Epidemiology of human immunodeficiency virus infection in women in the United States. *Obstetrics and Gynecology Clinics of North America, 17*(3), 523–544.

Evans, B.G., Catchpole, M.A., Heptonstall, J. (1993). Sexually transmitted diseases and HIV-1 infection among homosexual men in England and Wales. *British Medical Journal, 306*(6875), 426–428.

Eversley, R.B., Newstetter, A., Avins, A., et al. (1993a). Sexual risk and perception of risk for HIV infection among multiethnic family-planning clients. *American Journal of Prevention Medicine, 9*(2), 92–95.

Eversley, R.B., Policar, M., White, V., et al. (1993b). Self-reported sexually transmitted diseases among family planning clients: Ethnic differences in sexual risk behavior and HIV risk reduction. *Ethnicity and Disease, 3*(2), 181–188.

Feng, T., Anderson, J., Ofstead, L., et al. (1992, July). Obstetric and perinatal outcomes in HIV-infected pregnant women. Presented at the Eighth International AIDS Conference, Amsterdam, The Netherlands.

Fennema, J.S.A., van Ameijden, E.J.C., Coutinho, R.A. (1993). HIV prevalence among clients attending a sexually transmitted disease clinic in Amsterdam: The potential risk for heterosexual transmission. *Genitourinary Medicine, 69*(1), 23–28.

Finelli, L. Budd, J., Spitalny, K.C., et al. (1993). Early syphilis: Relationship to sex, drugs, and changes in high-risk behaviors from 1987–1990. *Sexually Transmitted Diseases, 20*(2), 89–95.

Flaskerud, J.H. (1992). HIV disease and levels of prevention. *Journal of Community Health Nursing, 9*(3), 137–150.

Flaskerud, J.H. (1994). Personal communication.

Flaskerud, J.H., Calvillo, E.R. (1991a). Beliefs about AIDS, health, and illness among low income Latina women. *Research in Nursing and Health, 14*, 431–438.

Flaskerud, J.H., Nyamathi, A. (1988). An AIDS education program for Vietnamese women. *New York State Journal of Medicine, 88*, 632–637.

Flaskerud, J.H., Nyamathi, A.M. (1989a). Black and Latina women's AIDS-related knowledge, attitudes, and practices. *Research in Nursing & Health, 12*, 339–346.

Flaskerud, J.H., Nyamathi, A.M. (1990). Effects of an AIDS education program on the knowledge, attitudes and practices of low income Black and Latina women. *Journal of Community Health, 15*(9), 343–355.

Flaskerud, J.H., Rush, C.E. (1989b). AIDS and traditional health beliefs and practices of Black women. *Nursing Research, 38*(4), 210–215.

Flaskerud, J.H., Thompson, J. (1991b). Beliefs about AIDS, health, and illness among low income White women. *Nursing Research, 40*(5), 266–271.

Flaskerud, J.H., Uman, G. (1993). Directions for focused AIDS education for Hispanic women. *Public Health Reports, 103*(3), 298–304.

Fleming, P.L., Ciesielski, C.A., Byers, R.H., et al. (1993). Gender differences in reported AIDS-indicative diagnoses. *Journal of Infectious Diseases, 168*(1), 61–67.

Folkman, S., Chesney, M., Pollack, L., et al. (1993). Stress, control, coping, and depressive mood in human immunodeficiency virus–positive and negative gay men in San Francisco. *The Journal of Nervous and Mental Disease, 181*(7), 409–416.

Friedman, S.R., Des Jarlais, D.C., Sterk, C.E. (1990). AIDS and the social relations of intravenous drug users. *The Milbank Quarterly, 68*(suppl. 1), 85–110.

Ginzburg, H.M. (1993). Federal response to needle-exchange programs. I. Historical perspective. *Pediatrics AIDS and HIV Infection: Fetus to Adolescents, 4*(1), 20–26.

Gollub, E.L., Stein, Z.A. (1993). Commentary: The new female condom—item 1 on a women's AIDS prevention agenda. *American Journal of Public Health, 83*(4), 498–500.

Gossop, M., Griffiths, P., Powis, B., et al. (1993). Severity of heroin dependence and HIV risk. I. Sexual behavior. *AIDS Care, 5*(2), 149–157.

Guillou, P.J. (1993). The effects of lipids on some aspects of the cellular immune response. *Proceedings of the Nutrition Society, 52*, 91–100.

Guydish, J.R., Abramowitz, A., Woods, W., et al. (1990). Changes in needle sharing behavior among intravenous drug users: San Francisco, 1986–1988. *American Journal of Public Health, 80*, 995–997.

Guydish, J., Bucardo, J., Young, M., et al. (1993). Evaluating needle exchange: Are there negative effects? *AIDS, 7*(6), 871–876.

Hague, R.A., Mok, J.Y.Q., Johnstone, F.D., et al. (1993). Maternal factors in HIV transmission. *International Journal of STD AIDS, 4*(3), 142–146.

Haram, S.K. (Nov. 12-15, 1993). Change in co-dependence and health promotion following participation in a program for family members of chemical dependents. Paper presented at the 1993 scientific sessions of the ANA Council of Nurse Researchers, Washington, D.C.

Hart, G.J., Dawson, R.M., Fitzpatrick, M., et al. (1993). Risk behavior, anti-HIV and anti–hepatitis B core prevalence in clinic and non-clinic samples of gay men in England, 1991–1992. *AIDS, 7*(6), 863–869.

Hein, K. (1993). "Getting real" about HIV in adolescents. *American Journal of Public Health, 83*(4), 492–494.

Hendriks, J.C.M., Medley, G.F., van Griensven, G.J.P., et al. (1993). The treatment-free incubation period of AIDS in a cohort of homosexual men. *AIDS, 7*(2), 231–239.

Hickey, M.S., Weaver, K.E. (1988). Nutritional management of patients with ARC or AIDS. *Gastroenterology Clinics of North America, 17*(3), 545–561.

HIV Frontline Update (March-April, 1994). Vitamins could slow AIDS onset. *HIV Frontline, 17*, 3.

Hoff, C., Peterson, R.D.A. (1989). Does exposure to HLA alloantigens trigger immunoregulatory mechanisms operative in both pregnancy and AIDS? *Life Sciences, 45*(23), iii-ix.

Holgrave, D.R., Valdiseri, R.O., Gerber, A.R., et al. (1993). Human immunodeficiency virus counseling, testing, referral, and partner notification services. *Archives of Internal Medicine, 153*, 1225–1230.

Ickovics, J.R., Rodin, J. (1992). Women and AIDS in the United States: Epidemiology, natural history, and mediating mechanisms. *Health Psychology, 11*(1), 1–16.

International Counterpart Forum, VIII International Conference on AIDS (1992, July). Strategies for HIV/ AIDS prevention and treatment educators. A report from the International Counterpart Forum, held during the Eighth International Conference on AIDS, Amsterdam, The Netherlands, pp. 1–16.

Ironson, G., LaPerriere, A., Antoni, M., et al. (1990). Changes in immune and psychological measures as a function of anticipation and reaction to news of HIV-1 antibody status. *Psychosomatic Medicine, 52*, 247–270.

Janssen, R.S., St. Louis, M.E., Satten, G.A., et al. (1992). HIV infection among patients in U.S. acute care hospitals: Strategies for the counseling and testing of hospital patients. *The New England Journal of Medicine, 327*(7), 445–448.

Jemmott, L.S. (Nov. 12-15, 1993). Perceived approval of sexual partner and HIV risk–associated behavior among Hispanic women: Implications for nursing. Paper presented at the 1993 scientific sessions of the ANA Council of Nurse Researchers, Washington, D.C.

Jewett, J.F., Hecht, F.M. (1993). Preventive health care for adults with HIV infection. *Journal of the American Medical Association, 269*(9), 1144–1153.

Kalichman, S.C., Hunter, T.L., Kelly, J.A. (1992). Perceptions of AIDS susceptibility among minority and nonminority women at risk for HIV infection. *Journal of Consulting and Clinical Psychology, 60*(5), 725–732.

Karan, L.D. (1989). AIDS prevention and chemical dependence treatment needs of women and their children. *Journal of Psychoactive Drugs, 21*(4), 395–399.

Kass, N.E., Faden, R.R., O'Campo, P., et al. (1992). Policy options for prenatal screening programs for HIV: The preferences of inner-city pregnant women. *AIDS & Public Policy Journal, 7*(4), 225–233.

Keet, I.P.M., Krijnen, P., Koot, M., et al. (1993). Predictors of rapid progression to AIDS in HIV-1 seroconverters. *AIDS, 7*(1), 51–57.

Keithley, J.K., Zeller, J.M., Szeluga, D.J., et al. (1992). Nutritional alterations in persons with HIV infection. *Image, 24*(3), 183–189.

Kelly, J.A., Murphy, D.A., Bahr, G.R., et al. (1993). Factors associated with severity of depression and high-risk sexual behavior among persons diagnosed with human immunodeficiency virus (HIV) infection. *Health Psychology, 12*(3), 215–219.

Kessler, R., Joseph, J., Ostrow, D., et al. (1989, June). Psychosocial cofactors in illness onset among HIV positive men. Presented at the 5th International AIDS Conference in Montreal, Quebec, Canada.

Killian, W.H. (1990, September). HIV counseling: Know the risks. *The American Nurse, 22*(8), 28.

Kim, M.V., Marmor, M., Dubin, N., et al. (1993). HIV risk-related sexual behaviors among heterosexuals in New York City: Associations with race, sex and intravenous drug use. *AIDS, 7*(3), 409-414.

Kippax, S., Crawford, J., Davis, M., et al. (1993). Sustaining safe sex: A longitudinal study of a sample of homosexual men. *AIDS, 7*(2), 257–263.

Kost, K., Forrest, J.D. (1992). American women's sexual behavior and exposure to risk of sexually transmitted diseases. *Family Planning Perspective, 24,* 244–245.

Koziol, D.E., Saah, A.J., Odaka, N., et al. (1993). A comparison of risk factors for human immunodeficiency virus and hepatitis B virus infections in homosexual men. *Annals of Epidemiology, 3*(4), 434–441.

Laga, M., Manoka, A., Kivuvu, M., et al. (1993). Non-ulcerative sexually transmitted diseases as risk factors for HIV-1 transmission in women: Results from a cohort study. *AIDS, 7*(1), 95–102.

Leach, C.T., Cherry, J.D., English, P.A., et al. (1993). The relationship between T-cell levels and CMV infection in asymptomatic HIV-1 antibody–positive homosexual men. *Journal of Acquired Immune Deficiency Syndromes, 6*(4), 407–413.

Learmont, J., Tivdall, B., Evans, L., et al. (1992). Long-term symptomless HIV-1 infection in recipients of blood products from a single donor. *Lancet, 340,* 863–867.

Lemp, G.F., Payne, S.F., Neal, D., et al. (1990). Survival trends for patients with AIDS. *Journal of the American Medical Association, 263*(3), 402–406.

Levy, J. (1993). The transmission of HIV and factors influencing progression to AIDS. *The American Journal of Medicine, 95,* 86–98.

Lifson, A.R., Rutherford, G.W., Jaffe, H.W. (1988). The natural history of human immunodeficiency virus infection. *The Journal of Infectious Diseases, 158*(6), 1360–1367.

Lindsay, M.K. (1993). A protocol for routine voluntary antepartum human immunodeficiency virus antibody screening. *American Journal of Obstetrics and Gynecology, 168*(2), 476–479.

Linn, J.G., Monnig, R.L., Cain, V.A., et al. (1993). Stages of illness, level of HIV symptoms, sense of coherence and psychological functioning in clients of community-based AIDS counseling centers. *Journal of the Association of Nurses in AIDS Care, 4*(2), 24–32.

Lovejoy, N.C., Paul. S., Freeman, E., et al. (1991). Potential correlates of self-care and symptom distress in homosexual/bisexual men who are HIV seropositive. *Oncology Nursing Forum, 18*(7), 1175–1185.

Lubeck, D.P., Bennett, C.L., Mazonson, P.D., et al. (1993). Quality of life and health service use among HIV-infected patients with chronic diarrhea. *Journal of Acquired Immune Deficiency Syndromes, 6,* 478–484.

Lyketsos, C.G., Hoover, D.R., Guccione, M., et al. (1993). Depressive symptoms as predictors of medical outcomes in HIV infection. *Journal of American Medical Association, 270,* 2563–2567.

Mascioli, E.A. (1993). Nutrition and HIV infection. *AIDS Clinical Care, 5*(11), 1.

Mann, J., Tarantola, D.J.M., Netter, T. (Eds.), (1992). *AIDS in the World: A Global Report.* Cambridge, MA: Harvard University Press.

Marion, L.N. (Nov. 12-15, 1993). Self and partner control/influence variables related to condom use: Divorced and separated women. Paper presented at the 1993 scientific sessions of the ANA Council of Nurse Researchers, Washington, D.C.

McCain, N.L. (Nov. 12-15, 1993). Correlates of stress in HIV-disease. Paper presented at the 1993 scientific sessions of the ANA Council of Nurse Researchers, Washington, D.C.

McCoy, H.V., Inciardi, J.A. (1993). Women and AIDS: Social determinants of sex-related activities. *Women and Health, 20*(1), 69–86.

McMahon, K.M. (1988). The integration of HIV testing and counseling into nursing practice. *Nursing Clinics of North America, 23*(4), 803–821.

Melbye, M., Smith, E. (1993). Preventing HIV spread in homo/bisexual men: How effective is it? Experience from the National Mandatory HIV Registry in Demark [letter]. *Journal of Acquired Immune Deficiency Syndromes, 6*(5), 536–537.

Menitove, J.E. (1990). Current risk of transfusion-associated human immunodeficiency virus infection. *Archives of Pathology and Laboratory Medicine, 114,* 330–334.

Meropol, N.J., Krause, P.R., Ratnoff, O.D., et al. (1989). Tendency to serious sequelae of infection with the human immunodeficiency virus in sibships with hemophilia. *Archives of Internal Medicine, 149,* 885–888.

Messiah, A., Bucquet, D., Mettetal, J.F., et al. (1993). Factors correlated with homosexually acquired human immunodeficiency virus infection in the era of "safer sex." *Sexually Transmitted Diseases, 20*(1), 51–58.

Metzger, D.S., Woody, G.E., McLellan, T., et al. (1993). Human immunodeficiency virus seroconversion among intravenous drug users in and out of treatment: An 18-month prospective follow-up. *Journal of Acquired Immune Deficiency Syndromes, 6,* 1049–1056.

Mintz, P.D. (1993). Participation of HIV-infected patients in autologous blood programs. *Journal of the American Medical Association, 269*(22), 2893–2894.

Mmiro, F., Ndugwa, C., Guay, L., et al. (1993). Effect of human immunodeficiency virus-1 infection on the outcome of pregnancy in Ugandan women. *Pediatrics AIDS and HIV Infection: Fetus to Adolescent, 4*(2), 67–73.

Mondanaro, J. (1990). Community-based AIDS prevention interventions: Special issues of women intravenous drug use—future directions for community-based prevention research. (NIDA Research Monograph No. 93, pp. 68-82.) Rockville, MD: National Institute on Drug Abuse.

Moore, P.S., Allen, S., Sowell, A.L., et al. (1993). Role of nutritional status and weight loss in HIV seroconversion among Rwandan women. *Journal of Acquired Immune Deficiency Syndromes, 6*, 611–616.

Munoz, A., Schrager, L.K., Bacellar, H., et al. (1993). Trends in the incidence of outcomes defining acquired immunodeficiency syndrome (AIDS) in multicenter AIDS cohort study: 1985–1991. *American Journal of Epidemiology, 137*(4), 423–438.

Nair, P., Alger, L., Hines, S., et al. (1993). Maternal and neonatal characteristics associated with HIV infection in infants of seropositive women. *Journal of Acquired Immune Deficiency Syndromes, 6*(3), 298–302.

Nanda, D., Minkoff, H.L. (1989). HIV in pregnancy: Transmission and immune effects. *Clinical Obstetrics and Gynecology, 32*(3), 456–466.

Nelson, K., Celentano, D.D., Suprasett, S., et al. (1993). Risk factors for HIV infection among young men in northern Thailand. *Journal of the American Medical Association, 270*(8), 955–960.

Newton-Nash, D.K., Flomenberg, P., Gill, J., et al. (1993, May). Cellular immune responses to hepatitis C. Fourth International Symposium on IICV, Tokyo, Japan.

Nieman, R.B., Fleming, J., Coker, R.J., et al. (1993). The effect of cigarette smoking on the development of AIDS in HIV-1 seropositive individuals. *AIDS, 7*(5), 705–710.

Nyamathi, A. (1992). A comparative study of factors affecting risk level of Black homeless women. *Journal of Acquired Immune Deficiency Syndromes, 5*, 222–228.

Nyamathi, A., Bennett, C., Leake, B., et al. (1993a). AIDS knowledge, perceived risk and high-risk behaviors among low and high acculturated Latina and African-American homeless and drug-addicted women. *American Journal of Public Health, 83*(1), 65–71.

Nyamathi, A., Lewis, C. (1991). Coping of African-American women at risk for AIDS. *Women's Health Issues, 1*(2), 53–62.

Nyamathi, A., Vasquez, R., (1989). The impact of poverty, homelessness, and drugs on Hispanic women at risk for HIV infection. *Hispanic Journal of Behavioral Sciences, 11*(4), 299–314.

Nyamathi, A., Wayment, H., Dunkel-Schetter, C. (1993b). Psychosocial correlates of emotional distress and risk behavior in African-American women at risk of HIV infection. *Anxiety, Stress, and Coping, 6*(2), 133–150.

Offir, J.T., Fisher, J.D., Williams, S.S., et al. (1993). Reasons for inconsistent AIDS-preventive behaviors among gay men. *Journal of Sex Research, 30*(1), 62–69.

Osborn, J.E. (1986). Co-factors and HIV: What determines the pathogenesis of AIDS? *Bio Essays, 5*(6), 287–289.

Osmond, D. (1990). Progression of AIDS in persons testing seropositive for antibody to HIV. In P.T. Cohen, M.A. Sande, & P.A. Volberding (Eds.), *The AIDS knowledge base* (pp. 1-1.16 to 8-1.1.6). Waltham, MA: Medical Publishing Group.

Ostrow, R.E.D., Whitaker, K., Frasier, K., et al. (1991). Racial differences in social support and mental health

in men with HIV infection: A pilot study. *AIDS Care, 3*(1), 55–62.

Otten, M.W., Zaidi, A.A., Wroten, J.E., et al. (1993). Changes in sexually transmitted disease rates after HIV testing and posttest counseling, Miami, 1988 to 1989. *American Journal of Public Health, 83*(4), 529–533.

Padian, N.S., O'Brien, T.R., Chang, Y., et al. (1993). Prevention of heterosexual transmission of human immunodeficiency virus through couple counseling. *Journal of Acquired Immune Deficiency Syndromes, 6*, 1043–1048.

Pappaioanou, M., Kashamuka, M., Behets, F., et al. (1993). Accurate detection of maternal antibodies to HIV in newborn whole blood dried on filter paper. *AIDS, 7*(4), 483–488.

Park, L.P., Margolick, J.B., Georgi, J.V., et al. (1993). Influence of HIV-1 infection and cigarette smoking on leukocyte profile in homosexual men. *Annals of New York Academy Science, 677*(March), 433–436.

Patijn, G.A., Strengers, P.F.W., Harvey, M., et al. (1993). Prevention of transmission of HIV by organ and tissue transplantation, HIV testing protocol and a proposal for recommendations concerning donor selection. *Transplant International, 6*(3), 165–172.

Petersen, L.R., Simonds, R.J., Koistinen, J. (1993). HIV transmission through blood, tissues, and organs. *AIDS, 7*(suppl. 1), S99–S107.

Peterson, J.L., Coates, T.J., Catania, J.A., et al. (1992). High-risk sexual behavior and condom use among gay and bisexual African-American men. *American Journal of Public Health, 82*(11), 1490–1494.

Phillips, A.N., Lee, C.A., Elford, J., et al. (1991). More rapid progression to AIDS in older HIV-infected people: The role of CD4$^+$ T-cell counts. *Journal on AIDS, 4*, 970–975.

Pleck, J.H., Sonenstein, F.L., Ku, L. (1993). Changes in adolescent males' attitudes toward the use of condoms, 1988–1991. *Family Planning Perspective, 25*(3), 106.

Quirk, M.E., Godkin, M.A., Schwenzfeier, E. (1993). Evaluation of two AIDS prevention interventions for inner-city adolescent and young adult women. *American Journal of Preventive Medicine, 9*(1), 21–26.

Richert, C.A., Peterman, T.A., Zaidi, A.A., et al. (1993). A method for identifying persons at high risk for sexually transmitted infections: Opportunity for targeting intervention. *American Journal of Public Health, 83*(4), 520–524.

Richman, K.M., Rickman, L.S. (1993). The potential for transmission of human immunodeficiency virus through human bites. *Journal of Acquired Immune Deficiency Syndromes, 6*(4), 402–406.

Rietmeijer, C.A.M., Penley, L.A., Cohn, D.L., et al. (1989). Factors influencing the risk of infection with human immunodeficiency virus in homosexual men, Denver, 1982–1985. *Sexually Transmitted Diseases, 16*(2), 95–102.

Rosenberg, M.J., Holmes, K.K. (1993). The World Health Organization Working Group on Virucides. Virucides in prevention of HIV infection: Research priorities. *Sexually Transmitted Diseases, 20*(1), 41–44.

Rosenblum, L.S., Buehler, J.W., Morgan, M.W., et al. (1993). Drug dependence: A leading diagnosis in hospitalized HIV-infected women. *Journal of Women's Health, 2*(1), 35–40.

Rothenberg, R., Woelfel, M., Stoneburner, R., et al. (1987). Survival with the acquired immunodeficiency syndrome: Experience with 5833 cases in New York City. *New England Journal of Medicine, 317*(21), 1297–1302.

Rowe, P.M. (1993). Resistance to HIV infection. *Lancet, 341*(8845), 624.

Sabin, C., Phillips, A., Elford, J., et al. (1993). The progression of HIV disease in a hemophilic cohort followed for 12 years. *British Journal of Hematology, 83*(2), 330–333.

Saracco, A., Musicco, M., Nicolos, A., et al. (1993). Man-to-woman sexual transmission of HIV: Longitudinal study of 343 steady partners of infected men. *Journal of Acquired Immune Deficiency Syndromes, 6*(5), 497–502.

Saunders, J. (1991–1995). Nursing, self-care and HIV disease. Research funded by the National Institute of Nursing Research, National Institutes of Health, Rockville, MD.

Schoenbach, V.J., Landis, S.E., Weber, D.J., et al. (1993). HIV seroprevalence in sexually transmitted disease clients in a low-prevalence Southern state: Evidence of sexual transmission. *Annals of Epidemiology, 3*(3), 281–288.

Schwartz, R.H. (1993). Syringe and needle exchange programs worldwide. I and II. *Southern Medical Journal, 86*(3), 318–322, 323–327.

Seage, G.R., III, Oddleifson, S., Carr, E., et al. (1993a). Survival with AIDS in Massachusetts, 1979 to 1989. *American Journal of Public Health, 83*(1), 72–78.

Seage, G.R., III, Mayer, K.H., Horsburgh, R., Jr. (1993b). Risk of human immunodeficiency virus infection from unprotected receptive anal intercourse increases with decline in immunologic status of infected partners. *American Journal of Epidemiology, 137*(8), 899–908.

Shayne, V.T., Kaplan, B.J. (1991). Double victims: Poor women and AIDS. *Women and Health, 17,* 21–37.

Sheppard, H.W., Lang, W., Ascher, M.S., et al. (1993). The characterization of non-progressors: Long-term HIV-1 infection with stable $CD4^+$ T-cell levels. *AIDS, 7*(9), 1159–1166.

Shor-Posner, G., Basit, A., Lu, Y., et al. (1993). Hypocholesterolemia is associated with immune dysfunction in early human immunodeficiency virus-1 infection. *The American Journal of Medicine, 94,* 515–519.

Siddiqui, N.S., Brown, L.S., Jr., Makuch, R.W. (1993). Short-term declines in CD4 levels associated with cocaine use in HIV-1 seropositive, minority injecting drug users. *Journal of the National Medical Association, 85*(4), 293–296.

Siegel, L. (1986). AIDS: Relationship to alcohol and other drugs. *Journal of Substance Abuse Treatment, 3,* 271–274.

Silvestre, A.J., Kingsley, L.A., Wehman, P., et al. (1993). Changes in HIV rates and sexual behavior among homosexual men, 1984–1988/92. *American Journal of Public Health, 83*(4), 578–580.

Solomon, G.F. (1991). Psychosocial factors, exercise, and immunity: Athletes, elderly persons, and AIDS patients. *International Journal of Sports Medicine, 15,* S50–S52.

Solomon, G.F., Temoshok, L., O'Leary, A., et al. (1987). An intensive psychoimmunologic study of long-surviving patients with AIDS. *Annals of New York Academy of Sciences, 496,* 647–655.

Solomon, L., Astemborski, J., Warren, D., et al. (1993). Differences in risk factors for human immunodeficiency virus type 1 seroconversion among male and female intravenous drug users. *American Journal of Epidemiology, 137*(8), 892–898.

Sonenstein, F.L., Pleck, J.H., Ku, L.C. (1989). Sexual activity, condom use and AIDS awareness among adolescent males. *Family Planning Perspective, 21,* 152–158.

Spitzer, M., Brennessel, D., Seltzer, V.L., et al. (1993). Is human papillomavirus–related disease an independent risk factor for human immunodeficiency virus infection? *Gynecology and Oncology, 49*(2), 243–246.

St. Louis, M.E., Kamenga, M., Brown, C., et al. (1993). Risk for perinatal HIV-1 transmission according to maternal immunologic, virologic, and placental factors. *Journal of the American Medical Association, 269*(22), 2853–2859.

Staff (1992, September). Women with AIDS: What is cause of lower survival? *AIDS Alert,* 142–143.

Stein, Z.A. (1990). HIV prevention: The need for methods women can use. *American Journal of Public Health, 80,* 460–462.

Sutin, D.G., Rose, D.N., Mulvihill, M., et al. (1993). Survival of elderly patients with transfusion-related acquired immunodeficiency syndrome. *Journal of the American Geriatrics Society, 41*(3), 214–216.

Swanson, J.M. (1992). Genital herpes and prevention of HIV infection: The report of a study-in-progress. *Journal of the Association of Nurses in AIDS Care, 3*(3), 30–36.

Swanson, J.M. (Nov. 12-15, 1993). Reduced sexual health risks and increased psychosocial adaptations in young adults with genital herpes: Effects of a psychoeducational intervention. Paper presented at the 1993 scientific sessions of the ANA Council of Nurse Researchers, Washington, D.C.

Task Force on Nutrition Support in AIDS (1989). Guidelines for nutrition support in AIDS. *Nutrition, 5*(1), 39–46.

Temoshok, L., O'Leary, A., Jenkins, S.R. (June, 1990). Survival time in men with AIDS: Relationships with psychological coping and autonomic arousal. Presented at the 6th International Conference on AIDS, San Francisco, CA.

Temple, M.T., Leigh, B.C., Schafer, J. (1993). Unsafe sexual behavior and alcohol use at the event level: Results of a national survey. *Journal of Acquired Immune Deficiency Syndromes, 6*(4), 393–404.

Tibaldi, C., Tovo, P.A., Ziarati, N., et al. (1993). Asymptomatic women at high risk of vertical HIV-1 transmission to their fetuses. *British Journal of Obstetrics and Gynecology, 100*(4), 334–337.

Tichy, A.M., Talashek, M.L. (1992). Older women: Sexually transmitted diseases and acquired immunodeficiency syndrome. *Nursing Clinics of North America, 27*(4), 937–949.

Turner, B.J., Denison, M., Eppes, S.C., et al. (1993). Survival experience of 789 children with the acquired immunodeficiency syndrome. *Pediatric Infection Disease Journal, 12*(4), 310–320.

Twu, S.J., Detels, R., Nelson, K., et al. (1993). Relationship of hepatitis B virus infection to human immunodeficiency virus type 1 infection. *The Journal of Infectious Diseases, 167,* 299–304.

Valdeserri, R.O., Moore, M., Gerber, A.R., et al. (1993). A study of clients returning for counseling after HIV testing: Implications for improving rates of return. *Public Health Reports, 108*(1), 12–18.

Vamvakas, E.H., Kaplan, H.S. (1993). Early transfusion and length of survival in acquired immunodeficiency syndrome: Experience with a population receiving medical care at a public hospital. *Transfusion, 33*(2), 111–118.

van den Hoek, A., van Haastrecht, H.J., Coutinho, R.A. (1990). Heterosexual behavior of intravenous drug users in Amsterdam: Implications for the AIDS epidemic. *AIDS, 4,* 449–453.

van der Graaf, M., Diepersloot, R. (1989). Sexual transmission of HIV: Routes, efficacy, cofactors, and prevention—a survey of the literature. *Infection, 17*(4), 210–215.

van Griensvan, G.J.P., Samuel, M.C., Winkelstein, W., Jr. (1993). The success and failure of condom use by homosexual men in San Francisco. *Journal of Acquired Immune Deficiency Syndromes, 6*(4), 430–431.

van Servellen, G., Padilla, G., Brecht, L., et al. (1993). The relationship of stressful life events, health status and stress-resistance resources in persons with AIDS. *Journal of the Association of Nurses in AIDS Care, 4*(1), 11–22.

Vlahov, D., Munoz, A., Anthony, J.G., et al. (1990). Association of drug injection patterns with antibody to human immunodeficiency virus type 1 among intravenous drug users in Baltimore. *Journal of Epidemiology, 132*, 847–856.

Waller, P.R., (Nov. 12-15, 1993). Predicting health promotion among gay men: Intervention implications. Paper presented at the 1993 scientific sessions of the ANA Council of Nurse Researchers, Washington, D.C.

Wara, D. (1993). Pediatric AIDS. II. Perinatal transmission and early diagnosis. *AIDS Clinical Care, 5*(3), 21–22.

Ward, B.J., Humphrey, J.H., Clement, L., et al. (1993). Vitamin A status in HIV infection. *Nutrition Research, 13*, 157–166.

Wardrop, K. (1993). A framework for health promotion—a framework for AIDS. *Canadian Journal of Public Health, 84*(suppl. 1), S9–S13.

Wayment, H.A., Newcomb, M.D., Hannemann, V.L. (1993). Female and male intravenous drug users not-in-treatment: Are they at differential risk for AIDS? *Sex Roles, 28*(1/2), 111–125.

Weatherburn, P., Davies, P.M., Hickson, F.C.I., et al. (1993). No connection between alcohol use and unsafe sex among gay and bisexual men. *AIDS, 7*(1), 115–119.

Winkelstein, W., Jr., Samuel, M.C., Hessol, N., et al. (1993). Factors associated with human immunodeficiency virus seroconversion in homosexual men in three San Francisco cohort studies, 1984–1989. *Journal of Acquired Immune Deficiency Syndromes, 6*(3), 303–312.

Wong, G. (1993). *HIV disease nutrition guidelines.* Chicago: Physicians Association for AIDS Care.

Worm, A.M., Gottschau, A. (1993). No change in incidence and prevalence of HIV among intravneous drug users in Copenhagen from 1985–1990. *Journal of Acquired Immune Deficiency Syndromes, 6*(7), 845–848.

Wright, J., Henry, S.B., Holzemer, W.L., et al. (1993). Evaluation of community-based nurse case management activities for symptomatic HIV/AIDS clients. *Journal of the Association of Nurses in AIDS Care, 4*(2), 37–47.

Yeung, S.C.H., Kazazi, F., Randle, C.G.M., et al. (1993). Patients infected with human immunodeficiency virus type 1 have low levels of virus in saliva even in the presence of periodontal disease. *Journal of Infectious Disease, 167*(4), 803–809.

Zhang, L.Q., MacKenzie, P., Cleland, A., et al. (1993). Selection for specific sequences in the external envelope protein of human immunodeficiency virus type 1 upon primary infection. *Journal of Virology, 67*(6), 3346–3356.

3 Pathophysiology of HIV-1, Clinical Course, and Treatment

Kathleen McMahon Casey

The human immunodeficiency virus type 1 (HIV-1), discovered in 1983, is considered to be the etiologic agent that causes AIDS. HIV-1 is a retrovirus belonging to the lentivirus family of viruses, which are generally known to result in neurotropic and lymphotropic viremic disease as a result of an indolent infection process characterized by a long clinical latency period (Libman, 1993). HIV-1 is one of five retroviruses, along with HIV type 2 (HIV-2) and human T-lymphotropic viruses types I, II, and IV (HTLV-I, HTLV-II, HTLV-IV), associated with human disease. Both HIV-1 and HIV-2 are considered to be the cause of AIDS. HTLV-I, which is predominantly found in southern Japan, the South Pacific, and parts of West Africa, as well as in the populations of African descent in the Western Hemisphere, is associated with chronic degenerative neurologic disease and is strongly implicated in T-cell leukemia/lymphoma (Madeleine et al., 1993; Selwyn & O'Connor, 1992). Although HTLV-II and HTLV-IV have been found in patients with leukemia and lymphoma, there is no evidence supporting the theory that these retroviruses are the direct cause of these illnesses (Gold, 1992). HIV-1 as a retrovirus has the ability to reverse the usual flow of genetic information with the enzyme reverse transcriptase, using viral RNA as a template for making DNA (Nash & Said, 1992).

Although both HIV-1 and HIV-2 are considered to be the etiologic agents of AIDS, the global distribution is markedly different (De Cock et al., 1993). Whereas HIV-1 is recognized as having spread worldwide, HIV-2 has been found predominantly in heterosexual populations in West Africa. De Cock and colleagues (1993) attributed the differences in the global spread of HIV-1 and HIV-2 to differences in transmissibility and duration of infectiousness. By 1991, there were only 18 reported cases of HIV-2 in the United States, and all were associated with immigration from, or travel to, West Africa (O'Brien et al., 1991). Sentinel surveillance studies conducted in cities in the United States where West African immigrants often settle have detected very few cases of HIV-2 disease (Onorato et al., 1993).

IMMUNOPATHOGENESIS

Life Cycle of HIV-1

Retroviruses are found in nearly all animal species. Infection can occur through sexual activities, through exposure to blood, and perinatally. The life cycle of HIV-1 includes the following components: (1) attachment of the virus to the host cell, (2) uncoating, followed by reverse transcription, (3) integration of newly synthesized DNA into the host cell DNA, with transcription and translation of the viral genetic message into viral protein (structural, regulatory, and functional), and (4) assembly, with release of virus out of the host cell (Gold, 1992; Grady, 1992). Researchers in basic science continue to work toward further understanding this life cycle process so that potential targets for antiviral therapy can be identified.

HIV-1 Structure and Genetic Composition

HIV-1 is composed of a central cylindrical core of diploid RNA surrounded by a spherical lipid envelope. Three structural components make up the viral genome and code for essential protein components. These genes are found on terminal repeat segments. The first, pol, is responsible for both the DNA polymerase and endonuclease that are located in the viral core. The second, gag, codes for p24, which is also found in the viral core and surrounds the viral RNA. It also codes for other core proteins such as p17, p9, and p7. Currently, p24 is measurable in patients' serum, and this test serves as a marker for viral replication. The third gene, called env, produces two glycoproteins that are part of the viral envelope and appear to be important in the recognition and attachment of HIV-1 to its CD4$^+$ lymphocyte target cell (Libman, 1993). HIV-1 also possesses genes that code for proteins that have important regulatory functions for the virus. Examples include tat (transactivator), rev (regulator of expression of virion proteins), nef (negative factor), vif (virion infectivity factor), vpu (required for efficient viral budding), and vpr (a weak activator of transcription) (Libman, 1993).

Mechanism of Infection

HIV-1 has specific tropism for CD4-positive cells, which include lymphocytes, monocytes, and macrophages. One infected T-lymphocyte expressing surface gp120 may bind to other CD4$^+$ cells (CD4 is the receptor for HIV-1 on T lymphocytes), forming a syncytium with up to 50 cells (Nash & Said, 1992). The pathophysiology of HIV-1 relates to this ability to infect human cells that possess CD4 membrane receptors. Clinically apparent disease with its immunodeficiency syndrome is a direct result of depletion of CD4$^+$ lymphocytes and infection of macrophages and monocytes. Other cell types, including epithelial gut cells, uterine cervical cells, and Langerhans cells of the skin, have also been identified as harboring HIV-1 infection (Libman, 1993).

Through the mechanism of binding site capability, HIV-1 fuses with the target cell's membrane, enters the host cell's cytoplasm, sheds its envelope coat, and releases its contents. Reverse transcription then occurs, creating viral DNA that exists in free form or

becomes integrated into the cellular DNA as a provirus. Infected cells can remain dormant. Cofactors may be important to their activation. Once activated, the gene products modulate viral progenesis with synthesizing of viral proteins. From these proteins, new virions are assembled that burst from the infected cell and circulate to a new receptor site (CD4) on another target cell. Although some types of host infected cells die with the budding forth of a new virion, macrophages and monocytes survive and therefore carry virus in their travels through the lymphoid and blood systems. This serves to protect the virus and enhance the opportunity for further infections to occur, leading to a compromised immune response. The functions of the macrophage and monocyte are compromised as well, leading to further immunosuppression. The virus gains access to the central nervous system via these infected macrophages, which cross the blood-brain barrier and cause damage (Libman, 1993).

Pathogenesis

CD4$^+$ helper T lymphocytes are the regulating cells within the immune system. These cells interact with monocytes, macrophages, cytotoxic T cells, natural killer cells, and B cells. Interactions between cells during HIV-1 infection can result in laboratory abnormalities, including (1) normal or decreased white blood cell counts, (2) decreasing lymphocyte values (total number and percentage of lymphocytes including CD4$^+$ cells), (3) dramatic changes in the CD4$^+$/CD8$^+$ ratio, (4) decreased CD4$^+$ function tests, (5) absent or decreased skin test reactivity (anergy), and (6) increased immunoglobulin levels (Grady & Vogel, 1993). Additionally, enhanced release of monokines, such as interleukin-2 (IL-2), tumor necrosis factor, and cachectin may explain the chronic fevers and wasting associated with HIV-1 disease. Involvement of alveolar macrophages may explain the high incidence of pulmonary infection seen in patients with AIDS (Nash & Said, 1992).

There is greater viral activity than had been previously appreciated in the lymphoid tissue during the clinically latent period (Tenner-Racz et al., 1993). Once virus is introduced into the body, it swiftly is disseminated via the bloodstream and the lymphoid organs are heavily seeded with virus (Pantaleo et al., 1993a). The follicular dendritic cells of bone marrow origin are instrumental in presenting virus to the CD4[+] cells. During this early period, the lymphoid system exerts control. The immune response by its tissues contain infection. It is only years later, after this protective system begins to wane, that virus is detectable in the blood by the usual method of p24 antigen detection. This recent discovery gives insight into the continuous active viral replication and destruction of the lymphoid microenvironment. It has led to discussions of the justification of earliest possible treatment and of the possibility of suppressing this early, vigorous, and harmful immune response with agents such as cyclosporine and Il-2 (Fauci, 1993a).

Newer concepts of HIV-1 pathogenesis are emerging. Previously it was identified that various HIV strains can be described as either rapid or slow, high or low, or syncytium inducing or not syncytium inducing. This distinction is important because these biologic features can determine tissue tropism (whether the virus goes to the bowel or brain) and the inherent ability to destroy the immune system. Levy (1993) proposed that as disease progresses the HIV-1 strains become more cytopathic, destroying CD4[+] cells very rapidly. Additionally, the author found that noncytopathic HIV-1 strains (e.g., HIV-1 SF162) that grow well in macrophages but do not kill CD4[+] lymphocytes in culture actually lead to a faster depletion of CD4[+] cells than do highly cytopathic strains (e.g., HIV-1 SF33). These data suggest that a relatively noncytopathic strain compromises the function of CD4[+] cells and produces a gradual but persistent loss of these cells with time by means other than direct cell killing.

The role of HIV-1 in the pathogenesis of AIDS continues to be discussed. Some scientists have stated that HIV-1 is probably a necessary but insufficient cause of AIDS (Duesberg, 1989; Staff, 1991; Wright, 1990). The principal hypothesis that is being investigated is the comorbid existence of other infectious agents that may play an active role in the pathogenesis of AIDS, with a focus on several species of mycoplasma. Although the exact pathogenic role of mycoplasma infection in the presence of HIV-1 is yet to be determined, it is believed that a synergistic, cytocidal effect on CD4[+] T cells may enhance the HIV-1 disease process (Lemaitre et al., 1992; Montagnier & Blanchard, 1993; Wang et al., 1992).

Factors Determining Disease Progression

Virus burden, the virulence of the infecting strain, race, sex, and age are factors that may determine the rate of progression (Gold, 1992). Susceptibility of the host may depend on a number of factors including genetic predisposition, the presence of the human leukocyte antigen specificity HLA-DR5, the size of the inoculum, and the route of exposure (Nash & Said, 1992). The host's immune status at the time of exposure may play a role. This status includes the effects of malnutrition and of chronic infections with viruses such as cytomegalovirus, Epstein-Barr virus, and the hepatitis viruses (Nash & Said, 1992). The role of cofactors in initial infection and viral replication continues to be studied.

Survival

Considerable attention has been directed toward the topic of increasing both survival rates and long-term survival in persons with HIV-1/AIDS. Tu and colleagues (1993) studied the survival differences and trends in patients with AIDS (after the diagnosis of AIDS) in the United States and found that injection drug users (IDUs) had a relatively shorter survival time than non-IDUs. After the diagnosis of *Pneumocystis carinii* pneumonia (PCP), non-IDUs survived approximately 15 months and IDUs survived approximately 12 months. After controlling for IDU status, the authors did not find much difference in survival among men who had sex with men, male heterosexuals, and female heterosexuals. Mortality rates since 1987 and after the diagnosis of PCP decreased by 28% for IDUs and 40% for non-IDUs. It has been hypothesized that increases in survival time are attributable to the introduction of antiretroviral therapy and PCP prophylaxis (Osmond et al., 1994; Lundgren et al., 1994). Long-term survival after an AIDS diagnosis—that is, more than 8 years—is considered rare (Tu et al., 1993).

In contrast, overall survival time with HIV-1 infection has been noted up to 15 years (Levy, 1993). According to Levy (1993) long-term survivors are described as "individuals living more than 8 years with HIV-1 infection (some now more than 15 years), show no symptoms of infection, and several have normal CD4$^+$ cell counts" (p. 1401). The author identifies the following characteristics found in long-term survivors: (1) low infectious virus load, (2) infection with a less cytopathic HIV-1 strain, (3) no enhancing antibodies, (4) TH1 cell response greater than TH2 cell response (TH1 and TH2 cells are subsets of CD4$^+$ cells), and (5) strong CD8$^+$ cell antiviral response. These features indicate that therapy to maintain TH1 cell responses and/or CD8$^+$ cell anti-HIV activity could achieve long-term survival in all HIV-infected individuals (Levy, 1993).

SEROLOGIC TESTING

Laboratory Tests to Detect HIV-1 Infection

The diagnosis of HIV-1 infection depends on the presence of virus or a serologic response to the virus (Gold, 1992). Testing serum for antibodies to HIV-1 is currently the most cost-effective and accurate method of screening for infection. Since March 1985, when the first serologic assay became approved as a response to the need to protect the nation's blood supply and blood product recipients, more methods have become available (Table 3–1). Of all available testing methods, the enzyme-linked immunosorbent assay, with Western blot confirmation, continues to be the testing method most widely used worldwide.

Table 3–1. HIV-1 Tests

 I. Virus culture techniques
    A. Peripheral blood mononuclear cells coculture for HIV-1
    B. Quantitative cell counts
    C. Quantitative plasma culture
 II. HIV antibody tests
    A. Enzyme-linked immunosorbent assay (ELISA)
    B. Western blot
    C. Radioimmunoprecipitation assay (RIPA)
    D. Indirect immunofluorescence assay (IFA)
 III. Antigen detection assays
    A. HIV p24 antigen test
    B. Acidified p24 antigen procedure
    C. Polyethylene glycol precipitation
 IV. Viral genome amplification tests
    A. Polymerase chain reaction (PCR) techniques
    B. Quantitative PCR

Data from Saag, M.S. (1992). AIDS testing: Now and in the future. In M.A. Sande & P.A. Volberding (Eds), *The Medical Management of AIDS* (3rd ed) (pp. 33–53). Philadelphia: W.B. Saunders.

Surrogate Markers

Blood tests with predictive ability are commonly used (Grady & Vogel, 1993). The most clinically useful tool to monitor progression of HIV-1 infection is the CD4$^+$ cell count. Many clinical trials have used this value as an entry criterion or end point for evaluation of a prospective therapy's relative worth. Despite its advantages and common usage, clinicians do not use a single result when making treatment decisions but rely on serial CD4$^+$ counts, because significant variations in laboratory reports can occur. There are diurnal variations, changes with acute viral infection or stress, and variations caused by nonstandardized laboratory methods such as the use of different machines, different antibodies, and different processing and shipping times.

Other surrogate markers are useful but in many instances are not readily available. The p24 antigen is easy to measure in serum, is easy to standardize, decreases with anti-HIV-1 therapies, and correlates with disease progression, but it is rarely detectable in symptom-free patients and those with high

CD4⁺ cell counts and does not predict clinical response to a therapy. Likewise, plasma viremia is quantifiable, is common in symptom-free patients, and correlates well with disease stage, but it is expensive and rarely available and its natural history is unclear. According to Saag (1992), from a clinical perspective the CD4⁺ cell count (and percentage) is the most readily available and widely used surrogate marker, although the use of p24 antigenemia and the determination of neopterin and beta-2 microglobulin levels are proving to be useful.

CLINICAL COURSE OF DISEASE

Pantaleo and colleagues (1993b) described the typical course of HIV-1 infection as (1) primary or initial infection with HIV-1, (2) followed by a prolonged period of clinical latency (median, 10 years) during which the individual is usually free of symptoms, (3) followed by clinically apparent disease with constitutional symptoms, and finally (4) the development of AIDS-indicator disease(s). The hallmarks of HIV-1 disease progression are the functional abnormalities and quantitative depletion of CD4⁺ T lymphocytes resulting in profound immunosuppression.

Primary Infection

In approximately 50% to 70% of individuals, primary infection develops within 3 to 6 weeks after the initial infection with HIV-1 (Tindall & Cooper, 1991). Contrary to popular belief, primary HIV-1 infection often produces clinically symptomatic illness, often compared to mononucleosis, and may be severe enough to warrant medical attention. Table 3–2 lists signs and symptoms that may accompany primary HIV-1 infection.

The initial burst of HIV-1 activity can produce an intense viremia that can result in drastically reduced CD4⁺ cell counts. A healthy, uninfected individual usually has 800 to 1,200 CD4⁺ cells per cubic millimeter (mm³) of blood. This initial attack can, in some instances, reduce the CD4⁺ cell count to less than 100 mm³ (or less than 7.5% of total lymphocytes), leaving the patient vulnerable to

Table 3–2. Clinical Manifestations of Primary HIV-1 Infection

I. Constitutional: fever, nausea, vomiting, fatigue, lymphadenopathy
II. Neurologic: headache, encephalopathy, neuropathy
III. Oral: thrush, pharyngitis
IV. Skin: rash, ulcers
V. Gastrointestinal tract: diarrhea, hepatomegaly
VI. Musculoskeletal: myalgia, arthralgia
VII. Hematopoietic: thrombocytopenia, leukopenia

Data from Clark, S.J., Saag, M.S., Don Decker, W., et al. (1991). High titers of cytopathic virus in plasma of patients with symptomatic primary HIV-1 infection. *New England Journal of Medicine, 324*(14), 954–960. Darr, E.S., Moudgil, T., Meyer, R.D., Ho, D.D. (1991). Transient high levels of viremia in patients with primary human immunodeficiency virus type 1 infection. *New England Journal of Medicine, 324*(14), 961–964.

the development of an opportunistic infection. In fact, primary infection may produce illness requiring hospitalization, and both esophageal candidiasis and PCP have been reported to occur in patients with primary HIV-1 infection (Tindall & Cooper, 1991; Vento et al., 1993).

Clinical Latency

In most cases primary infection is followed by a period of clinical latency in which the patient is virtually free of symptoms. This has recently been referred to as a clinically dichotomous situation because the levels of detectable viremia are low but the viral load and replication in lymphoid tissue are high (Pantaleo et al., 1993a). Although the clinical presentation of the infected individual usually does not include symptoms, this is a microbiologically active phase of disease characterized by a continual decline in the CD4⁺ cell counts and progression of illness. As HIV-1 disease progresses, clinically apparent disease manifests as symptomatic conditions that are associated with HIV-1 infection or are indicative of a defect in cell-mediated immunity or complicated by HIV-1 infection (Centers for Disease Control [CDC], 1992). HIV-1 often

Table 3–3. Conditions Presumed to be Caused By HIV-1 Infection

AFFECTED AREAS	MANIFESTATIONS
Central nervous system (Brew, 1992; Clark et al., 1991; Daar et al., 1991)	Aseptic meningitis and cranial neuropathy during primary infection; cognitive impairment; neuropathy
Eye (Farrell et al., 1988; Heinemann, 1992)	Uveitis
Heart (Andersen et al., 1988; Grody et al., 1990; Scully et al., 1992)	Cardiomyopathy; myocarditis
Lungs (Travis et al., 1992; White & Zaman, 1992)	Lymphocytic or nonspecific pneumonitis
Gastrointestinal tract (Kotler, 1993; Tanowitz et al., 1992)	Enteropathy; malabsorption
Kidneys (Nochy et al., 1993; Rao, 1991)	Glomerulosclerosis; glomerulonephritis; nephritis; nephrotic syndrome; uremia
Gynecologic system (Allen, 1990; Pomerantz et al. 1988)	Cervicitis
Musculoskeletal system (Buskila & Gladman, 1990)	Reiter's syndrome; psoriatic arthritis; arthritis; arthralgias
Skin (Berger, 1990)	Xerosis; seborrheic dermatitis; psoriasis; atopic dermatitis; hypersensitivity reactions
Hematologic system (Doweiko, 1993)	Anemia; granulocytopenia; thrombocytopenia
Endocrine system (Grinspoon & Bilezikian, 1992)	Adrenalitis; thyroiditis; lipid metabolism dysfunction; gonadal (male) dysfunction; pancreatitis

has a direct cytopathic effect on various parts of the body besides $CD4^+$ cells (Table 3–3). Symptomatic conditions, often seen in the later stages of illness, before the diagnosis of AIDS, are listed in Table 3–4.

Although there are direct correlations between deterioration in the immune system and clinically apparent disease, there are exceptions. Kaposi's sarcoma can occur at any point in the course of HIV-1 disease, as can progressive generalized lymphadenopathy and neurologic disease (Pantaleo et al., 1993b).

AIDS Indicator Diseases

The current surveillance case definition for AIDS in the United States contains 26 clinical conditions listed in Table 3–5 (CDC, 1987; 1992). Munoz and associates (1993) recently reviewed trends in the incidence of initial and secondary AIDS-defining illnesses from 1985 to 1991 among 2,627 homosexual

Table 3–4. Symptomatic Conditions in HIV-1–infected Adults and Adolescents

Bacillary angiomatosis
Candidiasis, oropharyngeal (thrush)
Candidiasis, vulvovaginal; persistent, frequent, or poorly responsive to therapy
Cervical dysplasia (moderate or severe/cervical carcinoma in situ)
Constitutional symptoms, such as fever (temperature $\geq 38.5°$ C) or diarrhea >1 month in duration
Hairy leukoplakia, oral
Herpes zoster (shingles) involving at least two distinct episodes or more than one dermatome
Idiopathic thrombocytopenia purpura
Listeriosis
Pelvic inflammatory disease, particularly if complicated by tuboovarian abscess
Peripheral neuropathy

Data from Centers for Disease Control and Prevention (1992). 1993 Revised classification system for HIV infection and expanded surveillance case definition for AIDS among adolescents and adults. *Morbidity and Mortality Weekly Report*, *41*(RR-17), 1–19.

Table 3–5. The 1993 AIDS Surveillance Case Definition

Candidiasis of bronchi, trachea, or lungs

Candidiasis, esophageal

Cervical cancer, invasive

CD4$^+$ T-lymphocyte count <200 mm^3 (<14%)

Coccidioidomycosis, disseminated or extrapulmonary

Cryptococcosis, extrapulmonary

Cryptosporidiosis, chronic intestinal (>1 month in duration)

Cytomegalovirus disease (other than liver, spleen, or nodes)

Cytomegalovirus retinitis (with loss of vision)

Encephalopathy, HIV related

Herpes simplex: chronic ulcer(s) (>1 month in duration) or bronchitis, pneumonitis, or esophagitis

Histoplasmosis, disseminated or extrapulmonary

Isosporiasis, chronic intestinal (>1 month in duration)

Kaposi's sarcoma

Lymphoma, Burkitt's (or equivalent term)

Lymphoma, immunoblastic (or equivalent term)

Lymphoma, primary, of brain

Mycobacterium avium complex or *Mycobacterium kansasii*, disseminated or extrapulmonary

Mycobacterium tuberculosis, any site (pulmonary or extrapulmonary)

Mycobacterium, other species or unidentified species, disseminated or extrapulmonary

Pneumocystis carinii pneumonia

Pneumonia, recurrent

Progressive multifocal leukoencephalopathy

Salmonella septicemia, recurrent

Toxoplasmosis of brain

Wasting syndrome caused by HIV

Data from Centers for Disease Control (1992). 1993 Revised classification system for HIV infection and expanded surveillance case definition for AIDS among adolescents and adults. *Morbidity and Mortality Weekly Report, 41*(RR-17), 1–19.

men with HIV-1 infection who were participating in the Multicenter AIDS Cohort Study. They reported significant decreases in the incidence of PCP as an initial AIDS-defining diagnosis that was expected in light of the proven efficacy of PCP prophylaxis. In contrast, they reported significant bacterial, fungal, and protozoal increases in other opportunistic infections, as well as increases in cytomegalovirus and herpes simplex virus infections and increases in Kaposi's sarcoma, lymphoma, and neurologic disease. It should be noted that this volunteer sample did not represent the general homosexual population and did not include IDUs and women. The authors concluded that research was needed to develop and test new strategies for curtailing or delaying the onset of opportunistic infections.

Caution should be exercised when reviewing the literature regarding the incidence of HIV-1–related comorbidity. Nahlen and colleagues (1993) conducted a retrospective review of 26,251 AIDS cases reported to the CDC with HIV-1 wasting as the only AIDS-indicator condition. Findings revealed that the wasting syndrome was more commonly reported as the only AIDS diagnosis among women, IDUs, sex partners of IDUs, black persons, and Hispanic persons. Comorbidity among AIDS-indicator diseases most strongly associated with wasting were isosporiasis, pulmonary candidiasis, esophageal candidiasis, HIV-1 encephalopathy, chronic mucocutaneous herpes simplex, and coccidioidomycosis. Careful analysis of data revealed that HIV-1 wasting varied most notably by geographic location, and the authors concluded that the differences noted were most probably related to differences in diagnostic and reporting practices and/or access to medical care: "In some geographic areas, a high prevalence of HIV-1 wasting syndrome may indicate lack of access to diagnostic procedures for opportunistic infections and malignancies in HIV-1 infected individuals" (Nahlen et al., 1993, p. 1187). The differences may also be related to treatment of these patients by less experienced clinicians (Stone et al., 1992).

Pillay and colleagues (1993) note that many symptoms in HIV-1–infected patients are never fully explored nor explained and that retrospective postmortem analysis of autopsy records documents a high prevalence of undiagnosed antemortem opportunistic infections. In many instances these infections were treatable.

Certain AIDS-related neoplasms have been associated with infectious agents. The role of Epstein-Barr virus in the lymphomagenesis of HIV-1–associated non-Hodgkin's lymphoma is currently under study (Mac-

Mahon et al., 1991; Samoszuk et al., 1993; Shibata et al., 1993). Kaposi's sarcoma research includes the possibility of an unidentified infectious pathogen that is spread sexually or through blood or that acts perinatally as a cofactor, as well as coinfection with human papillomavirus (HPV), acting as an oncogenic factor (Beral et al., 1990; Beral, 1991; Bowden et al., 1991; Friedman-Kien et al., 1990; Huang et al., 1992; Orlow et al., 1993). Coinfection with HPV and HIV-1 in women is believed to be associated with cervical carcinoma (CDC, 1990; Feingold et al., 1990; Franco, 1991; Keenlyside et al., 1993).

CLASSIFICATION SYSTEM FOR HIV-1/AIDS

Effective Jan. 1, 1993, the CDC implemented a new classification system for HIV-1 infection/AIDS in adults and adolescents (≥13 year of age) (CDC, 1992). The new system completely replaces the 1986 classification system and retains the 23 clinical conditions in the AIDS surveillance case definition published in 1987 (CDC, 1986; 1987). Three major changes occurred with the 1993 revision: (1) instead of simply identifying clinical categories, CD4+ T-lymphocyte counts were also emphasized; (2) a CD4+ T-cell count of less than 200 mm³ (<14% of total lymphocytes) was added to the AIDS case surveillance definition; and (3) three new AIDS-indicator

diseases were added, including pulmonary tuberculosis, recurrent pneumonia, and invasive cervical cancer (CDC, 1992). Table 3–6 presents the 1993 revised classification system.

CD4+ T-lymphocyte Categories

The three CD4+ T-lymphocyte categories are defined as follows: category 1, ≥500 cells mm³; category 2, 200 to 499 cells/mm³; category 3, <200 cells mm³. These categories correspond to CD4+ T-lymphocyte counts per microliter of blood and guide clinical and therapeutic actions in the management of HIV-1–infected adolescents and adults. The revised HIV-1 classification system also allows for the use of the percentage of CD4+ T-cells (see Table 5–5).

HIV-1–infected persons should be classified on the basis of existing guidelines for the medical management of HIV-1–infected persons. Thus the lowest accurate, but not necessarily the most recent, CD4+ T-lymphocyte count should be used for classification purposes.

Clinical Category A. Category A includes adults or adolescents who exhibit asymptomatic infection, persistent generalized lymphadenopathy, (PGL) or acute (primary) HIV-1 infection with accompanying illness or history of acute HIV-1 infection.

Table 3–6. 1993 Revised Classification System for HIV Infection and Expanded AIDS Surveillance Case Definition for Adolescents and Adults

CD4+ T CELL CATEGORIES	CLINICAL CATEGORIES*		
	(A) ASYMPTOMATIC, ACUTE (PRIMARY) HIV OR PGL	(B) SYMPTOMATIC, NOT (A) OR (C) CONDITIONS	(C) AIDS-INDICATOR CONDITIONS
(1) ≥500 mm³	A1	B1	C1
(2) 200-499 mm³	A2	B2	C2
(3) <200 mm³ AIDS-indicator T-cell count	A3	B3	C3

Data from Centers for Disease Control (1992). 1993 Revised classification system for HIV infection and expanded surveillance case definition for AIDS among adolescents and adults. *Morbidity and Mortality Weekly Report. 41*(RR-17), 1–19.
*See text for explanation.

Clinical Category B. Category B consists of symptomatic conditions in an HIV-1–infected adolescent or adult that are not included among conditions listed in clinical category C and that meet at least one of the following criteria: (a) the conditions are attributed to HIV-1 infection or are indicative of a defect in cell-mediated immunity, or (b) the conditions are considered by physicians to have a clinical course or to require management that is complicated by HIV-1 infection. Examples of conditions in clinical category B include, but are not limited to, those listed in Table 3–4.

For classification purposes, category B conditions take precedence over those in category A. For example, someone previously treated for oral or persistent vaginal candidiasis (and who has not developed a category C disease) but who is now free of symptoms should be classified in clinical category B.

Clinical Category C. Category C includes the clinical conditions listed in the AIDS surveillance case definition (see Table 3–5). For classification purposes, once a category C condition has occurred, the person will remain in category C. Chapter 4 discusses the AIDS-indicator diseases listed in category C.

The Revised System

According to the CDC (1992) the revised 1993 classification will provide uniform and simple criteria for categorizing conditions among adolescents and adults with HIV-1 infection and should facilitate efforts to evaluate current and future health care and referral needs for persons with HIV-1 infection. The addition of a measure of severe immunosuppression, as defined by a CD4$^+$ T-lymphocyte count of <200 mm^3 or a CD4$^+$ percentage of <14%, reflects the standard of immunologic monitoring for HIV-1–infected persons and will enable AIDS surveillance data to more accurately represent those who are recognized as having immunosuppression, who are in greatest need of close medical follow-up, and who are at greatest risk of having the full spectrum of severe HIV-1–related morbidity. The addition of three clinical conditions—pulmonary tuberculosis, recurrent pneumonia, and invasive cervical cancer—to AIDS surveillance criteria reflects the documented or potential importance of these diseases in the HIV epidemic. Two of these conditions (pulmonary tuberculosis and cervical cancer) are preventable if appropriate screening tests are linked with proper follow-up. The third, recurrent pneumonia, reflects the importance of pulmonary infections not included in the 1987 definition as leading causes of HIV-1–related morbidity and death. Successful implementation of expanded surveillance criteria will require the extension of existing safeguards to protect the security and confidentiality of AIDS surveillance information.

The European Center for the Epidemiological Monitoring of AIDS, representing 15 European surveillance systems, voted unanimously not to adopt the 1993 CDC AIDS case surveillance definition (Park, 1992). Although the group acknowledged the importance of monitoring CD4$^+$ cell counts, they provided five reasons for opposition to the new definition: (1) access to medical and social services varied between Europe and the United States (implying that services in Europe are available and are not contingent on entitlement criteria as in the United States); (2) the 1987 definition was sufficient and most people with AIDS who seek medical care would be reported; (3) those with access to CD4$^+$ cell counts would be overrepresented (as opposed to countries with limited access to this type of test) and distort the picture of the epidemic; (4) the new system would label HIV-1–infected, symptom-free people with the diagnosis of AIDS, which carries significant psychologic and social consequences; and (5) CD4$^+$ cell counting is not well standardized (Park, 1993). The group concluded that additional surveillance systems should be explored and considered.

DRUG THERAPY FOR HIV-1 INFECTION

The principal areas of drug research targeted specifically against HIV-1 disease (as opposed to AIDS-indicator diseases) include antiretroviral therapy, the use of vaccines, and immunomodulator therapy. Thus far the most quantifiable success in HIV-1 therapy has been achieved in antiretroviral therapy.

Antiretroviral Therapy

Preventing the spread of disease within the HIV-1–infected individual has been achieved with nucleoside analog reverse transcriptase inhibitors. Nucleoside analogs, such as zidovudine (azidothymidine [AZT]), didanosine (dideoxyinosine [ddI]), zalcitabine (dideoxycytidine [ddC]), and stavudine (didehydrodideoxythymidine [d4T]), can prevent the spread of HIV-1 to new cells but do not interfere with viral replication in infected cells (Hirsch & D'Aquila, 1993). Appendix III contains a discussion of these agents.

In 1993 the National Institutes of Health, U.S. Public Health Service, convened a panel of experts to make recommendations on the prescription of antiretroviral therapy for adult HIV-1–infected patients (Sande et al., 1993). Table 3–7 summarizes the clinical scenarios encountered in a primary care setting for HIV-1–infected individuals and the panel's recommendations regarding antiretroviral therapy. Stavudine was still under evaluation and is not included in the recommendations.

Until 1993, recommendations for initiating antiretroviral therapy were based on CD4$^+$ cell counts; when the counts fell to less than 500 mm^3, zidovudine therapy was initiated. Then, in April 1993, a preliminary report of the Concorde trial was published with results that had a major impact on the prescription of antiretroviral therapy for HIV-1 disease. The Concorde trial, a collaborative study of 1,762 HIV-1–infected individuals by researchers in Ireland, France, and the United Kingdom, took place between 1988 and 1991. The purpose of the study was to determine the benefits of initiating early (in symptom-free individuals) versus late (in individuals with symptoms) zidovudine therapy. The study results revealed no significant benefit from early versus late zidovudine therapy in terms of survival or disease progression (Aboulker & Swart, 1993, Concorde Coordinating Committee). However, several other studies have shown that early therapy for symptom-free individuals provided some benefit (Sande et al., 1993).

Aside from challenging the parochial approach to prescribing antiretroviral therapy on the basis of CD4$^+$ cell counts, the Concorde study forced clinicians to recognize the limitations of medical technology. According to Merle Sande:

> We also recognize that no 'average patient' exists. Some patients will do better, and others, worse, than the clinical studies would predict. Doctors and patients should work as a team to design a treatment strategy that is both clinically sound and appropriate for each individual patient's needs, priorities and circumstances of daily life (National Institute of Allergy and Infectious Diseases, 1993, June 25, p. 2).

Clinicians began to recognize that the plan of care for the HIV-1–infected individual, including the initiation of antiretroviral therapy, belonged to the client and that informed choices were ultimately to be made by the patient along with the clinician.

Adding to the dilemma in antiretroviral therapy was the known fact that after a time nucleoside analog therapy resulted in a resistant mutation in HIV-1 reverse transcriptase (St. Clair et al., 1991). According to Chang (1993), after approximately 1 year of monotherapy (single agent) with a nucleoside analog, suppression of HIV-1 activity becomes incomplete and results in diminished drug efficacy. Waning drug efficacy and drug resistance, along with dose-limiting toxic effects, have led researchers into clinical trials of combination antiretroviral therapy (Ragni, 1993). According to Ragni (1993):

> the rationale for this approach is that by combining drugs that are synergistic and non-cross-resistant, have no overlapping toxicity, and have different mechanisms of action, it may be possible to reduce drug toxicity, improve efficacy, delay or prevent resistance, and promote long-term survival (p. 15).

Combination therapy is prescribed in one of two ways. The first method is concurrent administration of two drugs, and the second

Table 3–7. Clinical Examples of Treatment Decisions Regarding the Use of Nucleoside Analogs

CLINICAL PRESENTATION	RECOMMENDATIONS
Asymptomatic; CD4$^+$ cell counts >500 mm^3 (>29%)	No therapy; continue clinical and immunologic monitoring every 6 months; consider initiating therapy if CD4$^+$ cell counts are rapidly declining
Asymptomatic; CD4$^+$ cell counts are between 200 mm^3 and 500 mm^3 (14%-28%) and no prior antiretroviral therapy	Two options: (1) initiate zidovudine therapy (at 600 mg/day in divided doses); (2) continue to monitor and do not start therapy
Symptomatic; CD4$^+$ cell counts between 200 mm^3 and 500 mm^3 (14%-28%) and no prior antiretroviral therapy	Initiate therapy (zidovudine, 600 mg/day in divided doses)
Asymptomatic; CD4$^+$ cell counts less than 200 mm^3 (<14%) and no prior antiretroviral therapy	Initiate therapy (zidovudine, 600 mg/day in divided doses)
Symptomatic; CD4$^+$ cell counts less than 200 mm^3 (14%) and no prior antiretroviral therapy	Initiate therapy (zidovudine, 600 mg/day in divided doses)
Tolerating zidovudine therapy and clinically stable; CD4$^+$ cell counts >300 mm^3 with no recent trend toward decline	Continue zidovudine therapy
Tolerating zidovudine therapy and clinically stable BUT showing evidence of further immunodeficiency (e.g., CD4$^+$ cell counts less than 300 mm^3)	Two options: (1) continue zidovudine therapy and monitor closely, or (2) switch to didanosine
Failing to respond to zidovudine and symptomatic; CD4$^+$ cell counts between 50 and 500 mm^3	Initiate alternative antiretroviral therapy
Failing zidovudine therapy; CD4$^+$ counts less than 50 mm^3	Initiate alternative antiretroviral therapy
Intolerant to zidovudine and asymptomatic; CD4$^+$ cell counts greater than 500 mm^3	Discontinue antiretroviral therapy and continue clinical observation and laboratory monitoring every 6 months
Intolerant to zidovudine and stable asymptomatic; CD4$^+$ cell counts between 50 and 500 mm^3	Initiate alternative antiretroviral monotherapy
Intolerant to zidovudine; CD4$^+$ cell counts are less than 50 mm^3	Two options: (1) initiate alternative antiretroviral therapy, or (2) discontinue all antiretroviral therapy (The reasons for this consideration are [1] toxic effects of antiretroviral agents are high in advanced disease, and [2] the quality of life may improve if therapy stops, but HIV titers may escalate.)

Data from Sande, M.A., Carpenter, C.C., Cobbs, G., et al. (1993). Antiretroviral therapy for adult HIV-infected patients. Recommendations from a state-of-the art conference. *Journal of the American Medical Association, 270*(21), 2583–2589.

method is to alternate the drugs on a weekly or monthly basis. Currently the combination of nucleoside analogs include zidovudine plus either didanosine or zalcitabine (Ragni, 1993).

Richman and colleagues (1994) reported the results of a study (N = 15) of combination therapy with zidovudine and zalcitabine to ascertain whether the simultaneous dosing would delay zidovudine resistance. On the basis of their findings, the authors concluded that zalcitabine did not appreciably delay the emergence of zidovudine resistance, and diminished susceptibility to zalcitabine was not observed with combination therapy in patients with advanced disease.

Combination therapy consisting of three drugs, zidovudine, didanosine, and nevirapine (a nonnucleoside inhibitor), are also under way (National Institute of Allergy and Infectious Diseases, 1993, May 21). Other nonnucleoside agents under investigation include reverse transcriptase inhibitors, such as nevirapine and pyridione, and agents known as protease inhibitors. Currently none of the three types of agents (nucleoside analogs, nonnucleoside agents, or protease inhibitors) have proved to be totally effective (Chang, 1993).

The implications of HIV-1 mutation and drug resistance extend beyond the complex issues of treatment failure for HIV-1–infected individuals. Erice and colleagues (1993) reported on an individual with primary HIV-1 infection caused by a virus already resistant to zidovudine. The newly infected person had a history of having sex with an HIV-1–infected individual who was receiving zidovudine therapy. It is probable that additional cases of newly HIV-1–infected, nucleoside analog–resistant patients will pose an additional challenge to the problems of antiretroviral therapy.

Immunomodulators

Immunopharmacology involves the study of the regulation of the immune system by pharmacologic agents and the development of methods to selectively modify immune function to treat human disease (Hadden & Smith, 1992). Immunosuppressive therapies with cytotoxic agents (radiation, glucocorticosteroids, cytotoxic drugs, antibody therapy, apheresis) are in common use. This area is undergoing intensive research. Cytokines were approved by the U.S. Food and Drug Administration beginning in 1989 (Wujcik, 1993), and clinical trials of interferons, interleukins, tumor necrosis factor, monoclonal antibodies, and other factors are in progress.

Considerable controversy has surrounded the efficacy of low-dose oral human interferon alfa (IFN-alfa) therapy. Koech and associates (1990), in a 6-week study of 40 patients with HIV disease treated with oral IFN-alfa, reported substantial increases in CD4$^+$ cell counts and a loss of HIV seropositivity (seroconversion) in eight patients. The Koech report was part of a multicenter clinical trial conducted in five African countries under the auspices of the African Regional Office of the World Health Organization (WHO). WHO (1990), in a review of the total sample (N = 108), found that none of the patients (including those reported by Dr. Koech and associates) had become seronegative during the trial. Data interpretation was considered difficult because of the uncontrolled nature of the trial (lack of standardization of enrollees and concomitant therapies). WHO (1990) concluded that no new conclusions could be drawn regarding the possible role of orally administered IFN-alfa in the treatment of HIV disease.

The National Institute of Allergy and Infectious Diseases (1992, April), in a review of orally administered IFN-alfa as therapy for HIV-1, concluded that "to date, the preponderance of data collected on CD4$^+$ cell counts and HIV disease serostatus from other low-dose oral IFN-alpha clinical trials appear to be in distinct contrast to the results reported by Dr. Koech et al. [1990] in their original publication and in follow-up reports" (p. 3). Continuing trials of orally administered IFN-alfa have not demonstrated significant changes in CD4$^+$ cell counts (American Foundation for AIDS Research, 1993).

Vaccines

Vaccine development against HIV-1 has three principal uses: (1) prevention of disease, (2) therapeutic effects for immunomodulation, and (3) perinatal vaccination. By 1993, more than 20 HIV-1–related vaccines had been entered into clinical trials to assess their safety (Fast & Walker, 1993). The majority of vaccines are composed of recombinant proteins such as the envelope glycoprotein precursor gp160 or the glycoprotein gp120.

Trials of preventive vaccines have been conducted in Europe, Japan, and the United

States, and although the results are yet to be completed, the vaccines appear to be safe and the trials have shown encouraging immunologic responses (Fast & Walker, 1993). The most prevalent misconception is that when used for preventive purposes, in uninfected volunteers, the vaccines will cause HIV disease/AIDS. According to Fast and Walker (1993), "the vaccines tested to date in seronegative volunteers can't cause HIV infection, although they would conceivably predispose to infection if the volunteer engages in high-risk activities" (p. S149).

Therapeutic vaccines for HIV-1–infected individuals are primarily for immunomodulating purposes to augment the immune responses of individuals already infected with HIV-1. The results thus far have demonstrated that the use of vaccines for HIV-1–infected individuals is safe and has resulted in an increase in both humoral and cellular immune responses to HIV-1 (stabilizing HIV-1 activity) and in increased CD4$^+$ cell counts (Cooney, 1993).

Perinatal vaccine trials of HIV-1–infected women began in the later half of 1993. Safety and efficacy data are not available. If these studies prove successful, further trials will be undertaken to determine whether HIV-1 vaccination will not only prevent vertical transmission of HIV-1 from mother to fetus but also slow or stop the decline in immune function that may occur in the mother during pregnancy (Fast & Walker, 1993).

Vaccine development is faced with both social and biologic obstacles. HIV-1 mutates rapidly, producing antigenetically heterogeneous virus, even within a single HIV-1–infected person; currently there are at least five known subgroups of HIV-1 (Letvin, 1993). Theoretically an effective vaccine should provide protection against all genetically diverse strains of HIV (Mascolini, 1993). "To date, however, protection has been achieved only against a virus identical in sequence to that used for immunization" (Letvin, 1993, p. 1404). Additional issues of costs, ethics in the clinical trial process, accessibility of the vaccines, duration of effectiveness, and spectrum of immunity provided by vaccines remain to be addressed.

CD4$^+$ T-LYMPHOCYTOPENIA WITHOUT HIV INFECTION

In July 1992, at the Eighth International Conference on AIDS, held in Amsterdam, the Netherlands, an ad hoc presentation was conducted to discuss cases of immunodeficiency that were not caused by either HIV-1 or HIV-2 (Moore & Ho, 1992). On Aug. 14, 1992, the CDC hosted a meeting at which more than 270 scientists exchanged information on this newly identified syndrome, which is now referred to as idiopathic CD4$^+$ T-lymphocytopenia (ICL). In an editorial, Fauci (1993b) summarized the characteristics of ICL: (1) it is rare; (2) it is not caused by HIV-1, HIV-2, HTLV-I, or HTLV-II; (3) it is heterogeneous; (4) it is clinically, epidemiologically, and immunologically different from HIV infection; and (5) it does not appear to be caused by a transmissible agent. ICL is diagnosed in patients if they have two or more CD4$^+$ T cell counts less than 300 mm^3 (less than 20% of the total number of lymphocytes), no evidence of HIV-1 or HIV-2 infection, and no defined cause or therapy that accounts for the low levels of CD4$^+$ T-cells (National Institute of Allergy and Infectious Diseases, 1993, Feb. 10).

Although ICL, as a clinical syndrome, was only recently identified, cases of opportunistic infections without a known cause of immunosuppression have been reported for decades, and it was not until the mid-1980s and the HIV epidemic that CD4$^+$ cell counts were routinely available (Fauci, 1993b). Confounding the issue is that many of the diseases seen in patients with ICL and AIDS are the same, such as PCP, toxoplasmosis, histoplasmosis, cryptococcosis, extrapulmonary infection with *Mycobacterium avium* complex, cytomegalovirus retinitis, and lymphoma (Duncan et al., 1993; Ho et al., 1993; Smith et al., 1993; Spira et al., 1993). Additionally, approximately one third of the patients with ICL have been noted to have some risk factor for HIV infection, although they are not infected with HIV (Fauci, 1993b). Soriano and associates (1992) summarized the etiologic factors associated with a low CD4$^+$ T-cell count (other than HIV-1 or HIV-2), including (1) infections caused by viruses (e.g., hepatitis, herpes, bacteria (e.g., tuberculosis), fungi (e.g., histoplasmosis, cryptococcosis), protozoa (e.g., leishmaniasis); (2) malnutrition; (3) drugs (e.g., corticosteroids); (4) congenital immune disorders; (5) autoimmune disorders; (6) proliferative disorders (e.g., thymoma); (7) common variable immunodeficiency; (8) pregnancy; and (9) old age.

NURSING RESEARCH RELATED TO HIV-RELATED DIAGNOSES

Summary of Research

Swanson and associates (1993a) identified the problem of AIDS dementia complex as a serious threat to the safety and quality of life of persons with HIV-1 disease. The authors noted in a review of the literature that although AIDS dementia complex may be readily apparent and diagnosed in later stages of disease, cognitive impairment may be manifested in earlier stages of HIV-1 infection and may interfere with understanding health teaching and with occupational performance.

Swanson and colleagues (1993b) conducted a descriptive correlational study of 141 persons with HIV-1 disease at the various stages of HIV-1 infection to characterize the cognitive and affective disorders present in this population across the spectrum of illness. Significant differences were found in the various stages of HIV-1 disease and performance on neuropsychologic testing declined with disease progression. In a discussion of the clinical implications for nursing, the authors noted that teaching methods needed to be adapted to match the cognitive limitations of HIV-1–infected individuals.

Research Needed

Additional considerations for nursing research include the following:

1. Prevention of certain opportunistic infections (e.g., salmonellosis and cryptosporidiosis)
2. Early identification of the signs, symptoms, and related variables (e.g., financial resources, lack of cooking facilities) associated with HIV wasting
3. Identification of which neuropsychologic tests are most useful in detecting cognitive impairment
4. Identification of community resources and access to gynecologic services for Papanicolaou smears to prevent invasive cervical cancer
5. Identification of nonpharmacologic methods to control and prevent secondary, recurrent opportunistic infections (e.g., *Candida* vulvovaginitis and thrush)

SUMMARY

The spectrum of HIV-1 disease is complex and highly variable among the populations and the individuals who are infected. The study of the pathogenesis of HIV-1 disease is evolving, and clinicians and scientists are continuously unmasking the actual effects of HIV-1 on the human body. Although significant amounts of knowledge have been gained since the identification of AIDS in 1981, definitive strategies to prevent infection with vaccines, or to treat the disease with antiretroviral agents or immunomodulators, are still forthcoming. The mutagenic properties of HIV-1 pose an impressive challenge to researchers as we approach the twenty-first century.

REFERENCES

Aboulker, J.P., Swart, A.M. (1993). Preliminary analysis of the Concorde trial. Concorde Coordinating Committee [letter]. *Lancet, 341*(8855), 1276.

Allen, M.H. (1990). Primary care of women infected with the human immunodeficiency virus. *Obstetrics and Gynecology Clinics of North America, 17*(3), 557–583.

American Foundation for AIDS Research (1993). Treatment for HIV infection. *AIDS/HIV Treatment Directory, 6*(3), 5–44.

Andersen, D.W., Virmani, R., Reilly, J.M., et al. (1988). Prevalent myocarditis at necropsy in the acquired immunodeficiency syndrome. *Journal of the American College of Cardiology, 11*(4), 792–793.

Beral, V. (1991). Epidemiology of Kaposi's sarcoma. *Cancer Surveys, 10*, 5–22.

Beral, V., Peterman, T.A., Berkelman, R.L., et al. (1990). Kaposi's sarcoma among persons with AIDS: A sexually transmitted infection? *Lancet, 335*(8682), 123–128.

Berger, T.G. (1990). Dermatologic manifestations of HIV infection. In P.T. Cohen, M.A. Sande, & P.A. Volberding (Eds.), *The AIDS knowledge base* (pp. 531.1–531.25). Waltham, MA: The Medical Publishing Group.

Bowden, F.J., McPhee, D.A., Deacon, N.J., et al. (1991). Antibodies to gp41 and nef in an otherwise HIV-negative homosexual man with Kaposi's sarcoma. *Lancet, 337*(8753), 1313–1314.

Brew, B.J. (1992). Central and peripheral nervous system abnormalities. *Medical Clinics of North America, 76*(1), 63–81.

Buskila, D., Gladman, D. (1990). Musculoskeletal manifestations of infection with human immunodeficiency virus. *Reviews of Infectious Diseases, 12*(2), 223–235.

Centers for Disease Control (1986). Classification system for human T-lymphotropic virus type III/lymphadenopathy associated virus infections. *Morbidity and Mortality Weekly Report, 35*(20), 334–339.

Centers for Disease Control (1987). Revision of the CDC surveillance case definition for acquired immunodeficiency syndrome. *Morbidity and Mortality Weekly Report, 36*(1S) 3S–15S.

Centers for Disease Control (1990). Risk for cervical disease in HIV infected women. *Morbidity and Mortality Weekly Report, 39*(47), 846–849.

Centers for Disease Control and Prevention (1992). 1993 Revised classification system for HIV infection and expanded surveillance case definition for AIDS among adolescents and adults. *Morbidity and Mortality Weekly Report, 41*(RR-17), 1–19.

Chang, H.E. (1993). Current understanding of HIV drug resistance. *PAACNOTES, 5*(9), 363–369, 395.

Clark, S.J., Saag, M.S., Don Decker, W., et al. (1991). High titers of cytopathic virus in plasma of patients with symptomatic primary HIV-1 infection. *New England Journal of Medicine, 324*(14), 954–960.

Concorde Coordinating Committee (1994). Concorde: MRC/ANRS randomized double-blind controlled trial of immediate and deferred zidovudine in symptom-free HIV infection. *Lancet, 343*(8902), 871–881.

Cooney, E.L. (1993). Therapeutic vaccines for HIV. *AIDS Clinical Care, 6*(8), 60–63.

Daar, E.S., Moudgil, T., Meyer, R.D., Ho, D.D. (1991). Transient high levels of viremia in patients with primary human immunodeficiency virus type 1 infection. *New England Journal of Medicine, 324*(14), 961–964.

De Cock, K.M., Adjorlolo, G., Ekpini, E., et al. (1993). Epidemiology and transmission of HIV-2: Why there is no HIV-2 pandemic. *Journal of the American Medical Association, 270*(17), 2083–2086.

Doweiko, J.P. (1993). Hematologic aspects of HIV infection. *AIDS, 7*(6), 753–757.

Duesberg, P.H. (1989). Human immunodeficiency virus and acquired immunodeficiency syndrome: Correlation but not causation. *Proceedings of the National Academy of Sciences, 86*(3), 755–764.

Duncan, R.A., von Reyn, C.F., Alliegro, G.M., et al. (1993). Idiopathic CD4⁺ T-lymphocytopenia: Four patients with opportunistic infections and no evidence of HIV infection. *New England Journal of Medicine, 328*(6), 393–398.

Erice, A., Mayers, D.L., Strike, D.G., et al. (1993). Brief report: Primary infection with zidovudine-resistant human immunodeficiency virus type-1. *New England Journal of Medicine, 328*(16), 1192–1193.

Farrell, P.L., Heinemann, M.H., Roberts, C.W., et al. (1988). Response of human immunodeficiency virus–associated uveitis to zidovudine. *American Journal of Ophthalmology, 106*(1), 7–10.

Fast, P.E., Walker, M.C. (1993). Human trials of experimental AIDS vaccines. *AIDS, 7*(suppl 1), 147–159.

Fauci, A.S. (1993a). Immunopathogenic mechanisms of HIV infection: Implications for therapeutic strategies [abstract No. PS-01-3]. *International Conference on AIDS, 9*(1), 9.

Fauci, A.S. (1993b). CD4⁺ T-lymphocytopenia without HIV infection: No lights, no camera, just facts [editorial]. *New England Journal of Medicine, 328*(6), 429–431.

Feingold, A.R., Vermund, S.H., Burk, R.D., et al. (1990). Cervical cytologic abnormalities and papillomavirus in immunodeficiency virus. *Journal of Acquired Immune Deficiency Syndromes, 3*(9), 896–903.

Franco, E.L. (1991). Viral etiology of cervical cancer: A critique of the evidence. *Review of Infectious Diseases, 13*(6), 1195–1206.

Friedman-Kien, A.E., Saltzman, B.R., Cas, Y.Z., et al. (1990). Kaposi's sarcoma in HIV-negative homosexual men [letter]. *Lancet, 335*(8682), 168–169.

Gold, J.W. (1992). HIV-1 infection: Diagnosis and management. *Medical Clinics of North America, 76*(1), 1–18.

Grady, C. (1992). HIV disease: Pathogenesis and treatment. In J.H. Flaskerud & P.J. Ungvarski (Eds.), *HIV/AIDS: A guide to nursing care* (2nd ed) (pp. 30–53). Philadelphia: W.B. Saunders.

Grady, C., Vogel, S. (1993). Laboratory methods for diagnosing and monitoring HIV infection. *Journal of the Association of Nurses in AIDS Care, 4*(2), 11–21.

Grinspoon, S.K., Bilezikian, J.P. (1992). HIV disease and the endocrine system. *New England Journal of Medicine, 327*(19), 1360–1364.

Grody, W.W., Cheng, L., Lewis, W. (1990). Infection of the heart caused by the human immunodeficiency virus. *American Journal of Cardiology, 66*(2), 203–206.

Hadden, J.W., Smith, D.L. (1992). Immunopharmacology, immunomodulation, and immunotherapy. *Journal of the American Medical Association, 268*(20), 2964–2969.

Heinemann, M.H. (1992). Ophthalmic problems. *Medical Clinics of North America, 76*(1), 83–97.

Hirsch, M.S., D'Aquila, R.T. (1993). Therapy for human immunodeficiency virus infection. *New England Journal of Medicine, 328*(23), 1686–1695.

Ho, D.D., Cao, Y., Zhu, T., et al. (1993). Idiopathic CD4⁺ T-lymphocytopenia immunodeficiency without evidence of HIV infection. *New England Journal of Medicine, 328*(6), 380–385.

Huang, Y.Q., Li, J.J., Rush, M.G., et al. (1992). HPV-16–related DNA sequences in Kaposi's sarcoma. *Lancet, 339*(8792), 515–518.

Keenlyside, R.A., Johnson, A.M., Mabey, C.W. (1993). The epidemiology of HIV-1 infection and AIDS in women. *AIDS, 7*(suppl 1), S83–S90.

Koech, D.K., Obel, A.O., Minowada, J., et al. (1990). Low dose oral alfa-interferon therapy for patients seropositive for human immunodeficiency virus type-1 (HIV-1). *Journal of Molecular Biotherapy, 2*(2), 91–95.

Kotler, D.P. (1993). Effect of malnutrition in the progression of AIDS. *HIV: Advances in Research and Therapy, 3*(3), 17–23.

Lemaitre, M., Henin, Y., Destouesse, F., et al. (1992). Role of mycoplasma infection in the cytopathic effect induced by human immunodeficiency virus type-1 in infected cell lines. *Infection and Immunity, 60*(3), 742–748.

Letvin, N.L. (1993). Vaccines against human immunodeficiency virus: Progress and prospects. *New England Journal of Medicine, 329*(19), 1400–2405.

Levy, J.A. (1992). Pathogenesis of HIV infection: Controversies and hypothesis. *HIV: Advances in Research and Therapy, 2*(2), 3–9.

Levy, J.A. (1993). HIV pathogenesis and long-term survival. *AIDS, 7*(11), 1401–1410.

Libman, H. (1993). Pathogenesis, natural history and classification of HIV infection. *Primary Care, 19*(1), 1–17.

Lundgren, J., Phillips, A., Pedersen, C., et al. (1994). Comparison of long–term prognosis of patients with AIDS treated and not treated with zidovudine. *Journal of the American Medical Association, 271*(14), 1088–1092.

MacMahon, E.M., Glass, J.D., Hayward, S.D., et al. (1991). Epstein-Barr virus related primary central nervous system lymphoma. *Lancet, 338*(8773), 969–973.

Madeleine, M.M., Wiktor, S.Z., Goedert, J.J., et al. (1993). HTLV-I and HTLV-II worldwide distribution: Reanalysis of 4,832 immunoblot results. *International Journal of Cancer, 54*(2), 255–260.

Mascolini, M. (1993). Cautious forecasts for HIV vaccines. *PAACNOTES, 5*(8), 322–326.

Montagnier, L., Blanchard, A. (1993). Mycoplasmas as cofactor in infection due to human immunodeficiency virus. *Clinical Infectious Diseases, 17*(suppl 1), S309–S315.

Moore, J.P., Ho, D.D. (1992). HIV-negative AIDS. *Lancet, 340*(8817), 475.

Munoz, A., Schrager, L.K., Bacellar, H., et al. (1993). Trends in the incidence of outcomes defining acquired immunodeficiency syndrome (AIDS) in the multicenter AIDS cohort study: 1985–1991. *American Journal of Epidemiology, 134*(4), 423–438.

Nahlen, B.L., Chu, S.Y., Nwanyanwu, O.C., et al. (1993). HIV wasting syndrome in the United States. *AIDS, 7*(2), 183–188.

Nash, G., Said, J.W. (Eds.) (1992). *Pathology of AIDS and HIV infection.* Philadelphia, PA: W.B. Saunders.

National Institute of Allergy and Infectious Diseases (1992, April). Low-dose oral interferon alpha as a therapy for human immunodeficiency virus infection (HIV-1): Completed and ongoing clinical trials [interim report]. In *Backgrounder.* Bethesda, MD: National Institutes of Health.

National Institute of Allergy and Infectious Diseases (1993, Feb. 10). Feature of CD4⁺ T cell suppression identified among people without HIV infection. *News from NIAID.* Bethesda, MD: National Institutes of Health.

National Institute of Allergy and Infectious Diseases (1993, May 21). NIAID opens combination therapy trial for HIV infection. *News from NIAID,* 1–3. Bethesda, MD: National Institutes of Health.

National Institute of Allergy and Infectious Diseases (1993, June 25). HIV therapy guidelines issued. *News from NIAID,* 1–4. Bethesda, MD: National Institutes of Health.

Nochy, D., Glotz, D., Dosquet, P., et al. (1993). Renal disease associated with HIV infection: A multicentric study of 60 patients from Paris hospitals. *Nephrology, Dialysis, Transplantation, 8*(1), 11–19.

O'Brien, T.R., Polm, C., Schable, C.A., et al. (1991). HIV-2 infection in an American. *AIDS, 5*(1), 85–88.

Onorato, I.M., O'Brien, T.R., Schable, C.A., et al. (1993). Sentinel surveillance for HIV-2 infection in high-risk U.S. populations. *American Journal of Public Health, 83*(4), 515–519.

Orlow, S.J., Cooper, D., Petrea, S., et al. (1993). AIDS-associated Kaposi's sarcoma in Romanian children. *Journal of the American Academy of Dermatology, 28*(3), 449–453.

Osmond, D., Charlebois, E., Lang, W., et al. (1994). Changes in AIDS survival time in two San Francisco cohorts of homosexual men, 1983 to 1993. *Journal of the American Medical Association, 271*(14), 1083–1087.

Panteleo, G., Graziosi, C., Demarest, J.F., et al. (1993a). HIV infection is active and progressive in lymphoid tissue during the clinically latent stage of disease. *Nature, 364*(6435), 291–292.

Pantaleo, G., Graziosi, C., Fauci, A.S. (1993b). The immunopathogenesis of human immunodeficiency virus infection. *New England Journal of Medicine, 328*(5), 327–335.

Park, R.A. (1992). European AIDS definition [news]. *Lancet, 339*(8794), 671.

Pillay, D., Lipman, M.C., Lee, C.A., et al. (1993). A clinicopathological audit of opportunistic viral infections in HIV-infected patients. *AIDS, 7*(7), 969–974.

Pomerantz, R.J., delaMonte, S.M., Donegan, S.P., et al. (1988). Human immunodeficiency virus (HIV) infection of the uterine cervix. *Annals of Internal Medicine, 108*(3), 321–327.

Ragni, M. (1993). Combination therapy with nucleoside analogues. *HIV: Advances in Research and Therapy, 3*(2), 15–22.

Rao, T.K. (1991). Human immunodeficiency virus (HIV) associated nephropathy. *Annual Review of Medicine, 42,* 391–401.

Richman, D.D., Meng, T., Spector, S.A., et al. (1994). Resistance to AZT and ddC during combination therapy in patients with advanced infection with human immunodeficiency virus. *Journal of Acquired Immune Deficiency Syndrome, 7*(2), 135–138.

Saag, M.S. (1992). AIDS testing: Now and in the future. In M.A. Sande & P.A. Volberding (Eds), *The medical management of AIDS* (3rd ed) (pp. 33–53). Philadelphia: W.B. Saunders.

Samoszuk, M., Nguyen, V., Shadon, F., Ramzi, E. (1993). Incidence of Epstein-Barr virus in AIDS-related lymphoma specimens. *Journal of Acquired Immune Deficiency Syndromes, 6*(8), 913–918.

Sande, M.A., Carpenter, C.C., Cobbs, G., et al. (1993). Antiretroviral therapy for adult HIV-infected patients: Recommendations from a state-of-the art conference. *Journal of the American Medical Association, 270*(21), 2583–2589.

Scully, R.E., Mark, E.J., McNeely, W.F., McNeely, B. (1992). Case records of the Massachusetts General Hospital: Case 44-1992. *New England Journal of Medicine, 327*(19), 1370–1376.

Selwyn, P.A., O'Connor, P.G. (1992). Diagnosis and treatment of substance users in HIV infection. *Primary Care, 19*(1), 119–156.

Shibata, D., Weiss, L.M., Hernandez, A.M., et al. (1993). Epstein-Barr virus–associated non-Hodgkin's lymphoma in patients infected with the human immunodeficiency virus. *Blood, 81*(8), 2102–2109.

Smith, D.K., Neal, J.J., Holmberg, S.D., et al. (1993). Unexplained opportunistic infections and CD4⁺ T-lymphocytopenia without HIV infection: An investigation of cases in the United States. *New England Journal of Medicine, 328*(6), 373–379.

Soriano, V., Hewlett, I., Heredia, A., et al. (1992). Idiopathic CD4⁺ T-lymphocytopenia [letter]. *Lancet, 340*(8819), 607–608.

Spira, T.J., Jones, B.J., Nicholson, J.K., et al. (1993). Idiopathic CD4⁺ T-lymphocytopenia: An analysis of five patients with unexplained opportunistic infections. *New England Journal of Medicine, 328*(6), 386–392.

Staff (1991). Mycoplasma and AIDS: What connection? [editorial]. *Lancet, 337*(8732), 20–22.

Stall, R., Wiley, J. (1988). A comparison of alcohol and drug use patterns of homosexual and heterosexual men: The San Francisco Men's Health Study. *Drug and Alcohol Dependence, 22*(1–2).

St. Clair, M.H., Martin, J.L., Tudor-Williams, G., et al. (1991). Resistance to ddI and sensitivity to AZT induced by a mutation in HIV-1 reverse transcriptase. *Science, 253*(5027), 1557–1559.

Stone, V.E., Seage, G.R., Hertz, T., et al. (1992). The relation between hospital experience and mortality for patients with AIDS. *Journal of the American Medical Association, 268*(19), 2655–2666.

Swanson, B., Cronin-Stubbs, D., Zeller, J.M., et al. (1993a). Characterizing the neuropsychological functioning of persons with human immunodeficiency virus (HIV) infection. Part I. Acquired immune deficiency syndrome complex: A review. *Archives of Psychiatric Nursing, 7*(2), 74–81.

Swanson, B., Cronin-Stubbs, D., Zeller, J.M., et al. (1993b). Characterizing the neuropsychological functioning of persons with human immunodeficiency virus (HIV) infection. Part II. Neuropsychological functioning of persons at different stages of HIV infection. *Archives of Psychiatric Nursing, 7*(2), 82–98.

Tanowitz, H.B., Simon, D., Wittner, M. (1992). Gastrointestinal manifestations. *Medical Clinics of North America, 76*(1), 45–62.

Tenner-Racz, K., Racz, P., Embretson, J., et al. (1993). Covert infection of CD4⁺ lymphocytes and macrophages in lymph nodes of HIV-infection demonstrated by a polymerase chain reaction (PCR) in situ method [abstract No. WS-A12-1]. *International Conference on AIDS, 9*(1), 28.

Tindall, B., Cooper, D.A. (1991). Primary infection: Host responses and intervention strategies. *AIDS, 5*(1), 1–14.

Travis, W.D., Fox, C.H., Devaney, K.O., et al. (1992). Lymphoid pneumonitis in 50 adult patients infected with the human immunodeficiency virus: lymphocytic interstitial pneumonitis versus nonspecific interstitial pneumonitis. *Human Pathology, 23*(5), 529–541.

Tu, X.M., Meng, X., Pagnano, M. (1993). Survival differences and trends in patients with AIDS in the United States. *Journal of Acquired Immune Deficiency Syndromes, 6*(10), 1150–1156.

Vento, S., DiPerri, G., Garofano, T., et al. (1993). *Pneumocystis carinii* pneumonia during primary HIV-1 infection. *Lancet, 342*(8862), 24–25.

Wang, R.Y., Shih, J.W., Grandinetti, T., et al. (1992). High frequency of antibodies to *Mycoplasma penetrans* in HIV-infected patients. *Lancet, 340*(8831), 1312–1316.

White, D.A., Zaman, M.K. (1992). Pulmonary disease. *Medical Clinics of North America, 76*(1), 19–44.

World Health Organization (1990, Sept. 14). *Multicenter clinical trial organized by the African Regional Office (AFRO) of the World Health Organization* [press release]. Geneva, Switzerland: World Health Organization.

Wright, K. (1990). Mycoplasma in AIDS spotlight. *Science, 248*(4956), 682–683.

Wujcik, D. (1993). An odyssey into biologic therapy. *Oncology Nursing Forum, 20*(6), 879–887.

Clinical Manifestations of AIDS in Adults

Peter J. Ungvarski and Jo Anne Staats

In the early years of the AIDS epidemic, the disease was considered essentially fatal and emphasis was placed on compassionate, low-technology care aimed at improving the quality rather than the length of life (Cotton, 1989). What many hoped to be a limited endemic among homosexual men in large urban centers in the United States has rapidly evolved into a major pandemic resulting in widespread human suffering and devastating socioeconomic consequences. (Lange & Tapper, 1993).

Although significant progress has been achieved in the development of antiretroviral agents to treat HIV infection and the prevention and treatment of AIDS-indicator diseases, new challenges and complications have emerged. The widespread and prolonged use of antibiotics has led to the emergence of drug-resistant organisms. Although probably anticipated by some, one of the more startling reports was that of a patient with infection caused by HIV already resistant to zidovudine (Erice et al., 1993.) Additionally, the resurgence of tuberculosis, including disease caused by drug-resistant strains of *Mycobacterium tuberculosis*, poses major public health problems beyond the limitations of the HIV-infected population.

In 1992 the Centers for Disease Control and Prevention (CDC) revised the classification system for diagnosing HIV infection and AIDS in adolescents and adults (see Chapter 3, Table 3–5). The expanded AIDS surveillance case definition resulted in a 204% increase in the number of AIDS cases reported in the first quarter of 1993, compared with the same period in 1992 (CDC, 1993a). In a report from the HIV clinic at Johns Hopkins Hospital, Baltimore, Md., the 1993 revision of the case definition of AIDS resulted in a doubling of prevalent AIDS cases, particularly among women and injection drug users (Chaisson et al., 1993). Patients meeting the 1993 cases definition were also more likely to be less immunocompromised and more likely to be free of symptoms.

As the number of individuals with a diagnosis of AIDS increases dramatically, so does the demand for health care services provided by knowledgeable health care professionals. Several studies have reported a significant increase in the mortality rate for AIDS patients at hospitals with less AIDS experience (Bennett et al., 1992; Stone et al., 1992; Turner & Ball, 1992). These data underscore the need for improved education of health care professionals responsible for caring for people with HIV disease/AIDS.

Nurses caring for people infected with HIV and those with a diagnosis of AIDS face a challenging situation. They must possess a clinical knowledge base of not only HIV disease but also the AIDS-related opportunistic infections and malignancies. These diseases are strange sounding, to say the least, and new to the nurse, who often feels powerless when confronted with providing nursing care in the presence of the unknown (Ungvarski, 1987). For example, how many nurses have cared for a person with progressive multifocal leukoencephalopathy? Therefore the goal of this chapter is to provide the information nurses require to provide care competently and comfortably for persons living with AIDS.

To understand the clinical aspects of the development of opportunistic infections (OIs) associated with AIDS, the reader should be aware of some generalizations that can be made about their presence in an HIV-infected person (Glatt et al., 1988; National Institute of Allergy and Infectious Diseases, 1990). OIs are caused by a diverse spectrum of pathogens, many of which are ubiquitous in nature and rarely cause disease in healthy hosts (persons with an intact immune system). In many cases, these infections are a secondary appearance of a previous primary infection or, in other words, a reactivation of a previously acquired pathogen. The OIs associated with AIDS are rarely curable and at best can be controlled during an acute episode; they require long-term suppressive therapy to prevent recurrence. Complicating the issue of long-term therapy is the resistance to standard therapies that some opportunistic pathogens develop.

A single OI is rare in persons with AIDS; concurrent or consecutive infections with different organisms are common. Infections associated with HIV, because of the coexisting immunodeficiency, are often severe and difficult to treat and require extended initial treatment regimens. Furthermore, many infections become disseminated, with a high density of organisms in the affected tissues. By understanding the epidemiologic characteristics of certain pathogens, the nurse can provide clients with information on preventing some of these infections. Progress in research on AIDS-related OIs has led to the development of prophylactic measures to prevent some infections.

Finally, clinicians responsible for caring for persons with advanced HIV disease and AIDS should be aware that the underlying immunodeficiency often results in an impaired inflammatory response, and the manifestations of infection such as fever may be greatly muted (Hibberd & Rubin, 1991). Therefore careful attention must be given to the subjective clinical findings presented by the patient, since an infectious process may be developing while the patient is afebrile.

The two most common neoplasms seen in HIV disease continue to be Kaposi's sarcoma and non-Hodgkin's lymphoma (Milliken & Boyle, 1993). In women, the predominant neoplastic disease associated with the diagnosis of AIDS is invasive cervical cancer, which is preventable by the proper recognition and treatment of cervical dysplasia (CDC, 1992a; 1992b). Other malignancies being more frequently reported in association with HIV infection are anogenital carcinoma and Hodgkin's disease (Milliken & Boyle, 1993).

The 1993 revised case definition for AIDS expanded the surveillance diagnostic categories by including a CD4$^+$ T-cell count of less than 200 mm^3 as an AIDS indicator condition, as well as by adding pulmonary tuberculosis, recurrent pneumonia, and invasive cervical cancer (CDC, 1992a). The following material focuses on the most frequently diagnosed AIDS-indicator diseases and their clinical manifestations, to assist the nurse in the development of the client's care plan. Appendix III contains a list of drugs frequently prescribed for AIDS-related conditions and the common side effects.

CANDIDIASIS

Epidemiology

Candida organisms are yeasts—that is, fungi—that exist predominantly in unicellular forms (Edwards, 1990). *Candida albicans* is ubiquitous in nature and has been found in soil, food, inanimate objects, and hospital environments. *Candida* is a commensal organism that can be found on teeth, gingiva, and skin, and in the oropharynx, vagina, and large intestine.

The majority of infections caused by *Candida* are endogenous and related to interruption of normal defense mechanisms. Examples of increased infection potential include naturally occurring immunocompromise with diseases such as diabetes mellitus; damaged or diseased skin or mucous membranes; invasive procedures such as insertion of intravenous cannulating devices and infusion-pressure monitoring equipment, Foley catheters, and drainage systems; immunosuppression related to therapy with drugs such as steroids, antibiotics; and acquired immunosuppression caused by disease such as HIV (Chernoff & Sande, 1990a; Edwards, 1990).

Human-to-human transmission is possible. Examples include congenital transmission in babies, in whom thrush develops after vaginal delivery; development of balanitis in uncircumcised men who do not wear a condom during intercourse with a woman who has *Candida* vaginitis; and nosocomial spread in hospital settings (Edwards, 1990).

Infections caused by *Candida* species are estimated to occur, at some time in the course of HIV disease, in 75% to 90% of the cases (Daar & Meyer, 1992; Rolston, 1993). Oropharyngeal candidiasis is frequently the initial indicator of HIV infection and has been noted to occur, in some patients, at the time of seroconversion to HIV (Pedersen et al., 1989; Rolston, 1993).

Pathogenesis

The likelihood of mucosal *Candida* infection increases with progressive cellular immunodeficiency associated with HIV disease and is often associated with a decreased number of circulating CD4$^+$ lymphocytes (Chaisson & Volberding, 1990; Tindall et al., 1989). Most clinicians now believe that oral candidiasis is an accurate predictor of disease progression and of the development of other AIDS-related infections (Barone et al., 1990; Greenspan et al., 1988).

The frequent use of broad-spectrum antibiotics to treat infections associated with HIV disease suppresses normal bacterial flora and allows *Candida* to proliferate, especially in the gastrointestinal tract (Chernoff & Sande, 1990a; Edwards, 1990). Skin alterations caused by poor nutrition, dehydration, poor hygiene, or indwelling catheters can also provide a portal of entry for *Candida*.

Most *Candida* infections in persons with HIV are mucocutaneous, whereas other fungal infections are disseminated. Candidemia, or disseminated infection, is seen in persons with HIV who have neutropenia because of antineoplastic and/or antiviral therapy, as well as in those with central venous access lines (Daar & Meyer, 1992; Rolston, 1993).

Clinical Presentation

Clinical presentation depends on the site of infection. The clinical presentation of thrush is creamy, curdlike, yellowish patches surrounded by an erythematous base and found on the buccal mucosa and tongue sur-

faces. The patches can be wiped off, leaving an erythematous or even bleeding mucosal surface. An atrophic form, seen occasionally, appears as smooth red patches on the hard or soft palate, buccal mucosa, or dorsal surface of the tongue (Greenspan et al., 1988). Thrush can be accompanied by angular cheilitis, which produces erythema, cracks, fissures, and maceration at the corners of the mouth (Berger, 1990).

Another oral form of candidiasis is *Candida* leukoplakia, which appears as white lesions on the buccal mucosa, tongue, or hard palate and cannot be wiped off (Greenspan et al., 1988). This can be confused with hairy leukoplakia. Oral candidiasis can be superimposed on other oral lesions such as herpes simplex and can cause secondary infections. Pindborg (1994) considers the term "thrush" to be unscientific and suggests clinicians use the term "pseudomembranous candidiasis" to describe oral candidiasis seen in HIV-infected individuals (p. 68). The author also divides the condition into the erythematous stage (often seen in symptom-free patients), pseudomembranous (seen in patients with AIDS), chronic (which is rare and seen on the margins of the tongue), and angular cheilitis.

Complaints of dysphagia in the individuals with HIV disease are most commonly associated with *C. albicans* (Cello, 1992). Thrush and esophageal candidiasis are not necessarily present concurrently; therefore the absence of thrush does not preclude the possibility that an HIV-infected person may have *Candida* esophagitis (Chernoff & Sande, 1990a; Gould et al., 1988). Cello (1992) defined the dysphagia associated with *Candida* esophagitis as difficulty in swallowing, with a sensation of food sticking. Although pain on swallowing (odynophagia) and episodic retrosternal pain without swallowing may be present with the complaint of dysphagia, they are more commonly associated with ulcerations of the esophagus caused by herpesvirus or cytomegalovirus (Cello, 1992; Gould et al., 1988).

Intertrigo can occur at any site where the proximity of skin surfaces provides a warm, moist environment. This cutaneous form of candidiasis can involve the groin, axillary vault, or areas surrounding the breasts and appears as a vivid red, slightly eroded eruption with a wrinkled surface coated by a white membrane (Berger, 1990; Edwards, 1990). *Candida* can proliferate in urine-soaked diapers and adult incontinence garments and underpads, beneath occlusive and wet dressings and condom catheters, around draining stomas and fistulas, and anywhere the skin stays moist continuously (Cuzzell, 1990). Clients with cutaneous candidiasis usually complain of burning and itching.

Candida infection of the nails is usually manifested as paronychia (inflammation of the tissues surrounding the nails) but can also involve the nail itself (Berger, 1990; Edwards, 1990). In addition to the inflamed appearance, the patient complains of tenderness in the area. Frequent exposure to water is a significant predisposing factor in *Candida* nail infection.

Vulvovaginal candidiasis is frequently the initial manifestation of HIV disease. Characterized by intense pruritus of the vulva and a curdlike vaginal discharge, this infection usually results in an erythematous vagina and labia and may extend into the perineum. Chronic refractory vaginal candidiasis may be an initial symptom of HIV disease. Women with HIV disease and unexplained oral and vaginal candidiasis are at risk for other opportunistic infections (Rhoads et al., 1987).

Although rare, disseminated candidiasis almost always occurs late in the course of AIDS. Other sites of *Candida* infection in HIV disease that have been reported include the trachea, bronchi, lungs, heart, central nervous system (CNS), eyes, joints, and testes (Daar & Meyer, 1992).

Diagnosis

Definitive diagnosis of candidiasis is made by gross inspection by endoscopy or at autopsy, or by microscopy on a specimen of affected tissues. Diagnosis by culture is unreliable because the distinction between infection and colonization, in body sites where *Candida* is normally present, is not always clear. Isolation of *Candida* from blood may also be questionable in a patient with an indwelling intravenous catheter, since transient candidiasis is possible and often clears without treatment once the device is removed (Chernoff & Sande, 1990a).

Treatment

Oropharyngeal or oral candidiasis is treated with clotrimazole troches, nystatin suspension, ketoconazole, and fluconazole. Generally, clotrimazole and nystatin are used initially, and if there is no response, systemic treatment with ketoconazole or fluconazole may be instituted. Studies have shown fluconazole to be more effective than ketoconazole (De Wit et al., 1989; Laine, et al., 1992). However, early sustained use of fluconazole for thrush can lead to the development of drug-resistant strains of *Candida* and preclude future use (especially if cryptococcosis develops) (Torres, 1993). These drugs are also recommended for the treatment of esophageal candidiasis. Cutaneous candidiasis may respond to topically applied clotrimazole, miconazole, or ketoconazole or to systemically administered ketoconazole or fluconazole. Topically applied imidazole may be used to treat candidiasis of the nails, and itraconazole may also be effective for this condition (Torres, 1993). Vaginal candidiasis is treated with clotrimazole or miconazole creams, tablets, or vaginal suppositories, and orally administered ketoconazole or fluconazole is prescribed for nonresponsive vaginitis. Several studies are investigating the effectiveness of using fluconazole to prevent vaginal candidiasis (American Foundation for AIDS Research, 1993). Amphotericin B with or without flucytosine is used to treat disseminated *Candida* infection, and ketoconazole and fluconazole may be used to treat resistant candidiasis.

Considerations for Nursing

Candidiasis should be considered a sentinel disease, and its presence without a plausible explanation should alert nurses to take careful histories and explore the possibilities of HIV disease. Nurses should be aware that mucocutaneous candidiasis is rarely cured and often becomes chronic or recurrent; therefore continual assessment for its presence is warranted. Equally important is the need to assess the client during each contact for cutaneous manifestations of candidiasis, especially in genital and perianal regions and under skin folds.

Nursing measures directed at preventing severe *Candida* infections include establishing an effective, routine regimen of oral hygiene; keeping skin surfaces dry and exposed to air as much as possible; teaching the client how to detect early signs and symptoms of infection; meticulously taking precautions, such as use of gloves, hand-washing techniques, and extreme care when handling and manipulating intravenous therapy equipment; and evaluating carefully the risk/benefit ratio when using occlusive dressings. Hilton and associates (1992), in a study of women with recurrent *Candida* vaginitis (who were not HIV infected), found that daily ingestion of 8 ounces of yogurt containing *Lactobacillus acidophilus* decreased both the colonization and the infection. Anecdotal reports from clinicians caring for patients with HIV/AIDS have noted an overall decrease in *Candida* infections when *L. acidophilus* in yogurt or capsule form is consumed daily.

CERVICAL CANCER (INVASIVE)

Epidemiology

Women infected with HIV have a high incidence of cervical intraepithelial neoplasia (CIN), also referred to as cervical dysplasia, the lesions that are a precursor to carcinoma of the cervix (CDC, 1990a). The progression of CIN to invasive cancer in immunocompetent women usually (1) is a slow process, taking several years, (2) on the average occurs between the ages of 45 and 50 years, and (3) when detected by Papanicolaou (Pap) smear in early stages, results in favorable treatment outcomes (Di Saia, 1990; Richart & Wright, 1993). However, the occurrence in HIV-infected women has been noted to be (1) more rapidly progressive, (2) more advanced, (3) more likely to occur between the ages of 16 and 48 years, (4) less responsive to standard treatments, and (5) given a poorer prognosis in comparison with uninfected women (Mai-

mon et al., 1990; 1993; Rellihan et al., 1990; Schwartz et al., 1991). Schäfer and colleagues (1991) reported that cervical dysplasia/neoplasia was seen in 41% of HIV-infected women compared with only 9% of uninfected intravenous drug users and 4% of the general clinic population.

Multifactorial risk factors for CIN and cervical cancer include (1) early age at first intercourse, (2) multiple sex partners, (3) sex with men with multiple sex partners, (4) cigarette smoking, (5) dietary deficiencies, (6) use of oral contraceptives, (7) immunosuppression, (8) low socioeconomic status, (9) lack of access to health care, (10) exposure to diethylstilbestrol in utero, and (11) a history of sexually transmitted diseases, especially infection with human papillomavirus (HPV) (CDC, 1990a; Fiengold et al., 1990; Franco, 1991; Reeves et al., 1989; Rubin & Lauver, 1990; Richart & Wright, 1993).

HIV may activate HPV, resulting in cellular abnormalities (Goldsmith, 1992). Vermund and colleagues (1991) found the rate of CIN to be 57% (14 of 27) for women coinfected with HIV and HPV, 18% (6 of 34) for women with either HIV or HPV, and 9% (3 of 35) for women who were not infected by either HIV or HPV.

Pathogenesis

Richart and Wright (1993) described CIN and carcinoma of the cervix as a continuum, progressing from mild dysplasia (grade I), to moderate dysplasia (grade II), to severe dysplasia and carcinoma in situ (grade III). The frequency and severity of cervical dysplasia have been correlated with the degree of immunosuppression as measured by $CD4^+$ cell counts, as well as coinfection with HPV (Schäfer et al., 1991; Vermund et al., 1991).

Clinical Presentation

The early stages of CIN have no symptoms and are usually discovered by Pap smears. Among HIV-infected women, 30% to 35% have abnormal Pap test results, which is five to eight times higher than normal (Marte, 1992). In addition, Maimon and colleagues

(1991) reported a high rate of false-negative Pap smears in HIV-infected women: only 3 of 32 women had abnormal cytologic findings on Pap smears, but 41% had CIN on colposcopy. The frequency and severity of CIN correlate with the degree of immunosuppression: the lower the CD4+ cell count, the higher the incidence of CIN (Maimon et al., 1990; Schäfer et al., 1991; Spinillo et al., 1992).

Early symptoms of carcinoma of the cervix include painless postcoital bleeding, metrorrhagia, and blood-tinged vaginal discharge. Ulceration and infection may lead to persistent vaginal discharge. As disease progresses, there may be abdominal, pelvic, back, or leg pain; anorexia; weight loss; anemia as a result of vaginal bleeding; and leg edema caused by obstruction of the lymph nodes. In cases of advanced disease, there may be hematuria or rectal bleeding because of involvement of the bowel and/or bladder (DiSaia, 1990; McMullin, 1992; Shell & Carter, 1987).

Diagnosis

The Pap smear is a screening tool to determine the presence of abnormal cells and/or visible lesions. Clients with abnormal Pap results are referred for cervical biopsy and colposcopy, which can be used to determine the presence of both HPV infection and CIN (Rubin & Lauver, 1990; Tinkle, 1990). If the client is not pregnant, an endocervical curettage will be done to obtain cervical cells.

If the lesion extends into the cervical canal and cannot be evaluated by colposcopy, conization will be done. Conization, or cone biopsy, is both a diagnostic and a treatment tool; it not only establishes the severity of CIN but also can remove a cone-shaped wedge of abnormal tissue (Bobak et al., 1993; DiSaia, 1990).

If biopsy reveals invasive cervical cancer, examination under anesthesia will be necessary to stage the disease and to determine the spread of disease beyond the cervix (DiSaia, 1990). Cervical cancer is staged according to the standards of the International Federation of Gynecology and Obstetrics. The disease will be staged from 0 to IV, depending on the extent of tissue and/or organ involvement. In addition, a complete diagnostic study will be performed by a gynecologic oncologist and a radiation oncologist so that suitable treatment can be planned.

Treatment

Treatments for CIN and cervical carcinoma in situ include CO_2 laser therapy, conization, cryosurgery, electrocautery, and simple hysterectomy. The loop electrocautery excision procedure is the newest procedure available.

Treatments for invasive cervical cancer depend on the stage of the disease. Treatments may include surgery, radiation, chemotherapy, or any combination of these modalities. Because cervical cancers are usually squamous cell carcinomas, chemotherapy has been less effective (Bobak et al., 1993). However, recent trials with cisplatin showed a response rate as high as 50% (DiSaia, 1990). In cases of rapidly progressing HIV disease, Schwartz and colleagues (1991) used cisplatin, vincristine, and bleomycin; Rellihan and colleagues (1990) used cisplatin, bleomycin, and mitomycin. Despite a course of chemotherapy and radiation treatments, both patients died within 5 months of diagnosis. Maimon et al. (1993) found that patients with CD4+ cell counts greater than 500/mm³ had a better response to therapy than those women with counts less than 500/mm³.

Considerations for Nursing

The combined diagnoses of HIV infection and gynecologic cancer have a profound physical and psychologic impact on a woman. Krouse (1985) and McMullin (1992) described a woman's response to the diagnosis of gynecologic cancer: shame and guilt about sexual activity, anger, hostility, depression, and social withdrawal. Individuals infected with HIV have similar reactions (see Chapter 11). Depending on the treatments ordered, a woman may also have to cope with major abdominal surgery and the side effects of radiation and/or chemotherapy.

In addition, treatment of invasive cervical cancer may affect a woman's sexuality and her image of herself. After a complete hysterectomy, a premenopausal woman loses her childbearing ability and undergoes surgically induced menopause. Radiation treatments may result in a decrease in vaginal lubrication and sensation, and/or vaginal narrowing caused by scar tissue. Not only do clients need information on safer sex guidelines, but they also need instructions on how to cope with vaginal narrowing and a loss of lubrication. There is a high potential for sexual dysfunction and disturbances of body image and self-esteem.

Unfortunately, many nurses still do not address sexual issues with their clients. When Jenkins (1988) studied women after gynecologic surgery, none had received sexual counseling from their nurses, and 88% believed that the nurse or the physician should broach the subject without the patient's having to ask. In a study of oncology nurses, Williams and associates (1986) found that a majority of the nurses surveyed did not believe that counseling about sexual issues was part of their role. If nurses are going to deal with the human responses to the dual diagnoses of AIDS and invasive cervical cancer, they need to become more comfortable discussing sexuality (see Chapters 2 and 5).

Invasive cervical cancer is preventable if women receive prompt diagnosis and treatment of cervical dysplasia (CDC, 1992a). All women should receive a regular Pap test, but it is imperative for HIV-infected women. Nurses need to be aware of the relationship between CIN and HIV infection so that they can educate women regarding their risk. Maimon and colleagues (1993) believe that all women less than 50 years of age who are given a diagnosis of invasive cervical cancer should receive counseling and testing for HIV. Given the prevalence of undiagnosed HIV infection in women, perhaps it is time to extend such counseling to all women in whom CIN has been diagnosed.

COCCIDIOIDOMYCOSIS

Epidemiology

Coccidioides immitis is a fungus that was originally identified in the United States as the etiologic agent of a self-limited disease seen frequently in California, known as San Joa-

quin Valley fever, or valley fever. *C. immitis* is endemic in certain parts of Arizona, California, Nevada, New Mexico, Texas, and Utah (CDC, 1993b). Infection can occur in persons residing outside coccidioidomycosis-endemic areas as a result of travel to these areas, laboratory exposure, or inhalation of contaminated fomites (e.g., soil, cotton, packing material, or museum artifacts) taken from areas with endemic disease (CDC, 1993b).

Active coccidioidomycosis is common among HIV-infected persons living in endemic areas, and evidence of prior infection, including a positive tuberculin skin-test result, does not appear to predict the development of active infection. Reactivation of previously acquired infection does occur in HIV-infected persons who have relocated to nonendemic areas (Galgiani & Ampel, 1990). Conversely, Bronnimann and associates (1987) reported cases of disseminated coccidioidomycosis in persons with HIV (PWHIV) shortly after the PWHIV moved to Tucson, Ariz. Although the estimated incidence in the United States is approximately 0.3% of AIDS patients, in Arizona coccidioidomycosis occurs in about 20% of PWHIV (Daar & Meyer, 1992).

Pathogenesis

After the spores are inhaled, the lungs become the primary site of infection. In the acute phase, purulent pulmonary infection may be present, followed by lesion fibrosis. As in tuberculosis, caseation may occur (Stevens, 1990). In an immunocompetent person, coccidioidomycosis is usually subclinical or subacute, and respiratory symptoms that develop are indistinguishable from ordinary upper respiratory tract infections (Stevens, 1990). In persons with HIV disease, coccidioidomycosis is disseminated and can involve extrapulmonary sites including the skin, meninges, lymph nodes, and liver (Fish et al., 1990).

Clinical Presentation

Clinical symptoms of coccidioidomycosis are usually nonspecific and include malaise, fever, weight loss, cough, and fatigue (Minamoto & Armstrong, 1988). Infection of the meninges, brain, and cerebellum, as well as peritonitis, has been reported (Byrne & Dietrich, 1989; Levy & Bredesen, 1988). Cutaneous manifestations are rare. Joint effusions and bone destruction, often seen with disseminated disease, have not been reported in persons with AIDS (Minamoto & Armstrong, 1988).

Diagnosis

The major problem in diagnosing coccidioidomycosis in PWHIV is the lack of suspicion of the disease (Stevens, 1990). This disease illustrates the need to include questions regarding travel in the clinical history taking of a person with or at risk for HIV disease. Persons with HIV disease who reside in or have traveled to endemic areas, as well as persons who have had positive skin test results for previous exposure, should be considered at risk for coccidioidomycosis. In the United States, endemic areas include Arizona, California, Nevada, New Mexico, Utah, and western Texas. Outside the United States, particular attention should be given to travel or previous residence in Mexico and Central and South America.

Definitive diagnosis of coccidioidomycosis is made by microscopy, culture, or direct examination of affected tissues or fluid from those tissues, including bronchoscopic specimens, blood, bone marrow, lymph nodes, urine, and liver specimens.

Treatment

As with most opportunistic infections associated with AIDS, treatment is not curative and lifelong suppressive therapy is required. For the initial phase of treatment, the drug of choice is usually amphotericin B, followed by a suppressive regimen with either amphotericin B or ketoconazole (Ampel et al., 1989; Armstrong, 1989; Minamoto & Armstrong, 1988). Trials of fluconazole for suppressive therapy are under way (American Foundation for AIDS Research, 1993). Problems with treatment of coccidioidomycosis in PWHIV include delayed diagnosis and a lack of effective and relatively nontoxic drugs (Armstrong, 1989).

Considerations for Nursing

Nurses should be aware of the geographic distribution of *C. immitis* and anticipate possible development of coccidioidomycosis in HIV-infected individuals who live in, have previously lived in, or may have traveled to these states. The importance of including travel and previous locales of residence in the history of clients with or at risk for HIV disease is self-evident in the case of coccidioidomycosis. HIV-infected persons should be advised against travel for pleasure to endemic areas.

CRYPTOCOCCOSIS

Epidemiology

Cryptococcus neoformans is a yeastlike fungus that is ubiquitous in nature and can be found worldwide. The organism is found in pigeon drippings and can be retrieved in nesting places, soil, fruit, and fruit juices. *C. neoformans* can remain viable for up to 2 years in desiccated pigeon feces (Davis, 1986). Neither person-to-person nor animal-to-person transmission has been documented. The disease is naturally acquired from the environment where the organism is aerosolized and inhaled. The severe cell-mediated immunodeficiency associated with HIV disease permits cryptococcosis to develop, causing meningitis or pneumonia, or both in most cases (Grant & Armstrong, 1988). Infection with *C. neoformans* is more common among intravenous drug users and ethnic minorities with AIDS and in the south central United States (Stansell & Sande, 1992; Chaisson & Volberding, 1990). This predisposition to cryptococcosis in these populations has not been explained (Stansell & Sande, 1992). Forthal and colleagues (1992) hypothesized that cigarette smoking, by impairing pulmonary defenses, may result in enhanced local replication and subsequent infection by *C. neoformans* in persons with AIDS.

Cryptococcosis is the most common life-threatening fungal infection associated with AIDS, and the third most common cause of CNS disease, after HIV encephalopathy and toxoplasmosis (Saag, 1993). Current estimates are that 5% to 13% of patients with AIDS acquire cryptococcosis (Coker et al., 1993; Levitz, 1991).

Pathogenesis

After being inhaled, the fungus settles in the lungs, where it can remain dormant or spread to other parts of the body, particularly the CNS. In a host with an intact immune system, the infection is usually contained, but in the presence of an immunodeficiency, the potential for extrapulmonary spread increases. Chernoff and Sande (1990b) speculated that cryptococcal infections in PWHIV probably result from reactivation of latent infection as the immune system is progressively destroyed.

Anticryptococcal factors present in normal serum are absent in cerebrospinal fluid, which therefore is a good growth medium for cryptococci and explains why the CNS is the predominant focus of infection (Stansell & Sande, 1992). Because the fungus usually infects the brain as well as the meninges, this disease is more appropriately referred to as cryptococcal meningoencephalitis than meningitis. Cryptococcus is responsible for three forms of infection: CNS, pulmonary, and disseminated.

Clinical Presentation

Pulmonary cryptococcosis may coexist with CNS and disseminated cryptococcal infection. Clark and colleagues (1990) suggested that the incidence of this form is high. Pulmonary infection may go undetected because initially it is often subclinical and asymptomatic (Chernoff & Sande, 1990b). Wasser and Talavera (1987) reported that the clinical presentation of patients with AIDS and primary pulmonary cryptococcosis included fever, cough, dyspnea, and pleuritic chest pain. In its most severe form, cryptococcosis can cause adult respiratory distress syndrome (Murray et al., 1988; Similowski et al., 1989).

The clinical presentation of CNS cryptococcosis is similarly elusive because of its characteristic waxing and waning course and insidious onset. No signs or symptoms are sufficiently characteristic to distinguish cryptococcal meningitis from other CNS infections seen with AIDS (Chuck & Sande, 1989). In addition, most cases of CNS cryptococcosis do not appear with classic signs of meningitis. In a study of 89 patients with AIDS and cryptococcal meningitis, Chuck and Sande (1989) found symptoms present in the following percentages of patients: fever, 65%; malaise, 76%; headaches, 73%; stiff neck, 22%; focal deficits, 6%; seizures, 4%; cough or dyspnea, 31%; and diarrhea, 21%. In the same group of patients, they found a temperature above 38.4° C (102° F) in only 56%, meningeal signs in 27%, alterations in mentation in 17%, and focal deficits in 15%.

Disseminated infection, or cryptococcemia, can involve numerous other sites in the body, including the bone marrow, kidneys, liver, spleen, lymph nodes, heart, oral cavity, and prostate (Daar & Meyer, 1992). Cutaneous infection, producing skin lesions, that often mimic molluscum contagiosum or Kaposi's sarcoma, has been reported in 10% to 15% of patients with cryptococcosis (Chernoff & Sande, 1990b; Concus et al., 1988; Jones et al., 1990; Miller, 1988). Although rare, cryptococcal arthritis, adrenalitis, and thyroiditis have also been reported (Daar & Meyer, 1992).

Diagnosis

The diagnosis of cryptococcal meningitis can be made by visualizing the fungus in cerebrospinal fluid with an India ink stain; detecting cryptococcal antigen in cerebrospinal fluid, urine, or serum; and culturing the fungus (Chernoff & Sande, 1990b). According to Chuck and Sande (1989), the most reliable methods of diagnosis are determining cryptococcal antigen titers and culturing blood and cerebrospinal fluid. Computed tomography of the head should be performed to rule out hydrocephalus and to look for focal lesions such as cryptococcomas, toxoplasmosis, or lymphoma (Chuck & Sande, 1989; Dismukes, 1988).

The client should be carefully examined for cryptococcus in other parts of the body such as the eye or skin. Chest roentgenograms are helpful in detecting cryptococcal pneumonia, especially in clients who have culture-positive sputum or bronchoscopic specimens (Chernoff & Sande, 1990b).

Treatment

Primary therapy for the initial cryptococcal infection includes amphotericin B, with or without flucytosine, or fluconazole. For the past 30 years, amphotericin B has been the mainstay of therapy for cryptococcal meningitis in immunocompetent individuals. Studies of immunosuppressed patients show a slightly less favorable response. Individuals treated with amphotericin B who have HIV infection and cryptococcal meningitis have a mortality rate in the acute stage of 10% to 40% (Powderly, 1992). Controversy exists over the effectiveness of the combination of amphotericin B and flucytosine (Powderly, 1992). Saag and colleagues (1992) studied the effectiveness of amphotericin B with or without flucytosine versus fluconazole in the treatment of acute cryptococcal meningitis. They found that mild cases of cryptococcal meningitis responded as well to fluconazole as to amphotericin, but the optimal therapy for patients with moderate to severe cryptococcal disease was inconclusive. Feinberg (1993) recommends high-dose amphotericin B therapy with or without flucytosine for the first 2 weeks of therapy. Liposomal amphotericin B is currently under investigation as a primary treatment for cryptococcosis (Coker et al., 1993).

As with many of the opportunistic infections associated with AIDS, initial treatment of the acute infection does not cure the patient; suppressive therapy is therefore necessary. Powderly and colleagues (1992) documented the superiority of daily oral fluconazole over weekly infusions of amphotericin B in long-term suppression of cryptococcal meningitis.

Considerations for Nursing

Because of the insidious onset of cryptococcal infection, as well as the waxing and waning presentation, persons with HIV disease often postpone medical evaluation. It may be significant others, family, or friends who notice personality or behavioral changes or cognitive impairment. Undetected CNS cryptococcosis can lead to seizures before help is sought. Without encouraging hypervigilant or hypochondriac behaviors, health care workers should stress to patients early in the course of HIV disease that it is infinitely better to ask questions or seek evaluation when symptoms appear than to wait until symptom severity increases.

For the person with AIDS and cryptococcosis, neuropsychiatric evaluation should be performed to detect the often subtle symptoms of cognitive impairment. Problems with short-term memory or calculations may lead to noncompliance with medication regimens and to recurrence during oral fluconazole therapy substituted for intravenous maintenance therapy.

The evaluation process associated with long-term suppressive therapy commonly includes lumbar punctures. Clients often experience fear and emotional trauma related to this procedure. Nurses should prepare clients adequately and support them during the procedure.

Cryptococcus is ubiquitous in nature, and infection is probably a reactivation of latent pulmonary foci. However, HIV-infected individuals should avoid places where exposure to *C. neoformans* is likely, such as pigeon roosts and areas where pigeons and other birds congregate in numbers (Chernoff & Sande, 1990b).

CRYPTOSPORIDIOSIS

Epidemiology

Cryptosporidium is a coccidian protozoan pathogen in man that has only recently received extensive study because of the high incidence of disease in persons with AIDS. Cryptosporidiosis was not identified in humans until 1976, and until 1982, only seven cases were reported in the literature (CDC, 1984). However, the identification of *Cryptosporidium* as a cause of infection in HIV-infected individuals has resulted in further study of this parasite, and it is now recognized as an important human enteric pathogen in both immunocompetent and immunosuppressed populations and a frequent cause of diarrhea (McGowan et al., 1993). Whether cryptosporidiosis in HIV-infected persons is a reactivation of a previous infection or is newly acquired has not been determined (Gellin & Soave, 1992).

The major modes of transmission of *Cryptosporidium* are from human to human or via contaminated water, although animal-to-human and human-to-animal transmissions have been reported (Soave & Sepkowitz, 1992). Human-to-human spread has been identified in attendees of day care centers, household contacts of infected persons, hospitalized patients, and health care workers. Waterborne transmission has been identified in travelers and swimmers and in contaminated community water supplies (*Cryptosporidium* is chlorine resistant) (CDC, 1991a; Soave & Sepkowitz, 1992). *Cryptosporidium* has been identified in rivers, reservoirs, and both treated and untreated sewage, and transmission through sexual activity, aerosolization, fomites, and contaminated food has been suggested but has not as yet been confirmed (Soave & Sepkowitz, 1992).

Although the parasite is known to be distributed throughout the world, the incidence of cryptosporidiosis as an AIDS-indicator disease varies. In the United States, studies of AIDS patients with diarrhea identified *Cryptosporidium* in 15% to 16% of the patients (Laughon et al., 1988; Smith et al., 1992). In Haiti and Africa, *Cryptosporidium* has been diagnosed in up to 50% of AIDS patients with diarrhea (Soave & Sepkowitz, 1992).

Pathogenesis

After ingestion of the organism, the most common site of infection is the small intestine, although, in immunocompromised individuals, cryptosporidia have been found throughout the gastrointestinal tract, including the pharynx, esophagus, stomach, duodenum, small intestine, appendix, colon, rectum, gallbladder, pancreas, bile, and pancreatic ducts,

and in the respiratory tract as well (Bartlett, 1993; Ma et al., 1984; Soave & Sepkowitz, 1992). Recent studies conclude that the severity and duration of illness in HIV-infected persons are related to the severity of immunosuppression in individuals with CD4$^+$ cell counts greater than 300 mm^3 (Flanigan et al., 1992; McGowan et al, 1993).

Clinical Presentation

The clinical presentation and severity of cryptosporidiosis in the HIV-infected person are variable, with some patients having unrelenting diarrhea whereas others have a brief episode of diarrhea and then become free of symptoms (McGowan et al., 1993). Symptoms of disease usually begin 5 to 14 days after exposure and typically consist of cramping abdominal pain, flatulence, diarrhea, and weight loss (Bartlett, 1993; Soave & Sepkowitz, 1992). Nausea, vomiting, myalgia, and fever may be present but are less common (Gellin & Soave, 1992).

In persons with HIV disease and severe immunoincompetence, the clinical presentation can include watery diarrhea (1 to 25 liters per day), profound weight loss, electrolyte imbalance, and severe dehydration (Soave & Sepkowitz, 1992). Right upper quadrant abdominal pain, nausea, and vomiting, in addition to enteritis, which indicates biliary cryptosporidiosis, have been documented in 15% of the cases (Gellin & Soave, 1992).

Diagnosis

The diagnosis of cryptosporidiosis is established by the detection of organisms in stool or tissue specimens. Anticryptosporidial immunoglobulins may be measured in persons with HIV disease but may not be useful in diagnosis because of compromised immunologic responses (Bartlett, 1993; Gellin & Soave, 1992).

Cryptosporidium infection can be microscopically identified in stool specimens with special staining techniques. They may also be identified through biopsy specimens of the gastrointestinal tract (Smith et al., 1992).

Treatment

No effective anticryptosporidial therapy exists. In immunocompetent individuals, the disease is self-limited and does not require therapy. Refractory cryptosporidiosis, as it occurs in most persons with AIDS, usually results in death from profound malabsorption, electrolyte imbalances, malnutrition, and dehydration. Anticryptosporidial agents that are under ongoing investigation and currently being used include paromomycin, letrazuril, and azithromycin (American Foundation for AIDS Research, 1993; Fichtenbaum et al., 1993; Smith et al., 1992). They all demonstrate some, but incomplete, effectiveness. Somatostatin, bovine colostrum, and atovaquone are also being studied.

At present, medical therapy is palliative and directed toward symptoms, focusing on fluid replacement, occasionally total parenteral nutrition, correction of electrolyte imbalance, and the prescription of analgesic, antidiarrheal, and antiperistaltic agents.

Considerations for Nursing

In the presence of unremitting cryptosporidiosis and the absence of an effective therapy, the primary focus of care is palliation, symptom control, and intensive nursing care. Nursing goals should include measures to minimize the physical discomforts associated with continuous explosive diarrhea (skin breakdown in the perianal, genital, gluteal, and upper thigh regions, and pain), as well as measures to help the patient cope with significant alterations in body image as a result of malnutrition, dehydration, and weight loss. Nurses caring for this client population need emotional support themselves to deal with such frustrations as never getting the bed clean for longer than a few minutes or having to leave the patient lying in fecal material to get medications.

Infection control measures should be carefully planned to prevent person-to-person transmission or transmission by fomites, not only in hospitals but in the home as well. Wearing of protective clothing and gloves during care, proper waste disposal, and meticulous hand washing, along with instructions to staff and significant others on enteric precautions, are imperative. Keeping the fecal waste contained is a never-ending challenge.

Fecal contamination of the environment can be problematic because *Cryptosporidium* is resistant to most disinfectants such as diluted bleach, iodophor, cresylic acid, benzalkonium chloride, and 5% formaldehyde (Gellin & Soave, 1992). Effective methods of disinfection include the use of full-strength bleach for more than 15 minutes, 5% ammonia for more than 15 minutes, and heat to greater than 65° C for 30 minutes (Current & Garcia, 1991).

Some clients are confronted with the decision of whether to accept insertion of indwelling infusion devices and total parenteral nutrition. Although some clients find this therapeutic modality attractive initially, it may prove frustrating to them once the therapy is started. Many soon discover that they are confined with the equipment, supplies, and an infusion pump, and that getting to the toilet with the equipment can be especially difficult.

Prevention of exposure includes teaching the importance of hand washing and of food and water safety, especially during travel (see Appendix IV). Counseling about such sexual practices as anilingus and avoiding direct contact with animal feces should also be provided.

CYTOMEGALOVIRUS DISEASE

Epidemiology

Cytomegalovirus (CMV) is ubiquitous in humans throughout the world. According to Adler (1992), although worldwide seropositivity for CMV varies with location, race, and socioeconomic status, nearly all individuals eventually become seropositive. The potential for infection is increased during two periods: the perinatal period through the preschool years, and later during sexually active years (Ho, 1990). In the first period, CMV can be acquired as intrauterine or congenital infection, via vaginal delivery through a contaminated cervix, from human milk by breastfeeding or from banked milk, by transmission from child to child in nurseries or day care centers, or among children within a family.

Infected children carry the virus in the respiratory tract and urine for long periods (Ho, 1990).

Drew and Erlich (1990a) identified several factors supporting heterosexual transmission in adults: (1) CMV does not spread from adults by ordinary, nonsexual contact; (2) the virus has been isolated from semen and cervical secretions; (3) the prevalence of CMV antibody more than doubles between the ages of 15 and 35, the years of the highest sexual activity; and (4) bidirectional transfer (from men to women and from women to men) has been documented. Kissing and spread through saliva are also a probable means of CMV transmission (Pagano & Lemon, 1986). Little information is available on CMV transmission and specific sexual practices, such as cunnilingus or fellatio, and virtually no studies of CMV transmission between lesbians have been reported. With the AIDS epidemic, specific activities between men have received considerable attention.

In 1981 investigators found a higher prevalence rate of CMV infection in homosexual men (Drew & Erlich, 1990a). This finding was confirmed in 1987 by Collier and associates. Of the numerous sexual practices among homosexual men studied, only receptive anal intercourse correlated with a higher incidence of CMV antibody or seroconversion. In 1988 Rabinowitz and colleagues reported for the first time a case of CMV proctitis after anal intercourse in an immunocompetent woman uninfected with HIV. This finding emphasizes that it is sexual practices, not sexual orientation, that may result in transmission of the disease.

Drew and Erlich (1990b) pointed out that reexposure, as by receptive anal intercourse without a condom in a man with long-standing seropositivity, can result in reinfection with exogenous strains of CMV (coexisting different isolates of CMV have been found in PWHIV). Double infections with CMV do occur in patients with AIDS. Alternative routes of CMV transmission include transfusion of blood products and transplantation of organs or tissues. Immunosuppressive drugs, corticosteroids, and cytotoxic drugs such as cyclophosphamide or azathioprine can permit reactivation of latent disease (Ho, 1990). Nelson and associates (1993) reported a higher incidence of CMV disease in PWHIV treated with corticosteroids.

With increased survival time in PWHIV, there has been a significant increase in CMV disease in the latter stages of HIV infection (Munoz et al., 1993). The most significant predictor of active CMV infection in persons with AIDS is a CD4$^+$ cell count <50 mm^3 (Katlama & Dickinson, 1993). According to Drew and colleagues (1992), although active CMV infection may cause life-threatening disease in 40% of PWHIV, autopsy and clinical studies indicate that 90% of PWHIV have active CMV infection during the course of the illness. The most prevalent form of active disease in PWHIV is CMV retinitis, seen in 25% of the patients, and gastrointestinal disease in 5% and pneumonia in 10% of the cases (Drew et al., 1992).

Pathogenesis

CMV causes disease in three ways: by directly destroying tissue in sites such as the brain, lungs, retina, and liver; by causing immunologic responses resulting in hemolytic anemia and thrombocytopenia; and by facilitating neoplastic transformation (Straus, 1990). According to Ho (1990), the site of latency is not precisely known but probably includes leukocytes. In immunologically normal adults, CMV is not detectable except in cervical secretions of some women and the semen of some men, with a higher incidence in homosexual men (Ho, 1990). Immunocompetent individuals may continue to shed the virus in body fluids for several months after recovering from acute CMV infection. Carriers, often chronic, include individuals with congenital or perinatal infection and immunocompromised hosts, such as transplant recipients and persons with HIV disease.

Clinical Presentation

Persons with HIV disease who have active CMV infection may remain free of symptoms or may exhibit various clinical manifestations such as chorioretinitis, pneumonitis, encephalitis, adrenalitis, colitis, esophagitis, cholangitis, and herpes (Drew et al., 1992). CMV ocular infection may result in complaints of painless visual loss (e.g., loss of a portion of the visual field, blurred vision, or the presence of floaters, either unilaterally or bilaterally) (Drew et al., 1992; Vinters & Ferreiro, 1990). Other ocular manifestations of CMV infection include panuveitis and conjunctivitis (Brown et al., 1988a; Daicker, 1988).

Pulmonary CMV infection is usually seen in combination with other opportunistic disease such as *Pneumocystis carinii* pneumonia, *Mycobacterium avium* complex infection, pyogenic bacterial infection, or *C. neoformans* infection (Wallace & Hannah, 1987). Drew and Ehrlich (1990b) noted that many of these clients respond to therapy directed at the concurrent infection (e.g., *Pneumocystis carinii* pneumonia), which raises the question of actual pathogenicity of pulmonary CMV. CMV pulmonary infection in a person with AIDS is often manifested as progressive shortness of breath, dyspnea on exertion, and a dry nonproductive cough, with or without fever (Drew et al., 1992; Jacobson & Mills, 1988). Other respiratory manifestations of CMV infection reported in persons with AIDS include fever and wheezing in a client with CMV bronchiolitis and hoarseness in a client with CMV infection of the laryngeal nerve (Small et al., 1989; Vasudevan et al., 1990).

When CMV and HIV coexist in the brain of a person with AIDS, the in vivo interaction may be the cause of the encephalitis (Wiley & Nelson, 1988). Regardless of whether HIV or CMV is causing the encephalitis, the clinical presentation is similar: personality changes, cognitive impairment, and motor impairment. Other CNS pathologic processes attributable to CMV include radiculomyelitis, ascending myelitis, and necrotizing spinal lesions.

Virtually all parts of the gastrointestinal tract, from the oral cavity to the perianal area, have been reported as infected with CMV. Esophageal ulceration with CMV is most often associated with odynophagia (Drew et al., 1992). CMV colitis is usually associated with weight loss, anorexia, and fever (Drew et al., 1992). The feces should be monitored regularly for hematochezia (blood), because the potential for hemorrhage, infarction, and perforation of the gastrointestinal tract exists. Other gastrointestinal sites reported to be infected with CMV in PWHIV include the liver, gallbladder, and pancreas (Cello, 1992).

CMV infection of the adrenal gland in PWHIV can produce such manifestations as postural hypotension and sodium deficits (Vinters & Ferreiro, 1990). CMV infection of the thyroid and pituitary glands has also been reported (Ferreiro & Vinters, 1988).

Vascular infection caused by CMV includes thrombophlebitis, cerebral venous thrombosis, and vascular cutaneous lesions that can be mistaken for Kaposi's sarcoma (Abrams & Farhood, 1989). Genitourinary CMV infection reported in persons with AIDS includes cystitis, endometritis, and infections of the cervix and testes (Benson et al., 1988; Brodman & Deligdisch, 1986; Brown et al., 1988b; Lucas et al., 1989; Nistal et al., 1990).

Diagnosis

Drew and Erlich (1990a) noted that CMV infection must be distinguished from CMV disease, because CMV can be isolated from blood, urine, semen, cervical secretions, or other body fluids in the absence of clinical illness. The diagnosis of CMV disease is based on microscopic identification of CMV inclusion bodies or positive results on culture of specimens from specific organs such as the brain, lung, liver, gastrointestinal tract, adrenal glands, and skin, or both, in the absence of other infectious agents.

The presumptive diagnosis of CMV chorioretinitis is usually based on loss of vision and characteristic findings of serial ophthalmoscopic examinations in a person with definitively diagnosed HIV disease. The diagnosis of CMV adrenalitis is usually presumptively based on the identification of adrenal insufficiency and isolation of CMV from the blood.

Treatment

Ganciclovir and foscarnet are the two drugs currently available and approved for the treatment of CMV retinitis. They are also used to treat CMV infections in other parts of the body. Both drugs require initial high-dose induction therapy followed by lower-dose maintenance therapy. Although both drugs have been reported to result in clinical improvement and despite lifelong suppressive therapy, some patients will have progression of disease (Studies of Ocular Complications of AIDS Research Group, 1992).

Dietrich and colleagues (1993) investigated the concurrent use of ganciclovir and foscarnet in a small group of patients who failed to respond to both ganciclovir and foscarnet as single agents. They found that concurrent use was effective in stabilizing progressive CMV disease and was well tolerated. Studies are being conducted with combining or alternating foscarnet and ganciclovir to decrease the risk of viral resistance (Katlama & Dickinson, 1993).

Concomitant use of zidovudine and ganciclovir results in severe neutropenia. Experiments are being conducted to test the efficacy of colony-stimulating factors to limit this effect (American Foundation for AIDS Research, 1993). Didanosine and zalcitabine have been used in place of zidovudine, with relative safety when ganciclovir is prescribed.

Studies comparing ganciclovir with foscarnet for CMV retinitis suggest that treatment with foscarnet offers a survival advantage (approximately 4 months) over therapy with ganciclovir (Studies of Ocular Complications of AIDS Research Group, 1992). The study also noted that the patients did not tolerate foscarnet as well as ganciclovir. Because many patients receiving foscarnet also continued with zidovudine therapy, the precise role of antiretroviral agents remained unclear with regard to the survival rates.

Several studies of oral ganciclovir therapy are ongoing to compare the efficacy of oral therapy with intravenous therapy. Intravitreous ganciclovir therapy, either by direct injection or the use of implantation sustained-release devices, is also under investigation (Anand et al., 1993). Both ganciclovir and foscarnet are used to treat extraocular CMV infection.

Considerations for Nursing

Active CMV disease occurring in the course of HIV illness can be physically and psychologically exhausting to the patient. This is true in the presence of CMV retinitis, when the threat of total blindness is ever present. Grieving over vision loss has the potential for impairing the individual's ability to participate actively in the activities of daily living. Many individuals will benefit from early referrals to organizations for the visually impaired, where they will discover assistive devices such as magnifying glasses and large-print reading materials, and focus on their abilities as opposed to their disabilities.

Throughout the HIV epidemic, concern has been expressed about the risk that health care workers, especially pregnant women caring for PWHIV, will acquire CMV infection. Balfour and Balfour (1986) studied graduates and nursing students caring for clients with a known high rate of CMV infection in renal transplant and hemodialysis services and neonatal intensive care units, and found that nurses who practice good personal hygiene are no more likely to acquire CMV than their peers in the community. Balcarek and colleagues (1990) studied employees at a children's hospital and found the incidence of CMV among them similar to the rate expected for the general population. Gerberding and associates (1987) and Gerberding (1989) found no evidence of increased risk of acquiring CMV from occupational exposure to PWHIV, even when exposure was for a long period. In fact, Gerberding (1989) pointed out that although the issue of CMV as an occupational hazard has stimulated controversy, occupational CMV transmission has yet to be documented in a health care worker, and advises that pregnant health care workers and sexual partners of pregnant women can safely provide care to persons with CMV infection by complying with the universal infection control guidelines.

Employers must recognize that the fear of an occupational CMV infection is very real among health care workers who wish to have children. They should also be aware that many nurses and physicians have outdated or erroneous information regarding the potential, versus the actual, transmission of CMV in a health care practice setting. Adler (1992) summarizes current knowledge that should be shared with concerned staff, including the following: (1) CMV does not survive in inanimate objects; (2) CMV can be readily inactivated by soap and water; (3) strict adherence to avoiding direct contact with blood and body fluids, as well as frequent and proper hand-washing techniques, will protect both staff and patients; (4) CMV infection from patients to staff occurs rarely, if at all, and has never been demonstrated; (5) pregnant women do not need to be tested for CMV because of the low incidence of infection; and (6) pregnant women should not be furloughed or transferred from assignments (because of the erroneous notion that their exposure to other patients would limit their potential exposure to CMV in other patient populations).

Additionally, although universal precautions do not apply to nasal secretions, urine, sputum, and so forth, unless they contain visible blood, all health care workers should wear gloves when the potential for contact with body fluids exists, and should practice strict hand-washing techniques to minimize contact with pathogens other than HIV. Finally, it is important to remember that CMV can be excreted in the blood, urine, and other body fluids in the absence of clinical illness (Drew & Erlich, 1990a). Caring for patients or specific diagnostic categories of patients does not mean that the potential for CMV exposure does not exist.

ENCEPHALOPATHY, HIV RELATED

Epidemiology

HIV encephalopathy is also referred to as AIDS dementia complex (ADC), HIV-1–associated dementia, subacute encephalopathy, and HIV or AIDS dementia. ADC is a neurobehavioral deficit that is a common neurologic complication of late-stage HIV infection (Bornstein et al., 1993). More recently the terms "HIV-1–associated minor cognitive/motor disorder" and "HIV-related cognitive impairment" have been applied to HIV-infected individuals with subtle or mild cognitive impairment that has not yet progressed to full-blown ADC (Boccellari et al., 1993). Although the precise incidence of ADC is under study, current estimates indicate that ADC will be diagnosed in 4% to 15% of HIV-infected persons (Britton, 1993; Egan, 1992).

Pathogenesis

Although there is agreement that HIV is present early in the course of infection, as evidenced by detection of HIV in cerebral spinal fluid, there is limited evidence that early brain invasion occurs (Britton, 1993). The neuropathology in affected patients appears to be subcortical, involving the white matter in the brain, the spinal cord, and subcortical gray matter with significant neuronal damage (Boccellari et al., 1993; Simpson, 1993).

Price and associates (1988b) proposed that the neurologic manifestations of HIV infection require immunosuppression severe enough to allow for rampant viral activity resulting in increased viral load. However, Grant and Heaton (1990) suggested that although HIV-related CNS dysfunction tends to be correlated with immune system disease, immunosuppression is not necessary for the development of neurologic complications. The risk of having ADC has been correlated inversely with hemoglobin levels and body weight, and an increased mortality rate has been found among demented patients (Britton, 1993). Janssen and associates (1992) suggested that age (very young or old) is associated with the development of ADC.

Clinical Presentation

Clinical symptoms of ADC include cognitive dysfunction (inability to concentrate, decreased memory, slowness in thinking), motor deficits (leg weakness, ataxia, clumsiness), and behavioral changes (apathy, reduced spontaneity, social withdrawal) (Price et al., 1988b).

In a small number of patients, the initial or predominant feature of ADC is agitated organic psychosis ranging from irritability, hyperactivity, and anxiety without an identifiable cause to mania or delirium (Price et al., 1988a). Boccellari and colleagues (1988) reported hyperactivity, euphoria, and grandiose delusions, increasing the possibility of a secondary mania in persons with ADC and no previous psychiatric history.

Left undiagnosed or untreated, ADC progresses slowly as a predominant component, and the individual becomes increasingly apathetic and indifferent to his or her illness. Progression of motor abnormalities can lead to paraparesis and bladder and bowel incontinence. At the end stages, the person with ADC usually lies in bed with a vacant stare, minimally responsive to the environment, incontinent, and unable to walk (Price et al., 1988b).

Diagnosis

Diagnosis of ADC may initially be overlooked, especially in an acute care setting, where examination of the mental status of a person with AIDS is not a priority, given the plethora of physical problems requiring attention. In addition, a differential diagnosis is required to distinguish ADC from opportunistic infections or neoplasms of the CNS, metabolic abnormalities, and psychiatric illnesses. ADC may also be confused with multiple sclerosis, Parkinson's disease, or Alzheimer's disease (Price et al., 1988a; Weiler et al., 1988). Weiler (1989) pointed out that ADC in elderly persons may increase significantly in the coming years because of a greater number of patients with AIDS older than 50 years of age. This author also noted a tendency to discount AIDS as a possible diagnosis because of a patient's age.

Diagnosis of ADC begins with a history, presence of neurologic signs and symptoms indicating cognitive, motor, and behavioral dysfunction, and serologic evidence of exposure to HIV. Computed tomography and magnetic resonance imaging should be performed to look for cerebral atrophy and white matter disease, and cerebrospinal fluid analysis can show elevated protein levels and pleocytosis, as well as rule out other infections or neoplasms (Price et al., 1988a; Berger & Levy, 1993). Results of a preliminary study suggest that magnetic resonance spectroscopy may be able to detect biochemical changes in brains

of HIV-infected individuals early in the course of disease (Staff, 1993).

Treatment

Thus far, the most dramatic response to treatment has been with zidovudine. Persons with HIV disease and AIDS treated with zidovudine have shown improvement in cognitive functions, including memory, attention, and general mental speed, as well as improvement in motor skills (Schmitt et al., 1988; Yarchoan et al., 1988). The possibility that zidovudine may prevent ADC by inhibiting viral replication may explain the declining incidence of ADC because widespread use of this drug began in some countries (Portegies et al., 1989; Vago et al., 1993). Portegies and associates (1993) reported that ADC rarely developed during zidovudine therapy in HIV-infected individuals with symptoms. There is evidence that higher doses of zidovudine (1000 mg/day) are more effective in the treatment of ADC (Simpson, 1993). Yarchoan and colleagues (1990) noted improvement in a small number of patients with ADC who are taking didanosine. CNS stimulants such as methylphenidate and dextroamphetamine have also been used with favorable results (Angrist et al., 1991; Fernandez et al., 1988). Cognitive stimulation therapy should be provided along with medication.

Considerations for Nursing

Because of the time spent with HIV-infected clients in the provision of nursing care, nurses are key clinicians in detecting the subtle signs and symptoms of ADC. Clients with HIV disease commonly complain about problems with memory, concentration, and maintaining their train of thought. Nurses begin to notice this when they find themselves repeating information previously discussed with the client, or when the client cannot pay attention to conversations with them.

Simple numeric calculations can be difficult for clients and can lead to financial miscalculations and errors in self-medication; this should not be confused with a lack of basic arithmetic skills resulting from a limited education or learning disabilities. Clients may take longer to complete routine activities of daily living and may omit details, resulting in a disheveled appearance. They may watch television less and read less because of inability to follow the plot or characters or to interpret written meanings. The nurse may recognize problems with memory and comprehension when an evaluation of the outcomes of teaching shows that minimal or no learning has taken place.

Nurses in community-based settings or clinics may notice missed appointments or inability to comply with prescribed medication regimens. The latter may especially create problems if the client is supposed to take zidovudine every 4 hours to control and reduce ADC or is receiving antibiotic therapy for infectious processes such as tuberculosis.

Many clients are aware of changes in cognitive abilities and become embarrassed or ashamed. In an attempt to hide symptoms, they may talk less and withdraw socially. Lovers, spouses, and significant others are helpful in noticing these behaviors, especially in individuals who deny the existence of any problem. Suicide risk increases with the development of dementia related to fear and experience of losing cognitive capacity (Forstein, 1992; Glass, 1988).

Early motor impairment may be discrete, and patients may not notice that they frequently drop things or that hand activities such as eating and writing are slower and less precise. Significant changes in writing a signature can lead to problems with checks and legal documents. Disturbances in gait, coordination, and balance can lead to tripping and falling. Initially this may be passed off as clumsiness; however, the nurse will notice the client reflexively exercising more caution when walking.

For clients who cannot take or do not respond to zidovudine, the nursing care plan should include client safety and preparation of the significant others for the cognitive, motor, and behavioral changes that will occur. Health teaching should be directed toward the care partner, and the care plan should include respite for the care partner, to prevent phys-

ical and psychologic exhaustion. Referrals for home care and emotional support should also be made.

HERPES SIMPLEX VIRUS DISEASE

Most people think of herpes as a synonym for a cold sore or genital lesion. However, the name is derived from a family of viruses called Herpetoviridae, which has several members including (1) herpes simplex virus type 1 (HSV-1), which causes cold sores and eye infections; (2) herpes simplex virus type 2 (HSV-2), which causes genital herpes; (3) varicella-zoster virus (VZV), the cause of chickenpox and shingles; (4) Epstein-Barr virus (EBV), the cause of infectious mononucleosis; (5) cytomegalovirus (CMV), which causes mononucleosis; (6) human herpes virus type 6, the cause of roseola; and (7) herpes B virus (sometimes referred to as human herpes virus type 7 or simian herpes B virus), which causes skin lesions or brain infection (Straus, 1990).

A major biologic feature of the herpesviruses is the phenomenon of latency and reactivation. After initial or primary infection with any of the seven herpesviruses, they remain lifelong latent viruses in humans and have the potential to reactivate, producing recurrent or secondary infections. Sites of latency include sensory nerve ganglia for HSV-1, HSV-2, VZV, and herpes B virus; monocytes, neutrophils, or lymphocytes for CMV; B lymphocytes and salivary glands for EBV; and lymphocytes for human herpes virus type 6 (Straus, 1990).

Epidemiology

Herpes simplex viruses are ubiquitous and have a worldwide distribution. Humans appear to be the only natural host. The primary mode of transmission is direct contact with oral secretions (HSV-1) or genital secretions (HSV-2). Transmission of HSV-1 can occur in the genital area by oral-sexual contact or autoinoculation (i.e., touching a cold sore and then touching the genital area), and HSV-2 can be transmitted orally by similar modes. Although transmission is facilitated during contact with a person with active infection (lesions present), it can also occur as a result of contact with symptom-free excretors (Hirsch, 1990; Rooney et al., 1986).

Serologic studies indicate that exposure to HSV-1 commonly occurs in early childhood and that the risk of infection is related to socioeconomic conditions such as overcrowding (Corey & Spear, 1986; Erlich & Mills, 1990). A different pattern of infection occurs with HSV-2. Except in infants born to mothers with vaginal lesions, HSV-2 infection risk usually begins at puberty with the onset of sexual activity and increases with the number of different sexual partners (Corey & Spear, 1986; Erlich & Mills, 1990). Higher rates of HSV-2 prevalence have been found in prostitutes, sexually active homosexual men (who have higher rates than sexually active heterosexual men), adults of lower socioeconomic status, and persons attending sexually transmitted disease clinics (Corey & Spear, 1986). Although latent HSV may reactivate in persons with HIV disease, causing severe recurrent disease, Safrin and colleagues (1991a) did not find an increase in the frequency or severity of HSV infection in this population despite severe immunosuppression.

HSV that is resistant to acyclovir is being diagnosed with increased frequency, possibly because of the escalating use of acyclovir prophylaxis for HSV (Cockerell, 1993). Current estimates of acyclovir-resistant HSV in HIV-infected persons are not available.

Pathogenesis

Primary exposure to HSV at mucosal surfaces or abraded skin permits entry of the virus and initiation of replication. The virus is then transported along nerve pathways. Although uncommon in immunocompetent individuals, the finding of multiple strains of the same HSV subtype in an immunocompromised person suggests that exogenous infection with different strains of the same subtype is possible (Corey & Spear, 1986).

After resolution of the primary infection, HSV becomes latent within sensory nerve ganglia, usually the trigeminal, sacral, and vagal ganglia. Once latency is established, the virus may be reactivated at any time and may replicate and travel along sensory epithelial surfaces, resulting in acute HSV infection (Erlich & Mills, 1990; Hirsch, 1990).

Clinical Presentation

Orolabial HSV infection in adults with HIV disease, usually because of recurrent disease, frequently appears as painful vesicular lesions that rapidly coalesce and rupture, producing ulcers on the lips, tongue, pharynx, or buccal mucosa (Drew et al., 1992). Fever, pharyngitis, and cervical lymphadenopathy may be present.

HSV genital infection is usually manifested by small papules that evolve into fluid-filled vesicles that are painful and tender to the touch (Drew et al., 1992). Inguinal lymphadenopathy may be present, and dysuria may be a complaint even if the urethra is not infected (Drew et al., 1992). After the vesicles ulcerate, healing takes place during a period of several weeks. Carpenter and associates (1991) found severe genital HSV disease to be the AIDS-defining diagnosis in 18% to 44% of women in whom AIDS developed.

Perianal and anorectal HSV infection and HSV proctitis may also be seen in HIV infected persons. The result can be localized pain, itching, pain on defecation, tenesmus, constipation, sacral radiculopathy, impotence, and neurogenic bladder (Drew et al., 1992).

HSV esophagitis can occur in the absence of oropharyngeal HSV lesions and may be confused with *Candida* esophagitis (Drew et al., 1992). Initial presentation may include dysphagia, which if untreated can result in odynophagia and retrosternal pain.

Although rare, HSV encephalitis can occur as a life-threatening complication in HIV disease. A subacute illness may begin with headache, meningismus, and personality changes, or an acute onset may show fever, headache, nausea, lethargy, confusion, cranial nerve deficits, and seizures (Drew et al., 1992).

Diagnosis

The optimal method of laboratory diagnosis of HSV is direct culture of material from the suspected lesion. When the specimen is obtained by scraping or swabbing, care should be taken to avoid contamination with stool, blood, alcohol, or detergent, because these substances can inactivate the virus and result in a negative culture result (Erlich & Mills, 1990). A transport medium should be used to prevent viral drying. According to Erlich and Mills (1990), serologic tests for HSV are of little practical importance because HSV antibody prevalence rates in PWHIV are known to be high; these tests are likewise of little use in differentiating HSV-1 from HSV-2. HSV encephalitis is difficult to diagnose, and in the absence of brain biopsy, empiric antiviral therapy is usually initiated (Drew et al., 1992).

Treatment

Primary therapy for HSV infection is acyclovir, which is available in intravenous, oral, and topical preparations. Intravenously administered acyclovir is used for severe HSV infections and is specifically indicated for HSV encephalitis. Orally administered acyclovir, in suspension or capsules, may be used for either acute HSV infection or long-term suppressive therapy. Topical acyclovir ointment is used to relieve subjective symptoms of skin lesions and to reduce viral shedding. Engel and colleagues (1990) reported success in treating acyclovir-resistant HSV-2 infection in PWHIV by administering high doses of acyclovir by continuous infusion for 6 weeks. This was done after treatment failure when acyclovir had been given orally and intravenously in traditional divided doses. Foscarnet has also been used for successful treatment of acyclovir-resistant HSV-2 infection (Erlich et al., 1989; Safrin et al., 1991b).

Considerations for Nursing

The health history of an HIV-infected person is important to determine the potential for recurrent HSV infection. The individual's knowledge of HSV transmission, as well as prevention related to specific sexual behaviors such as condom use and oral sex, should be assessed. Practicing safer sex should be reviewed with all HIV-infected persons to prevent transmission or acquisition of sexually transmitted diseases. HIV-infected clients

sometimes assume that if they have sex with another HIV-infected person, they can do whatever they want and no longer need to practice safer sex. Health teaching should stress that the rate of HSV infection is high in HIV-infected persons and that even if no HSV lesions are visible, symptom-free excretors can pass on the virus (Drew et al., 1992; Hirsch, 1990).

Nursing care of external lesions is directed at preventing secondary infections and autoinoculation, especially from genital and perianal lesions to other parts of the body. This is a problem in persons with HIV disease, who for any number of reasons may have impaired cognitive function. The burning, itching, and tingling sensations associated with mucocutaneous lesions invite scratching. Acyclovir ointment can reduce these sensations. When acyclovir ointment is used on an area that will be covered with clothing or that comes in direct contact with bed linen, the area should be covered with an impervious dressing so that the ointment is not absorbed by clothing and stays on the lesion(s). Dressing the lesions of confused and disoriented individuals may be necessary to prevent autoinoculation.

The risk of nosocomial transmission of HSV-1 and HSV-2 from infected patients, most often causing herpetic whitlow, is well documented (Henderson, 1990). Nurses should wear gloves during physical examination of a new client because they cannot predict what types of mucocutaneous lesion may be present. Gloves should also be worn for any procedures that involve oral or genital secretions, such as mouth care, suctioning, urinary catheter procedures, or vaginal care. Meticulous hand washing should be performed, and skin-to-lesion contact should be avoided as much as possible.

HISTOPLASMOSIS

Epidemiology

Histoplasma capsulatum is a fungus that is part of the intestinal flora of birds and bats and exists in its native habitat, the soil (Loyd et al., 1990). The major endemic areas in the United States are the middle, central, and south central states. Endemic areas have a higher incidence of progressive disseminated histoplasmosis (PDH) as an opportunistic infection in persons with HIV disease (Kurtin et al., 1990). PDH has also been reported in persons from nonendemic areas such as New York City who have long been removed from endemic areas such as the Caribbean or South America (Salzman et al., 1988).

Pathogenesis

H. capsulatum spores are inhaled, enter the bloodstream via the alveoli, and migrate throughout the reticuloendothelial system, including the liver, spleen, and lymph nodes. Infection with *H. capsulatum* in persons with HIV disease is due to reactivation of a previous infection or reinfection of persons living in endemic areas (Chernoff, 1990; Fels, 1988; Loyd et al., 1990).

Clinical Presentation

The predominant signs and symptoms associated with PDH are fever, weight loss, abdominal pain, diarrhea, cough, fatigue, lymphadenopathy, hepatomegaly, splenomegaly, oral ulcers, and skin lesions (Johnson et al., 1989; Neubauer & Bodensteiner, 1992; Wheat et al., 1990). Common laboratory abnormalities include anemia, leukopenia, and thrombocytopenia (Daar & Meyer, 1992; Neubauer & Bodensteiner, 1992). Other signs and symptoms may indicate adrenalitis, meningitis, retinitis, and genitourinary involvement (Chernoff, 1990; Zighelboim et al., 1992).

Diagnosis

Diagnostic delays may be encountered when clinicians omit travel history as part of the client's health history. HIV-infected patients with constitutional signs and symptoms at presentation, who have lived or traveled to endemic areas, should be examined for PDH. Definitive diagnosis of histoplasmosis is made by microscopy (history or cytology, culture, or detection of antigen in a specimen obtained directly from the tissues affected or from a fluid from those tissues) (CDC, 1992a).

The possibility of histoplasmosis under-

scores the need to include travel in the health history of a person with HIV disease. Smith and colleagues (1989), in their presentation of the first case of disseminated histoplasmosis in a person with AIDS in Europe, emphasized the importance of a detailed history, including travel, in clinical evaluation.

According to Johnson and associates (1989), bone marrow biopsy and culture, examination and culture of pulmonary tissue and secretions, and blood culture were the most common initial means of establishing the diagnosis. Roentgenograms of the chest are unreliable and have shown no abnormalities in up to 30% of individuals with disseminated histoplasmosis. In an HIV-infected person, disseminated histoplasmosis at a site other than or in addition to the lungs or cervical or hilar lymph nodes fulfills the CDC criteria for a diagnosis of AIDS (CDC, 1992a).

Treatment

The primary agent used to treat PDH has been amphotericin B, followed by lifetime suppressive therapy with either ketoconazole or amphotericin B. Newer agents being utilized include itraconazole and fluconazole (Katlama & Dickinson, 1993; Sharkey-Mathis et al., 1993; Wheat et al., 1993).

Considerations for Nursing

The diagnosis of histoplasmosis can be delayed if travel history of an HIV-infected person is not documented. Clients who were born in or have lived in endemic areas or who have relocated in large cities such as New York, Boston, or San Francisco may be overlooked for latent histoplasmosis infection. It seems prudent, on the basis of epidemiologic data, to advise HIV-infected individuals against travel for pleasure to endemic areas.

ISOSPORIASIS

Epidemiology

Isospora belli is a coccidian protozoan parasite that is widely distributed throughout the animal kingdom and is endemic to parts of Chile, Africa, and Southeast Asia (Soave &

Sepkowitz, 1992). Sorvillo and colleagues (1990) reported a 25% increase in 1989 in cases of isosporiasis in persons with AIDS, primarily Latino immigrants from Mexico and Central America. The mode of transmission, although as yet unconfirmed, is thought to be direct contact with infected animals, humans, or contaminated water (Gellin & Soave, 1992). Isosporiasis has been reported in fewer than 0.2% of all AIDS cases in the United States and in up to 15% of patients with AIDS in Haiti (Gellin & Soave, 1992).

Pathogenesis

After ingestion, *Isospora* cysts infect the small intestine and result in malabsorption and a nonbloody, watery diarrhea. Restrepo and associates (1987) reported disseminated, extraintestinal isosporiasis in a person with AIDS.

Clinical Presentation

The clinical features of isosporiasis resemble those of cryptosporidiosis, with the exception of less frequent bowel movements: 8 to 10 per day in isosporiasis compared with 6 to 26 per day in cryptosporidiosis (Wofsy, 1990). Characteristics of this illness include profuse watery, nonbloody diarrhea; cramping abdominal pain; nausea; anorexia; weight loss; weakness; occasional vomiting; and a low-grade fever (Smith & Janoff, 1988; Wofsy, 1990). Clinical illness ranges from self-limiting enteritis or chronic diarrhea in immunocompetent individuals to chronic or relapsing disease in PWHIV (Soave & Weikel, 1990). Severe debilitating dehydration may occur (Pape et al., 1989). Steatorrhea (fat in feces) caused by malabsorption can be seen in stool specimens.

Diagnosis

Diagnosis of isosporiasis is by identification of the *Isospora* oocysts in fecal specimens. Several specimens, as well as specimen concentration techniques, may be required to confirm the diagnosis, since *Isospora* oocysts may be shed only intermittently and in small numbers (Soave & Weikel, 1990). Pape and colleagues (1989) recommended that a minimum of four stool examinations be performed for patients with AIDS and chronic diarrhea.

Treatment

The effective treatment of isosporiasis in PWHIV is a 7-10 course of trimethoprim-sulfamethoxazole (TMP-SMX) (Gellin & Soave, 1992; Pape et al., 1989). For prevention of relapse, chronic suppressive therapy with TMP-SMX or sulfadoxine-pyrimethamine is prescribed; pyrimethamine can be prescribed for persons allergic to sulfonamides (Gellin & Soave, 1992; Pape et al., 1989). Other agents that have been used to treat isosporiasis include roxithromycin, metronidazole, quinacrine, and nitrofurantoin (Gellin & Soave, 1992).

Considerations for Nursing

Food and water precautions should be advised for all HIV-infected persons to avoid infection such as isosporiasis (see Appendix IV). This is especially important with travel to tropical and subtropical climates. Additional health teaching for persons with isosporiasis includes avoidance of sexual practices such as anilingus, which may predispose others to infection with *Isospora* or reexpose the client. The importance of indefinite continuation of suppressive therapy must also be emphasized.

Although nosocomial transmission has not been reported, the use of gloves and other barrier precautions, along with meticulous hand washing, is essential to prevent health care workers and significant others from acquiring isosporiasis. Frequent routine cleaning of the infected person's environment with standard disinfectant and cleaning agents is essential.

KAPOSI'S SARCOMA

Epidemiology

Variations in the epidemiologic patterns, clinical manifestations, and course of Kaposi's sarcoma (KS) are classified as four types:

(1) classic, or non-HIV–related, KS; (2) African, or endemic, KS; (3) KS associated with iatrogenic immunosuppression, sometimes referred to as renal transplant KS; and (4) epidemic, or HIV-related, KS (Friedman-Kien et al., 1989; Krigel & Friedman-Kien, 1988). The most notable characteristics distinguishing epidemic, or HIV-related, KS from the other three types are its fulminant, widely disseminated course and shorter survival. The histopathologic features of KS are essentially the same for all four variations (Friedman-Kien et al., 1989). The following discussion is limited to the HIV-related, or epidemic, form of KS.

Although KS has been noted to occur in adults of all risk categories and in children, the predominant incidence has been in men who have sex with men. This has led to extensive investigation of possible cofactors that may predispose an HIV-infected individual to KS. One hypothesis is that there was a relationship between recreational drug use, specifically nitrate inhalants ("poppers") and the development of KS in the presence of HIV infection (Haverkos, 1990). However, further study of nitrate inhalants as a cofactor for KS has not been supported (Beral et al., 1992; Lifson et al., 1990; Messiah et al., 1989).

Another area of investigation has been the role of CMV in the development of KS in persons with HIV disease. However, this role remains uncertain because scientists have been unable to demonstrate direct infection of KS tissue and because some patients with HIV and KS show no evidence of current or previous CMV infection (Heyer et al., 1990; Mitsuyasu, 1993). Additionally, theories regarding the genetic predisposition to KS in the presence of HIV have not been supported (Friedman-Kien et al., 1989). More recently, scientific inquiry has focused on the theory that an infectious pathogen, transmitted through blood, sexually, or perinatally, may act as a cofactor in the development of AIDS-related KS (Beral et al., 1990; Beral, 1991; Bowden et al., 1991; Friedman-Kien et al., 1990; Orlow et al., 1993). Huang and associates (1992) suggested that human papillomavirus infection may have a role in the pathogenesis of KS. Epidemiologic data suggest that specific sexual practices (i.e., anilingus and fecal-oral contact) may serve as a mode of transmission of an infectious agent and may lead to the development of KS (Beral et al., 1990, 1992; Beral, 1991).

Other theories regarding the origins of AIDS-related KS include (1) the immune surveillance theory, that the immune system is unable to detect and prevent a spontaneous neoplasm; (2) the HIV theory, that HIV has a direct oncogenic potential; and (3) the circulating endothelial growth factors theory, that KS is not a true malignancy but a stimulated response to HIV disease, in which lymphatic endothelial cells proliferate (Heyer et al., 1990).

Pathogenesis

Although some studies suggest a vascular endothelial cell origin of KS, theories about lymphatic endothelial cell origin are consistent with the clinical distribution of KS lesions along cutaneous lymphatic drainage channels, as well as lymphedema frequently seen in persons with AIDS-related KS (Heyer et al., 1990). KS is a multicentric process that can occur in the lymphatic endothelium at any site, including internal organs; however, the first lesions often appear subtly on the face or head or in the oral cavity. In most cases, KS progresses rapidly and is detected because of the appearance of new lesions on mucocutaneous surfaces and the viscera (Heyer et al., 1990).

The development of KS, unlike the development of most opportunistic infections seen in AIDS, is not directly linked to immunosuppression. KS can develop in an individual with HIV disease and a relatively normal $CD4^+$ cell count. Conversely, a relationship exists between degree of immunosuppression and aggressive presentation and survival (Heyer et al., 1990; Mitsuyasu, 1993).

Clinical Presentation

KS is manifested cutaneously as subcutaneous, painless, nonpruritic tumor nodules that are usually pigmented and violaceous (red to blue), nonblanching, and palpable

(Heyer et al., 1990). Discrete patch-stage lesions appear early in some individuals and may be mistaken for bruises, purpura, or diffuse cutaneous hemorrhages (Friedman-Kien et al., 1989). The patches can then form into plaques and eventually coalesce and form nodular tumors. New multifocal lesions may appear at any time, and characteristic sites include the tip of the nose, eyelid, hard palate, posterior pharynx, glans penis, thigh, and sole of the foot (Heyer et al., 1990). Although rare, skin breakdown over the tumors can occur and can bleed, necrose, and become painful. Lymphedema can occur in the face, penis, scrotum, and lower extremities. The client is usually aware of its presence and points it out when being examined. The consistency of fluid collection is usually firm and nonpitting (Heyer et al., 1990).

Gastrointestinal KS is often clinically inapparent, although signs and symptoms of obstruction may be present; in some cases, enteropathies from small bowel involvement are noted, and very rarely bleeding occurs (Friedman, 1988; Mitsuyasu, 1988). Pulmonary KS may be indistinguishable from pneumonia and may be manifested as fever, as well as cough, dyspnea, and wheezing if the tumors are causing airflow obstruction; hemoptysis has also been reported (Ognibene & Shelhamer, 1988). KS of the central nervous system is rare, and reported symptoms are transient hemiparesis and dizziness (So et al., 1988).

Diagnosis

Although many clinicians state that KS lesions are readily recognized, and the CDC revised definition of AIDS in 1987 included the presumptive diagnosis of KS (based on the characteristic gross appearance of any erythematous or violaceous placque-like lesion on skin or mucous membrane), numerous mucocutaneous lesions that are manifestations of other conditions can be easily confused with epidemic KS. The CDC (1987; 1992a) has cautioned clinicians against making a presumptive diagnosis if they have seen only a few cases of epidemic KS. In addition,

a presumptive diagnosis should be made only when laboratory evidence supports the diagnosis of HIV, because KS in homosexual men who are at risk for HIV infection but who are HIV-seronegative has been reported (Bowden et al., 1991; Friedman-Kien et al., 1990). Definitive diagnosis is by tissue biopsy to establish a histologic diagnosis.

In 1989 the Oncology Subcommittee of the AIDS Clinical Trials Group, sponsored by the National Institutes of Health, proposed a new staging classification based on tumor bulk, immune function, and the presence of systemic illness (Krown et al., 1989). This system essentially predicts a favorable prognosis for individuals with tumors confined to skin or lymph nodes or with minimal oral disease; CD4$^+$ cell counts of more than 200 cells/mm^3; no history of thrush, opportunistic infection, or constitutional symptoms; and a Karnofsky performance status score of 70 or better. Poor prognosis is associated with tumor-related edema or extensive ulceration of the viscera; a CD4$^+$ cell count of less than 200 cells/mm^3; a history of thrush, opportunistic infections, or neurologic or constitutional disease; and a Karnofsky performance status score of less than 70.

Treatment

When treatment options are evaluated, many factors must be considered: the extent and location of lesions, the presence of KS-related symptoms (pain, edema, cough, gastrointestinal bleeding), and the stage of HIV infection. KS patients with a CD4$^+$ cell count greater than 200 cells/mm^3 and no HIV-related symptoms have a better prognosis.

Kaplan (1990), noting that treatment is not indicated for all persons with AIDS-related KS, identified subgroups of patients for whom the goals of therapy are palliative and cosmetic. Indications for palliation include painful or uncomfortable intraoral or pharyngeal lesions that interfere with nutrition, respiratory tumors that may cause airway obstruction, lymphedema related to KS, plantar lesions that interfere with ambulation, and containment of rapidly progressive disease.

Treatment plans often include a variety of options for local and systemic therapies. Radiation therapy is commonly used for persons with single or locally symptomatic areas. Intralesional therapy with vinblastine or interferon alfa may be used for cosmetic purposes on small cutaneous lesions, and laser therapy and cryotherapy have also been used on small, isolated KS lesions (Kaplan, 1990; Esplin & Levine, 1991).

For individuals with rapidly progressive disease or advanced, widespread symptomatic disease, systemic therapy with antineoplastic agents may be appropriate. Single or combination agents used for systemic therapy include bleomycin, doxorubicin, etoposide, vinblastine, vincristine, mitoxantrone, and doxorubicin. Used as a single agent, vinblastine, vincristine, and etoposide may be up to 70% effective (Chism, 1993). Bleomycin, doxorubicin, and epirubicin are also frequently used as single agents (Krown et al., 1992a). Doxorubicin, bleomycin, and vincristine are commonly combined in a chemotherapeutic regimen. Studies are currently evaluating the effectiveness of liposomal doxorubicin and liposomal daunorubicin (American Foundation for AIDS Research, 1993; Chism, 1993; Fischl et al., 1993).

Bone marrow suppression, nausea, vomiting, fever, diarrhea, and hair loss are the major side effects associated with chemotherapy and may aggravate HIV-related symptoms. Two colony-stimulating factor (CSF) drugs, granulocyte-macrophage CSF and granulocyte CSF, are frequently used to counteract bone marrow suppression and allow for continuation of chemotherapy.

Interferon alfa has been approved for the treatment of KS in patients with a CD4[+] cell count greater than 200 cells/mm[3]. Two to 3 months of treatment may lead to tumor regression in those patients who lack B cell–related symptoms (American Foundation for AIDS Research, 1993). Krown and colleagues (1992b) demonstrated the effectiveness of the combination of interferon alfa and zidovudine in a select group of patients with HIV infection and KS.

Considerations for Nursing

Many clinical issues surrounding the development of epidemic KS may cause confusion, not only among clients and significant others, but also among nurses. First, KS can develop at any time during the course of HIV disease and does not necessarily result from immunosuppression. Therefore KS can develop in an HIV-infected client who is in a relatively good state of health as evidenced by lymphocyte subset studies. Second, clients and staff who have heard of long-term survivors of AIDS (most of whom have epidemic KS) may become complacent, believing that the course of the disease is indolent. All clients with KS must be monitored regularly for clinical progression, immunosuppression, and the development of opportunistic infections. Third, some nurses may think that not seeking active treatment is fatalistic and need assistance in understanding the indicators for therapy. Finally, some nurses, especially in areas with a low incidence of HIV disease, think that KS develops in all clients with AIDS and are not aware of the decreasing incidence of this AIDS-related malignancy.

Clients with external KS lesions usually have alterations in body image, as well as the potential for developing ineffective coping strategies. Whenever clients with facial KS lesions look in the mirror, or at the facial expression of someone new, they see a reflection that reminds them of their illness. Referrals to support groups, especially groups of persons with AIDS-related KS, can be invaluable in helping clients adjust to the diagnosis and develop positive coping strategies. Learning to cover lesions with makeup (best results are achieved with theatrical makeup) can also contribute immensely to the client's self-esteem and sense of well-being.

Another insufficiently addressed problem is sexual dysfunction related to dermal KS lesions, especially on the abdomen, genitals, or upper aspect of the thighs. Clothing that the client and sexual partner find arousing and erotic may help to eliminate some of the related performance problems. Colored condoms may cover penile lesions and allow more normal sexual activities. This is an especially important consideration because KS is often diagnosed early in HIV disease, when, in the absence of clinically symptomatic illness, the individual is sexually active.

LYMPHOMA, NON-HODGKIN'S

Epidemiology

Non-Hodgkin's lymphoma (NHL) may occur in any population at risk for HIV infection, and the clinical and pathologic aspects of disease appear similar among these groups (Levine, 1992; Milliken & Boyle, 1993). Approximately 3% of persons with HIV infection have been found to have NHL at the time of diagnosis of AIDS, and NHL develops in others after AIDS diagnosis (Gail et al., 1991). Advances in HIV- and AIDS-related therapies have resulted in prolongation of survival and an increase in the incidence of NHL (Levine, 1992). NHL tends to occur late in the course of HIV infection and is related to progressive immunosuppression (Levine, 1992; Munoz et al., 1993).

Pathogenesis

The lymphomas are cancers of the immune system. In all forms of lymphatic cancer, lymph tissue cells begin growing abnormally and spread to other organs. According to Kaplan (1990), the NHLs are a heterogeneous group of malignancies that range from indolent to fulminant in their disease course. NHLs can originate as a malignancy of T cells, but the vast majority occur as B-cell malignancies. NHLs are commonly classified according to pathologic and morphologic characteristics and are divided into three categories: low-grade, intermediate-grade, and high-grade lymphomas. Although low-grade NHL occurs in HIV-infected persons, it is not considered to be HIV related because its incidence is not increased in these patients (Milliken & Boyle, 1993).

Lymph node–based NHL is uncommon in persons with AIDS, in whom 80% to 90% of the NHL is extranodal disease involving the CNS, gastrointestinal tract, bone marrow, and liver (Levine, 1992). Other sites of NHL in persons with AIDS include the gallbladder, orbit, jaw, rectum, earlobe, popliteal fossa, heart, lung, skin, pancreas, subcutaneous and soft tissue, epidural spaces, appendix, gingiva, parotid gland, and paranasal sinuses (Kaplan, 1990; Levine, 1992). The role of Epstein-Barr virus in the pathogenesis of lymphomas in AIDS patients is under investigation (Mac-Mahon et al., 1991; Samoszuk et al., 1993).

Clinical Presentation

At presentation, approximately 74% of patients with NHL have nonspecific symptoms consisting of unexplained fever, drenching night sweats, or weight loss greater than 10% of their total body weight (Doll & Ringenberg, 1989; Levine, 1992). Differential diagnosis is required to exclude opportunistic infections with a similar clinical presentation, such as cytomegalovirus and mycobacterial infection, as well as HIV wasting.

In up to 25% of persons with HIV disease and NHL, the lymphoma is confined to the CNS (Formenti et al., 1989; Rosenblum et al., 1988). The most common symptoms are confusion, lethargy, and memory loss. Other symptoms include hemiparesis, aphasia, seizures, cranial nerve palsies, headache, numbness of the chin, and stiff neck (Kaplan, 1990; Levine, 1992).

Diagnosis

Aside from noninvasive radiographic techniques, such as computed tomographic scanning, magnetic resonance imaging, ultrasonography, and gallium scanning, bone marrow aspiration and lumbar puncture are usually included in the diagnostic evaluation (Levine, 1992). The diagnosis of CNS lymphoma is complicated. NHL cannot be differentiated from other CNS infections, such as toxoplasmosis, on the basis of computed tomographic scanning or magnetic resonance imaging (Kaplan, 1990). To avoid brain biopsy, the patient may have to undergo empiric treatment for toxoplasmosis. Definitive diagnosis of NHL is by histologic tissue examination.

Treatment

Kaplan and Northfelt (1992) emphasized that treatment should be individualized and recommend the following: (1) standard-dose chemotherapy may be appropriate for patients with good immune function and without a prior opportunistic infection; (2) a lower-dose treatment regimen might be selected for the patient with more severe immunologic compromise, a marginal Karnofsky performance scale score, and a history of opportunistic infection; and (3) for some severely ill patients, therapy may be withheld altogether. According to Milliken and Boyle (1993), chemotherapy often fails to induce remission, is complicated by the development of an opportunistic infection, is poorly tolerated in the presence of bone marrow dysfunction, and may exacerbate the immunosuppression induced by HIV and lead to earlier death.

Since no standard regimen for treating NHL associated with AIDS has been established, therapy must be individualized. Successful therapy has been associated with a low-dose modification of the combination of methotrexate, bleomycin, doxorubicin, cyclophosphamide, vincristine, and dexamethasone (m-BACQD regimen, modified) (Levine, 1992). Regimens using a combination of chemotherapy, antiretroviral agents, prophylaxis for *Pneumocystis carinii* pneumonia and the use of colony-stimulating factors (mainly granulocyte CSF) offer promise for decreasing morbidity and mortality rates and are currently being investigated (Milliken & Boyle, 1993). Brain radiotherapy for CNS lymphoma has demonstrated successful response (Baumgartner et al., 1990). Despite advances in therapy for AIDS-related NHL, responses are usually short in duration and have not had a major impact on survival (Kaplan & Northfelt, 1992).

Considerations for Nursing

Persons with HIV disease and NHL may require the nurse's assistance in making decisions about therapy. Questions regarding risk versus benefit, survival, and adverse effects of chemotherapy and irradiation are common, especially if the client has been learning about HIV disease. A client's demands for concrete statistics and survival data can be frustrating for both the client and the nurse because a standard treatment approach has not been established.

MYCOBACTERIUM AVIUM COMPLEX DISEASE

Epidemiology

Mycobacterium avium-intracellulare is ubiquitous and has been isolated from soil, water, animals, birds, and foodstuffs such as eggs and nonpasteurized dairy products. *M. avium-intracellulare* is often referred to as atypical mycobacterial infection and is noncommunicable, with little evidence of person-to-person transmission (Sanders & Horowitz, 1990). *M. avium-intracellulare* appears to have little virulence in the normal host.

Mycobacterium avium complex (MAC) causes disseminated disease in up to 40% of patients with HIV disease in the United States (Chaisson et al., 1992; Havlik et al., 1992; Horsburgh et al., 1991). Studies of MAC in HIV-infected individuals indicate that the infection appears as a result of primary acquisition of the organism rather than reactivation of a previous infection, except in the southeastern part of the United States, where preexisting exposure to MAC is common (Chaisson & Volberding, 1990; Horsburgh, 1991). The primary risk factor for development of MAC infection is a CD4$^+$ T-cell count of less than 100 mm^3, and infection is rare in patients with higher counts (Horsburgh, 1991).

Pathogenesis

MAC is acquired orally or inhaled, with the gastrointestinal tract or respiratory tract, respectively, acting as a portal of entry. In persons with HIV infection, colonization can progress to dissemination. In the respiratory tract, focal pneumonia can occur but is relatively uncommon, occurring in about 4% of the cases (Ruf et al., 1990). Localized gastrointestinal tract infection may involve the esophagus, duodenum, and small or large intestine (Horsburgh, 1991). Dissemination can involve the blood, bone marrow, liver, spleen, and lymph nodes, and the organism has been recovered from the eye, brain, meninges, cerebrospinal fluid, skin, tongue, heart, lung, stomach, thyroid, breast, parathyroid, adrenal glands, kidneys, pancreas, prostate gland, testis, and urine (Horsburgh, 1991; Klatt et al., 1987; Pitchenik & Fertel, 1992; Wallace & Hannah, 1988).

Clinical Presentation

The most common clinical features are unexplained systemic symptoms of fever, with or without night sweats, weight loss, and debilitation (Chaisson et al., 1992; Hawkins et al., 1986; Modilevsky et al., 1989; Wallace & Hannah, 1988). Other symptoms include chronic diarrhea, abdominal pain, anemia, malabsorption resembling Whipple's disease, extrahepatic biliary obstruction, and intraabdominal lymphadenopathy (Horsburgh, 1991; Pitchenik & Fertel, 1992). Although rare, clinical symptoms of MAC may be present and may include pneumonia, arthritis, skin lesions, pericarditis, meningitis, endophthalmitis, osteomyelitis, and infection of the lymph nodes and rectal mucosa in association with Kaposi's sarcoma (Pitchenik & Fertel, 1992).

Diagnosis

Definitive diagnosis of MAC infection is established by culture of any sterile site, but blood, bone marrow, and lymph nodes are the most likely sites of involvement (CDC, 1987; 1992a; Klatt et al., 1987; Wallace & Hannah, 1988). MAC infection may be misdiagnosed as HIV wasting syndrome because the presenting symptoms are similar.

Treatment

Essential concepts basic to treatment are that MAC, unlike tuberculosis, is not communicable to the general population, the efficacies of current drug therapy are modest, and MAC is less often fatal than tuberculosis

when left untreated (Pitchenik & Fertel, 1992). The decision to treat a person with HIV disease and MAC is highly individual and takes into account several factors including (1) the severity of illness, (2) the general state of health, (3) the potential for drug adverse effects or intolerance, (4) the presence of concurrent infections or diseases and the required therapy, and (5) potential adverse reactions with incompatible agents (Sanders & Horowitz, 1990; Small & Hopewell, 1990). Clement (1990) recommended that individuals with constitutional symptoms, bacteremia, bone marrow dysfunction, gastrointestinal disease, or active pulmonary disease be treated and that persons with renal or hepatic dysfunction or no symptoms be excluded from treatment. Although the goals of treatment are to reduce bacterial load and reduce symptoms to improve the quality of life, consideration must be given to the significant toxicity of the multiple drug regimens required to treat MAC infection.

Treatment regimens vary and can include anywhere from two to six drugs, including azithromycin, amikacin, clarithromycin, clofazimine, ethambutol, ciprofloxacin, rifampin, rifabutin, cycloserine, ethionamide, and streptomycin (Horsburgh, 1991; Katlama & Dickinson, 1993; Pitchenik & Fertel, 1992).

Since MAC infection in association with HIV disease occurs in significant numbers of individuals and results in substantial mortality rates as well as reduced survival time, the CDC (1993c) recommends that patients with HIV infection and a $CD4^+$ T-cell count of <100 mm^3 should receive prophylaxis against MAC with rifabutin. Results of controlled trials of rifabutin prophylaxis against MAC in patients with HIV disease have demonstrated a reduction in the frequency of disseminated infection (Nightengale et al., 1993).

Considerations for Nursing

Many health care workers are unaware that the genus *Mycobacterium* is one of the most widely distributed bacterial genera and contains approximately 19 medically important species, of which MAC is one (Sanders & Horowitz, 1990). Therefore it is not unusual for staff members hearing the word *Mycobacterium* to institute acid-fast bacillus (AFB) precautions that would prevent person-to-person airborne transmission, which is appropriate with *M. tuberculosis* but unnecessary with MAC infection. Staff education is essential so that unnecessary isolation precautions are not instituted. Explaining to the staff that MAC is not spread from person to person and is often referred to as an atypical, noncommunicable disease may help.

Drug interactions are frequently encountered with antimycobacterial agents. Both rifabutin and rifampin have approximately 33 potential drug interactions. An important drug-drug interaction of rifabutin is that it decreases the effectiveness of oral contraceptives and may lead to menstrual irregularities and pregnancy (Szoka & Edgren, 1988). Therefore women must be informed and assisted in selecting alternative forms of birth control when taking rifabutin.

MYCOBACTERIAL TUBERCULOSIS

Epidemiology

The number of cases of tuberculosis (TB) reported annually in the United States decreased steadily from 1954 to 1983, and then the trend dramatically reversed, the incidence increasing by 3% in 1986, by 5% in 1989, and by 6% in 1990 (Barnes et al., 1991). TB is not evenly distributed throughout all segments of the United States. Although New York City represents 3% of the nation's population, it accounts for the highest incidence of TB in the United States, or 14% of the nation's cases (New York State Department of Health, AIDS Institute, 1993). Worldwide estimates are that 1.7 billion persons, one third of the world's population, are infected with *Mycobacterium tuberculosis,* resulting in 8 million new cases of TB and 2.9 million deaths annually (Arachi, 1991).

The most potent risk factor for the development of TB is coinfection with HIV (Barnes et al., 1991). Groups known to have a higher

prevalence of TB infection include medically underserved populations (including some African Americans, Latinos, Asians and Pacific Islanders, American Indians, and Alaskan Natives), homeless persons, current or former prison inmates, alcoholics, injection drug users, elderly persons, foreign-born persons from areas of the world with a high prevalence of TB (e.g., Asia, Africa, the Caribbean, and Latin America), and contacts of persons with active TB (CDC, 1990b). Groups with a higher risk of progression from latent TB infection to active disease include persons with certain medical conditions including HIV infection, silicosis, postoperative recovery from gastrectomy or jejunoileal bypass surgery, body weight less than 10% below the ideal, chronic renal failure, diabetes mellitis, therapy-induced immunosuppression, hematologic disorders (e.g., leukemia and lymphomas), and certain malignancies; persons who have been infected with TB in the past 5 years; children less than 5 years of age; and persons with fibrotic lesions on chest x-ray film (CDC, 1990b).

Among the increasing number of tuberculosis cases, large outbreaks of multiple drug–resistant TB (MDR-TB) have recently been reported (Edlin et al., 1992; Fischl et al., 1992; Frieden et al., 1993; Pearsen et al., 1992). The principal causes of MDR-TB are thought to be attributed to the ingestion of single antituberculosis agents for prolonged periods or erratic compliance with therapy (Barnes & Barrows, 1993). The majority of patients reported with MDR-TB are HIV infected, and nearly all the patients have organisms that are resistant to both isoniazid and rifampin. Many of the outbreaks of MDR-TB have been associated with nosocomial transmission, affecting health care workers as well as patients. Factors contributing to these outbreaks include (1) delayed diagnosis of TB, (2) delayed recognition that the TB was in fact MDR-TB, with resultant prolonged ineffective therapy and prolonged periods of infectiousness, (3) delayed initiation and adequate duration of TB isolation, (4) inadequate ventilation in TB isolation rooms, (5) lapses in TB isolation practices, and (6) inadequate precautions for cough-inducing procedures (Barnes & Barrows, 1993).

Pathogenesis

M. tuberculosis is carried in airborne particles, known as droplet nuclei, that can be generated when persons with pulmonary or laryngeal TB sneeze, cough, speak, or sing. The particles are estimated to be approximately 1 to 5 microns in size, and normal air currents keep them airborne and can spread them throughout a room or building (Wells, 1955). Infection occurs when a susceptible person inhales the droplet nuclei and they reach the alveoli of the lungs. Once in the alveoli, the organisms spread throughout the body. Usually within 2 to 10 weeks after initial infection, the immune response limits the multiplication and spread of the tubercle bacilli. However, some of the bacilli remain dormant and viable for many years. This is referred to as latent TB infection, and these persons have positive results on a purified protein derivative (PPD) skin test. They have no symptoms of active TB (disease) and are not infectious. The estimated lifetime risk in these individuals for the development of active TB is approximately 10% (Barnes et al., 1991).

HIV infection is considered to be the strongest risk factor for the progression from latent TB infection to active TB disease, with an estimated 8% to 10% per year (Selwyn et al., 1989). Persons with HIV who become newly infected with TB have an even greater risk for the development of active TB (Edlin et al., 1992; Dooley et al., 1992). The most notable clinical feature of tuberculosis in HIV-infected persons is the high frequency of extrapulmonary disease, usually with concomitant pulmonary tuberculosis (Barnes et al., 1991; Barnes & Barrows, 1993).

Clinical Presentation

Clinically apparent TB can precede, coincide with, or follow a diagnosis of AIDS. Consistent with the nature of clinical problems associated with HIV disease, the clinical features vary with the degree of immuno-suppression; the more severe the $CD4^+$ lymphopenia, the more atypical the clinical presentation (Chaisson & Volberding, 1990).

Fever, weight loss, night sweats, and fatigue may be the initial complaints, but these symptoms, along with lymphadenopathy, are present in other diseases associated with HIV disease. Whereas dyspnea, chills, hemoptysis, and chest pain may occur with pulmonary TB infection, extrapulmonary disease occurs in 40% to 75% of individuals with a dual diagnosis of HIV disease and TB (CDC, 1989a). Extrapulmonary sites or fluids that may show evidence of TB in HIV-infected persons include lymph nodes, bones, joints, bone marrow, liver, spleen, cerebrospinal fluid, skin, gastrointestinal mucosa, CNS, mass lesions (tuberculoma), urine, and blood or tuberculosis bacteremia (Jacobson, 1992).

Diagnosis

Persons with HIV infection may have suppressed reactions to tuberculin skin testing because of anergy, especially with low $CD4^+$ T-cell counts. In the presence of anergy, they will have a negative tuberculin skin test result whether or not they are infected with *M. tuberculosis*. Persons with HIV infection should be evaluated for anergy in conjunction with PPD testing (see Chapter 5, Table 5–4).

In most cases of HIV infection, a chest x-ray film will suggest mycobacterial disease; however, in some instances the chest x-ray film may appear normal, even in the presence of TB, or may reveal interstitial infiltrates similar to those seen with *Pneumocystis carinii* pneumonia (PCP) (Barnes et al., 1991). Acid-fast smears and culture examination of three sputum specimens collected on different days are the main diagnostic test for pulmonary TB. Sputum smears that fail to demonstrate acid-fast bacilli do not exclude the diagnosis of TB. In HIV-infected persons with pulmonary TB, sputum smears may be less likely to reveal acid-fast bacilli (Klein et al., 1989). A positive result on culture of sputum or another clinical specimen, with organisms identified as *M. tuberculosis,* provides a definitive diagnosis of TB. Conventional laboratory methods used to identify *M. tuberculosis* may require 4 to 8 weeks for results. New techniques for the diagnosis of TB include radiometric culture methods, combined with a DNA probe for an *M. tuberculosis*– specific ribosomal RNA sequence, which allows for the identification of *M. tuberculosis* in 1 to 3 weeks (Barnes & Barrows, 1993). The most promising diagnostic method is the polymerase chain reaction for mycobacterial DNA (Barnes & Barrows, 1993).

Treatment

Currently the CDC (1993d) recommends that a four-drug regimen with isoniazid, rifampin, pyrazinamide, and either streptomycin or ethambutol be used for initial empiric treatment of TB. When adherence with the regimen is assured, such as with directly observed therapy (DOT), the four-drug regimen usually results in effective treatment and a rapid sputum conversion. The four-drug regimen can also be administered in a DOT program, either three times a week from the beginning of therapy or twice a week after a 2-week induction phase of daily therapy (CDC, 1993d). Patients who are treated with the four-drug regimen, but who default on therapy, are more likely to be cured and not relapse than patients on a three-drug regimen (CDC, 1993d). Institutions (e.g. health care and correctional facilities) that have had outbreaks of MDR-TB, or that are resuming therapy for a person with a prior history of anti-TB therapy, may need to use five- or six-drug regimens as initial therapy. The CDC (1993d) offers an alternative regimen in areas where the resistance to isoniazid occurs in less than 4% of the TB cases. The initial therapy may be limited to isoniazid, rifampin, and pyrazinamide.

All persons with TB from whom *M. tuberculosis* has been isolated should have drug-susceptibility testing performed on their first isolate; these results should be reported to the local health department. Drug susceptibility testing will provide the basis for determination of the continuation phase of therapy and identify drug resistance. The treatment of patients with MDR-TB should be determined in consultation with physicians experienced in the treatment of MDR-TB. Second-line medications that may be prescribed for treatment include ciprofloxacin, ofloxacin, kanamycin, amikacin, capreomycin, ethionamide, cycloserine, para-aminosalicylic acid, and/or clofazimine.

Treatment of HIV-infected persons should continue for a total of 9 months and for at least 6 months after sputum conversion (CDC, 1989a). Regimens used for pulmonary TB and extrapulmonary TB are similar. However, therapy may be extended in disseminated disease, miliary disease, disease involving the bones or joints, or tuberculosis lymphadenitis. Treatment regimens for pregnant women should be adjusted because streptomycin may cause congenital deafness and because pyrazinamide teratogenicity has not been determined. Second-line medications that may not be safe in pregnancy include kanamycin, amikacin, capreomycin, ciprofloxacin, ofloxacin, ethionamide, cycloserine, and clofazimine (New York City Department of Health, 1992).

Chemoprophylaxis to prevent the development of active TB should be provided to HIV-infected persons or those likely to be at risk for HIV infection who refuse testing, who have a tuberculin skin test lesion at least 5 mm in diameter, who are close contacts of infectious TB patients, who were previously untreated after a positive PPD test result, and whose chest x-ray films suggest previous untreated TB (CDC, 1991b). Chemoprophylaxis for persons exposed to MDR-TB is a complex issue that should be determined by an expert medical consult; it will usually involve identifying the source patient so that the drug susceptibility pattern can be evaluated.

Mahmoadi and Iseman (1993) studied the records of 35 MDR-TB patients to identify medical mismanagement practices that deviated from established guidelines and determine the impact of these practices on the development of MDR-TB and adverse medical sequelae. Medical mismanagement was detected in 80% of the cases, with an average of 3.93 errors noted per patient record. The most common errors were the addition of a single drug to a failing regimen, failure to identify preexisting or acquired drug resistance, initiation of an inadequate primary regimen, failure to identify and address noncompliance, and inappropriate isoniazid preventive therapy.

Bacille Calmette-Guérin (BCG) is not routinely recommended for use in the United States. Although limited data suggest that the vaccine may be safe for use in HIV-infected, symptom-free children, it is not recommended for HIV-infected adults (CDC, 1993e).

Considerations for Nursing

Health teaching for the person with newly diagnosed HIV and TB should include an explanation of the disease, the treatment plan, and the importance of completing the full course of therapy. Additionally, assessment should include evaluation of the patient's understanding of the teaching provided, individual needs and preferences, living conditions and employment, and factors that may impede the ability of a patient to comply with the prescribed regimen (e.g., cognitive impairment, profound fatigue, and continued drug or alcohol abuse). Before discharge from the hospital, every patient should be evaluated for the need for DOT, and appointments for follow-up should be scheduled. In areas where DOT programs have not been established, a referral for home visits from a visiting nurse should be considered. Patients not receiving DOT therapy who miss appointments or display other nonadherent behaviors should be reported to the local health department.

In addition to monitoring the patient's compliance with the prescribed medication regimen, the nurse should evaluate the clinical response (signs and symptoms) to therapy. Additionally, the nurse should determine whether the client has had frequent loose stools and/or diarrhea, which may be related to malabsorption. Berning and colleagues (1992) reported malabsorption of antituberculosis medications in a person living with AIDS, in association with loose stools with a high fecal fat content.

PNEUMOCYSTOSIS

Epidemiology

Pneumocystis carinii is a ubiquitous organism with a worldwide distribution. It exists in human lungs and has been identified in the lungs of rats, rabbits, guinea pigs, dogs, mice, goats, sheep, cattle, monkeys, foxes, shrews, swine, and cats (Hughes, 1982). Although the organism can be found in the air, on food, and in water, transmission appears to be by the airborne route (Hughes, 1982). Seroepidemiologic studies have indicated that the most healthy children have acquired *P. carinii* infection by 4 years of age (Hopewell, 1992). Approximately 80% of the population has detectable antibodies to *P. carinii*, indicating primary infection early in life (Phair et al., 1990).

The most common respiratory complication in patients with AIDS is opportunistic pneumonia caused by *P. carinii* (Weinberger, 1993). Since 1987 the incidence of PCP has decreased significantly. The decrease has been attributed to the introduction of antiviral therapy and the initiation of standard prophylactic strategies to prevent PCP. Without PCP prophylaxis, it is estimated that 75% of PWHIV will have PCP during the course of their illness (Phair et al., 1990).

Pathogenesis

According to Walzer (1990), *P. carinii* has such low virulence that the initial infection in an immunocompetent person is suppressed by normal host defense mechanisms and causes no observable damage. In immunocompromised hosts, PCP is usually a reactivation of a latent infection as a result of childhood exposure (Hopewell, 1992). Hughes (1982) demonstrated that the organism is communicable and that horizontal transmission may occur from sources of infection to susceptible persons (e.g., persons who are immunodeficient).

HIV-infected individuals are at greatest risk for PCP when the CD4$^+$ T-cell count is <200 mm^3 or <20% of total circulating lymphocytes, or when they have had a previous episode of PCP (Phair et al., 1990). Although

P. carinii infection is generally confined to the lungs, extrapulmonary pneumocystosis can occur. Hematogenous dissemination from a pulmonary site has involved infection in the skin, external auditory canal, meninges, eye, plural space, lymph nodes, heart, spleen, and liver (Hopewell, 1992).

Clinical Presentation

According to Hopewell (1992), clients usually have fever, fatigue, and weight loss for several weeks to months before respiratory symptoms develop. Thrush, indicative of severe immunocompromise, is usually present, along with a $CD4^+$ cell count less than 200 cells/mm^3. The initially mild presentation and insidious onset are characteristic of PCP in persons with HIV disease (Levine & White, 1988). The most common symptoms are fever; shortness of breath, usually manifested initially as dyspnea on exertion and later noted also at rest; and cough, which usually starts out dry and nonproductive and later becomes productive (Hopewell, 1992; Levine & White, 1988).

The initial cough may be productive in clients who smoke or have bacterial bronchitis or pneumonia. In the presence of severe immunocompromise, the body's host defense mechanisms are severely impaired and fever may not be present. Kales and colleagues (1987), in a review of 140 patients with AIDS and PCP, noted the presence of fever in 86%. In 6% to 7% of the clients the initial presentation of PCP is asymptomatic (Levine & White, 1988).

Diagnosis

HIV-infected individuals treated with zidovudine and pentamidine aerosol prophylaxis may have a decrease in the severity of PCP if it does develop, resulting in subtle symptom presentation (Hopewell, 1992). None of the regimens used for PCP prophylaxis have been shown to be completely protective against PCP for HIV-infected persons (Masur, 1992). Additionally, HIV-infected individuals who have not been receiving health care follow-up or PCP prophylaxis or both may have marked symptoms and advanced pneumonia at presentation.

Chest x-ray findings usually reveal diffuse interstitial or alveolar infiltrates, or both, but atypical findings range from normal chest x-ray films to the presence of a localized infiltrate, nodule, cavity, or pneumothorax (Weinberger, 1993). Arterial blood gas studies may reveal hypoxemia, hypocapnia, and an increase in the alveolar/arterial oxygen gradient, especially with exercise (Hopewell, 1990).

Definitive diagnosis of PCP is by identification of *P. carinii* by microscopy. Specimens are usually obtained by induced sputum procedures or by bronchoscopy. Presumptive diagnosis can be made based on (1) a history of dyspnea on exertion or nonproductive cough of recent onset (within the past 3 months); (2) chest x-ray evidence of diffuse bilateral interstitial infiltrates or gallium scan evidence of diffuse bilateral pulmonary disease; (3) arterial blood gas analysis showing an arterial oxygen tension of less than 70 mm Hg or a low respiratory diffusing capacity (less than 80% of predicted values); and (4) no evidence of bacterial pneumonia (CDC, 1992a). The detection of *P. carinii* in extrapulmonary sites is difficult, and even repeated biopsies may fail to yield a definitive diagnosis (Ravalli et al., 1990).

Treatment

The drugs of choice for the treatment of PCP are either TMP-SMX or pentamidine isethionate (Weinberger, 1993). Other agents that may be prescribed include trimethoprim-dapsone, clindamycin-primaquine, or atovaquone. The newest drug approved to treat moderate to severe PCP is trimetrexate glucuronate, which has antineoplastic and antifolate as well as antiprotozal activities (Feinberg et al., 1992; Voelker, 1994).

Intubation and mechanical ventilation may improve the chance of survival for PWHIV with PCP associated with respiratory failure (Efferen et al., 1989). Adjunctive corticosteroid therapy for moderate to severe

PCP reduces the mortality rate and the need for mechanical ventilation (Nielsen et al., 1992; Weinberger, 1993). However, the use of corticosteroids in patients with advanced immunosuppression caused by HIV infection may result in increased incidence of cytomegalovirus disease (Nelson et al., 1993).

Primary prophylaxis (to prevent an initial episode of PCP) is indicated for HIV-infected patients if their CD4$^+$ cell count is <200 mm^3 or CD4$^+$ cells are <20% of total lymphocytes (U.S. Public Health Service, 1993). Because of variations in repeated CD4$^+$ cell counts, some experts advise considering PCP prophylaxis in patients with higher CD4$^+$ cell counts (e.g., between 200 and 250 mm^3) (Bozzette et al., 1990). Other considerations for the initiation of prophylaxis include the presence of HIV-related thrush and unexplained fevers as well as rapidly declining CD4$^+$ cell counts (U.S. Public Health Service, 1993). Secondary prophylaxis (to prevent a recurrence of PCP) is an absolute necessity for patients with a history of PCP.

The preferred drugs for prophylaxis are orally administered TMP-SMX or aerosol preparations of pentamidine administered with the Respirgard II jet nebulizer (Marquest) or the Fisons ultrasonic handheld nebulizer (Fisoneb, Fisons). Other regimens that are being studied but are not as yet recommended include aerosol administration of pentamidine by other nebulization devices, intermittent parenteral administration of pentamidine, and oral administration of dapsone-pyrimethamine, sulfadoxine with pyrimethamine, clindamycin-primaquine, a quinoline, and atovaquone (U.S. Public Health Service, 1993). Intolerance to TMP-SMX and aerosol administration of pentamidine may require that one of these regimens be employed. Oral dapsone therapy has recently been recommended as an alternative to the use of TMP-SMX and pentamidine (El-Sadr et al., 1994).

Considerations for Nursing

Nurses should understand clearly that PCP or disseminated pneumocystosis may still develop in persons receiving primary or secondary PCP prophylaxis. Therefore HIV-infected individuals should be taught to pay attention to signs and symptoms of infection development, even when they are afebrile, and to seek medical advice. The causes of prophylactic therapy failure include poor compliance, unusual or erratic pharmacokinetics, or resistance by pathogens to a specific drug (Masur, 1992). Pentamidine aerosol therapy results in minimal systemic absorption of the drug and provides minimal prophylaxis against extrapulmonary pneumocystosis.

Clinicians administering pentamidine aerosol therapy should be aware that occupational hazards include considerable environmental contamination by the aerosol delivery system and/or coughing by the patient during the procedure. Environmental contaminants include droplets containing pentamidine and infectious microorganisms aerosolized from the patient's lungs (U.S. Public Health Service, 1993).

PNEUMONIA, RECURRENT

Epidemiology

Selwyn and colleagues (1988) conducted the first prospective study of HIV-infected persons without AIDS. They studied a group of injection drug users who were enrolled in a methadone treatment program and found a markedly increased incidence of bacterial pneumonia associated with HIV infection in injection drug users without AIDS. Their clinical data as well as data from other studies have shown a higher mortality rate among this group (Farizo et al., 1992; Polsky et al., 1986; Witt et al., 1987). It is believed that needle sharing, environmental conditions associated with exposure to respiratory pathogens, and cofactors such as heavy alcohol use and inadequate nutrition may predispose patients to bacterial pneumonia (Farizo et al., 1992).

Streptococcus pneumoniae and *Haemophilus influenzae* are the most common causes of bacterial pneumonia in persons with HIV infection (Farizo et al., 1992; Selwyn et al., 1992). These organisms are also the most frequent cause of community-acquired pneumonia in immunocompetent individuals. Other causes of bacterial pneumonia include *Branhamella catarrhalis, Legionella pneumophila,* and *Nocardia asteroides. Pseudomonas aeruginosa* pneumonia is often associated with end-stage disease, previous use of multiple antibiotics, and frequent hospitalizations (Zuger, 1992).

The AIDS Surveillance Data Project found that individuals with a CD4$^+$ T-lymphocyte count less than 200 cells/mm^3 had a five times greater chance of having one episode of bacterial pneumonia in a 12-month period than an HIV-infected person with a CD4$^+$ T-cell count more than 200 cells/mm^3 (CDC, 1992a). In addition, the risk of having multiple episodes of bacterial pneumonia in a 12-month period is 20 times higher in the group with a lower CD4$^+$ cell count (CDC, 1992a).

Pathogenesis

Microorganisms that cause bacterial pneumonia reach the lungs by (1) direct inhalation of the organism, (2) aspiration of secretions from the mouth and nasopharynx, (3) spread by the blood to the lungs from another site, and (4) penetration of the lung tissue (Reynolds, 1991).

As HIV infection progresses, it has an adverse effect on humoral immunity and B-cell function. Defects in B-cell function lead to failure to develop antibody responses to microorganisms. It is believed that this adverse effect by HIV leads to repeated episodes of bacterial pneumonia in the HIV-infected individual. Community-acquired pneumonias generally occur earlier in the course of HIV infection, whereas nosocomial infections are also associated with higher morbidity and mortality rates.

Clinical Presentation

The presentation of bacterial pneumonia in the person with HIV infection may differ from that in the immunocompetent individual. There may be a more abrupt onset, with fever, cough with purulent sputum, and systemic toxic effects. With pneumococcal pneumonia and a significantly decreased CD4$^+$ cell count, there may be more bacteremia, more empyema, and a higher mortality rate. It is

common to see concurrent bacterial pneumonia and PCP. Bacterial pneumonia may also be difficult to differentiate from PCP (Magnenat et al., 1991; Selwyn et al., 1992).

Diagnosis

As of January 1993, recurrent bacterial pneumonia was included in the CDC definition of AIDS (CDC, 1992a). Recurrent bacterial pneumonia is defined as two or more episodes of bacterial pneumonia within 1 year, regardless of the CD4$^+$ cell count.

The chest radiograph is the first diagnostic procedure performed. In an immunocompetent individual the chest radiograph frequently shows dense segmental or lobar consolidation. Diffuse interstitial infiltrates are more typically seen with persons with HIV infection and bacterial pneumonia (Zuger, 1992). The majority of patients with HIV infection and bacterial pneumonia do have an atypical chest radiograph initially (Magnenat et al., 1991).

Microscopic examination and culture of respiratory secretions are essential to determine the appropriate treatment. The specimen should also be obtained before antimicrobial therapy is instituted. If the patient is unable to produce sputum, then sputum induction is indicated. Bronchoscopy with bronchial-alveolar lavage is useful in identifying the organisms if less invasive diagnostic tests are unsuccessful (Magnenat et al., 1991).

Treatment

Empiric antimicrobial therapy should be started while laboratory studies are awaited. If a community-acquired organism is suspected, a drug active against *S. pneumoniae* and *H. influenzae* should be used. It may be possible to treat this type of pneumonia with oral antibiotic therapy on an outpatient basis.

A pneumonia that develops during hospitalization is probably caused by a gram-negative bacilli or *Staphylococcus aureus*. A broad-spectrum antibiotic should be started until there is an identification of the organism. When results of cultures and sensitivities are available, the treatment can be changed to an antimicrobial agent appropriate for the identified organism. Additional treatment measures include fluids, antipyretic drugs, airway suction or postural drainage, and bronchodilators for bronchospasm (Reynolds, 1991).

Pneumococcal vaccination is recommended by the CDC (1989b). Rose and colleagues (1993) concluded after analyzing the effectiveness of pneumococcal vaccine in HIV-infected individuals that it is a reasonable prevention strategy at all stages of immunodeficiency.

Considerations for Nursing

Any patient with a newly acquired cough should be encouraged to see his or her physician. Intervention in the early stages may allow for outpatient treatment with orally administered antibiotics.

For a hospitalized patient, a new cough or fever should be evaluated for the presence of TB as well as pneumonia. After an initial intravenous course of antibiotics, patients may complete their antibiotic therapy orally on an outpatient basis.

Patients should be instructed in the importance of completing antibiotics as prescribed. Discontinuation of the drug may lead to relapse. In addition, patients with a new cough should be strongly discouraged from taking antibiotics that they may have left from previous treatments. It should be explained to them that antibiotics are not interchangeable; they are specific for specific organisms. By taking unprescribed antibiotics, they may initially mask the symptoms and cause delay in the identification of the organism, which may lead to a more severe episode of pneumonia.

PROGRESSIVE MULTIFOCAL LEUKOENCEPHALOPATHY

The Papovaviridae are a family of viruses that contain two genera, papillomavirus and polyomavirus. Papillomavirus is associated with infection of surface epithelia, which produces benign tumors or warts (Dix & Bredesen, 1988; Lehrich, 1990). Polyomaviruses include three types: the J.C. virus, the B.K. virus (both labeled with the initials of the name of the patient from whom they were first isolated), and simian virus 40 (SV40). The J.C. virus is associated with progressive multifocal leukoencephalopathy (PML), and the B.K. virus causes hemorrhagic cystitis in immunocompromised individuals (Chaisson & Griffin, 1990). The SV40 virus, which causes asymptomatic latent infection in rhesus monkeys, was accidentally introduced into large numbers of people immunized against the poliovirus between 1955 and 1961 (Chaisson & Griffin, 1990; Dix & Bredesen, 1988). No evidence that this exposure produced illness has been found, although seroconversion to SV40 was detectable in 20% of vaccine recipients (Chaisson & Griffin, 1990; Dix & Bredesen, 1988). Thus far, SV40 has been recovered from the brains of two patients with PML, neither of whom had received the SV40-contaminated polio vaccine or been exposed to monkeys (Dix & Bredesen, 1988).

Epidemiology

The J.C. virus is distributed worldwide. Both the J.C. and B.K. viruses cause childhood infection without a recognized disease syndrome, as evidenced by the fact that 50% of children by 6 years of age demonstrate seroconversion to these viruses (Chaisson & Griffin, 1990). By 9 years of age, essentially all people have been infected by the B.K. virus, and by middle adulthood, 80% to 90% of the population has become infected with the J.C. virus (Chaisson & Griffin, 1990). Evidence suggests that the appearance of PML in persons with HIV disease is associated with the phenomenon of latency and reactivation of the J.C. virus related to immunosuppression. PML is diagnosed in approximately 4% of patients with AIDS (Worley & Price, 1992).

Pathogenesis

The kidney is considered the site of latent J.C. virus infection, as evidenced by the presence of the virus in urine; hematogenous spread by lymphocytes to the brain is suspected (Chaisson & Griffin, 1990). PML is a subacute demyelinating disease of the CNS. Multiple lesions develop in white matter of the cerebrum, and sometimes in the brain stem or cerebellum, resulting in focal neurologic deficits. The disease progresses rapidly, often leads to dementia, blindness, and paralysis, and in most cases results in death within 1 year (Dix & Bredesen, 1988). Berger and Mucke (1988) reported prolonged survival (more than 30 months) after diagnosis in two individuals with AIDS and PML.

Clinical Presentation

Berger and colleagues (1987) found that initial manifestations of PML included extremity weakness, cognitive dysfunction, visual loss, gait disturbance, limb incoordination, headache, and speech or language disturbance. In addition, they found that the spectrum of neurologic illness most often included spastic hemiparesis, visual field loss, and altered mentation throughout the course of the disease.

Symptoms attributable to cerebellar involvement include ataxia, limb dysmetria, and dysarthria. Cortical infection manifestations include aphasia, apraxia, Gerstmann's syndrome, prosopagnosia, left-sided neglect, and impaired spatial orientation. Berger and colleagues (1987) concluded that some of these symptoms may be attributable to coexisting HIV encephalitis, because PML is a disease of white matter.

Diagnosis

The physician is faced with a differential diagnosis including CNS toxoplasmosis, primary CNS lymphoma, PML, and AIDS-dementia complex, cryptococcal meningitis, and other CNS opportunistic infections and neoplasms. Although computed tomographic scanning, magnetic resonance imaging, angiography, and electroencephalography may contribute to diagnosis, a definitive diagnosis of PML requires microscopic examination of brain tissue, usually obtained by stereotactic biopsy (Berger & Levy, 1993; Ragland, 1993).

Treatment

No form of therapy for PML has been efficacious. Attempted therapies have included the use of prednisone, acyclovir, and adenine arabinoside administered both intravenously and intrathecally; cytosine arabinoside; platelets matched by human leukocyte antigen (HLA); HLA-matched lymphocytes; and zidovudine (Berger et al., 1987; Dix & Bredesen, 1988; Ragland, 1993). Case reports and small trials have demonstrated some benefit from prolonged use of cytosine arabinoside, administered either intravenously or intrathecally or by both routes (Ragland, 1993). There have also been isolated reports of spontaneous remission of PML (Berger & Levy, 1993; Ragland, 1993).

High-dose zidovudine therapy has also been reported to be beneficial. It is theorized that immune function may be enhanced by blockage of the synergistic effect of HIV and PML (Ragland, 1993).

Considerations for Nursing

PML requires intensive nursing care and places demands on the staff. Medicine has little to offer as far as treatment is concerned. Assessment and planning should take into account the psychologic trauma encountered by families, lovers, spouses, and significant others, as well as nursing staff, as they watch an ambulatory, communicative, social human being become bedbound, bowel and bladder incontinent, and devoid of interaction with surroundings. In the end stages of the disease, quadriplegia and coma often appear (Lehrich, 1990). With the support of significant others, many individuals can be safely cared for with the assistance of a home care or hospice program. In some cases the lack of these support systems or the burdens of care make a skilled nursing facility more appropriate for long-term care.

SALMONELLOSIS

Epidemiology

Salmonellae are gram-negative bacteria that can be pathogenic to both animals and man. *Salmonella* is the most commonly reported cause of food-borne outbreaks in the United States, accounting for 15,162 cases of illness, 1,734 hospitalizations, and 53 deaths between 1985 and 1992 (CDC, 1993b). The incidence of salmonellosis among persons with AIDS has been estimated to be 100-fold greater than among the general population (Sperber & Schleupner, 1987).

In humans, *Salmonella* is usually acquired by ingestion of contaminated food or water (Hook, 1990). Other reported modes of acquisition include ingestion of contaminated medications or diagnostic agents; direct fecal-oral spread, especially with sexual activities that include anilingus with an infected person; transfusion of contaminated blood products; and inadequately sterilized fiberoptic instruments used in upper gastrointestinal tract endoscopic procedures (Hook, 1990).

Although *Salmonella* may be transmitted from person to person, infection in animals is the principal source of nontyphoidal *Salmonella* in humans. *Salmonella* has been found in chickens, turkeys, ducks, cows, pigs, turtles, cats, dogs, mice, guinea pigs, hamsters, doves, pigeons, parrots, starlings, sparrows, cowbirds, sheep, seals, donkeys, lizards, and snakes (Hook, 1990). With the exclusion of *Salmonella typhi*, of which humans are the only known reservoirs, almost all *Salmonella* species produce disease in both animals and humans. Significant sources of human infection are chickens, turkeys, ducks, and their eggs, which may contain not only surface contamination but also infected yolks (Hook, 1990). In 1990, dramatic increases in *Salmonella enteritidis* infection associated with contaminated eggs in New England and the mid-Atlantic states were reported (CDC, 1990c).

Meats, especially beef and pork, and raw and powdered milk are often implicated in outbreaks of *Salmonella* infection (Hook, 1990). Raw meat and poultry, purchased in retail markets, are frequently contaminated with *Salmonella,* and food handlers are more likely to be symptom-free carriers of *Salmonella* than are members of the general population (Hook, 1990).

Other sources of *Salmonella* include pets, especially turtles; waterborne outbreaks involving *S. typhi*, also called typhoid fever; ingested items contaminated with animal ma-

nure (this caused a marijuana-associated outbreak in 1981); nosocomial spread from person to person by the hands or clothing of hospital staff; and fomites such as dust, patient care equipment, and furniture (Hook, 1990).

Hidden culprits in disease transmission may include cultural beliefs and practices. Riley and colleagues (1988) reported salmonellosis in Hispanic persons ingesting rattlesnake capsules. The ingestion of rattlesnake meat or dried powder is a well-described Mexican folk remedy. Pharmacies in Hispanic neighborhoods in Mexico and southern California sell the capsules under a variety of names: *vibra de cascabel, pulvo de vibora,* and *carne de vibora.*

Pathogenesis

The development of disease after *Salmonella* ingestion is related to the virulence of the organism, inoculum size, and the host defenses. In HIV-infected individuals with severe cell-mediated immunodeficiency, infection can become disseminated. *Salmonella* passes through the stomach and begins multiplying in the small intestine. Small inocula of *Salmonella* may be inactivated by gastric pH, but larger inocula may survive and cause infection (Chaisson et al., 1990). *Salmonella* can then pass through the intestinal mucosa to the large lymphatic vessels and, through hematogenous spread, can infect any organ. Jacobs and colleagues (1985) isolated *Salmonella* in cultures of specimens from lungs, heart, brain, liver, spleen, kidneys, and bone marrow of persons with AIDS and salmonellosis. Destruction of the gastrointestinal mucosa in persons with AIDS, resulting from concurrent lesion-producing infections with such agents as cytomegalovirus, *Candida,* and herpes simplex, can also provide easy access for salmonellae to enter the bloodstream (Chaisson et al., 1990).

Clinical Presentation

In immunocompetent individuals, salmonellosis symptoms are most often confined to the gastrointestinal tract, but persons with HIV disease appear to lack localizing signs indicating salmonellosis (Chaisson et al.,

1990). Nonspecific signs and symptoms include fever (seen in virtually all cases), chills, sweats, weight loss, diarrhea, and anorexia (Chaisson et al., 1990).

Diagnosis

Diagnosis of *Salmonella* infection is based on bacterial culture. Because many persons with HIV disease and salmonellosis have *Salmonella* bacteremia, routine blood cultures can provide the diagnosis. Stool cultures may yield the organism in individuals with blood cultures negative for *Salmonella*. Despite treatment, cultures may continue to yield the organism (Chaisson et al., 1990). Recurrent *Salmonella* bacteremia despite appropriate treatment has been reported (Nadelman et al., 1985; Sperber & Schleupner, 1987).

Treatment

Although treatment of nontyphoid salmonellosis is usually unnecessary in immunocompetent individuals, it is required in persons with HIV disease (Chaisson et al., 1990). Antibiotic selection depends on drug sensitivities; however, ampicillin and chloramphenicol are most often used. Despite the efficacy of TMP-SMX, Chaisson and colleagues (1990) recommended that the drug combination not be used because of the possibility of allergic reactions and the potential need for them later to treat PCP. Other agents employed to treat salmonellosis in HIV disease include third-generation cephalosporin, amoxicillin, ciprofloxacin, and nonfloxacin. Because chronic infection and relapse are common in persons with HIV disease, suppressive therapy, usually with the above-named antibiotics, is necessary to prevent recurrence. Some individuals, even while continuing suppressive therapy, may have recurrent infection and may require retreatment with intravenous antibiotic therapy.

Considerations for Nursing

Because *Salmonella* infection is preventable, HIV-infected persons should be taught how to avoid infection as soon as the diagnosis of HIV disease is known. See Appendix IV for information on food safety, water safety, pet care, and travel. When taking a health history, the nurse should include cultural practices that may expose the client to pathogens, such as exposure to animal blood or ingestion of raw animal products.

Nurses should be aware of the need to wear gloves and practice meticulous hand washing when handling fecal material, especially from HIV-infected persons with diarrhea of unknown cause. They should also be aware of the role that clothing may have in *Salmonella* transmission and should wear a plastic apron or disposable gown when providing care to a client with fecal incontinence. The plan of care should include environmental cleaning to reduce the potential for transmission of fomites. Although enteric precautions are employed when the diagnosis is known, the potential problem of *Salmonella* infection exists before the definitive diagnosis is made. Therefore barrier precautions should be practiced routinely.

TOXOPLASMOSIS

Epidemiology

Toxoplasma gondii is an obligate protozoan that causes toxoplasmosis in humans and domestic animals. Infection with *T. gondii* occurs worldwide, and the organism infects herbivorous, carnivorous, and omnivorous animals. Although the definitive hosts of *Toxoplasma* are members of the cat family, not all cats are infected. McCabe and Remington (1990) noted that excretion of *Toxoplasma* oocysts has been reported in approximately 1% of the cats in diverse parts of the world. Although cats are considered of primary importance in transmission of the infection, toxoplasmosis has been found in locales without cats, and a low prevalence of infection has been reported in areas with cats (McCabe & Remington, 1990). Wallace and associates (1993) studied 723 HIV-infected adults to determine whether cat ownership contributed to the risk of toxoplasmosis, and found that cat ownership/exposure did not appear to be a risk factor for seroconversion.

The prevalence of *Toxoplasma* tissue cysts in meat consumed by humans is high. Although tissue cysts are rarely found in beef, as much as 25% of lamb and pork samples tested have been shown to contain the cysts (McCabe & Remington, 1990). Cockroaches, flies, earthworms, snails, and slugs may serve as transport hosts for the oocyst, and ingestion of vegetables containing cysts probably accounts for *Toxoplasma* seropositivity in vegetarians (McCabe & Remington, 1990). Oocysts have also been found in nonpasteurized goat's milk and in eggs. The major means of transmission of *Toxoplasma* to humans is through ingestion of meats and vegetables containing oocysts (McCabe & Remington, 1990; Remington & McLeod, 1992). The only evidence of human-to-human transmission is from mother to fetus when the mother has acquired infection during pregnancy. Rarer documented sources of infection include accidental self-inoculation by laboratory workers, transfusion of infected whole blood or white blood cells, and organ transplantation (McCabe & Remington, 1990).

Serologic surveys to detect *T. gondii* have demonstrated that 15% to 68% of adults in the United States and more than 90% of the adults in some European countries, most notably France and Germany, have previously acquired the infection (Gellin & Soave, 1992). Toxoplasmosis is currently estimated to occur in 3% to 40% of all patients with AIDS (Porter & Sande, 1992).

Approximately 30% to 38% of HIV-infected patients with serologic evidence of infection with *T. gondii* will develop toxoplasmosis (Gellin & Soave, 1992; Israelski et al., 1993). However, Porter and Sande (1992) found that one in every six (N = 115) patients in whom CNS toxoplasmosis developed did not have serologic evidence of infection.

Prophylaxis with TMP-SMX, used to prevent PCP, may also confer some protection against toxoplasmosis. Ruskin and LaRiviene (1991), in a study of the efficacy of TMP-SMX prophylaxis for PCP, found that toxoplasmosis did not occur in any of the patients receiving the drug.

Pathogenesis

After entering the body, usually by ingestion, *Toxoplasma* replicates, disseminates via the blood and lymphatic vessels, and causes asymptomatic or mildly symptomatic infection in an immunocompetent host. In an immunodeficient host, such as a person with HIV disease, regardless of whether the infection is primary or secondary (reactivation), the organism rapidly causes focal or diffuse meningoencephalitis with cellular necrosis (McCabe & Remington, 1990; Reinis-Lucey et al., 1990). Jautzke and colleagues (1993) studied 80 autopsy cases to identify extracerebral toxoplasmosis in other organs and demonstrated infection in cardiac muscle, lungs, liver, pancreas, gastrointestinal tract, adrenal glands, lymph nodes, and testis.

Clinical Presentation

Despite the severity of infection, the symptoms of toxoplasmosis in a person with AIDS may be vague and nonspecific and are sometimes ignored (Reinis-Lucey et al., 1990). In a review of the literature by Israelski and Remington (1988), 44% to 56% of the patients complained of headache and 60% had altered mental status manifested as confusion, lethargy, delusional behavior, frank psychosis, global cognitive impairment, anomia, and coma; the presence of fever varied from a low of 10% of the cases to 74%. The most common focal neurologic deficit is hemiparesis; others include aphasia, ataxia, visual field loss, cranial nerve palsies, dysmetria, and motor disorders. In approximately one third of AIDS patients with toxoplasmosis, seizures are the initial reason for seeking medical attention (Israelski et al., 1990). Symptoms attributable to extracerebral toxoplasmosis include diarrhea, adrenal insufficiency, peritonitis, orchitis, pneumonia, myocarditis, hepatitis, and gastric outlet obstruction (Gellin & Soave, 1992). Babies of HIV-infected women who have no history of *T. gondii* infection during pregnancy have been noted to have congenital toxoplasmosis (Mitchell et al., 1990).

Diagnosis

In the presence of HIV disease, the appearance of neurologic symptoms can suggest any number of opportunistic infections and neoplastic processes. The physician must direct the clinical diagnosis not only toward establishing the presence of toxoplasmosis but also toward clearly ruling out other infections such as cryptococcal meningitis, progressive multifocal leukoencephalopathy, herpes simplex encephalitis, mycobacterial encephalitis, HIV disease of the CNS, and neoplasms such as primary lymphoma of the brain and Kaposi's sarcoma.

In most cases, toxoplasmosis in clients with laboratory-confirmed HIV disease is diagnosed presumptively according to guidelines suggested by the CDC (1987). These guidelines include (1) recent onset of focal neurologic abnormality consistent with intracranial disease or a reduced level of consciousness, (2) brain imaging evidence of a lesion having a mass effect (on computed tomography or nuclear magnetic resonance imaging) or whose radiographic appearance is enhanced by injection of contrast medium, and (3) serum antibody to *Toxoplasma* or successful response to therapy for toxoplasmosis (CDC, 1987; 1992a). However, Porter and Sande (1992) did report that the absence of detectable serum antibodies to *Toxoplasma* cannot exclude a diagnosis of cerebral toxoplasmosis.

Treatment

The mainstay of therapy for toxoplasmosis in PWHIV has been the combination of pyrimethamine and sulfadiazine (or trisulfapyrimidines). Symptoms usually diminish within 8 to 10 days, and abnormalities on computed tomographic scanning resolve between the first and fourth weeks of therapy (Reinis-Lucey et al., 1990). Adjunctive therapy may include dexamethasone for abscesses associated with a severe mass effect, phenytoin for infection-induced seizure, and folinic acid to ameliorate the bone marrow toxicity of pyrimethamine (Reinis-Lucey et al., 1990). Israelski and Remington (1988) emphasized that folic acid should not be used because it inhibits the action of pyrimethamine (i.e., the destruction of *Toxoplasma* by blocking folic acid metabolism of the organism).

PWHIV who take sulfadiazine and pyrimethamine for toxoplasmosis have a high incidence of adverse reactions. Severe adverse reactions necessitating discontinuation of this regimen during the initial treatment phase may occur in 40% to 60% of the patients (Haverkos, 1987; Israelski & Remington, 1988; McCabe & Remington, 1990). Usually an alternative regimen is selected. Alternative regimens include cessation of sulfadiazine and continuation of pyrimethamine alone or with the addition of clindamycin. Dannemann and associates (1992) found clindamycin with pyrimethamine to be effective therapy for toxoplasmosis encephalitis in persons with AIDS. Although clindamycin appears to be effective for toxoplasmosis chorioretinitis, it does not penetrate the CNS well and should not be used alone for CNS toxoplasmosis (Reinis-Lucey et al., 1990).

As with most opportunistic infections in PWHIV, suppressive therapy is necessary because cure is not possible. Agents employed are pyrimethamine with or without sulfadiazine, pyrimethamine-sulfadoxine, and clindamycin.

There has been interest in toxoplasmosis prophylaxis. Carr and colleagues (1992) evaluated the effectiveness of low-dose TMP-SMX prophylaxis for toxoplasmosis encephalitis and found it to be effective. Investigation continues in using TMP-SMX prophylactically in individuals with AIDS who have CD4$^+$ T-cell counts less than 100 mm^3.

Considerations for Nursing

Whether infection with *T. gondii* in a person with AIDS is due to primary or secondary infection (reactivation of latent infection) is often unknown. Because the *Toxoplasma* antibody status of the most persons with HIV disease is unknown and probably some have not been infected, and because toxoplasmosis may be a preventable disease, clients should be taught about prevention of *Toxoplasma* infection as early as possible in the course of HIV disease. See Appendix IV for information on food safety, water safety, pet care, and travel.

For the person with AIDS and toxoplasmosis, emphasis on health teaching, follow-up, and evaluation of compliance with a suppressive therapy regimen is essential to prevent relapse. Factors that may impede compliance, such as cognitive impairment or continuation or resumption of alcohol or drug use, should be assessed when individualized follow-up is planned. Often a significant other is asked to assume some responsibility for suppressive therapy, since the client may be unable to do so. Porter and Sande (1992) found that 60% of patients who stopped suppressive therapy had a relapse, and 22% who continued suppressive therapy had recurrent disease.

WASTING SYNDROME CAUSED BY HIV

Epidemiology

According to King (1990), prospective and retrospective studies have demonstrated that 91% to 100% of PWHIV lose weight. Weight loss in PWHIV in the United States is more often sporadic than the unremitting weight loss seen in Third World countries, where treatment for AIDS-related diseases and HIV are not available (Grunfeld, 1992). Sharkey and associates (1992) found that a decrease in the CD4$^+$ T-cell count correlated positively with a decrease in weight. Precise estimates of the incidence of HIV wasting may be difficult to determine. Nahlen and colleagues (1993), in a study of 26,251 persons with AIDS reported to the CDC between 1987 and 1991, found individuals at risk of being injection drug users more likely to be reported with wasting syndrome. However, careful analysis revealed that the identification of HIV wasting in persons with AIDS was probably related to geographic variations in diagnostic and reporting practices and to differences in access to medical care.

Pathogenesis

Mechanisms of weight loss and malnutrition, seen in HIV disease, can be re-lated to reduced food intake, malabsorption of nutrients, and altered metabolism of nutrients (Life Sciences Research Office [LSRO], 1990). Factors related to reduced food intake include anorexia, oral or esophageal lesions, nausea and/or vomiting, diarrhea, neurologic or psychiatric conditions, fatigue, inadequate finances, lack of facilities to store and prepare food, lack of knowledge about nutrition, disinterest in diet and weight loss, and side effects of medications.

Nutritional malabsorption is related to injury to the small intestine and, in some instances, disease of the digestive organs. Kotler (1992) identified three categories of intestinal disease: primary infection of the enterocytes (e.g., cryptosporidiosis, isosporiasis); secondary involvement from systemic or disseminated disorders (e.g., cytomegalovirus infection or Kaposi's sarcoma); and inflammatory bowel disease (e.g., intestinal infection caused by HIV).

Metabolic changes may be related to alterations in cytokine activities as a result of HIV or other infections (Kotler, 1992). Hypermetabolic states, in the presence of active secondary infections, have shown weight loss averaging 5% of body weight in 28 days (Grunfeld, 1992). Changes in measures of nutritional status seen in HIV disease include nutrients such as protein, amino acids, lipids, folate, vitamins B_{12} and B_6, zinc, selenium, copper, and iron (LSRO, 1990).

Clinical Presentation

The most common symptoms seen in HIV wasting syndrome are anorexia, diarrhea, nausea and/or vomiting, oral lesions, dysphagia, taste and/or smell changes, physical limitations, neuropsychiatric symptoms including HIV encephalopathy, medication interactions and/or side effects, and allergies and/or intolerance (Newman, 1992). Additional symptoms that may be noted are odynophagia, steatorrhea, abdominal pain, and polyuria, polydypsia, and polyphagia, along with neuropathy, indicating the presence of diabetes.

Diagnosis

Diagnosis of HIV is made only with a definitive diagnosis of HIV infection based on laboratory confirmation. The criteria for the diagnosis of HIV wasting syndrome include profound involuntary weight loss of >10% of baseline body weight plus either chronic diarrhea (at least two loose stools per day for ≥30 days), or chronic weakness and documented fever (for ≥30 days, intermittent or constant) in the absence of a concurrent illness or condition other than HIV infection that could explain the findings (e.g., neoplasm, tuberculosis, enteritis) (CDC, 1992a).

Treatment

While disease-specific causes of weight loss are being investigated, symptom control is a primary concern (Cimoch, 1992). Agents used to treat nausea and vomiting include phenothiazine derivatives, benzquinamide hydrochloride, trimethobenzamide hydrochloride, hydroxyzine, metoclopramide, scopolamine, dronabinol, and ondansetron hydrochloride. Treatment of anorexia includes the use of megestrol acetate or dronabinol. Management of diarrhea includes the use of antimotility agents (e.g., loperamide hydrochloride, diphenoxylate/atropine), luminal-acting agents (e.g., fiber, kaolin, pectin), and hormonal agents such as octreotide.

Oral supplements most frequently used for treatment of weight loss include Ensure, Sustacal, and Resource (Cimoch, 1992). For patients with fat malabsorption, Lipisorb and Isosource may be prescribed. Newer products that are designed to help modulate the immune system, currently under study for efficacy, include Immun-Aid, Alitra Q, and Impact. Elemental products that may be prescribed are Opti, Vital High Nitrogen, and Vivonex T.E.N. Chlebowski and colleagues (1993) demonstrated the benefits of nutritional support by prescribing an enterotropic peptide-based formula (a nutritional supplement known as Advera) versus standard enteral formulas in the treatment of HIV-infected patients. In addition to maintaining weight, the patients who received this supplement had significantly reduced hospitalizations.

Because of the risk, expense, and inconvenience, parenteral nutrition is usually considered a final option except for severe malnutrition associated with disease involving the entire small intestine and malabsorption, in which total parenteral nutrition is indicated (LSRO, 1990; Task Force on Nutrition Support in AIDS, 1989). Parenteral products such as amino acids, lipids, and glutamine are expensive and have not been proved efficacious in the treatment of HIV-related malnutrition (Cimoch, 1992).

Considerations for Nursing

Nutrition counseling and education should be provided as soon as HIV is diagnosed (see Appendix IV). Although weight loss is a common occurrence in HIV disease, it should not be casually accepted as a consequence of the disease process. Kotler and colleagues (1989) provided important evidence that maintaining body mass can prolong survival in AIDS. Strategies to maximize food intake include substituting calorie containing and nutrient-dense foods and beverages for low- or no-calorie foods and beverages; increasing the number and/or size of feedings daily; fortifying foods with caloric- and protein-containing ingredients; using caloric-containing condiments; modifying the diet according to tolerance; and adding nutritional supplements as indicated (Newman, 1992).

NURSING RESEARCH RELATED TO AIDS-INDICATOR DISEASES

Nursing research specific to AIDS-indicator diseases is virtually nonexistent. Ragsdale (1993) in a review of the literature suggests that collaborative nursing research is needed especially in the areas of physiologic responses to illness and the related nursing care. Considerations for future nursing research include the following:

1. Descriptive studies identifying physiologic responses associated with each of the AIDS diagnoses

2. Qualitative research using focus groups to identify individual responses to the AIDS-indicator diseases

3. Identification of the comorbidities of AIDS-indicator diseases and the associated signs and symptoms, with exploration of gender differences

4. Identification of self-care strategies that PWHIV employ to cope with various AIDS-indicator diseases

5. Identification of the costs of nursing care for PWHIV

6. Comparison of diagnostic differences between nurse practitioners, physician's assistants, and physicians in regard to AIDS-indicator diseases

SUMMARY

A current definition of nursing is the diagnosis and treatment of human responses to actual or potential health problems (American Nurses' Association, 1980). Therefore nursing a client with a diagnosis of AIDS means that the nurse must have full knowledge of the pathologic nature of HIV disease, as well as the common AIDS-related diseases (Ungvarski, 1987). Without this knowledge, the identification of the client's biobehavioral responses becomes difficult, limiting the effectiveness of the nurse-client relationship and the nursing process. As the complexities of HIV disease and advances in its treatment continue to evolve, the nurse will be challenged to maintain an up-to-date knowledge base.

REFERENCES

Abrams, J., Farhood, A.I. (1989). Infection-associated vascular lesions in acquired immunodeficiency syndrome patients. *Human Pathology, 20*(10), 1025–1026.

Adler, S. (1992). Hospital transmission of cytomegalovirus. *Infectious Agents and Disease, 1*(1), 43–49.

American Foundation for AIDS Research (1993). Opportunistic infections and related disorders. *AIDS/HIV Treatment Directory, 4*(4), 1–108.

American Nurses' Association (1980). *Nursing: A social policy statement.* Kansas City, MO: The Association.

Ampel, N.M., Wieden, M.A., Galgiani, J.N. (1989). Coccidioidomycosis: Clinical update. *Review of Infectious Diseases, 11*(6), 897–911.

Anand, R., Nightingale, S.D., Fish, R.H., et al. (1993). Control of cytomegalovirus retinitis using sustained release of intraocular ganciclovir. *Archives of Ophthalmology, 111*(February), 223–227.

Angrist, B., d'Hollosy, M., Satriano, J., et al. (1991). Central nervous system stimulants as symptomatic treatment for AIDS-related neuropsychiatric impairment. *Journal of Clinical Psychopharmacology, 12*(4), 268–272.

Arachi, A. (1991). The global tuberculosis situation and the new control strategy of the World Health Organization. *Tubercle, 72,* 1–6.

Armstrong, D. (1989). Problems in management of opportunistic fungal diseases. *Review of Infectious Diseases, 11*(suppl 7), S1591–S1599.

Balcarek, K.B., Bagley, R., Cloud, G., et al. (1990). Cytomegalovirus infection among employees of a children's hospital: No evidence for increased risk associated with patient care. *Journal of the American Medical Association, 263*(6), 840–844.

Balfour, C.L., Balfour, H.H. (1986). Cytomegalovirus is not an occupational risk for nurses in renal transplant and neonatal units: Results of a prospective study. *Journal of the American Medical Association, 256*(14), 1909–1914.

Barnes, P.F., Barrows, S.A. (1993). Tuberculosis in the 1990s. *Annals of Internal Medicine, 119*(5), 400–410.

Barnes, P.F., Block, A.B., Davidson, P.T., Snider, D.E. (1991). Tuberculosis in patients with human immunodeficiency virus infection. *New England Journal of Medicine, 324*(23), 1644–1650.

Barone, R., Ficarra, G., Gaglioti, D., et al. (1990). Prevalence of oral lesions among HIV-infected intravenous drug abusers and other risk groups. *Oral Surgery, Oral Medicine and Oral Pathology, 69*(2), 169–172.

Bartlett, J.A. (1993). Cryptosporidiosis. *PAACNOTES, 5*(3), 110–112.

Baumgartner, J., Rachlin, J., Beckstead, J., et al. (1990). Primary central nervous system lymphomas: Natural history and response to radiation therapy in 55 patients with acquired immune deficiency syndrome. *Journal of Neurosurgery, 73*(2), 206–211.

Bennett, C.L., Adams, J., Gertler, P., et al. (1992). Relation between hospital experience and in-hospital mortality for patients with AIDS-related *Pneumocystis carinii* pneumonia: Experience from 3,126 cases in New York City in 1987. *Journal of Acquired Immune Deficiency Syndromes, 5*(9), 856–864.

Benson, M.C., Kaplan, M.S., O'Toole, K., et al. (1988). A report of cytomegalovirus cystitis and a review of other genitourinary manifestations of the acquired immune deficiency syndrome. *Journal of Urology, 140*(1), 153–154.

Beral, V. (1991). Epidemiology of Kaposi's sarcoma. *Cancer Surveys, 10,* 5–22.

Beral, V., Bull, D., Darby, S., et al. (1992). Risk of Kaposi's sarcoma and sexual practices associated with fecal contact in homosexual or bisexual men with AIDS. *Lancet, 339*(8794), 632–635.

Beral, V., Peterman, T.A., Berkelman, R.L., et al. (1990). Kaposi's sarcoma among persons with AIDS: A sexually transmitted infection? *Lancet, 335*(8682), 123–128.

Berger, J.R., Kaszovitz, B., Post, M.J., et al. (1987). Progressive multifocal leukoencephalopathy associated with human immunodeficiency virus infection: A review of the literature with a report of sixteen cases. *Annals of Internal Medicine, 107*(1), 78–87.

Berger, J.R., Levy, R.M. (1993). The neurologic complications of human immunodeficiency virus infection. *Medical Clinics of North America, 77*(1), 1–23.

Berger, J.R., Mucke, L. (1988). Prolonged survival and partial recovery in AIDS associated progressive multifocal leukoencephalopathy. *Neurology, 38*(7), 1060–1065.

Berger, T. (1990). Dermatologic manifestations of AIDS. In P.T. Cohen, M.A. Sande, & P.A. Volberding (Eds.), *The AIDS knowledge base* (pp. 531.1, 531.25). Waltham, MA: Medical Publishing Group.

Berning, S.F., Huitt, G., Iseman, M.D., et al. (1992). Malabsorption of antituberculosis medications by a patient with AIDS [letter]. *New England Journal of Medicine, 327*(25), 1817–1818.

Bobak, I.M., Jensen, M.D., Lowdermilk, D.L. (1993). *Maternity and gynecologic care* (5th ed.). St. Louis, MO: Mosby–Year Book.

Boccellari, A.A., Dilley, J.W., Chambers, D.B., et al. (1993). Immune function and neuropsychological performance in HIV-1–infected homosexual men. *Journal of Acquired Immune Deficiency Syndromes, 6*(6), 592–601.

Boccellari, A., Dilley, J.W., Shore, M.D. (1988). Neuropsychiatric aspects of AIDS dementia complex: A report on a clinical series. *Neurotoxicology, 9*(3), 381–389.

Bornstein, R.A., Nasrallah, H.A., Para, M.F., et al. (1993). Neuropsychological performance in symptomatic and asymptomatic HIV infection. *AIDS, 7*(4), 519–524.

Bowden, F.J., McPhee, D.A., Deacon, N.J., et al. (1991). Antibodies to gp41 and nef in an otherwise HIV-negative homosexual man with Kaposi's sarcoma. *Lancet, 337*(8753), 1313–1314.

Bozzette, S.A., Sattler, F.R., Chiu, J., et al. (1990). A controlled trial of early adjunctive treatment with corticosteroids for *Pneumocystis carinii* pneumonia in the acquired immunodeficiency syndrome. *The New England Journal of Medicine, 323*(21), 1451–1457.

Britton, C.B. (1993). The neurology of HIV infection: Clinical, pathogenetic and treatment perspectives. *AIDS, 7*(suppl 1), S218–S223.

Brodman, M., Deligdisch, L. (1986). Cytomegalovirus endometritis in a patient with AIDS. *Mount Sinai Journal of Medicine, 53*(8), 673–675.

Bronnimann, D.A., Adam, R.D., Galgiani, J.N., et al. (1987). Coccidioidomycosis in the acquired immunodeficiency syndrome. *Annals of Internal Medicine, 106*(3), 372–379.

Brown, H.H., Glasgow, B.J., Holland, G.N., et al. (1988a). Cytomegalovirus infection of the conjunctiva in AIDS. *American Journal of Ophthalmology, 106*(1), 102–104.

Brown, S., Senekjian, E.K., Montag, A.G. (1988b). Cytomegalovirus infection of the uterine cervix in a patient with acquired immunodeficiency syndrome. *Obstetrics and Gynecology, 71*(3, Pt. 2), 489–491.

Byrne, W.R., Dietrich, R.A. (1989). Disseminated coccidioidomycosis with peritonitis in a patient with acquired immunodeficiency syndrome: Prolonged survival associated with positive skin test reactivity to coccidioidin. *Archives of Internal Medicine, 149*(4), 947–948.

Carpenter, C.C., Mayer, K.H., Stein, M.D., et al. (1991). Human immunodeficiency virus infection in North American women: experience with 200 cases and a review of the literature. *Medicine, 70*(5), 307–325.

Carr, A., Tindall, B., Brew, B.J., et al. (1992). Low-dose trimethoprim-sulfamethoxazole prophylaxis for toxoplasmic encephalitis in patients with AIDS. *Annals of Internal Medicine, 117*(2), 106–111.

Cello, J.P. (1992). Gastrointestinal tract manifestations of HIV infection. In M.A. Sande & P.A. Volberding (Eds.), *The medical management of AIDS* (3rd ed.) (pp. 176–192). Philadelphia, PA: W.B. Saunders.

Centers for Disease Control (1984). Update: Treatment of cryptosporidiosis in patients with acquired immunodeficiency syndrome (AIDS). *Morbidity and Mortality Weekly Report, 33*(9), 117–119.

Centers for Disease Control (1987). Revision of the CDC surveillance case definition for acquired immunodeficiency syndrome. *Morbidity and Mortality Weekly Report, 36*(No. 1S), 3S–15S.

Centers for Disease Control (1989a). Tuberculosis and human immunodeficiency virus infection: Recommendations of the Advisory Committee for the Elimination of Tuberculosis (ACET). *Morbidity and Mortality Weekly Report, 38*(14), 236–238, 243–250.

Centers for Disease Control (1989b). Immunization practices advisory committee (ACIP). Pneumococcal polysaccharide vaccine. *Morbidity and Mortality Weekly Report, 38*, 64–68, 73–76.

Centers for Disease Control (1990a). Risk for cervical disease in HIV infected women. *Morbidity and Mortality Weekly Report, 39*(47), 846–849.

Centers for Disease Control (1990b). Screening for tuberculosis and tuberculosis infection in high-risk populations and the use of preventive therapy for tuberculosis infection in the United States. *Morbidity and Mortality Weekly Report, 39*(RR-8), 1–12.

Centers for Disease Control (1990c). Update: *Salmonella enteritidis* infections and grade A shell eggs—United States, 1989. *Morbidity and Mortality Weekly Report, 38*(51-52), 877–882.

Centers for Disease Control (1991a). Waterborne-disease outbreaks. *Morbidity and Mortality Weekly Report, 40*(SS-3), 1–22.

Centers for Disease Control (1991b). Purified protein derivative (PPD)–tuberculin anergy and HIV infection: Guidelines for anergy testing and management of anergic persons at risk of tuberculosis. *Morbidity and Mortality Weekly Report, 40*(RR-5), 27–33.

Centers for Disease Control and Prevention (1992a). Revised classification system for HIV infection and expanded surveillance case definition for AIDS among adolescents and adults. *Morbidity and Mortality Weekly Report, 41*(RR-17), 1–19.

Centers for Disease Control and Prevention (1992b, October). *Addendum to the proposed expansion of the AIDS surveillance case definition.* Atlanta, GA: CDC.

Centers for Disease Control and Prevention (1993a). Impact in the United States of expanding the AIDS surveillance case definition, first quarter, 1993. *HIV/AIDS Prevention, 4*(2), 3.

Centers for Disease Control and Prevention (1993b). Coccidioidomycosis—United States, 1991–1992. *Morbidity and Mortality Weekly Report, 42*(2), 21–24.

Centers for Disease Control and Prevention (1993c). Recommendations on prophylaxis and therapy for disseminated *Mycobacterium avium* complex for adults and adolescents infected with human immunodeficiency virus. *Morbidity and Mortality Weekly Report, 42*(No. RR-9), 17–20.

Centers for Disease Control and Prevention (1993d). Initial therapy for tuberculosis in the era of multidrug resistance. *Morbidity and Mortality Weekly Report, 42*(RR-7), 1–8.

Centers for Disease Control and Prevention (1993e). Recommendations of the Advisory Committee on Immunization Practices (ACIP): Use of vaccines and immune globulins in persons with altered immunocompetence. *Morbidity and Mortality Weekly Report, 42*(RR-4), 1–18.

Centers for Disease Control and Prevention (1993f). Outbreaks of *Salmonella enteritidis* gastroenteritis—California, 1993. *Morbidity and Mortality Weekly Report, 42*(41), 793–797.

Chaisson, R.E., Griffin, D.E. (1990). Progressive multifocal leukoencephalopathy in AIDS. *Journal of the American Medical Association, 264*(1), 79–82.

Chaisson, R.E., Moore, R.D., Richman, D.D., et al. (1992). Incidence and natural history of *Mycobacterium avium* complex infections in patients with advanced human immunodeficiency virus disease treated with zidovudine. The Zidovudine Epidemiology Study Group. *American Review of Respiratory Disease, 146*(2), 285–289.

Chaisson, R.E., Sande, M.A., Gerberding, J.L. (1990). Salmonella. In P.T. Cohen, M.A. Sande, & P.A. Volberding (Eds.), *The AIDS knowledge base* (611.1–611.6). Waltham, MA: Medical Publishing Group.

Chaisson, R.E., Stanton, D.L., Gallant, J.E., et al. (1993). Impact of the 1993 revision of the AIDS case definition on the prevalence of AIDS in a clinical setting. *AIDS, 7*(6), 857–862.

Chaisson, R.E., Volberding, P.A. (1990). Clinical manifestations of HIV infection. In G.L. Mandell, R.G. Douglas, Jr., & J.E. Bennett (Eds.), *Principles and practice of infectious diseases* (3rd ed.) (pp. 1059–1092). New York: Churchill Livingstone.

Chernoff, D. (1990). Histoplasmosis. In P.T. Cohen, M.A. Sande, & P.A. Volberding (Eds.), *The AIDS knowledge base* (pp. 634.1–634.4). Waltham, MA: Medical Publishing Group.

Chernoff, D., Sande, M.A. (1990a). Candidiasis. In P.T. Cohen, M.A. Sande, & P.A. Volberding (Eds.), *The AIDS knowledge base* (pp. 632.1–632.6). Waltham, MA: Medical Publishing Group.

Chernoff, D., Sande, M.A. (1990b). Cryptococcosis. In P.T. Cohen, M.A. Sande, & P.A. Volberding (Eds.), *The AIDS knowledge base* (pp. 633.1–633.8). Waltham, MA: Medical Publishing Group.

Chism, J. (1993). Kaposi's sarcoma (KS) treatment overview. *Treatment Issues, 7*(1), 1–5.

Chlebowski, R.T., Beall, G., Grosvenor, M., et al. (1993). Long-term effects of early nutritional support with new enterotropic peptide–based formula versus standard enteral formula in HIV-infected patients: Randomized prospective trial. *Nutrition, 9*(6), 507–512.

Chuck, S.L., Sande, M.A. (1989). Infections with *Cryptococcus neoformans* in the acquired immunodeficiency syndrome. *New England Journal of Medicine, 321*(12), 794–799.

Cimoch, P. (1992). Current agents for the management of wasting and malnutrition in HIV/AIDS. In G. Nary (Ed.), *Nutrition and HIV/AIDS* (vol. 1) (pp. 27–32). Chicago, IL: PAAC Publishing.

Clark, R.A., Greer, D.L., Valainis, G.T., et al. (1990). *Cryptococcus neoformans* pulmonary infection in HIV-1–infected patients. *Journal of Acquired Immune Deficiency Syndromes, 3*(5), 480–484.

Clement, M. (1990). Patient care queries: What is the recommended therapy for *Mycobacterium avium* complex (MAC) infection? *AIDS Clinical Care, 2*(2), 14.

Cockerell, C.J. (1993). Update on cutaneous manifestations of HIV infection. *AIDS, 7*(suppl 1), S213–S218.

Coker, R.J., Vivani, M., Gazzard, B.G., et al. (1993). Treatment of cryptococcosis with liposomal amphotericin B (AmBisome) in 23 patients with AIDS. *AIDS, 7*(6), 829–835.

Collier, A.C., Meyers, J.D., Corey, L., et al. (1987). Cytomegalovirus infection in homosexual men: Relationship to sexual practices, antibody to human immunodeficiency virus, and cell-mediated immunity. *American Journal of Medicine, 82*(3), 593–601.

Concus, A.P., Helfand, R.F., Imber, M.J., et al. (1988). Cutaneous cryptococcosis mimicking molluscum contagiosum in a patient with AIDS [letter]. *Journal of Infectious Diseases, 158*(4), 897–898.

Corey, L., Spear, P.G. (1986). Infection with herpes simplex viruses. *New England Journal of Medicine, 314*(11), 686–691.

Cotton, D.I. (1989). Improving survival in acquired immunodeficiency syndrome: Is experience everything [editorial]? *Journal of the American Medical Association, 261*(20), 3016–3017.

Current, W.L., Garcia, L.S. (1991). Cryptosporidiosis. *Clinical Microbiology Reviews, 4*(3), 325–358.

Cuzzell, J.Z. (1990). Clues: itching and burning skin folds. *American Journal of Nursing, 90*(1), 23–24.

Daar, E.S., Meyer, R.D. (1992). Bacterial and fungal infections. *The Medical Clinics of North America, 76*(1), 173–203.

Daicker, B. (1988). Cytomegalovirus panuveitis with infection of corneotrabecular endothelium in AIDS. *Ophthalmologia, 197*(4), 169–175.

Dannemann, B.R., McCutchan, A., Israelski, D.M. (1992). Treatment of toxoplasmic encephalitis in patients with AIDS: A randomized trial comparing pyrimethamine plus clindamycin to pyrimethamine plus sulfadiazine. *Annals of Internal Medicine, 116*(1), 33–43.

Davis, C.E. (1986). Cryptococcus. In A.I. Braude (Ed.), *Infectious diseases and medical microbiology* (2nd ed.) (pp. 564–571). Philadelphia, PA: W.B. Saunders.

De Wit, S., Weerts, D., Goosens, H., Clumeck, N. (1989). Comparison of fluconazole and ketoconazole for oropharyngeal candidiasis in AIDS. *Lancet, 1*(8641), 746–748.

Dietrich, D.J., Pales, M.A., Lew, E.A., et al. (1993). Concurrent use of ganciclovir and foscarnet to treat cytomegalovirus infection in AIDS patients. *The Journal of Infectious Diseases, 167*(May), 1184–1188.

DiSaia, P.J. (1990). Malignant lesions of the uterine cervix. In J.R. Scott, P.J. DiSaia, C.B. Hammond, & W.N. Spellacy (Eds.), *Danforth's Obstetrics and Gynecology* (6th ed.) (pp. 995–1012). Philadelphia, PA: J.B. Lippincott.

Dismukes, W.E. (1988). Cryptococcal meningitis in patients with AIDS. *Journal of Infectious Disease, 157*(4), 624–628.

Dix, R.D., Bredesen, D.E. (1988). Opportunistic viral infections in acquired immunodeficiency syndrome. In M.L. Rosenblum, R.M. Levy, & D.E. Bredesen (Eds.), *AIDS and the nervous system* (pp. 221–261). New York: Raven Press.

Doll, D.C., Ringenberg, O.S. (1989). Lymphomas associated with HIV infection. *Seminars in Oncology Nursing, 5*(4), 255–262.

Dooley, S.W., Villarino, M.E., Lawrence, M., et al. (1992). Nosocomial transmission of tuberculosis in a hospital unit for HIV-infected patients. *Journal of the American Medical Association, 267*(19), 2632–2635.

Drew, W.L., Bukles, W., Erlich, K.S. (1992). Management of herpesvirus infections (CMV, HSV, VZV). In M.A. Sande & P.A. Volberding (Eds.), *The medical management of AIDS* (3rd ed.) (pp. 359–382). Philadelphia: W.B. Saunders.

Drew, W.L., Erlich, K.S. (1990a). Cytomegalovirus epidemiology. In P.T. Cohen, M.A. Sande, & P.A. Volberding (Eds.), *The AIDS knowledge base* (pp. 643.1–643.4). Waltham, MA: Medical Publishing Group.

Drew, W.L., Erlich, K.S. (1990b). Cytomegalovirus as a cofactor in AIDS. In P.T. Cohen, M.A. Sande, & P.A. Volberding (Eds.), *The AIDS knowledge base* (pp. 644.1–644.2). Waltham, MA: Medical Publishing Group.

Edlin, B.R., Tokars, J.I., Grieco, M.H., et al. (1992). An outbreak of multidrug-resistant tuberculosis among hospitalized patients with acquired immunodeficiency syndrome. *The New England Journal of Medicine, 326*(23), 1514–1521.

Edwards, J.E. (1990). Candida species. In G.L. Mandell, R.G. Douglas, Jr., & J.E. Bennett (Eds.), Principles and practice of infectious diseases (3rd ed.) (pp. 1943–1958). New York: Churchill Livingstone.

Efferen, L.S., Nadarajah, D., Palat, D.S. (1989). Survival following mechanical ventilation for *Pneumocystis carinii* pneumonia in patients with acquired immunodeficiency syndrome: A different perspective. *American Journal of Medicine, 87*(4), 401–404.

Egan, V. (1992). Neuropsychological aspects of HIV infection. *AIDS Care, 4*(1), 3–10.

El-Sadr, W., Oleske, J.M., Agins, B.D., et al. (1994, January). *Evaluation and management of early HIV infection. Clinical Practice Guideline,* No. 7 (AHCPR Publication No. 94-0572). Rockville, MD: Agency for Health Care Policy and Research, Public Health Service, U.S. Department of Health and Human Services.

Engel, J.P., Englund, J.A., Fletcher, C.V., et al. (1990). Treatment of resistant herpes simplex virus with continuous infusion acyclovir. *Journal of the American Medical Association, 263*(12), 1662–1664.

Erice, A., Mayers, D.L., Strike, D.G., et al. (1993). Brief report: Primary infection with zidovudine-resistant human immunodeficiency virus type 1. *The New England Journal of Medicine, 328*(6), 1163–1165.

Erlich, K.S., Jacobson, M.A., Koehler, J.E., et al. (1989). Foscarnet therapy for severe acyclovir-resistant herpes simplex virus type-2 infections in patients with the acquired immunodeficiency syndrome (AIDS). *Annals of Internal Medicine, 110*(9), 710–713.

Erlich, K.S., Mills, J. (1990). Herpes simplex virus. In P.T. Cohen, M.A. Sande, & P.A. Volberding (Eds.), *The AIDS knowledge base* (pp. 642.1–642.16). Waltham, MA: Medical Publishing Group.

Esplin, J.A., Levine, A.M. (1991). HIV-related neoplastic disease: 1991. *AIDS, 5*(suppl 2), S203–S210.

Farizo, K.M., Buehler, J.W., Chamberland, M.E., et al. (1992). Spectrum of disease in persons with human immunodeficiency infection in the United States. *Journal of the American Medical Association, 267*(13), 1798–1805.

Feinberg, J. (1993). Fluconazole versus amphotericin B for acute cryptococcal meningitis: The pendulum swings back. *AIDS Clinical Care 5*(5), 39–43.

Feinberg, J., McDermott, C., Nutter, J. (1992). Trimetrexate (TMTX) salvage therapy for PCP in AIDS patients with limited therapeutic options [abstract No. PoB 3297]. *International Conference on AIDS, 8*(2), B136.

Feingold, A.R., Vermund, S.H., Burk, R.D., et al. (1990). Cervical cytologic abnormalities and papillomavirus in women infected with human immunodeficiency virus. *Journal of Acquired Immune Deficiency Syndromes, 3*(9), 896–903.

Fels, A.O. (1988). Bacterial and fungal pneumonias. *Clinics in Chest Medicine, 9*(3), 449–457.

Fernandez, F., Adams, F., Levy, J.K., et al. (1988). Cognitive impairment due to AIDS-related complex and its response to psychostimulants. *Psychosomatics, 29*(1), 38–46.

Ferreiro, J., Vinters, H.V. (1988). Pathology of the pituitary gland in patients with the acquired immunodeficiency syndrome (AIDS). *Pathology, 20*(3), 211–215.

Fichtenbaum, C.J., Ritchie, D.J., Powderly, W.G. (1993). Use of paromomycin for treatment of cryptosporidiosis in patients with AIDS. *Clinical Infectious Diseases, 16*(February), 298–300.

Fischl, M.A., Krown, S.C., O'Boyer, K.D., et al. (1993). Weekly doxorubicin in the treatment of patients with AIDS-related Kaposi's sarcoma. *Journal of Acquired Immune Deficiency Syndromes, 6*(3), 259–264.

Fischl, M.A. Uttamchardani, R.B., Daikos, G.L., et al. (1992). An outbreak of tuberculosis caused by multiple-drug resistant tubercle bacilli among patients with HIV infection. *Annals of Internal Medicine, 117*(3), 177–183.

Fish, D.G., Ampel, N.M., Galgiani, J.N., et al. (1990). Coccidioidomycosis during human immunodeficiency virus infection. *Medicine (Baltimore), 69*(6), 384–391.

Flanigan, T., Whalen, C., Turner, J., et al. (1992). *Cryptosporidium* infection and CD4 counts. *Annals of Internal Medicine, 116,* 840–842.

Formenti, S.C., Gill, P.S., Lean, E., et al. (1989). Primary central nervous system lymphoma in AIDS: Results of radiation therapy. *Cancer, 15*(63), 1101–1107.

Forstein, M. (1992). The neuropsychiatric aspects of HIV infection. *Primary Care Clinics in Office Practice, 19*(1), 97–117.

Forthal, D., Gordon, R., Larsen, R., et al. (1992). Cigarette smoking increases the risk of developing cryptococcal meningitis [abstract No. PoB 3172]. *International Conference on AIDS, July 19-24, 8*(2), B115.

Franco, E.L. (1991). Viral etiology of cervical cancer: A critique of the evidence. *Review of Infectious Diseases, 13*(6), 1195–1206.

Freedberg, R.S., Gindea, A.J., Dieterich, D.T., et al. (1987). Herpes simplex pericarditis in AIDS. *New York State Journal of Medicine, 87*(5), 304–306.

Frieden, T.R., Sterling, T., Pablos-Merdez, A., et al. (1993). The emergence of drug-resistant tuberculosis in New York City. *The New England Journal of Medicine, 328*(8), 521–526.

Friedman, S.L. (1988). Gastrointestinal and hepatobiliary neoplasms in AIDS. *Gastroenterology Clinics of North America, 17*(3), 465–486.

Friedman-Kien, A.E., Ostreicher, R., Saltzman, B. (1989). Clinical manifestations of classical, endemic African, and epidemic AIDS-associated Kaposi's sarcoma. In A.E. Friedman-Kien (Ed.), *Color atlas of AIDS* (pp. 11–48). Philadelphia: W.B. Saunders.

Friedman-Kien, A.E., Saltzman, B.R., Cos, Y.Z., et al. (1990). Kaposi's sarcoma in HIV-negative homosexual men [letter]. *Lancet, 335*(8682), 168–169.

Gail, M.H., Pluda, J.M., Rabkin, C.S., et al. (1991). Projections of the incidence of non-Hodgkin's lymphoma related to acquired immunodeficiency syndrome. *Journal of the National Cancer Institute, 83*(10), 695–701.

Galgiani, J.N., Ampel, N.M. (1990). Coccidioidomycosis in human immunodeficiency virus–infected patients. *Journal of Infectious Diseases, 162*(5), 1165–1169.

Gellin, B., Soave, R. (1992). Coccidian infections in AIDS: Toxoplasmosis, cryptosporidiosis and isosporiasis. *The Medical Clinics of North America, 76*(1), 205–234.

Gerberding, J.L. (1989). Risks to health care workers from occupational exposure to hepatitis B virus, human immunodeficiency virus, and cytomegalovirus. *Infectious Disease Clinics of North America, 3*(4), 735–745.

Gerberding, J.L., Bryant-LeBlanc, C.E., Nelson, K., et al. (1987). Risk of transmitting the human immunodeficiency virus, cytomegalovirus, and hepatitis B virus to health care workers exposed to patients with AIDS and AIDS-related conditions. *Journal of Infectious Diseases, 156*(1), 1–8.

Glass, R.M. (1988). AIDS and suicide [editorial]. *Journal of the American Medical Association, 259*(9), 1369–1370.

Glatt, A.E., Chirgwin, K., Landesman, S.H. (1988). Treatment of infections with human immunodeficiency virus. *The New England Journal of Medicine, 318*(22), 1439–1448.

Goldsmith, M.F. (1992). Specific HIV-related problems of women gain more attention at a price affecting more women. *Journal of the American Medical Association, 268*(14), 814–816.

Gould, E., Kory, W.P., Raskin, J.B., et al. (1988). Esophageal biopsy findings in the acquired immunodeficiency syndrome (AIDS): Clinicopathologic correlation in 20 patients. *Southern Medical Journal, 81*(11), 1392–1395.

Grant, I.H., Armstrong, D. (1988). Fungal infections in AIDS: Cryptococcosis. *Infectious Disease Clinics of North America, 2*(2), 457–464.

Grant, I., Heaton, R.K. (1990). Human immunodeficiency virus type 1 (HIV-1) and the brain. *Journal of Consulting and Clinical Psychology, 58*(1), 22–30.

Greenspan, J.S., Greenspan, D., Winkler, J.R. (1988). Diagnosis and management of the oral manifestations of HIV infection and AIDS. *Infectious Disease Clinics of North America, 2*(2), 373–385.

Grunfeld, C. (1992). Metabolic disturbances, anorexia, and wasting in HIV/AIDS. In G. Nary (Ed.), *Nutrition and HIV/AIDS* (Vol. 1) (pp. 9–15). Chicago: PAAC Publishing.

Haverkos, H.W. (1987). Assessment of therapy for *Toxoplasma* encephalitis: The TE Study Group. *American Journal of Medicine, 82*(5), 907–914.

Haverkos, H.W. (1990). The search for cofactors in AIDS, including analysis of the association of nitrate inhalant abuse and Kaposi's sarcoma. *Progress in Clinical and Biological Research, 325*, 93–102.

Havlik, J.A., Horburgh, C.R., Metchoch, B., et al. (1992). Disseminated *Mycobacterium avium* complex infection: Clinical identification and epidemiologic trends. *Journal of Infectious Diseases, 165*(3), 577–580.

Hawkins, C.C., Gold, J.W., Whimbey, E., et al. (1986). *Mycobacterium avium* complex infections in patients with the acquired immunodeficiency syndrome. *Annals of Internal Medicine, 105*(2), 184–188.

Henderson, D.K. (1990). Nosocomial herpes virus infections. In G.L. Mandell, R.G. Douglas, Jr., & J.E. Bennett (Eds.), *Principles and practice of infectious diseases* (3rd ed.) (pp. 2236–2245). New York: Churchill Livingstone.

Heyer, D.M., Kahn, J.O., Volberding, P.A. (1990). HIV-related Kaposi's sarcoma. In P.T. Cohen, M.A. Sande, & P.A. Volberding (Eds.), *The AIDS knowledge base* (pp. 713.1–713.19). Waltham, MA: The Medical Publishing Group.

Hibberd, P.L., Rubin, R.H. (1991). Fever in the immunocompromised host. In P.A. Mackowiak (Ed.), *Fever: Basic mechanisms and management* (pp. 197–218). New York: Raven Press.

Hilton, E., Isenberg, H.D., Alperstein, P., et al. (1992). Ingestion of yogurt containing *Lactobacillus acidophilus* as prophylaxis for candida vaginitis. *Annals of Internal Medicine, 116*(5), 353–357.

Hirsch, M.S. (1990). Herpes simplex virus. In G.L. Mandell, R.G. Douglas, Jr., & J.E. Bennett (Eds.), *Principles and practice of infectious diseases* (3rd ed.) (pp. 1144–1153). New York: Churchill Livingstone.

Ho, M. (1990). Cytomegalovirus. In G.L. Mandell, R.G. Douglas, Jr., & J.E. Bennett (Eds.), *Principles and practice of infectious diseases* (3rd ed.) (pp. 1159–1172). New York: Churchill Livingstone.

Hook, E.W. (1990). Salmonella species (including typhoid fever). In G. L. Mandell, R.G. Douglas, Jr., & J.E. Bennett (Eds.), *Principles and practice of infectious diseases* (3rd ed.) (pp. 1700–1716). New York: Churchill Livingstone.

Hopewell, P.C. (1990). *Pneumocystis carinii* pneumonia. In M.A. Sande & P.A. Volberding (Eds.), *The medical management of AIDS* (2nd ed.) (pp. 209–240). Philadelphia: W.B. Saunders.

Hopewell, P.C. (1992). *Pneumocystis carinii* pneumonia: Current concepts. In M.A. Sande & P.A. Volberding (Eds.), *The medical management of AIDS* (3rd ed.) (pp 261–283). Philadelphia: W.B. Saunders.

Horsburgh, C.R. (1991). *Mycobacterium avium* complex infection in the acquired immunodeficiency syndrome. *The New England Journal of Medicine, 324*(19), 1332–1338.

Huang, Y.Q., Li, J.J., Rush, M.G., et al. (1992). HPV-16–related DNA sequences in Kaposi's sarcoma. *Lancet, 339*(8792), 515–518.

Hughes, W.T. (1982). Natural mode of acquisition for de novo infection with *Pneumocystis carinii*. *The Journal of Infectious Diseases, 145*(6), 842–848.

Israelski, D.M., Chmiel, J.S., Poggensee, L., et al. (1993). Prevalence of *Toxoplasma* infection in a cohort of homosexual men at risk for AIDS and toxoplasma encephalitis. *Journal of Acquired Immune Deficiency Syndromes, 6*(4), 414–418.

Israelski, D.M., Dannemann, B.R., Remmington, J.S. (1990). Toxoplasmosis in patients with AIDS. In M.A. Sande & P.A. Volberding (Eds.), *The medical management of AIDS* (2nd ed.) (pp. 241–264). Philadelphia: W.B. Saunders.

Israelski, D.M., Remington, J.S. (1988). Toxoplasmosis encephalitis in patients with AIDS. In M.A. Sande & P.A. Volberding (Eds.), *The medical management of AIDS* (pp. 193–211). Philadelphia: W.B. Saunders.

Jacobs, J.L., Gold, J.W., Murray, H.W., et al. (1985). *Salmonella* infections in patients with the acquired immunodeficiency syndrome. *Annals of Internal Medicine, 102*(2), 186–188.

Jacobson, M.A. (1992). Mycobacterial diseases: Tuberculosis and disseminated *Mycobacterium avium* complex infection. In M.A. Sande & P.A. Volberding (Eds.), *The medical management of AIDS* (3rd ed.) (pp. 284–296). Philadelphia: W.B. Saunders.

Jacobson, M.A., Mills, J. (1988). Serious cytomegalovirus disease in the acquired immunodeficiency syndrome (AIDS): Clinical findings, diagnosis, and treatment. *Annals of Internal Medicine, 108*(4), 585–594.

Janssen, R.S., Nwanyanwu, O.C., Selik, R.M., Stehr-Green, J.K. (1992). Epidemiology of human immunodeficiency virus encephalopathy in the United States. *Neurology, 42*(8), 1472–1476.

Jautzke, G., Sell, M., Thalmann, U., et al. (1993). Extracerebral toxoplasmosis in AIDS: Histological and immunohistological findings based on 80 autopsy cases. *Pathology, Research and Practice, 189*(4), 428–436.

Jenkins, B. (1988). Patients' reports of sexual changes after treatment for gynecological cancer. *Oncology Nursing Forum, 15*(3), 349–354.

Johnson, P.C., Hamill, R.J., Sarosi, G.A. (1989). Clinical review: Progressive disseminated histoplasmosis in the AIDS patient. *Seminars in Respiratory Infections, 4*(2), 139–146.

Jones, C., Orengo, I., Rosen, T., et al. (1990). Cutaneous cryptococcosis simulating Kaposi's sarcoma in the acquired immunodeficiency syndrome. *Cutis, 45*(3), 163–167.

Kales, C.P., Murren, J.R., Torres, R.A., et al. (1987). Early predictors of in-hospital mortality for *Pneumocystis carinii* pneumonia in the acquired immunodeficiency syndrome. *Archives of Internal Medicine, 147*(8), 1413–1417.

Kaplan, L.D. (1990). The malignancies associated with AIDS. In M.A. Sande & P.A. Volberding (Eds.), *The medical management of AIDS* (2nd ed.) (pp. 339–364). Philadelphia: W.B. Saunders.

Kaplan, L.D., Northfelt, D.W. (1992). Malignancies associated with AIDS. In M.A. Sande & P.A. Volberding (Eds.), *The medical management of AIDS* (3rd ed.) (pp. 399–429). Philadelphia: W.B. Saunders.

Katlama, C., Dickinson, G.M. (1993). Update on opportunistic infections. *AIDS, 7*(suppl 1), S185–S194.

King, A.B. (1990). Malnutrition in HIV infection: Prevalence, etiology and management. *PAAC Notes, 2*(3), 122–129.

Klatt, C., Jensen, D.F., Meyer, P.R. (1987). Pathology of *Mycobacterium avium-intracellulare* infection in acquired immunodeficiency syndrome. *Human Pathology, 18*(7), 709–714.

Klein, N.C., Duncason, F.P., Lenox, T.H., et al. (1989). Use of mycobacterial smears in the diagnosis of pulmonary tuberculosis in AIDS/ARC patients. *Chest, 95*(6), 1190–1192.

Kotler, D. (1992). Causes and consequences of malnutrition in HIV/AIDS. In G. Nary (Ed.), *Nutrition and HIV/AIDS* (Vol. 1) (pp. 5–8). Chicago: PAAC Publishing.

Kotler, D.P., Tierney, A.R., Altilio, D., et al. (1989). Body mass repletion during ganciclovir treatment of cytomegalovirus infections in patients with acquired immunodeficiency syndrome. *Archives of Internal Medicine, 149*(4), 901–905.

Krigel, R., Friedman-Kien, A.E. (1988). Kaposi's sarcoma in AIDS: Diagnosis and treatment. In V.T. DeVita Jr., S. Hellman, & S.A. Rosenberg (Eds.), *AIDS: Etiology, diagnosis, treatment and prevention* (pp. 245–261). Philadelphia: J.B. Lippincott.

Krouse, H.J. (1985). A psychological model of adjustment in gynecologic cancer patients. *Oncology Nursing Forum, 12*(6), 45–49.

Krown, S.E., Metroka, C., Wernz, J.C. (1989). Kaposi's sarcoma in the acquired immunodeficiency syndrome: A proposal for uniform evaluation, response, and staging criteria. *Journal of Clinical Oncology, 7*(9), 1201–1207.

Krown, S.E., Myskowski, P.L., Pardes, J. (1992a). Kaposi's sarcoma. *Medical Clinics of North America, 76*(1), 235–252.

Krown, S.E., Paredes, J., Bundow, D., et al. (1992b). Interferon-alpha, zidovudine, and granulocyte-macrophage colony-stimulating factor: A phase I AIDS Clinical Trials Group study in patients with Kaposi's sarcoma associated with AIDS. *Journal of Clinical Oncology, 10*(8), 1344–1351.

Kurtin, P.J., McKinsey, D.S., Gupta, M.R., et al. (1990). Histoplasmosis in patients with acquired immunodeficiency syndrome: Hematologic and bone marrow manifestations. *American Journal of Clinical Pathology, 93*(3), 367–372.

Laine, L., Dretler, R.H., Conteas, C.N., et al. (1992). Fluconazole compared with ketoconazole for the treatment of *Candida* esophagitis in AIDS. *Annals of Internal Medicine, 117*(8), 655–660.

Lange, J.M., Tapper, M.L. (1993). Clinical treatment. *AIDS, 7*(suppl 1), S171–S172.

Laughon, B.E., Druckman, D.A., Vernon, A., et al. (1988). Prevalence of enteric pathogens in homosexual men with and without acquired immune deficiency syndrome. *Gastroenterology, 94*, 984–993.

Lehrich, J.R. (1990). JC, BK, and other polyomaviruses (progressive multifocal leukoencephalopathy). In G.L. Mandell, R.G. Douglas, Jr., & J.E. Bennett (Eds.), *Principles and practice of infectious diseases* (3rd ed.) (pp. 1200–1203). New York: Churchill Livingstone.

Levine, A. (1992). AIDS-associated malignant lymphoma. *The Medical Clinics of North America, 76*(1), 253–268.

Levine, S.J., White, D.A. (1988). *Pneumocystis carinii*. *Clinics in Chest Medicine, 9*(3), 395–423.

Levitz, S.M. (1991). The ecology of *Cryptococcus neoformans* and the epidemiology of cryptococcosis. *Reviews of Infectious Diseases, 13*(6), 1163–1169.

Levy, R.M., Bredesen, D.E. (1988). Central nervous system dysfunction in acquired immunodeficiency syndrome. In M.L. Rosenblum, R.M. Levy, & D.E. Bredesen (Eds.), *AIDS and the central nervous system* (pp. 29–63). New York: Raven Press.

Life Sciences Research Office, Federation of American Societies for Experimental Biology (1990, November). *Nutrition and HIV Infection.* Washington, DC: Center for Food Safety and Applied Nutrition, Food and Drug Administration, U.S. Department of Health and Human Services.

Lifson, A.R., Darrow, W.W., Hessol, N.A., et al. (1990). Kaposi's sarcoma in a cohort of homosexual and bisexual men: Epidemiology and analysis for cofactors. *American Journal of Epidemiology, 131*(2), 221–231.

Loyd, J.E., DesPrez, R.M., Goodwin, R.A., Jr. (1990). *Histoplasma capsulatum.* In G.L. Mandell, R.G. Douglas, Jr., & J.E. Bennett (Eds.), *Principles and practice of infectious diseases* (3rd ed.) (pp. 1989–1998). New York: Churchill Livingstone.

Lucas, S.B., Parr, D.C., Wright, E., et al. (1989). AIDS presenting as cytomegalovirus cystitis. *British Journal of Urology, 64*(4), 429–430.

Ma, P., Villanueva, T.G., Kaufman, D., et al. (1984). Respiratory cryptosporidiosis in acquired immune deficiency syndrome. *Journal of the American Medical Association, 252*(10), 1298–1301.

MacMahon, E.M., Glass, J.D., Hayward, S.D., et al. (1991). Epstein-Barr virus related primary central nervous system lymphoma. *Lancet, 338*(8773), 969–973.

Magnenat, J., Nicod, L.P., Auckenthaler, R. (1991). Mode of presentation and diagnosis of bacterial pneumonia in human immunodeficiency virus–infected patients. *American Review of Respiratory Disease, 144*(4), 917–922.

Mahmoudi, A., Iseman, M.D. (1993). Pitfalls in the care of patients with tuberculosis: Common errors and their association with the acquisition of drug resistance. *Journal of the American Medical Association, 270*(1), 65–68.

Maimon, M., Fruchter, R.G., Serur, E., et al. (1990). Human immunodeficiency virus infection and cervical neoplasia. *Gynecologic Oncology, 38*, 377–382.

Maimon, M., Fruchter, R.G., Guy, L., et al. (1993). Human immunodeficiency virus infection and invasive cervical carcinoma. *Cancer, 71*(2), 402–406.

Maimon, M., Tarricone, N., Vieira, J., et al. (1991). Colposcopic evaluation of human immunodeficiency virus–seropositive women. *Obstetrics and Gynecology, 78*(1), 84–88.

Marte, C. (1992). Cervical dysplasia in HIV-infected women. *PAACNOTES, 4*(8), 391–393.

Masur, H. (1992). Prevention and treatment of pneumocystis pneumonia. *The New England Journal of Medicine, 327*(26), 1853–1860.

McCabe, R.E., Remington, J.S. (1988). Toxoplasmosis: The time has come. *The New England Journal of Medicine, 318*(5), 313–315.

McCabe, R.E., Remington, J.S. (1990). *Toxoplasma gondii.* In G.L. Mandell, R.G. Douglas, Jr., & J.E. Bennett (Eds.), *Principles and practice of infectious diseases* (pp. 2090–2103). New York: Churchill Livingstone.

McGowan, I., Hawkins, A., Weller, I. (1993). The natural history of cryptosporidial diarrhea in HIV-infected patients. *AIDS, 7*(3), 349–354.

McMullin, M. (1992). Holistic care of the patient with cervical cancer. *Nursing Clinics of North America, 27*(4), 847–858.

Messiah, A., Rozenbaum, W., Vittecoq, D., et al. (1989). Possible correlation between exposure to AIDS risk factors, clinical presentation in AIDS, and subsequent prognosis. *European Journal of Epidemiology, 5*(3), 336–342.

Miller, J.S. (1988). Cutaneous cryptococcus resembling molluscum contagiosum in a patient with acquired immunodeficiency syndrome. *Cutis, 41*(6), 411–412.

Milliken, S., Boyle, M.J. (1993). Update on HIV and neoplastic disease. *AIDS, 7*(suppl 1), S203–S209.

Minamoto, G., Armstrong, D. (1988). Fungal infections in AIDS: Histoplasmosis and coccidioidomycosis. In M.A. Sande & P.A. Volberding (Eds.), *The medical management of AIDS* (pp. 213–223). Philadelphia: W.B. Saunders.

Mitchell, C.D., Erlich, S.S., Mastrucci, M.T., et al. (1990). Congenital toxoplasmosis occurring in infants perinatally infected with human immunodeficiency virus 1. *Pediatric Infectious Disease Journal, 9*(7), 512–518.

Mitsuyasu, R.T. (1988). Kaposi's sarcoma in the acquired immunodeficiency syndrome. *Infectious Disease Clinics of North America, 2*(2), 511–523.

Mitsuyasu, R.T. (1993). New developments in the pathogenesis of Kaposi's sarcoma. *PAACNOTES, 5*(2), 66–69.

Modilevsky, T., Sattler, F.R., Barnes, P.F. (1989). Mycobacterial diseases in patients with human immunodeficiency virus infection. *Archives of Internal Medicine, 149*(10), 2201–2205.

Munoz, A., Schrager, L.K., Bacellar, H., et al. (1993). Trends in the incidence of outcomes defining acquired immunodeficiency syndrome (AIDS) in the multicenter AIDS cohort study: 1985–1991. *American Journal of Epidemiology, 137*(4), 423–438.

Murray, R.J., Becker, P., Furth, P., et al. (1988). Recovery from cryptococcemia and the adult respiratory distress syndrome in the acquired immunodeficiency syndrome. *Chest, 93*(6), 1304–1306.

Nadelman, R.B., Mathur-Wagh, U., Yancovitz, S.R., et al. (1985). *Salmonella* bacteremia associated with the acquired immunodeficiency syndrome (AIDS). *Archives of Internal Medicine, 145*(11), 1968–1971.

Nahlen, B.L., Chu, S.Y., Nwanyanwu, C., et al. (1993). HIV wasting syndrome in the United States. *AIDS, 7*(2), 183–188.

Nanda, D., Minkoff, H.L. (1992). Pregnancy and women at risk for HIV infection. *Primary Care Clinics in Office Practice, 19*(1), 157–169.

National Institute of Allergy and Infectious Diseases (1990, May). HIV associated opportunistic infections: NIAID-supported clinical research. *OI Backgrounder.* Bethesda, MD: The Institute.

Nelson, M.R., Erskine, D., Hakins, D.A., et al. (1993). Treatment with corticosteroids: A risk for the development of clinical cytomegalovirus disease in AIDS. *AIDS, 7*(3), 375–378.

Neubauer, M.A., Bodensteiner, D.C. (1992). Disseminated histoplasmosis in patients with AIDS. *Southern Medical Journal, 85*(12), 1166–1170.

Newman, C.F. (1992). The role of nutritional assessments and nutritional plans in the management of HIV/AIDS. In G. Nary (Ed.), *Nutrition and HIV/AIDS* (Vol. 1) (pp. 57–106). Chicago: PAAC Publishing.

New York City Department of Health (1992). Tuberculosis treatment. *CH1: City Health Information, 11*(5), 1–4.

New York State Department of Health, AIDS Institute (1993, Spring). *Focus on AIDS in New York State.* New York: The Department.

Nielsen, T.L., Schattenkerk, J.K., Jensen, B.N., et al. (1992). Adjunctive corticosteroid therapy for *Pneumocystis carinii* pneumonia in AIDS: A randomized European multicenter open label study. *Journal of Acquired Immune Deficiency Syndromes, 5*(7), 726–731.

Nightengale, S.D., Cameron, D.W., Gerdin, M.D., et al. (1993). Two controlled trials of rifabutin prophylaxis against *Mycobacterium avium* complex infection in AIDS. *The New England Journal of Nursing, 329*(12), 828–833.

Nistal, M., Regadera, J., Paniagua, R., Rodriguez, M.C. (1990). Nuclear bodies (spheroidea) in Sertoli cells of a man with acquired immunodeficiency syndrome (AIDS) and testicular infection by cytomegalovirus. *Ultrastructural Pathology, 14*(1), 21–26.

Ognibene, F.P., Shelhamer, J.H. (1988). Kaposi's sarcoma. *Clinics in Chest Medicine, 9*(3), 459–465.

Orlow, S.J., Cooper, D., Petrea, S., et al. (1993). AIDS-associated Kaposi's sarcoma in Romanian children. *Journal of the American Academy of Dermatology, 28*(3), 449–453.

Pagano, J.S., Lemon, S.M. (1986). The herpesviruses. In A.I. Braude (Ed.), *Infectious diseases and medical microbiology* (2nd ed.) (pp. 470–481). Philadelphia: W.B. Saunders.

Pape, J.W., Verdier, R.I., Johnson, W.D., Jr. (1989). Treatment and prophylaxis of *Isospora belli* infection in patients with the acquired immunodeficiency syndrome. *The New England Journal of Medicine, 320*(16), 1044–1047.

Pearsen, M.L., Jereb, J.A., Frieden, T.R., et al. (1992). Nosocomial transmission of multidrug-resistant *Mycobacterium* tuberculosis. *Annals of Internal Medicine, 117*(3), 191–196.

Pedersen, C., Lindhart, B.O., Jensen, B.L., et al. (1989). Clinical course of primary HIV infection: Consequences for course of infection. *British Medical Journal, 299*(6692), 154–157.

Phair, J., Munoz, A., Detels, R., et al. (1990). The risk of *Pneumocystis carinii* pneumonia among men infected with human immunodeficiency virus type 1. *The New England Journal of Medicine, 322*(3), 161–165.

Pindborg, J.J. (1994). The use of the term "thrush" [letter]. *Journal of Acquired Immune Deficiency Syndromes, 7*(1), 98.

Pitchenik, A.E., Fertel, D. (1992). Tuberculosis and non-tuberculosis mycobacterial disease. *The Medical Clinics of North America, 76*(1), 121–171.

Polsky, B., Gold, J.W.M., Whimbey, C., et al. (1986). Bacterial pneumonia in patients with acquired immunodeficiency syndrome. *Annals of Internal Medicine, 104*(1), 38–41.

Portegies, R., de Gans, J., Lange, J.M., et al. (1989). Declining incidence of AIDS dementia complex after introduction of zidovudine treatment. *British Medical Journal, 299*(6703), 819–821.

Portegies, P., Enting, R.H., de ans, J., et al. (1993). Presentation and course of AIDS dementia complex: 10 years of follow-up in Amsterdam, the Netherlands. *AIDS, 7*(5), 669–675.

Porter, S.B., Sande, M.A. (1992). Toxoplasmosis of the central nervous system in the acquired immunodeficiency syndrome. *The New England Journal of Medicine, 327*(23), 1643–1648.

Powderly, W.G. (1992). Therapy for cryptococcal meningitis in patients with AIDS. *Clinical Infectious Diseases, 14*(suppl 1), S54–S58.

Powderly, W.G., Saag, M.S., Clod, G.A., et al. (1992). Controlled trial of amphotericin B to prevent relapse of cryptococcal meningitis in patients with acquired immunodeficiency syndrome. *The New England Journal of Medicine, 326*(12), 793–798.

Price, R.W., Brew, B., Sidtis, J., et al. (1988a). The brain in AIDS: Central nervous system HIV-1 infection and the AIDS dementia complex. *Science, 239*(4840), 586–592.

Price, R.W., Sidtis, J., Rosenblum, M. (1988b). The AIDS dementia complex: Some current questions. *Annals of Neurology, 23*(suppl), S27–S33.

Rabinowitz, M., Bassan, I., Robinson, M.J. (1988). Sexually transmitted cytomegalovirus proctitis in a woman. *American Journal of Gastroenterology, 83*(8), 885–887.

Ragland, J. (1993). Progressive multifocal leukoencephalopathy. *AIDS Clinical Care, 5*(3), 17–19.

Ragsdale, D. (1993). A call for help: Collaborative nursing research. *Journal of the Association of Nurses in AIDS Care, 4*(2), 48–52.

Ravalli, S., Garcia, R.L., Vincent, R.A., et al. (1990). Disseminated *Pneumocystis carinii* infection in the acquired immunodeficiency syndrome. *New York State Journal of Medicine, 90*(3), 155–157.

Reeves, W.C., Rawls, W.E., Brintan, L.A. (1989). Epidemiology of genital papillomaviruses and cervical cancer. *Reviews of Infectious Diseases, 11*(3), 426–439.

Reinis-Lucey, C., Sande, M.A., Gerberding, J.L. (1990). Toxoplasmosis. In P.T. Cohen, M.A. Sande, & P.A. Volberding (Eds.), *The AIDS knowledge base* (pp. 656.1–656.15). Waltham, MA: Medical Publishing Group.

Rellihan, M.A., Dooley, D.P., Burke, T.W., et al. (1990). Rapidly progressing cervical cancer in a patient with human immunodeficiency virus infection. *Gynecologic Oncology, 36*, 435–438.

Remington, J.S., McLeod, R. (1986). Toxoplasmosis. In A.I. Braude (Ed.), *Infectious diseases and medical microbiology* (2nd ed.) (pp. 1521–1535). Philadelphia: W.B. Saunders.

Remington, J.S., McLeod, R. (1992). Toxoplasmosis. In S.L. Gorback, J.G. Bartlett, & N.R. Blacklow (Eds.), *Infectious Diseases* (pp. 1328–1343). Philadelphia: W.B. Saunders.

Restrepo, C., Macher, A.M., Radany, E.H. (1987). Disseminated extra-intestinal isosporiasis in a patient with acquired immunodeficiency syndrome. *American Journal of Clinical Pathology, 87*(4), 536–542.

Reynolds, H.Y. (1991). Pneumonia and lung abscess. In J.D. Wilson, E. Braunwald, K.J. Isselbacher, et al. (Eds.), *Harrison's principles of internal medicine* (12th ed.) (pp. 1064–1069). New York: McGraw-Hill.

Rhoads, J.L., Wright, D.C., Redfield, R.R., et al. (1987). Chronic vaginal candidiasis in women with human immunodeficiency virus infection. *Journal of the American Medical Association, 257*(22), 3105–3107.

Richart, R.M., Wright, T.C. (1993). Controversies in the management of low-grade cervical intraepithelial neoplasia. *Cancer, 71*(4 suppl), 1413–1421.

Riley, K.B., Antoniskis, D., Maris, R., et al. (1988). Rattlesnake capsule–associated *Salmonella arizona* infections. *Archives of Internal Medicine, 148*(5), 1207–1210.

Rolston, K.V. (1993). Candidiasis. *PAACNOTES, 5*(2), 54–56.

Rooney, J.F., Felser, J.M., Ostrove, J.M., et al. (1986). Acquisition of genital herpes from an asymptomatic sexual partner. *The New England Journal of Medicine, 314*(24), 1561–1564.

Rose, D.N., Schechter, C.B., Sacks, H.S. (1993). Influenza and pneumococcal vaccination of HIV-infected patients: A policy analysis. *The American Journal of Medicine, 94*(2), 160–168.

Rosenblum, M.L., Levy, R.M., Bredesen, D.E., et al. (1988). Primary central nervous system lymphomas in patients with AIDS. *Annals of Neurology, 23*(suppl), S13–S16.

Rubin, M.M., Lauver, D. (1990). Assessment and management of cervical intraepithelial neoplasia. *Nurse Practitioner, 15*(9), 23–31.

Ruf, B., Jautzke, G., Schurmann, D., et al. (1990). Clinical aspects and pathology of mycobacterial infections in AIDS: Pulmonary and extrapulmonary manifestations. *Pneumologie, 44*(suppl 1), 502–503.

Ruskin, J., LaRiviene, M. (1991). Low dose co-trimoxazole for prevention of *Pneumocystis carinii* pneumonia in human immunodeficiency virus disease. *Lancet, 337*(8739), 468–471.

Saag, M.S. (1993). Cryptococcal meningitis. *PAACNOTES, 5*(1), 34–37.

Saag, M.S., Powderly, W.G., Cloud, G.A., et al. (1992). Comparison of amphotericin B with fluconazole in the treatment of acute AIDS-associated cryptococcal meningitis. *The New England Journal of Medicine, 326*(2), 83–89.

Sadeghi, S.B., Sadeghi, A., Robboy, S.J. (1988). Prevalence of dysplasia and cancer of the cervix in a nationwide Planned Parenthood population. *Cancer, 61*, 2359–2361.

Safrin, S., Ashley, R., Houlihan, C., et al. (1991a). Clinical and serologic features of herpes simplex virus infection in patients with AIDS. *AIDS, 5*(9), 1107–1110.

Safrin, S., Crumpacker, C., Chatis, P., et al. (1991b). A controlled trial comparing foscarnet with vidarabine for acyclovir-resistant mucocutaneous herpes simplex in the acquired immunodeficiency syndrome. *The New England Journal of Medicine, 325*(8), 551–555.

Salzman, S.H., Smith, R.L., Aranda, C.P. (1988). Histoplasmosis in patients at risk for the acquired immunodeficiency syndrome in a nonendemic setting. *Chest, 93*(5), 916–921.

Samoszuk, M., Nguyen, V., Shadan, F., Ramzi, E. (1993). Incidence of Epstein-Barr virus in AIDS-related lymphoma specimens. *Journal of Acquired Immune Deficiency Syndromes, 6*(8), 913–918.

Sanders, W.E., Horowitz, E.A. (1990). Other mycobacterium species. In G.L. Mandell, R.G. Douglas, Jr., & J.E. Bennett (Eds.), *Principles and practice of infec-*

tious diseases (3rd ed.) (pp. 1914–1926). New York: Churchill Livingstone.

Schäfer, A., Friedmann, W., Mielke, M., et al. (1991). The increased frequency of cervical dysplasia-neoplasia in women infected with the human immunodeficiency virus is related to the degree of immunosuppression. *American Journal of Obstetrics and Gynecology, 164*(2), 593–599.

Schmitt, F.A., Bigley, J.W., McKinnis, R., et al. [AZT Collaborative Working Group] (1988). Neuropsychological outcome of zidovudine (AZT) treatment of patients with AIDS and AIDS-related complex. *The New England Journal of Medicine, 319*(24), 1573–1578.

Schwartz, L.B., Carcangiu, M.L., Bradham, L., Schwartz, P.E. (1991). Rapidly progressive squamous cell carcinoma of the cervix coexisting with human immunodeficiency virus infection: Clinical opinion. *Gynecologic Oncology, 41*, 255–258.

Selwyn, P.A., Alcalus, P., Hartel, D., et al. (1992). Clinical manifestations and predictors of disease progression in drug users with human immunodeficiency virus infection. *The New England Journal of Medicine, 237*(24), 1697–1703.

Selwyn, P.A., Feingold, A.R., Hartel, D., et al. (1988). Increased risk of bacterial pneumonia in HIV-infected intravenous drug users without AIDS. *AIDS, 2*(4), 267–272.

Selwyn, P.A., Hartel, D., Lewis, V.A., et al. (1989). A prospective study of the risk of tuberculosis among intravenous drug users with human immunodeficiency virus infection. *The New England Journal of Medicine, 320*(9), 545–550.

Sharkey, S.J., Sharkey, K.A., Sutherland, L.R., et al. (1992). Nutritional status and food intake in human immunodeficiency virus infection. *Journal of Acquired Immune Deficiency Syndromes, 5*(11), 1091–1098.

Sharkey-Mathis, P.K., Velez, J., Fetchick, R., et al. (1993). Histoplasmosis in the acquired immunodeficiency syndrome (AIDS): Treatment with intraconazole and fluconazole. *Journal of Acquired Immune Deficiency Syndromes, 6*(7), 809–819.

Shell, J.A., Carter, J. (1987). The gynecological implant patient. *Seminars in Oncology Nursing, 3*(1), 54–66.

Similowski, T., Datry, A., Jais, P., et al. (1989). AIDS-associated cryptococcosis causing adult respiratory distress syndrome. *Respiratory Medicine, 83*(6), 513–55.

Simpson, D.M. (1993). HIV and the nervous system. *PAACNOTES, 5*(1), 14, 15, 37.

Small, P.M., Hopewell, P.C. (1990). *Mycobacterium avium* complex. In P.T. Cohen, M.A. Sande, & P.A. Volberding (Eds.), *The AIDS knowledge base* (pp. 621.1–621.4) Waltham, MA: Medical Publishing Group.

Small, P.M., McPhaul, L.W., Sooy, C.D., et al. (1989). Cytomegalovirus infection of the laryngeal nerve presenting as hoarseness in patients with acquired immunodeficiency syndrome. *American Journal of Medicine, 86*(1), 108–110.

Smith, E., Franzmann, M., Mathiesen, L.R. (1989). Disseminated histoplasmosis in a Danish patient with AIDS. *Scandinavian Journal of Infectious Diseases, 21*(5), 573–575.

Smith, P.D., Janoff, E.N. (1988). Infectious diarrhea in human immunodeficiency virus infection. *Gastroenterology Clinics of North America, 17*(3), 587–598.

Smith, P.D., Quinn, T.C., Strober, W., et al. (1992). Gastrointestinal infections in AIDS. *Annals of Internal Medicine, 116*(1), 63–77.

So, Y.T., Choucair, A., Davis, R.L., et al. (1988). Neoplasms of the central nervous system in acquired immunodeficiency syndrome. In M.L. Rosenblum, R.M. Levy, & D.E. Bredesen (Eds.), *AIDS and the nervous system* (pp. 285–300). New York: Raven Press.

Soave, R., Sepkowitz, K.A. (1992). *Cryptosporidium, Isospora, Dientamoeba.* In S.L. Gorbach, J.G. Bartlett, & N.R. Blacklow (Eds.), *Infectious diseases* (pp. 1996–1999). Philadelphia: W.B. Saunders.

Soave, R., Weikel, C.A. (1990). *Cryptosporidium* and other protozoa including *Ispospora, Sarcocystis, Balantidium coli,* and *Blastocystis.* In G.L. Mandell, R.G. Douglas, Jr., & J.E. Bennett (Eds.), *Principles and practice of infectious diseases* (3rd ed.) (pp. 2122–2130). New York: Churchill Livingstone.

Sorvillo, F., Lieb, L., Iwakoshi, K., et al. (1990). *Isospora belli* and the acquired immune deficiency syndrome [letter]. *The New England Journal of Medicine, 322*(2), 131.

Sperber, S.J., Schleupner, C.J. (1987). Salmonellosis during infection with human immunodeficiency virus. *Reviews of Infectious Diseases, 9*(5), 925–934.

Spinillo, A., Tenti, P., Zappatore, R., et al. (1992). Prevalence, diagnosis, and treatment of lower genital neoplasia in women with human immunodeficiency virus infection. *European Journal of Obstetrics and Gynecology, 43*, 235–241.

Staff (1993). Magnetic resonance spectroscopy may offer early look at HIV disease–mediated changes in the brain. *Journal of the American Medical Association, 269*(9), 1084.

Stansell, J.D., Sande, M.A. (1992). Cryptococcal infections in AIDS. In M.A. Sande & P.A. Volberding (Eds.), *The medical management of AIDS* (3rd ed.) (pp. 297–310). Philadelphia: W.B. Saunders.

Stevens, D.A. (1990). *Coccidioides immitis.* In G.L. Mandell, R.G. Douglas, Jr., & J.E. Bennett (Eds.), *Principles and practice of infectious diseases* (3rd ed.) (pp. 2008–2017). New York: Churchill Livingstone.

Stone, V.E., Seage, G.R., Hertz, T., Epstein, A.M. (1992). The relation between hospital experience and mortality for patients with AIDS. *Journal of the American Medical Association, 268*(19), 2655–2661.

Straus, S.E. (1990). Introduction to Herpetoviridiae. In G.L. Mandell, R.G. Douglas, Jr., & J.E. Bennett (Eds.), *Principles and practice of infectious diseases* (3rd ed.) (pp. 1139–1144). New York: Churchill Livingstone.

Studies of Ocular Complications of AIDS Research Group (1992). Mortality in patients with the acquired immunodeficiency syndrome treated with either foscarnet or ganciclovir for cytomegalovirus retinitis. *The New England Journal of Medicine, 326*(4), 213–219.

Szoka, P.R., Edgren, R.A. (1988). Drug interactions with oral contraceptives: Compilation and analysis of an adverse experience database. *Fertility and Sterility, 49*(5, suppl 2), 31S–38S.

Task Force on Nutrition Support in AIDS (1989). Guidelines for nutrition support in AIDS. *Nutrition, 5*(1), 39–46.

Tindall, B., Hing, M., Edwards, P., et al. (1989). Severe clinical manifestations of primary HIV infection. *AIDS, 3*(11), 747–749.

Tinkle, M.B. (1990). Genital human papillomavirus infection: A growing health risk. *Journal of Obstetrics, Gynecologic, and Neonatal Nursing, 19*(6), 501–507.

Torres, G. (1993). Opportunistic infections overview. *Treatment Issues, 7*(8), 1–5.

Turner, B.J., Ball, J.K. (1992). Variations in inpatient mortality for AIDS in a national sample of hospitals. *Journal of Acquired Immune Deficiency Syndromes, 5*(10), 978–987.

Ungvarski, P.J. (1987). Demystifying AIDS: Educating nurses for care. *Nursing and Health Care, 8*(10), 570–573.

U.S. Public Health Service Task Force on Antipneumocystis Prophylaxis in Patients with Human Immunodeficiency Virus Infection (1993). Recommendations for prophylaxis against *Pneumocystis carinii* pneumonia for persons with human immunodeficiency virus. *Journal of Acquired Immune Deficiency Syndromes, 6*(1), 46–55.

Vago, L., Castagna, A., Lazzarin, A., et al. (1993). Reduced frequency of HIV-induced brain lesions in AIDS patients treated with zidovudine. *Journal of Acquired Immune Deficiency Syndromes, 6*(1), 42–45.

Vasudevan, V.P., Mascarenhas, D.A., Klapper, P., et al. (1990). Cytomegalovirus necrotizing bronchiolitis with HIV infection. *Chest, 25*(3), 311–312.

Vermund, S.H., Kelley, K.F., Klein, R.S., et al. (1991). High risk of human papillomavirus infection and cervical squamous intraepithelial lesions among women with symptomatic human immunodeficiency virus infection. *American Journal of Obstetrics and Gynecology, 165*(2), 392–398.

Vinters, H.V., Ferreiro, J.A. (1990). CMV: What is its effect on AIDS patients, and how do you treat it? *AIDS Medical Report, 3*(5), 43–56.

Voelker, R. (1994). More choices for treating AIDS-related pneumonia. *Journal of the American Medical Association, 271*(3), 176–177.

Wallace, J.M., Hannah, J. (1987). Cytomegalovirus pneumonitis in patients with AIDS: Findings in an autopsy series. *Chest, 92*(2), 198–203.

Wallace, J.M., Hannah, J.B. (1988). *Mycobacterium avium* complex infection in patients with acquired immunodeficiency syndrome: A clinicopathologic study. *Chest, 93*(5), 926–932.

Wallace, M.R., Rossetti, R.J., Olson, P.E. (1993). Cats and toxoplasmosis risk in HIV-infected adults. *Journal of the American Medical Association, 269*(1), 76–77.

Walzer, P.D. (1990). *Pneumocystis carinii*. In G.L. Mandell, R.G. Douglas, Jr., & J.E. Bennett (Eds.), *Principles and practice of infectious diseases* (3rd ed.) (pp. 2103–2110). New York: Churchill Livingstone.

Wasser, L., Talavera, W. (1987). Pulmonary cryptococcosis in AIDS. *Chest, 92*(4), 692–695.

Weiler, P.G. (1989). AIDS and dementia. *Generations: Journal of the American Geriatric Society, 36*(2), 139–141.

Weiler, P.G., Mungas, D., Pomerantz, S. (1988). AIDS as a cause of dementia in the elderly. *Journal of the American Geriatric Society, 36*(2), 16–18.

Weinberger, S.E. (1993). Recent advances in pulmonary medicine [second of two parts]. *The New England Journal of Medicine, 328*(20), 1462–1470.

Wells, W.F. (1955). *Airborne contagion and air hygiene; an ecological study of droplet infections.* Cambridge, MA: Harvard University Press.

Wheat, L.J., Connolly-Stringfield, P.A., Baker, R.L., et al. (1990). Disseminated histoplasmosis in the acquired immune deficiency syndrome: Clinical findings, diagnosis and treatment, and review of the literature. *Medicine (Baltimore), 69*(6), 361–374.

Wheat, J., Hafner, R., Wulfsohn, M., et al. (1993). Prevention of relapse of histoplasmosis with intraconazole in patients with the acquired immunodeficiency syndrome. *Annals of Internal Medicine, 118*(8), 610–616.

Wiley, C.A., Nelson, J.A. (1988). Role of human immunodeficiency virus and cytomegalovirus in AIDS encephalitis. *American Journal of Pathology, 133*(1), 73–81.

Williams, H.A., Wilson, M.E., Hongladarom, G., McDonnell, M. (1986). Nurses' attitudes toward sexuality in cancer patients. *Oncology Nursing Forum, 13*(2), 39–43.

Witt, D.J., Craven, D.C., McCabe, W.R. (1987). Bacterial infections in adult patients with the acquired immune deficiency syndrome (AIDS) and the AIDS-related complex. *The American Journal of Medicine, 82*(5), 900–906.

Wofsy, C.B. (1990). *Isospora belli*. In P.T. Cohen, M.A. Sande, & P.A. Volberding (Eds.), *The AIDS knowledge base* (pp. 657.1–657.4). Waltham, MA: The Medical Publishing Group.

Worley, J.M., Price, R.W. (1992). Management of neurologic complications of HIV-1 infection and AIDS. In M.A. Sande & P.A. Volberding (Eds.), *The medical management of AIDS* (3rd ed.) (pp. 193–217). Philadelphia: W.B. Saunders.

Yarchoan, R., Pluda, J.M., Thomas, R.V, et al. (1990). Long-term toxicity/activity profile of 2',3'-dideoxyinosine in AIDS or AIDS-related complex. *Lancet, 336*(8714), 526–529.

Yarchoan, R., Thomas, R.V., Grafman, J., et al (1988). Long-term administration of 3'-azido-2',3'-dideoxythymidine to patients with AIDS-related neurological disease. *Annals of Neurology, 23*(suppl), S82–S87.

Zighelboim, J., Goldfarb, R.A., Mody, D., et al. (1992). Prostatic abscess due to *Histoplasma capsulatum* in a patient with the acquired immunodeficiency syndrome. *Journal of Urology, 147*(1), 166–168.

Zuger, A. (1992). Bacterial infection in AIDS. Part I. *AIDS Clinical Care, 4*(9), 69–71.

5 Nursing Management of the Adult Client

Peter J. Ungvarski and Joan Schmidt

The primary goal of the nurse caring for clients with infection caused by HIV is the protection and/or enhancement of health. This is achieved through the nursing diagnosis and treatment of human responses, both physical and psychologic, to actual or potential health problems related to HIV infection, and by assisting the client in making informed health choices.

The scope of nursing practice in the context of the spectrum of HIV disease can be categorized into primary, secondary, and tertiary prevention activities. Primary prevention strategies include health appraisal of all clients, irrespective of their reason(s) for care, to identify behaviors or experiences that may have exposed the individual to HIV in the past or that will, without behavior change, potentially expose them in the future. On the basis of clinical findings, the nurse will then be required to assist clients (those who express an interest) in accessing the HIV testing process and to provide them with information to reduce the potential risk of HIV infection. Secondary prevention strategies include the baseline assessment of the person newly identified as infected, with teaching to promote and protect the client's health and planning for follow-up care. Tertiary prevention strategies include the diagnosis and treatment of human responses encountered by clients with advanced, symptomatic HIV disease, including the associated AIDS-indicator diseases.

Discussion of the nursing care needs of adults in this chapter focus on pathophysiologic (physical) responses to HIV disease. Chapter 11 contains a detailed discussion of the psychologic aspects of nursing care.

PRIMARY PREVENTION

The primary-prevention category of nursing care focuses on an organized, systematic approach to health appraisal to (1) identify individuals with risk behaviors associated with HIV transmission, (2) detect signs and symptoms that may indicate the presence of HIV disease or a related illness that is indicative of AIDS, (3) determine the need for health teaching to reduce the risk of acquiring HIV infection, and (4) determine the need for secondary and/or tertiary prevention strategies.

Social History

Although no one would dispute the fact that HIV infection is a preventable disease, current data suggest that HIV prevention efforts in the United States are sorely lacking. According to the Centers for Disease Control and Prevention (CDC), (1993a), while death rates from most other leading causes of death in the United States declined or remained relatively stable, by 1992 HIV infection became the leading cause of death in more than 60 cities in the United States among men between the ages of 25 and 44 years.

Sexual activity, as a principal mode of HIV transmission, accounts for 62% of all AIDS cases among adults and adolescents in the United States (CDC, 1993, October). From a broader perspective, clinicians should be aware that approximately 12 million newly acquired sexually transmitted diseases (STDs) occur each year in the United States (Barringer, 1993). These data underscore the need for primary prevention strategies through sexual history taking and counseling, but currently available information suggests that this is not happening.

Surveys of U.S. physicians indicate that sexual history taking is not part of routine practice and in fact is done with less than 25% of their health assessments of clients (Ferguson et al., 1991; Gemson et al., 1991). A study of nurses' AIDS-related knowledge found that 91.3% (N = 1,019) do not usually take a sexual history (van Servellen et al., 1988). Confounding the issue is the fact that studies of knowledge, attitude, and practices of physicians, nurses, and other health care professionals reveal significant knowledge gaps in the basic pathophysiologic aspects of HIV disease (Gemson et al., 1991; Henry et al., 1993; Passannante et al., 1993).

Human sexuality is inextricably woven into the fabric of all human beings, and the promotion of sexual health is a legitimate, essential function of both physicians and nurses (Fogel, 1990). Sexual history taking should be included in any detailed health assessment and extend beyond simply looking for HIV-related sexual risk behaviors. Sexual history taking may be uncomfortable for both the client and the clinician, and questions may delve into areas that both perceive as socially unacceptable. The client may be reluctant to discuss sexual activities in the presence of judgmental attitudes, rejecting responses from the clinician for fear of discrimination if confidentiality is breached (Hecht & Soloway, 1993a).

Sexual history taking should be inclusive and detailed and should be performed universally with all clients. The concept of high-risk groups is obsolete. A major pitfall to avoid with sexual history taking is to make assumptions regarding sexual behaviors of clients based on preconceived ideas of certain lifestyles. All gay men are not at risk for HIV infection. Even gay men with multiple sexual partners, if they practice mutual masturbation exclusively, are unlikely to acquire HIV infection.

The concept of monogamy is likewise elusive. Individuals, both men and women, have little control over the sexual activities of their partners. The biased perception that casual sex intrinsically increases the risk of HIV, versus monogamy, can be misleading. Rodrigues and Moreno (1991) noted that HIV transmission can and does occur in women in a stable relationship or marriage. Smeltzer and Whipple (1991) pointed out that women are often unaware of the risks of HIV infection because they may not associate themselves with so-called high-risk groups but may in fact participate in high-risk behaviors.

AIDS in persons older than 50 years of age accounts for 8% of the cases in women and 11% of the cases in men (CDC, 1993, October). The incidence of both AIDS and STDs is increasing in older Americans (Tichy & Talashek, 1992; Wallace et al., 1993). Sexual history taking should not be omitted because of age. The failure to identify HIV infection in older clients has led to the misdiagnosis of Alzheimer's disease in the presence of HIV dementia and has delayed diagnosis of pneumonia caused by *Pneumocystis carinii* in elderly individuals (Fillit et al., 1990; Hargreaves et al., 1988; Weiler et al., 1988). Hinkle (1991) concluded that health care professionals have been guilty of complacency when it comes to screening and educating the elderly population regarding HIV infection.

A prerequisite to effective sexual history taking is self-evaluation and values clarification of individual attitudes toward various sexual behaviors (Andrist, 1988; Fogel, 1990). This necessary step, along with first practicing sexual history taking with colleagues, is helpful if the nurse is going to maintain a nonjudgmental demeanor during the actual interview process and avoid a shocked expression in response to answers given. Nurses should examine their feelings and responses regarding oral sex, anal sex, masturbation, homosexuality, heterosexuality, bisexuality, transvestism, transsexualism, casual sex, prostitution, use of birth control methods and devices, and sexual encounters outside of alleged monogamous relationships. It should be emphasized that the nurses taking the sexual history do not in any way relinquish their own values in the process of acknowledging the values of others (Hogan, 1980).

Andrist (1988) and Kelly and Holman (1993) offered some helpful suggestions for nurses taking sexual histories. The nurse should begin by ensuring privacy; should appear warm, open, and empathetic; and should maintain eye contact. Introduce the topic by making a general statement that concerns about sexual issues are universal. Assist the client in identifying risk-related sexual activities and explore how much knowledge the client has regarding the HIV-related risk behaviors of their sexual partner(s). Finally, offer information that specifically addresses the client's concerns. Printed material that is sexually explicit and directed toward specific lifestyles is available from most nonprofit, community-based AIDS organizations.

Exploration of the use of mood-affecting agents should be conducted objectively, and assumptions regarding the direct, causal effects of alcohol or drugs on risky sexual behavior should be avoided. Temple and colleagues (1993) found that although sexual encounters with new partners were more likely to involve alcohol, the presence of alcohol in the event was not significantly associated with risky sexual behaviors. The authors concluded that the relationship between drinking and risky sex is the result of a complex interaction among personality, situational, and behavioral factors. Weiner and associates (1992) reported that cocaine and crack-cocaine users who primarily perform oral sex were more likely to become infected with HIV than those who primarily perform vaginal intercourse. The authors speculated that crack smoking itself, possibly through oral trauma caused by the heat of the crack pipe, may be a factor in making fellatio a risky behavior. Other problems noted to be associated with crack use were hypersexuality, trading sex for drugs, and impaired judgment leading to inconsistent condom use.

It is important to use open-ended questions to obtain accurate information on substance use. Given the psychologic defense mechanisms that substance users employ, direct questions such as "Do you use drugs?" are too threatening and unlikely to yield truthful responses (Blum, 1987). Although many standard assessment forms place alcohol and drug use in the section with tobacco, it may be better to ask about substance use

during the dietary assessment: "What do you usually eat in a day? What do you drink? Could you tell me about your use of alcohol and drugs?" Nurses need to know which substances are being used and the route of administration, but knowing the amounts of use is not necessary unless the client is being admitted for detoxification.

Questions of drug use will lead to questions about needle exposure. Although some exposures, such as those of an intravenous heroin addict, are obvious, other types of needle exposure may put people at risk, such as tattooing done on the streets or needle sharing among individuals who self-administer estrogens intramuscularly because they plan eventually to have transsexual surgery. In the early years of the AIDS epidemic, epidemiologic studies in Haiti traced HIV transmission to dirty needles used by untrained persons to give intramuscular injections (Pape & Johnson, 1989).

Using the health history to identify persons at risk for HIV disease should also include occupational history and accidental exposure to blood, needles, or instruments (Hecht & Soloway, 1993a). Attempting to sort out which occupations may be at risk might be difficult. Although the more obvious individuals include physicians, nurses, laboratory workers, and phlebotomists, selectively questioning persons in only a few occupations may overlook others such as police officers, paramedics, and sanitation workers. Questioning should therefore include all individuals to be as inclusive as possible.

Travel history and exploration of potential risk of exposure should be questioned. Emphasizing the need to explore travel, Rowbottom (1993) noted that STDs and HIV were being diagnosed in an increasing number of Australians after international travel. More recently, reports from the World Health Organization indicated that contaminated injection equipment in health care settings in Romania and the former Soviet Union (Mann, Tarantola, & Netter, 1992) was a primary source of large-scale epidemics of HIV disease. Along with travel history, immigration history is equally important.

Medical History and Review of Systems

When reviewing the client's medical history, the nurse should note the presence of recurrent infections such as bacterial infections or recurrent vaginal candidiasis. These types of conditions may reflect an underlying immunodeficiency, especially if they did not respond well to treatment.

The last part of the health history, the review of systems, is a detailed look for signs and symptoms of HIV disease and possibly of an associated AIDS-indicator disease. After completion, a careful review of the history with the client should conclude with questions regarding whether the client is satisfied with the history or wishes to change any areas. This will provide the basis for nursing care planning and health teaching. Table 5–1 provides a detailed outline for taking a health history. When all findings are summarized, the process concludes with a discussion of HIV testing, the client's responses to testing, and whether or not the client wishes assistance in obtaining testing. Chapter 2 discusses the issues and process of HIV testing.

All clinicians should avoid speculating with the client on the probability of positive or negative test results based on the health history findings. This is especially important when, for example, the sexual history reveals obscure or rare experiences with possible exposure to HIV and when the review of symptoms alludes to an underlying immunodeficiency. It has recently been reported that idiopathic CD4$^+$ T-lymphocytopenia, or profound depletion of CD4$^+$ T lymphocytes in the absence of HIV infection, has occurred in approximately one third of individuals described to have had some risk factor for HIV infection (Fauci, 1993).

SECONDARY PREVENTION

Secondary prevention strategies should be implemented as soon as a diagnosis is made and is confirmed by laboratory testing (see Appendix I). Activities include an initial workup consisting of a detailed physical examination and laboratory evaluation, and provision of health information that supports and protects the health of the client (see Appendix IV).

Physical Examination

The physical examination findings are as diversified as the spectrum of HIV disease. Findings range from normal in a symptom-free HIV-infected person, to evidence of the presence of an opportunistic disease or infection that is associated with a diagnosis of AIDS. HIV-related conditions have demonstrated to date the ability of HIV to affect virtually every anatomic structure and organ site (Hernandez, 1990). Therefore a complete physical examination should be performed, and any deviations from normal findings should be considered significant in relation to HIV infection. The early detection of complications related to HIV disease are often treatable, and treatment can sometimes prevent or slow progressions to more serious disease (Hecht & Soloway, 1993a). Table 5–2 outlines the elements of a baseline physical examination of the person with HIV infection.

Laboratory Testing

Initial laboratory testing of the HIV-infected person is important not only to establish baseline data on the newly diagnosed individual but also to determine disease progression, as a means of identifying complications of HIV disease, and to provide possible evidence of drug toxicity (Bartlett, 1993). Because of the limited information available on which to base recommendations for the routine use of most of these tests, as well as for the frequency with which they should be ordered, there is no consensus regarding these issues (Hecht & Soloway, 1993b). Table 5–3 outlines initial laboratory screening and reflects the current opinions found in the literature.

The complete blood cell count is necessary to identify three common problems in HIV disease: anemia, thrombocytopenia, and leukopenia. From a nursing perspective, client complaints about being tired or having profound fatigue may often be related to varying

Table 5–1. Primary Prevention: Health History Taking to Identify Persons at Risk for HIV Disease

A. Social history
1. Sexual activities
   a. Absolutely safe behavior: abstinence or mutually monogamous with a noninfected partner
   b. Very safe behavior: noninsertive sexual practices
   c. Probably safe behavior: insertive sexual practices with the use of condoms and spermicide
   d. Risky behavior: everything else
   e. Use of condoms (both male and female), including application, removal, use of lubricants, and difference in condom efficacy
   f. Engaging in sex with multiple partners.
   g. Use of mood-affecting drugs before or during sexual activities
   h. Determination of whether HIV disease has been diagnosed in anyone with whom the client has had sex
2. Use of mood-affecting drugs
   a. Drugs such as alcohol, marijuana, cocaine, crack, LSD, methaqualone (Quaalude), amphetamines, barbiturates, tranquilizers, amyl or butyl nitrate (called "poppers"), and heroin
   b. Route of administration: oral, inhalation (including sniffing, snorting, and smoking), intravenous, or subcutaneous ("skin popping")
   c. Any current or previous treatment for substance abuse
3. Needle exposure
   a. Use of drugs via intravenous route, and sharing of needles, syringes, and other drug paraphernalia
   b. Other needle-exposure activities such as application of tattoos, acupuncture, treatment by "folk doctors" or other unlicensed individuals, or sharing of prescribed drugs between friends
   c. Determination of whether HIV disease has been diagnosed in anyone with whom client has shared needles
4. Occupational history
   a. Client's occupation and responsibilities in relation to risk potential for HIV exposure
   b. Any exposure of the client to HIV
   c. The type of health care follow-up that the client has pursued since exposure
   d. The client's knowledge level regarding the signs and symptoms of seroconversion and the need for follow-up
5. Travel
   a. Within the past 10 years
   b. Sexual activities when traveling in areas where the number of AIDS cases is high, such as New York, California, New Jersey, Texas, or Florida, or countries such as Haiti or Zaire
   c. Treatment of illnesses while traveling
   d. Immigration history and potential exposures in country of origin
B. Medication history: current or previous use of medication that suppresses the immune system, such as steroids; current treatment of chemical dependence if applicable
C. Medical history
1. Major diseases including (but not limited to) tuberculosis; hepatitis A, B, C, or D; mononucleosis; and hemophilia; receiving treatment with clotting replacements such as factor VIII
2. Treatment for psychiatric/emotional disorders
3. Transfusion donor or recipient
D. Surgical history
E. Childhood illnesses, including (but not limited to) varicella; immunization history
F. Sexually transmitted diseases (STDs), including (but not limited to) syphilis; gonorrhea; amebiasis; herpes simplex (herpes labialis or herpes genitalis); *Giardia lamblia* enteritis; and *Chlamydia* infection
G. Review of systems
1. General: a comment from the client concerning a self-appraisal of their current state of health should be elicited
2. Skin: eruptions, lesions, itching, dryness, redness, rashes, lumps, color changes, changes in hair or nails
3. Head: headaches, lightheadedness, other sensations
4. Eyes: blurred vision, diplopia, loss of visual fields, "floaters"

Table 15–1. Primary Prevention: Health History Taking to Identify Persons at Risk for HIV Disease *Continued*

5. Ears: impaired hearing, tinnitus
6. Nose and sinuses: obstruction, pain, discharges, nosebleed, chronic infections
7. Mouth and throat: creamy white patches, lesions, bleeding gums, dysphagia, odynophagia, changes in taste, sore throat
8. Respiratory tract: dyspnea with or without certain activities, coughing, wheezing, chest pain, "cold" or "flulike" symptoms; date and results of last chest x-ray examination and tuberculin test
9. Cardiovascular system: chest pain, palpitations, edema, known hypertension or hypotension
10. Gastrointestinal tract: changes in appetite, involuntary weight loss, abdominal pain or cramping, changes in bowel habits, loose stools, diarrhea, blood in stool, rectal and perianal pain and itching
11. Genitourinary system: dysuria, nocturia, pain, itching, discharges, lesions
12. Gynecologic concerns: changes in menstruation, dyspareunia, vaginal discharge, breast abnormalities, obstetric history, abortions, chronic infections
13. Musculoskeletal system: arthralgia, myalgia
14. Neurologic and emotional concerns: loss of memory, nervousness, personality changes, confusional states, stiff neck, photophobia, tremors, paresthesias, seizures, syncope
15. Endocrine system: polyuria, polyphagia, polydipsia, fevers, night sweats
16. Hematopoietic changes: lymphadenopathy, bruising or bleeding, history of anemia

Table 5–2. Secondary Prevention: Baseline Physical Examination of the HIV-infected Client

A. General: weight, height, temperature, respiratory rate, pulse, blood pressure
B. Neurologic examination
   1. Cerebral functions: impaired cognitive functions, decreased level of consciousness, anger, inattentiveness, depression, denial
   2. Cranial nerve (CN) examination
      a. CN II (optic nerve): papilledema, white retinal spots, yellow-white retinal infiltrates, retinal hemorrhage, visual field deficiencies, blurred vision
      b. CNs III, IV, VI (oculomotor, trochlear, abducens nerves): impaired extraocular movements, unequal pupils, diplopia, ptosis, nystagmus
      c. CN V (trigeminal nerve): photophobia
      d. CN VII (facial nerve): hemiparesis
      e. CN VIII (acoustic nerve): tinnitus, vertigo, impaired hearing
      f. CNs IX, X (glossopharyngeal and vagus nerves): dysphagia, dysarthria
   3. Motor examination: motor weakness, hemiparesis, paraparesis
   4. Sensory examination: dysesthesias, paresthesias, areas of anesthesia
   5. Cerebellar examination: ataxia, dysmetria, tremors
   6. Reflexes: abnormal reflexes, positive Babinski's sign
   7. Meningeal signs: nuchal rigidity, Brudzinski's sign, Kernig's sign
C. Mouth and throat examination: lesions, discoloration, exudates
D. Cardiovascular examination
   1. Heart: disturbances in cardiac rate and rhythm, presence of pericardial friction rub
   2. Peripheral vascular system: edema, decrease in peripheral pulse(s)
E. Respiratory examination: tachypnea, lag of excursion on palpation, dullness to percussion, presence of rales (crackles) or rhonchi (wheezes)
F. Lymphatic examination: lymphadenopathy
G. Abdominal examination: masses, tenderness, hepatomegaly, splenomegaly, hyperactive bowel sounds
H. Breast examination: lesions, masses, discoloration, tenderness, discharges
I. Examination of genitalia (both men and women) and perianal region: lesions, discharges
J. Musculoskeletal examination: pain on range of motion, evidence of muscle wasting
K. Skin examination: lesions or discolorations, dryness, thinning of hair, alopecia

Table 5–3. Initial Laboratory Studies for the HIV-infected Person

TESTS	PURPOSE	COMMENTS
Complete blood cell count with differential count	Detect anemia, leukopenia, or thrombocytopenia	Complications frequently seen in HIV disease
Multichannel chemistry panel	May reveal renal, liver, metabolic, or nutritional disease	
Urinalysis	May reveal renal, liver, metabolic, or nutritional disease	
Tuberculin skin test (Mantoux test) with anergy panel	Detect disease or infection caused by *M. tuberculosis*	Anergy testing is recommended with two skin test controls, using *Candida,* mumps, or tetanus toxoid; testing is annual unless client is anergic for 2 consecutive years; anergic clients should be evaluated initially by chest x-ray examination
Chest x-ray examination	Screen for asymptomatic respiratory disease (e.g., tuberculosis)	Repeat for signs and symptoms of pulmonary disease for clients newly identified as having positive PPD results, and for newly identified anergic clients
Pregnancy test	To detect pregnancy when the client's menstrual history and physical examination indicate	
Papanicolaou (Pap) test	To detect cervical dysplasia or neoplasia	For abnormal or uninterpretable results, a colposcopy should be performed
Venereal Disease Research Laboratory (VDRL) test or rapid plasma reagin (RPR) screening test	To screen for untreated cases of syphilis	High rates of coinfection in HIV population; false-negative and false-positive results, although rare, do occur; clients with negative results who are sexually active should be tested yearly; clients with positive results should have fluorescent treponemal antibody absorption (FTA-ABS) test performed for confirmation
Gonorrhea culture	To detect infection	Screen all women (even if free of symptoms); culture of specimens from men with symptoms; evaluation should include possibility of pharyngeal and/or rectal infection
Chlamydia culture	To detect infection	Screen all women (even if free of symptoms); test all men with symptoms; sexual partners should be evaluated
Hepatitis B panel	To detect infection (acute or prior)	Prevalence of past exposure is high in most HIV-infected populations in U.S.; if result is negative and a client is at a continued risk of having HBV infection, vaccination is recommended

Table 5–3. Initial Laboratory Studies for the HIV-infected Person *Continued*

TESTS	PURPOSE	COMMENTS
Toxoplasmosis serologic test	To identify previously exposed individuals and assess risk of development of acute disease	Some HIV-infected clients, although previously infected with *Toxoplasma,* may have negative test results (see text)
CD4$^+$ T-cell count/percentage and CD4$^+$/CD8$^+$ ratio	To assess degree of immunodeficiency	Absolute numbers may vary significantly from test to test; percentage is considered a more stable numeric value and more reliable
Serologic tests for potential opportunistic pathogens	To detect antibodies to pathogens, which indicates previous infections	Not routinely performed (see text)

Data from AIDS Institute (1992, December). HIV medical evaluation and preventive care. In *Protocols for the medical care of HIV infection* (2nd ed.). Albany, NY: New York State Department of Health. Bartlett, J.G. (1993). Routine laboratory testing in asymptomatic infection. *PAACNOTES: The Newsjournal of the Physicians in AIDS Care,* 5(5), 192–197. Hecht, F.M., Soloway, B. (1993). Laboratory tests for monitoring HIV infection. In D.J. Cotton & J.H. Friedland (Eds.), *HIV infection: a primary care approach* (rev. ed.) (pp 16–18). Waltham, MA: Massachusetts Medical Society.

degrees of anemia. The increasing severity of anemia may also lead to shortness of breath and impaired cognition. Decreasing platelet counts will increase the propensity for bleeding. Therefore clinicians should always monitor the use of commonly used over-the-counter medications, such as aspirin, that could further complicate the clinical picture. Depending on the severity of the problem, ensuing leukopenia may require more stringent advice to protect the client against infection. These three frequently coexisting problems are often aggravated by the toxic and other side effects of prescribed medications, and careful monitoring is required.

Baseline information on liver and kidney function from serum chemistry studies will often dictate, later in the course of disease, which medications will be chosen to treat the complications of HIV disease. Once again, clinicians should be aware, not only of the over-the-counter medications the client is taking, but also of the self-prescribed drugs they are obtaining through such suppliers as buyers' clubs (see Chapter 12). Because of the malaise often experienced by persons with HIV infection, it is not uncommon for individuals to take drugs such as acetaminophen routinely (on a daily basis), just to get through the day. Unknowingly, they may be taking, in combination with certain prescribed medications, drugs that may increase the potential for hepatotoxic effects.

Persons with HIV disease are particularly vulnerable to reactivation of latent tuberculosis (TB) infections and to disease caused by new TB infections. The potential for TB transmission is increased when HIV-infected persons are placed in congregate living arrangements such as hospitals, prisons, residences, and shelters. The current resurgence of TB in the United States is largely related to the HIV epidemic (Barnes et al., 1991). Since 1986 the CDC has recommended that HIV-infected individuals who have not had a prior reaction to purified protein derivative (PPD) undergo tuberculin testing annually. This applies to all HIV-infected persons. Clinicians should avoid attempting to distinguish individuals at risk for TB as a basis for determining who should be tested. This point is emphasized by recent studies in which TB caused by tubercle bacilli resistant to multiple drugs was diagnosed in persons not typically recognized to have a high prevalence of TB and in patients without traditional risk factors for drug-resistant TB (Fischl et al., 1992; Pearsen et al., 1992).

Because some HIV-infected persons may have suppression of cellular hypersensitivity mediated by T lymphocytes, referred to as anergy, they may not react to a tuberculin skin test, even in the presence of mycobacterial infection or disease. Therefore the testing of individuals with known or suspected HIV infection should include the use of anergy testing of delayed-type hypersensitivity (DTH) skin test antigens, as a control, at the time the tuberculin skin test is administered (CDC, 1991a) (Table 5–4). Chapter 4 contains a detailed discussion of tuberculosis, including drug-resistant infection and disease.

Initial screening for STDs such as syphilis, gonorrhea, and/or *Chlamydia* infection is appropriate for HIV-infected persons to detect occult disease. Many HIV-infected women come from populations with a high incidence of *Chlamydia* infection and gonorrhea (U.S. Preventive Services Task Force, 1989a; 1989b). The need for repeated testing for these diseases is determined by the clinician and by the client's current history of sexual activities. However, because the client may not always provide complete or accurate information, some clinicians may choose to screen routinely for these STDs in all sexually active individuals.

Gynecologic abnormalities such as vaginal candidiasis, infection with human papillomavirus, cervical intraepithelial neoplasia, and pelvic inflammatory disease tend to occur in higher rates in HIV-infected women (Jewett & Hecht, 1993). Therefore the routine evaluation of women for these problems is warranted. Papanicolaou tests should be performed at least on an annual basis (CDC, 1990a). Chapter 8 discusses the course of HIV disease in women and the related nursing care.

CD4$^+$ T-lymphocyte counts are the most widely used laboratory method of evaluating persons with HIV infection (CDC, 1992a; Stein et al., 1992). The CD4$^+$ T-lymphocyte counts are considered a surrogate marker to determine HIV-related immune dysfunction and disease progression, and are used to guide treatment decisions such as instituting antiretroviral therapy and prophylaxis for certain opportunistic infections. Problems that exist with the interpretation of the absolute CD4$^+$ T-cell count include interlaboratory variability, diurnal variations, and intercurrent variations (Bartlett, 1993; CDC, 1992b; Malone

Table 5–4. Guidelines for Tuberculin and Anergy Testing and HIV Infection

1. All persons with HIV infection should receive a purified protein derivative (PPD)–tuberculin skin test (5TU, PPD by Mantoux method).
2. Because of the occurrence of anergy to PPD among persons with HIV infection who are at risk of having tuberculosis, persons with HIV infection should also be evaluated for delayed-type hypersensitivity (DTH) anergy at the time of PPD testing.
3. Companion testing with two DTH antigens (*Candida,* mumps, or tetanus (toxoid) administered by the Mantoux method is recommended. However, a multipuncture device that administers a battery of DTH antigens may be used.
4. Any induration to a DTH antigen measured at 48 to 72 hours is considered evidence of DTH responsiveness; failure to elicit a response is considered evidence of anergy.
5. Those persons with a positive (>5 mm induration) PPD reaction are considered to be infected with *M. tuberculosis* and should be evaluated for isoniazid preventive therapy after active tuberculosis has been excluded.
6. Persons who manifest a DTH response but have a negative PPD reaction are, in general, considered not to be infected with *M. tuberculosis.*
7. Anergic persons with a negative reaction to tuberculin, whose risk of acquiring a tuberculosis infection is estimated to be ≥10%, should also be considered for isoniazid preventive therapy after active tuberculosis is excluded. This group should include known contacts of patients with infectious tuberculosis, injection drug users, prisoners, homeless persons, migrant laborers, and persons born in countries in Asia, Africa, and Latin America (with high rates of tuberculosis).
8. Although CD4$^+$ T-cell counts should be performed as a part of the evaluation and management of persons with HIV infection, this measurement is not a substitute for anergy evaluation.

Data from Centers for Disease Control and Prevention (1991). Purified protein derivative (PPD)–tuberculin anergy and HIV infection: Guidelines for anergy testing and management of anergic persons at risk of tuberculosis. *Morbidity and Mortality Weekly Report, 40*(RR-5), 33.

et al., 1990). According to Murphy and Chmiel (1992), a more consistent measurement is the percentage of lymphocytes that are CD4$^+$ T cells (Table 5–5). Hecht and So-

Table 5–5. Absolute Numbers of CD4+ T-cell Counts and Equivalent CD4+ T-cell Percentage

CD4+ T-CELL COUNT (mm³)	CD4+ T-CELL PERCENTAGE (%)
≥500	≥29
200–499	14–28
<200	<14

Data from Centers for Disease Control and Prevention (1992). 1993 Revised classification system for HIV infection and expanded surveillance case definition for AIDS among adolescents and adults. *Morbidity and Mortality Weekly Report, 41*(RR-17), 1–19.

loway (1993b) recommended that evaluation of surrogate markers include the absolute CD4+ T-cell count, the CD4+ T-cell percentage, and the CD4+/CD8+ ratio. Clinical decisions should never be based on one laboratory report but on baseline data, trends, and changes.

Careful explanations of CD4+ T-cell measurements must be provided for the client. Hypervigilant behaviors regarding their CD4+ T-cell counts may develop in some individuals. Variations in absolute numbers because of laboratory reporting differences, as well as intrapersonal variations, must be explained. Many HIV-infected individuals have friends who are also infected, attend HIV support groups, and exchange information. Lack of an understanding of CD4+ T-cell count variables can lead to unnecessary anxiety and worry. Other markers of immune status, such as serum concentrations of neopterin, beta$_2$-microglobulin, HIV p24 antigen, soluble interleukin-2 receptors, and immunoglobulin A, and reactions to DTH skin tests, may be useful in the evaluation of HIV-infected patients but are not strongly predictive of HIV disease progression, as are CD4+ T-cell counts (CDC, 1992a).

Routine serologic testing to detect antibodies to previously acquired pathogens is not routinely performed (Bartlett, 1993). For example, serologic evidence of prior infection with herpes simplex virus is found in up to 80% to 90% of HIV-infected adults (Bartlett, 1993). Seroprevalence studies of non-HIV-infected populations in the United States indicate that 40% to 60% of the population has

had infection with cytomegalovirus (Cheeseman, 1992). Similarly, serologic testing for previous infection with *Cryptococcus neoformans, Histoplasma capsulatum,* or *Coccidioides* has not proved useful in identifying patients at risk but may be useful in assessment of clinical disease (Bartlett, 1993; Dismukes, 1988; Galgiani & Ampel, 1990; Wheat et al., 1992). Although most physicians continue to advocate testing for serologic evidence of toxoplasmosis early in HIV disease, Porter and Sande (1992) found that one in every six patients (N = 115) with toxoplasmosis did not have detectable anti-*Toxoplasma* IgG antibodies. Therefore a negative serologic status does not exclude the potential diagnosis of toxoplasmosis in persons with AIDS. Many clinicians however, continue to perform annual tests for *Toxoplasma* infection in unexposed patients.

Immunizations

In general, persons with HIV infection should not receive live-virus or live-bacteria vaccines (CDC, 1993b). However, because limited studies of both patients with and those without symptoms of HIV infection who have received measles-mumps-rubella (MMR) vaccine have not documented serious or unusual adverse events, MMR vaccination is recommended when indicated (Onorato et al., 1988; Sprauer et al., 1993). Regardless of prior vaccination status, all HIV-infected individuals who are exposed to measles should receive immune globulin. Other live, attenuated vaccines such as oral polio vaccine (OPV), bacille Calmette-Guérin (BCG), typhoid vaccine, and smallpox vaccine should not be administered to HIV-infected individuals. Yellow fever vaccine should be given to HIV-infected persons only when potential exposure cannot be avoided (CDC, 1993b).

The use of killed or inactivated vaccines in HIV-infected persons in most cases is relatively safe. The CDC (1993b) recommends that the decision to administer *Haemophilus influenzae* type b (Hib) conjugate vaccine should be based on the patient's risk of Hib disease and the effectiveness of the vaccine. Steinhart and associates (1992), although they did not recommend routine use, suggested that because Hib vaccine is safe and inexpensive, administration of the vaccine to HIV-infected people may be worthwhile.

Routine administration of influenza vaccine is recommended (CDC, 1993b). This vaccine is given annually, usually in November (AIDS Institute, 1992; Hecht & Soloway, 1993c). Opposing reports on the effects of influenza immunization in the presence of HIV-1 viral load were published in 1993. Whereas O'Brien and colleagues (1993) reported that influenza immunization may stimulate HIV-1 replication, Yerly and associates (1993) found no detectable effect on HIV-1 viral load after immunization. Current recommendations are that influenza immunization be offered to HIV-infected individuals.

Since Schuchat and colleagues (1991) identified an increased risk of pneumococcal disease, pneumococcal vaccine is recommended for HIV-infected persons. Revaccination 6 years after the initial dose is recommended for high-risk individuals such as HIV-infected persons (CDC, 1991b).

Initial laboratory evaluation of all HIV-infected persons should include screening for hepatitis B virus (HBV). If HBV antigen and core antibody are not detected, administration of HBV vaccine is recommended, especially in the case of injection drug users (AIDS Institute, 1992; Bartlett, 1993; CDC, 1991b; Hecht & Soloway, 1993b). Because of the expense of the vaccine, laboratory screening should be performed first. After administration of HBV vaccine, antibody response should be tested, and those who have not responded should be vaccinated with one to three additional doses (CDC, 1993b).

Other vaccines containing killed or inactivated antigens, such as diphtheria-tetanus-pertussis vaccine, enhanced inactivated polio vaccine, meningococcal vaccine, rabies vaccine, cholera vaccine, plague vaccine, and anthrax vaccine, may be used for the same indications as for persons with healthy immune systems (CDC, 1993b). In general, it should be noted that response rates to vaccinations are lower in the HIV-infected individual and that declines in response appear to be related to progressive immunodeficiency (Hecht & Soloway, 1993c).

HIV-infected people may benefit from protection by passive immunization through the use of immune globulin preparations (CDC, 1993b). Immune globulin is recommended to prevent measles after exposure. Individuals with symptomatic HIV infection should receive immune globulin regardless of their previous vaccination status, because measles vaccine may not be effective in such patients and the disease may be severe. Immune globulin should also be used when the person with HIV disease has been exposed to hepatitis A.

Varicella-zoster immune globulin (VZIG) is indicated for severely immunocompromised persons after significant exposure to chickenpox or herpes zoster. Significant exposure is defined as household contact, close contact indoors for more than 1 hour, sharing of the same hospital room, or prolonged direct, face-to-face contact such as occurs with nurses or physicians who care for infected patients (CDC, 1993b).

Other immune globulins should be administered for the same indications and in the same doses as for immunocompetent persons. These preparations include hepatitis B immune globulin (HBIG), vaccinia immune globulin (VIG), tetanus immune globulin (TIG), and human rabies immune globulin (HRIG).

Health Teaching

The primary purpose of health teaching is to assist the client with decision making regarding health protection in the presence of HIV disease. Although some clients may choose to improve their own health by adopting all suggestions provided by the nurse, many will not, and others will select only a few areas in which to initiate change. It is important to remember that the choice belongs to the individual client, not the clinician.

Goal setting should be an endeavor on which client and clinician can mutually agree. Motivation for change can be assessed by asking the client which areas that were covered in the health teaching session the client would like to change, as well as which topics are of no interest (Kelly et al., 1991). According to Redland and Stuifbergen (1993), success in achieving goals is increased when the goals are somewhat flexible, short term, and realistic for the individual's life situation. Teaching should also include the planning of relapse prevention. The clinician and client should discuss how to handle relapses as well as how to handle choices to stressful situations.

Basic to planning care is the nurse's knowledge that infection is the leading cause of morbidity in immunodeficient persons. The depressed activity of the $CD4^+$ T cells in persons with HIV infection leaves them vulnerable to a variety of infections. Infection prevention should therefore be considered a pragmatic necessity rather than an abstract concept. The vulnerability of persons with HIV infection to opportunistic infections is increased when they are treated with antimicrobial or antineoplastic agents, many of which induce leukopenia and cause cellular or mucosal damage. Critical to infection development in the person with HIV infection is an interaction of multiple predisposing factors, such as (1) local colonization of potentially pathogenic organisms from normal flora or the environment, (2) local damage to the integument or mucosa that allows entry of these organisms, and (3) a decrease in the number of $CD4^+$ T cells that results in rapid progression of the infectious process. Thus health protection on a secondary level focuses on maintaining or improving the individual's level of wellness through health teaching, as well as on instructing the client about ways to avoid spreading HIV to others (see Appendix IV).

Many infectious complications seen in HIV-infected clients can be prevented (Filice & Pomeroy, 1991). Health teaching that results in behavioral changes in the client are the primary strategy for infection prevention. For example, following food and water safety teaching can prevent such diseases as cryptosporidiosis, salmonellosis, campylobacteriosis, isosporiasis, giardiasis, and toxoplasmosis. Following safer-sex guidelines can reduce the risk that the client will acquire a variety of STDs. Maintaining a regular schedule of health care follow-up screening for tuberculosis and receiving an annual influenza vaccination can reduce the potential for disease.

If the client permits, the nurse should include the client's lover, spouse, friends, or family (whomever the client designates as significant others) in health teaching and should provide printed materials for use as a reference source. This approach is especially indicated when teaching is implemented soon after the initial diagnosis of HIV infection. Weisman (1979) best described this period as one of existential plight. The overwhelming impact of the initial diagnosis precipitates psychologic turmoil that can last for weeks. Although clients are unlikely to retain much of the information given at this time, this contact may be the only one that the nurse will have with the client. Providing printed material and sharing information with the client and significant others will at least ensure that the information has been made available. It is also important at this time that the nurse provide a printed schedule and information for health care follow-up, together with a list of community-based organizations for professional and peer support.

Follow-up

Health care follow-up for an individual whose HIV disease has just been diagnosed should be scheduled immediately, rather than waiting until problems develop. Continuous monitoring of clinical status is also important if antiretroviral therapy and chemoprophylaxis for opportunistic infections are to be instituted at the appropriate time. Symptom-free clients should be seen at 6- to 12-month intervals, and clients with symptoms should be seen at 1- to 3-month intervals, depending on the severity of illness (AIDS Institute, 1992). Follow-up testing should be performed at this time (see Table 5–6).

Physical assessment at follow-up visits should be inclusive, with particular attention given to (1) general appearance, including weight changes, evidence of muscle wasting, and adenopathy; (2) eye examination for visual impairment and exudates; (3) oral examination for lesions and/or thrush; (4) skin examination for general condition and for lesions; (5) neurologic examination for mental status and sensorimotor changes; and (6) pelvic-genitourinary examination.

Table 5–6. Planning Clinical Follow-up for the HIV-infected Person

ASSESSMENT PARAMETERS	CLIENTS WITH NO SYMPTOMS	CLIENTS WITH SYMPTOMS
History/physical examination	Every 6 to 12 months	Every 1 to 3 months
Complete blood cell count with differential count	Annually	Every 3 to 6 months
Multichannel chemistry panel	Annually	Every 3 to 6 months
Urinalysis	Annually	Every 3 months
Tuberculin testing (purified protein derivative [PPD])	Annually	Annually
Papanicolaou (Pap) smear	Every 6 to 12 months	Every 6 to 12 months (some clinicians recommend every 3 to 6 months in HIV-infected women with symptoms)
VDRL test	Annually if client is sexually active	Annually if client is sexually active
Gonorrhea/*Chlamydia* test	Every 6 to 12 months if client is sexually active	Every 3 to 6 months if client is sexually active
Toxoplasmosis serologic test	Annually, for nonexposed patients	Annually, for nonexposed patients
CD4$^+$ T-cell count/percentage and CD4$^+$/CD8$^+$ ratio	Every 6 to 12 months	Every 3 months

Data from AIDS Institute (1992, December). HIV medical evaluation and preventive care. In *Protocols for medical care of HIV infection* (2nd ed.). Albany, NY: New York State Department of Health. Bartlett, J.G. (1993). Routine laboratory testing in asymptomatic infection. *PAACNOTES: The Newsjournal of the Physicians in AIDS Care*, 5(5), 192–197. Hecht, F.M., Soloway, B. (1993). Laboratory tests for monitoring HIV infection. In D.J. Cotton & J.H. Friedland (Eds.), *HIV infection: a primary care approach* (rev. ed.) (pp. 16–18). Waltham, MA: Massachusetts Medical Society.

Updated history should include a review of systems (signs and symptoms) and notation of any illness that has occurred since the last visit, where the patient was treated, and how the problem was managed. Evaluation of health teaching performed in the past or currently needed should be performed at follow-up visits.

During the course of the follow-up treatment, decisions will have to be made as HIV disease progresses. Perhaps one of the most important decisions to be made concerns the issue of antiretroviral therapy. Before 1993, the guidelines for antiretroviral therapy were very specific. However, at the Ninth International Conference on AIDS, held in Berlin, Germany, in June 1993, clinical investigators and practioners reviewed all available research and concluded that the efficacy of current antiviral therapy was questionable in many respects (Cotton, 1993). The questions raised centered around the extent to which zidovudine impedes early disease progression,

the efficacy of other nucleoside analogs such as didanosine and zalcitabine, and the likelihood that newer drugs under study would hold more promise. Confounding the issue of evaluating all published trial results were the facts, reported by Choi and colleagues (1993), that monitoring CD4$^+$ T-cell counts alone may not tell the true story and that CD4$^+$ T-cell percentages are a preferred surrogate marker (most studies reported only CD4$^+$ T-cell counts as a marker of antiretroviral therapy efficacy).

After the Berlin conference, an independent panel of experts convened at the National Institute of Allergy and Infectious Diseases (NIAID) and released preliminary recommendations on the use of antiretroviral drugs in the care of adults with HIV infection. The recommendations covered (1) the initiation of antiretroviral therapy, (2) changing therapy in patients tolerating initial therapy, (3) therapy in patients intolerant to zidovudine, and (4) therapy in patients with disease progression despite zidovudine therapy (Staff, 1993). A less publicized underpinning of these meetings was the acknowledgment that there is no "typical" patient, that each person is unique, and that any clinical decision regarding antiretroviral therapy should be made by both the patient and the clinician (NIAID, 1993). Chapter 3 discusses the details of current recommendations regarding antiretroviral therapy.

Additional treatment decisions include the initiation of chemoprophylactic therapy to prevent opportunistic infections. Current recommendations include prophylactic therapy to prevent *Pneumocystis carinii* pneumonia in HIV-infected persons with $CD4^+$ T-cell counts less than 200 mm^3, and prophylaxis for disseminated *Mycobacterium avium* complex infection in HIV-infected individuals with $CD4^+$ T-cell counts less than 100 mm^3 (CDC, 1992c, 1993c). Guidelines for prophylaxis against both of these opportunistic infections are contained in Chapter 4.

Medication Management

Managing increasing numbers of prescribed medications can be difficult for persons with HIV (PWHIV). In a study of the nursing care needs of PWHIV admitted to a home care program, Hurley and Ungvarski (1994), noted that the number of medications ordered in the sample (N = 244) ranged from 0 to 18 per patient, with an average of 6.4 medications prescribed for each subject. Forty percent of the subjects lacked the ability to self-medicate and needed either supervision or reminders, help with administration, or complete preparation and administration. Additionally, many of the patients did not have the prescribed medications in the home.

The problem of noncompliance, in the case of medication management related to the treatment of pulmonary tuberculosis, extends beyond the welfare of the individual patient. In this situation, noncompliance may not only result in significant morbidity and death but also may lead to the development of drug resistance and the spread of disease. Mahmoudi and Iseman (1993) identified the failure to recognize and deal with noncompliance with the prescription of medications as a major pitfall in the care of patients with tuberculosis.

An additional issue of concern is undercompliance, in which case an individual willing to take the prescribed medication decides to reduce the dosage and/or the dosing schedule. Undercompliance may be revealed when the client seeks confirmation from the clinician that such an activity is acceptable.

Stephenson and colleagues (1993) identified three key areas in the assessment of patient compliance. First is the attendance at and participation in appointments made for health care follow-up (missed appointments should be noted). Second is the lack of responsiveness to usually (or previously) adequate doses of medication. Further assessment is needed to distinguish problems with therapy from those related to compliance. Third is direct measure of medication consumption with laboratory evaluation. The authors acknowledged that the latter is available only for a small number of medications and is not always reliable, as well as being time-consuming and expensive.

Careful questioning, the most widely used method of assessing compliance, can often detect noncompliant individuals. Stephenson and associates (1993) suggested specific strategies that should be used in the self-report interview, including (1) asking the patient to tell exactly what medications they are taking and when they are taking them, (2) using a nonjudgmental, nonthreatening approach, and stating that many people have difficulty taking their medications, (3) opening the discussion with whether or not the client ever has problems with taking medications, and (4) if the patient acknowledges problems, asking how many times, during the previous day or week, doses have been missed.

Techniques to monitor medication compliance such as pill counts, drug levels, and pill monitors pose ethical questions because they invade privacy and question the patient's autonomy. These techniques can be used when the reasons for monitoring assessments have been provided and the patient has been informed of their use (Stephenson et al., 1993).

Assessment should include not only the individual client but also the significant others and/or family members and the living environment to identify potential conflicts with prescribed medication regimens (Weitzel, 1992). Cultural beliefs regarding the taking of prescribed medications may affect compliance. Care partners worried about side effects of certain drugs may withhold them or reduce the dose and/or frequency. Homes where individuals are abusing substances may result in sharing of, or stealing, narcotic analgesics or tranquilizers. Lack of a refrigerator may preclude the ability to properly store some medications, and lack of finances may result in the patient's picking and choosing which medications can be obtained.

Finally, the discrete, subtle, and often underdiagnosed problem of cognitive impairment can contribute significantly to compliance capabilities. Clinicians should consider the multifaceted nature of medication management when evaluating the outcomes of prescribed therapy.

TERTIARY PREVENTION

The tertiary level of nursing care is concerned with minimizing the disabilities that result from advancing HIV disease, and includes individuals with symptoms as well as persons with a definitive diagnosis of AIDS. The primary focus is on symptom control so that the quality of life can be maintained or improved for clients in the later stages of the illness trajectory.

Giardino and Wolf (1993) noted that symptoms serve as intervention foci for nurses in planning the care of patients and emphasized that patients' subjective experiences with symptoms and their desire for specific treatment may contrast sharply with nurses' objective assessment of both the presence and severity of symptoms. Symptoms are the subjective phenomena regarded as indicators of a condition departing from normal function. Signs are defined as objective indicators of disease that are verifiable by physical findings or by the results of technology (Giardino & Wolf, 1993).

For measurement of symptoms, numerous instruments have been developed and tested for reliability and validity. The problem with many tools is that they are of limited usefulness in the clinical setting in which most nurses work, given the time constraints associated with the delivery of nursing care. Additionally, many tools are not user friendly and require training to use them properly.

Giardino and Wolf (1993), in a review of symptom experiences and nursing, identified several useful tools that may be used for symptom assessment. The Duke–University of North Carolina Health Profile (DUHP) measures adults' ongoing health status in the primary care setting and assesses symptom experience, physical function, and emotional and social function (Parkerson et al., 1981). The DUHP, considered too lengthy, was revised by Parkerson and colleagues (1990) into the Duke Health Profile (DUKE) and is considered useful in monitoring health as an outcome of health promotion interventions. The briefest, yet most effective, measure of wellness and dysfunction is a modified version of the DUHP, the mini-DUHP (Blake & Vandiver, 1986). McCorkle and Young (1978) developed the Symptom Distress Scale (SDS) to measure the degree of physical distress that the patient experiences with nausea, insomnia, pain, fatigue, cough, changes in appetite, bowel habits, concentration, appearance, breathing, and outlook. Rhodes and associates (1986) adopted the SDS for use in evaluating nausea and vomiting associated with chemotherapy. The Cornell Medical Index (CMI) is also considered to be a reliable measure of the patient's perception of illness and the reported presence of symptoms (Abramson et al., 1965; 1966).

The most convenient tool for symptom assessment is the Visual Analog Scale (VAS) (Freud, 1923). It is a self-reporting measure of subjective experiences of symptoms. The VAS provides a rapid way for the patient to identify the severity of the symptom and to monitor trends in symptom presentation and symptom control evaluation (Gift, 1989; Freud, 1923). The vertical scale has been found to be more sensitive when symptoms are measured and easier for patients to use (Gift et al., 1986).

The nursing care plans presented are organized according to symptoms that may be identified by the patient, significant other, and/or clinician. Nursing treatments and interventions are directed at symptom control, and, in many cases, symptom management targets the subjective experience rather than the underlying condition (Giardino & Wolf, 1993).

Although nursing interventions specific to the identified symptoms seen in PWHIV have not been studied, it is reasonable to expect that symptom strategies developed empirically for other patient populations may be effective. For example, the topic of dyspnea and the related nursing care is based on research conducted on patients with lung disease, cardiac disease, and cancer. Much of the knowledge gained regarding fever has been conducted with afebrile individuals or individuals with febrile conditions associated with neurologic disorders. An exception is the topic of weight loss, which has been studied extensively in PWHIV.

SYMPTOM: *Fever*

Etiology:

A. Chronic HIV infection
B. Secondary opportunistic infection(s)
C. Malignancy
D. Autoimmune disorders
E. Diarrhea
F. Dehydration
G. Allergic response to medications (drug fever)
H. Infections of intravenous lines, catheters, drains, and incisions

Nursing Assessment:

A. Subjective data
   1. History of symptom
   2. Associated symptom
   3. Twenty-four hour dietary history, including fluid intake
   4. Medical and surgical history
   5. Current drug therapy

B. Objective data
   1. Vital signs
   2. Mental status, including alertness, cognition, and orientation
   3. Skin assessment, including integrity, temperature, turgor, appearance, and signs of injury or infection
   4. Assessment for dehydration, including the preceding, plus fluid intake and output estimates, and assessment of urine color, quantity, and consistency

NOTE WELL: Mackowiak and associates (1993), in a study of normal body temperatures, suggested that 37.2° C (98.9° F) in the early morning and 37.7° C (99.9° F) overall should be regarded as the upper limit of the normal body temperature range in healthy adults aged 40 years or younger. This study used an electronic digital thermometer measuring oral temperatures.

C. Assessment tools (Holtzclaw, 1992)
   1. In euthermia and low-grade fever, oral or axillary modes can be used
   2. Rectal temperature, although often undesirable, is more reliable than oral in afebrile persons (no studies are available that investigated linear relationships between rectal and other measures in febrile patients)
   3. Statistically significant differences have been found in electronic thermometer readings when the probe is placed in the posterior sublingual versus front sublingual regions; negligible differences were seen when mercury thermometers were used (Erickson, 1980)
   4. Continuous pulmonary artery and tympanic membrane temperatures are ideal
   5. Hot and cold liquids can influence oral temperatures for as long as 9 minutes
   6. Although oxygen administration has no effect on oral temperature, tachypnea and mouth breathing can cause lower readings (Dressler et al., 1983)
   7. Liquid crystal "stick on" patches to measure temperature are inaccurate in febrile patients (Ilsley et al., 1983)

8. Use the same instrument, technique, and placement for each measurement to ensure that trends in temperature change are accurately detected

NOTE WELL: It is important for clinicians to remember that because of the underlying immunodeficiency resulting in an impaired inflammatory response, clinical manifestations of infection, including fever, may be greatly muted (Hibberd & Rubin, 1991).

Nursing Diagnoses:

High risk for altered body temperature; high risk for fluid volume deficit

Goals:

After discussing the finding of assessment and the nursing diagnosis, the client and/or care partner and the nurse will select interventions to:

A. Control fever
B. Replace fluid loss

Considerations for Nursing Care and Health Teaching:

A. Nonpharmacologic interventions (Holtzclaw, 1992)
   1. Promote heat loss by:
      a. Allowing heat to escape from trunk by applying a sheet and a loosely woven blanket
      b. If no skin lesions are present and patient is ambulatory, immerse in a tub bath with water temperature at 39° C (102.2° F); avoiding chilling when emerging from bath
   2. Avoid counterproductive treatments such as:
      a. Tepid water sponge bathing, which causes defensive vasoconstriction (this has not been shown to be an effective coolant in fever, it can cause shivering, and it is also distressful) (Morgan, 1990; Newman, 1985)
      b. Alcohol sponging causes vasoconstriction, shivering, and toxic fumes, and may be absorbed cutaneously, causing hypoglycemia

(McCarthy, 1991; Morgan, 1990; Newman, 1985)
   3. Holtzclaw (1992) recommended that the use of cooling blankets and ice packs be reserved for conditions in which core temperature is rising uncontrollably to potentially damaging levels (Goodman and Knochel [1991] suggested that hypothermia blankets and similar devices not be used in interleukin-1–mediated temperature elevations [pyrogenic fever], because the associated shivering is counterproductive to core temperature reduction)
   4. Prevent febrile shivering
      a. Keep patient in a warm room to avert shivering (Palmes & Park, 1965)
      b. Avoid fanning bedcovers, skin exposure, or rapid removal of clothing that might cause chilling
   5. Control febrile shivering by wrapping the arms from fingertips to axillae and the legs from toes to groin with three layers of terrycloth toweling (Abbey et al., 1973; Caruso et al., 1992; Holtzclaw, 1990a; 1990b)
B. Increase caloric and fluid intake
   1. Provide a plan for six feedings distributed over a 24-hour period
   2. Provide high-protein, high-calorie nutritional supplements, especially in the presence of anorexia
   3. Provide at least 2 to 2.5 liters of fluid to drink daily
   4. Record intake and output
C. Maintain comfort and safety
   1. Provide dry clothes and bed linens; use cotton materials rather than synthetics
   2. Use emollient creams for dry skin
   3. Monitor mental status frequently, especially when client is febrile
   4. Evaluate client's need for assistance with all activities of daily living
D. For chronic recurrent night fever and night sweats:
   1. Suggest that client take the antipyretic agent of choice before going to sleep
   2. Have a change of bedclothes nearby in case a change is necessary
   3. Keep a plastic cover on the pillow

4. Place a towel over the pillow in case of profuse diaphoresis
5. Keep liquid at bedside to drink

E. Pharmacologic treatment should include consideration of the following:
1. Clinicians should assess the client's patterns of use of aspirin, nonsteroidal antiinflammatory agents, and acetaminophen
2. Follow-up should include comparing patterns of use of these agents with laboratory evaluation of hepatic and hematologic abnormalities, as well as interactions with other agents
3. Although concern has been expressed about concomitant administration of zidovudine and acetaminophen, Steffe and associates (1990) and Sattler and colleagues (1991) found no significant interaction between the two drugs; however, Shriner and Goetz (1992) reported severe hepatotoxic effects in a patient taking both drugs and cautioned clients to be aware of this potential problem, especially in patients who are malnourished and have hepatic disease
4. Aspirin and other nonsteroidal antiinflammatory agents may have an immunomodulating effect on $CD4^+$ T cells (Armistead, 1992; Macilwain, 1993); however, use of these agents may be contraindicated in severe hematologic abnormalities such as thrombocytopenia

Referrals:

A. Clinical nurse specialist (CNS) in HIV disease
B. Dietitian
C. Visiting nurse

Evaluation:

The client will:

A. Identify appropriate measures to be taken in the presence of fever
B. Demonstrate the ability to initiate and maintain adequate hydration and nutrition
C. Demonstrate the ability to take and record the temperature accurately

SYMPTOM: *Fatigue*

Etiology:

A. Chronic HIV infection
B. Secondary opportunistic infection(s) or malignancies
C. Anemia
D. Malnutrition
E. Diarrhea
F. Prolonged immobility
G. Psychologic factors
H. Situational factors

Nursing Assessment:

A. Subjective data
1. History of symptoms
2. Associated symptoms (e.g., anxiety, depression, dyspnea)
3. Current ability to perform activities of daily living safely and to exercise
4. Factors that increase fatigue (e.g., weather, alcohol, bathing)
5. Medical and surgical history
6. Current drug therapy
7. Nutrition history

B. Objective data
1. Assess activity tolerance by taking vital signs before and immediately after the performance of an activity such as bathing, dressing, or ambulating
2. Assess client for associated signs and symptoms such as pallor, diaphoresis, or complaints of dyspnea or dizziness

C. Assessment tools
1. Symptom Distress Scale (SDS) (McCorkle & Young, 1978)
2. Visual Analog Scale to Measure Fatigue Severity (VAS-F) (Lee et al., 1991)
3. Piper Fatigue Scale (PFS) (Piper et al., 1989)
4. Pearson and Byars' Fatigue Feeling Tone Scale (Pearson & Byars, 1956)

Nursing Diagnosis:

Fatigue

Goals: (Hart et al., 1990)

After discussing and validating the findings of assessment and nursing diagnosis, the client and/or care partner and nurse will select interventions to:

A. Increase self-awareness of fatigue, associated symptoms, environmental factors affecting fatigue, and activity tolerance
B. Identify the importance of resting when needed
C. Develop a plan for activity and rest
D. Accept assistance when needed
E. Develop a lifestyle that keeps client involved in activities of daily living (ADL), independent, and socially active

Considerations for Nursing Care and Health Teaching (Gift & Pugh, 1993; Hart et al., 1990; Piper, 1993):

A. Promote self-care and self-awareness
1. Have client keep a daily fatigue diary for at least 1 week to identify sources of fatigue and appropriate interventions, as well as patterns of peak fitness
2. Use an assessment tool to evaluate fatigue
B. Promote adequate sleep
1. Increase the amount of sleep
2. Reduce the amount of sleep cycle interruptions by:
   a. Preparing for sleep
   b. Keeping needed items at bedside (e.g., iced water, urinal, towel to absorb perspiration)
   c. See "Insomnia"
C. Encourage adequate nutrition
1. Substances such as coffee, tobacco, or alcohol may, in some individuals, increase fatigue
2. Abstain from or curtail foods that the client may be sensitive to
3. See "Weight Loss"
D. Promote rest and activity
1. Assist the patient in pacing of activities
   a. Plan a written 24-hour schedule for ADL that alternates short activities with rest periods
   b. Assist in identifying activity priorities such as eating breakfast and then resting before bathing in the morning, as opposed to the reverse

c. Evaluate the individual's needs and point out ways to conserve energy, such as:
   (1) Sitting down while dressing, shaving, or preparing food
   (2) Sitting in a shower chair while bathing
   (3) Using disposable items for eating so that no cleanup is needed
2. Write up a plan, progressing from daily to weekly, for rest and activities
3. Always plan activities ahead of time
4. Several short periods of rest may be more effective than fewer long rest periods
5. Plan an exercise schedule (physiologic immobilization may lead to increased fatigue as a result of decreased endurance)
   a. Plan exercise at peak energy times (after a rest period)
   b. Follow exercise with rest
   c. Have physical therapist assess the client and plan an exercise program
   d. Aerobic exercise, which increases endurance, has been shown to reduce fatigue (MacVicar & Winningham, 1986; Pardue, 1984; Thayer, 1987)
E. Additional natural techniques (discussed in Chapter 12) that may be of benefit include:
1. Progressive muscle relaxation
2. Acupressure
3. Massage
4. Reflexology
5. Imagery and visualization
6. Autogenic relaxation
7. Reframing and positive affirmations
8. Therapeutic touch
9. Social support and support groups

Referrals:

A. Physical therapist
B. Occupational therapist
C. CNS in HIV disease or rehabilitation
D. Visiting nurse
E. Community-based AIDS program that provides visitors, or "buddies"

Evaluation:

The client will:

A. Identify causative factors that increase fatigue

B. Demonstrate the ability to plan a schedule of paced activity for a 24-hour period

C. Demonstrate the ability to participate in a program of exercise

D. Verbalize a decrease in the fatigue experienced for a 24-hour period

SYMPTOM: *Weight Loss*

Etiology (Grunfeld, 1992; King, 1990; Kotler et al., 1989; Kotler 1992):

A. Increased nutrient requirements resulting from primary systemic infection with HIV or secondary systemic (opportunistic) infection, causing:
  1. Hypermetabolism
  2. Fever
  3. Catabolism

B. Decreased food intake resulting from side effects of medication or systemic infection, causing:
  1. Anorexia
  2. Nausea
  3. Vomiting
  4. Alterations in taste

C. Oral or esophageal infection, causing:
  1. Impaired chewing
  2. Difficulty in swallowing

D. Decreased assimilation of food because of primary intestinal infection with HIV or secondary (opportunistic) gastrointestinal infection, causing:
  1. Malabsorption
  2. Diarrhea

E. Inability to obtain food because of:
  1. Fatigue
  2. Lack of money
  3. Distance from shopping
  4. Lack of utilities to store and prepare food

F. Lack of knowledge of the importance of nutrition in HIV infection and its impact on survival

G. Neuropsychiatric problems such as:
  1. Depression
  2. Impaired cognition
  3. Paralysis

Nursing Assessment (Bradley-Springer, 1991; Lindsey, 1993; Newman, 1992; Task Force on Nutrition Support in AIDS, 1989):

A. Subjective data
  1. Medical and surgical history, including signs and symptoms, stage of HIV infection, opportunistic infections and/or neoplasms, and related therapy
  2. Medication profile, including prescribed medications, over-the-counter medications, alternative therapies, and recreational drugs
  3. Diet history, including food patterns, tolerances and allergies, cultural preferences, and knowledge of nutrition
  4. Mental status, including cognitive impairment, anxiety, and depression
  5. Resources to buy, store, and prepare food
  6. Related signs and symptoms such as dyspnea and/or fatigue
  7. Social supports

B. Objective data
  1. Height and weight
  2. Anthropometric measurements
  3. Examination of skin, hair, nails, and oral cavity
  4. Examination of cranial nerves I (olfactory), V (trigeminal), IX (glossopharyngeal), and X (vagus)
  5. Evaluation of ability to feed self
  6. Laboratory data including blood cell count and serum albumin level

C. Assessment tool: nutritional diary, recorded for at least 1 week to identify patterns and problems (should include related symptoms)

Nursing Diagnosis:

Altered nutrition: less than body requirements

Goals (Task Force on Nutrition Support in AIDS, 1989):

After discussing and validating the findings of

assessment and the nursing diagnosis, the client and/or care partner and the nurse will select interventions to:

A. Preserve lean body mass
B. Provide adequate levels of all nutrients

Considerations for Nursing Care and Health Teaching (Newman, 1992; Life Sciences Research Office, 1990; Task Force on Nutrition Support in AIDS, 1989):

A. Minimize factors contributing to anorexia
  1. For alterations in the sense of smell:
     a. Hyperosmia (increased sense of smell): avoid cooking odors by keeping windows open and the home well aerated; encourage meals that include cold foods
     b. Hyposmia (decreased sense of smell): use spices such as basil, oregano, rosemary, thyme, cloves, mint, cinnamon, or lemon juice to enhance smell
  2. For alterations in sense of taste (especially related to distaste for red meat):
     a. Marinate meat before cooking in commercial marinade, wine, or vinegar
     b. As substitutes for red meat, use other protein sources such as eggs, peanut butter, tofu, cheeses, poultry, or fish
  3. For persons living alone or experiencing fatigue or depression:
     a. Eat small meals frequently throughout the day; try to eat "by the clock"
     b. Include high-calorie snacks and/or commercially prepared supplements (liquids or bars)
     c. Indulge desires for favorite foods
     d. Consume more nutrient-dense foods and beverages, rather than filling up on low-calorie items
     e. Drink liquids a half hour before eating instead of with meals
     f. Prepare meals (such as soups or casseroles) ahead of time so that they can be divided into individual servings and frozen until ready to use
     g. Keep easy-to-prepare foods on hand, such as frozen dinners, canned foods, and eggs
     h. Make food presentation and service appealing
     i. Encourage dining with friends or family in pleasant surroundings
     j. Get family members and friends involved in meal preparation; the warm atmosphere that they can provide may stimulate the patient's appetite
     k. Utilize home food delivery service (e.g., Meals on Wheels programs)
     l. Direct the patient to support services in the community; sources of information on available food programs may include outpatient dietitians at local hospitals or public health department nutritionists
     m. Carry powdered forms of liquid dietary supplements because they may be easier to carry than ready-to-use forms in cans
  4. See "Nausea"

B. Minimize factors related to difficulty in chewing, dysphagia (difficulty in swallowing), or odynophagia (painful swallowing)
  1. Avoid:
     a. Rough foods such as raw fruits and vegetables
     b. Spicy, acidic, or salty foods
     c. Alcohol or tobacco
     d. Excessively hot or cold foods
     e. Sticky foods such as peanut butter and slippery foods such as gelatin, bologna, and elbow macaroni
  2. Encourage:
     a. Eating foods at room temperature
     b. Choosing mild foods and drinks (e.g., apple juice rather than orange juice)
     c. Eating dry-grain foods such as breads, crackers, and cookies after softening in milk, tea, or other mild beverage
     d. Eating nonabrasive, easy-to-swallow foods such as ice cream,

pudding, well-cooked eggs, noo-
dle dishes, baked fish, and soft
cheese
   e. Eating popsicles to numb pain
   f. Using straw when drinking
   g. Tilting head back or moving it forward to make swallowing easier
C. Minimize factors related to inability to obtain food:
  1. Evaluate financial resources and the
need for referral for Medicaid, food
stamps, and other services
  2. Evaluate the home and the client's ability to prepare and obtain food, looking
for such factors as:
   a. Absence of cooking facilities (e.g.,
living in a shelter or hotel for homeless persons)
   b. Need for alternative housing arrangements
  3. Explore community resources that
provide free meals
D. Discuss nutritional requirements for persons with HIV disease, including:
  1. High-protein sources and ways to increase protein intake by:
   a. Adding skim milk powder to regulate whole milk
   b. Preparing canned creamed soups
with heavy cream instead of water
or milk
   c. Increasing intake of peanut butter
and eating it on whole-wheat bread
   d. Adding pasteurized processed
cheeses to soups and vegetables
   e. Eating hard-boiled eggs for snacks
  2. Increasing caloric intake by:
   a. Using extra peanut butter, cream
cheese, sugar, honey, sour cream,
and mayonnaise
   b. Substituting heavy creams for milk
in coffee, tea, soups, and other
foods
   c. Eating sweets for snacks
   d. Drinking commercially prepared
liquid dietary supplements
   e. Making a liquid nutritional supplement at home by mixing:
    (1) A 1-quart packet of powdered
milk with
    (2) One quart of whole milk and

    (3) Four packets of a flavored in-
stant breakfast mix
    NOTE: This powdered pack-
age recipe is significantly easier
to travel with than ready-to-use
canned preparations.
   f. Eating small, frequent meals instead of a few large meals
  3. Reviewing a balanced diet selection for
a 24-hour menu plan
E. Review essential elements of a low-micro-
bial diet and food safety and preparation
(see Appendix IV)
F. See "Diarrhea"

NOTE WELL: The nutritional teaching
should, as much as possible, follow the client's
usual pattern of food intake rather than expecting the client to follow a totally new, unfamiliar prescription for meal planning.

Referrals:

A. Dietitian
B. Social worker
C. CNS in HIV disease
D. Visiting nurse
E. Community-based AIDS program that
provides meals

Evaluation:

The client will:

A. Demonstrate weight maintenance or gain
B. Identify factors related to anorexia, difficulty in chewing, dysphagia, or odynophagia
C. Identify sufficient resources to obtain and
prepare food—or social work intervention has been established to obtain food
stamps or public assistance
D. Identify means of increasing protein and
calorie intake
E. Identify key concepts in planning a low-
microbial diet
F. Select a balanced 24-hour menu

SYMPTOM: *Nausea*

Etiology:

A. Opportunistic infections either in the gastrointestinal tract or disseminated

B. Neoplasms in the gastrointestinal tract
C. Side effects of medications
D. Associated with pain, anorexia, vomiting, fear, and anxiety (Grant, 1987)
E. Psychologically induced when the individual is exposed to noxious odors, tastes, sights
F. Anticipatory nausea and vomiting, a learned phenomenon in which nausea and/or vomiting precedes the administration of a chemotherapeutic agent (Briscoe, 1989; Duigon, 1986; Pratt et al., 1984)

Nursing Assessment:

A. Subjective data
 1. History of symptom
 2. Associated symptoms
 3. Current drug therapy
 4. Nutrition history
 5. Impact of symptom on ADL
 6. Factors that increase or decrease symptom
B. Objective data
 1. Height and weight
 2. Vital signs
 3. Anthropometric measurements
 4. Laboratory tests for serum albumin, total protein, and transferrin values; complete blood cell count with differential cell count; and serum electrolyte values (to detect malnutrition and dehydration)
C. Assessment tools
 1. Rhodes Index of Nausea and Vomiting (INV) Form 2 (Rhodes et al., 1986)
 2. Morrow Assessment of Nausea and Emesis (MANE) (Morrow, 1984)
 3. Adapted Symptom Distress Scale (ASDS) Form 2 (Rhodes, 1990)
 4. Self-care journal (SCJ) (Rhodes, 1990)

Nursing Diagnosis:

Knowledge deficit of effective strategies to manage nausea

Goals:

After discussing the findings of assessment and the nursing diagnosis, the client and/or care partner and the nurse will select interventions to:

A. Manage nausea
B. Maintain adequate nutrition and hydration

Considerations for Nursing Care and Health Teaching:

A. Nonpharmacologic interventions (Jablonski, 1993; Rhodes, 1990)
 1. Relaxation using videotape with soothing music, environmental sounds, and images of nature have been used effectively (Burish & Carey, 1984; Lyles et al., 1982; Redd, 1984)
 2. Distraction or relaxation, including:
  a. Rest, reading, or relaxation tapes
  b. Television
  c. Music
  d. Exercise
  e. Games
  f. Imagery
  g. Laughter or humor
  h. Conversations or storytelling
  i. Massage
  j. Therapeutic touch
 3. Nutritional suggestions for controlling nausea, including (Life Sciences Research Office, 1990):
  a. Eat larger meals at times when feeling better; reschedule meals if nausea consistently occurs at the same time of day
  b. Avoid favorite foods during nausea to prevent development of taste aversions for these foods
  c. Eat saltier foods
  d. Avoid very sweet foods
  e. Avoid greasy or fatty foods
  f. Try cold entrees rather than hot ones; they are less aromatic and often better tolerated
  g. Eat smaller portions of food throughout the day
  h. Stay out of the kitchen while food is being prepared if food odors provoke nausea
  i. Eat dry foods, such as toast or crackers, especially if nausea occurs in the morning (unless oral or esophageal lesions are present or salivary flow is impaired)
  j. Eat soft, bland foods that are easier

to tolerate, such as rice, soft-cooked or poached eggs, apple juice, nectars, and custards

    k. Time meals and medications to avoid anticipatory vomiting

    l. Take an antiemetic drug before meals

    m. Replace fluid and salt by consuming broths, ginger ale, and juices if vomiting occurs

    n. Drink fluids through a straw, and between meals rather than with meals

    o. Chew foods thoroughly and eat slowly

    p. Rest after meals, but avoid reclining or lying down immediately after eating

  4. See "Weight Loss"

B. Pharmacologic treatment should include the following considerations:

  1. For severe nausea, it may be more effective to take an antiemetic agent on a regularly scheduled basis rather than only as needed

  2. Because of the continuous development of new antiretroviral therapies to treat HIV infection, information on drug interactions is often limited

  3. Benzodiazepines that may be used as antiemetics may alter the pharmacokinetics of zidovudine, potentially increasing toxicity (Burger et al., 1993)

  4. The use of a cannabinoid such as dronabinol for antiemetic purposes may be of benefit in HIV-infected individuals, because it may also act as an appetite stimulant and result in weight gain (Plasse et al., 1991)

Referrals:

A. Dietitian
B. CNS in HIV disease
C. Visiting nurse

Evaluation:

The client will:

A. Identify causative factors
B. Identify appropriate management strategies
C. Report decreasing episodes of nausea

SYMPTOM: *Diarrhea*

Etiology:

A. Gastrointestinal infection caused by:

  1. Bacteria (e.g., *Salmonella, Shigella, Mycobacterium avium-intracellulare, Campylobacter*)

  2. Fungi (e.g., *Candida*)

  3. Protozoa (e.g., *Cryptosporidium, Isospora belli, Microsporidium, Entamoeba histolytica, Giardia*)

  4. Viruses (e.g., cytomegalovirus, herpes simplex virus, adenovirus, astrovirus, picornavirus)

B. Kaposi's sarcoma in the gastrointestinal tract
C. Gastrointestinal reaction to medications
D. Lactose intolerance
E. Inappropriate dietary intake
F. Intolerance to dietary supplements with a high osmolarity

Nursing Assessment:

A. Subjective data

  1. Usual pattern of elimination

  2. Usual pattern of nutrition

  3. Food intolerance, especially lactose intolerance as evidenced by cramping, flatulence, and diarrhea when they consume milk or milk products (Roberts, 1993)

  4. History of diarrhea

  5. Associated symptoms

  6. Current drug therapy

  7. Sexual activities involving anal intercourse or oral-anal contact

  8. Current and past medical and surgical findings

B. Objective data

  1. Observation of fecal material (for steatorrhea)

  2. Assessment of mucocutaneous surfaces (hydration status)

  3. Assessment of blood pressure for orthostatic hypotension

  4. Auscultation and palpation of abdomen

  5. Examination of perianal region

  6. Baseline serum albumin, total iron-binding capacity, blood urea nitrogen, and creatinine levels (Roberts, 1993)

C. Assessment tool: Record of intake and output

Nursing Diagnoses:

Diarrhea; high risk for fluid volume deficit

Goals:

After discussing and validating the findings of assessment and the nursing diagnosis, the client and/or care partner and the nurse will select interventions to:

A. Reduce symptoms and facilitate the restoration of usual bowel patterns
B. Prevent associated complications such as dehydration and skin breakdown

Considerations for Nursing Care and Health Teaching:

A. Low-residue, high-protein, high-calorie diet (Culhane, 1984; Task Force on Nutrition Support in AIDS, 1989)
   1. Diet includes:
      a. Cottage cheese, cream cheese, and mild processed cheeses
      b. Cooked eggs
      c. Boiled low-fat milk, yogurt, and buttermilk
      d. Clear broth and bouillon
      e. Baked, broiled, or roasted fish, poultry, or lean ground beef
      f. Gelatin, pudding, custard
      g. Cooked Cream of Wheat or Cream of Rice cereal
      h. Bananas, applesauce, peeled apples, apple juice, grape juice, or avocados
      i. White bread, toast, or crackers made from refined flour
      j. Noodles, pasta, or white rice, cooked vegetables such as baked potatoes, carrots, squash, peas, green or wax beans
      k. Cream soups
   2. Diet excludes:
      a. Whole-grain bread, whole-grain cereals, or brown rice
      b. Nuts, seeds, popcorn, pretzels, potato chips, and similar snacks
      c. Fried foods
      d. Fresh fruits (except those listed previously), dried fruits

e. Raw vegetables and fresh salads
      f. Rich pastries
      g. Strong spices such as chili powder or curry
      h. Foods that increase flatus such as cabbage, broccoli, and onions
      i. Coffee, tea, colas, chocolate
      j. Carbonated beverages
      k. Alcohol beverages
      l. Tobacco
B. Hydrate with at least 2.5 to 3 liters of fluid per day, including:
   1. Water
   2. Gatorade
   3. Noncarbonated drinks or soda that has been opened and is relatively "flat" (with minimum carbonation left)
   4. Caffeine-free drinks
   5. Diluted fruit juices
C. Provide small, frequent meals and dietary supplements
D. Avoid foods that are very hot, very cold, or spicy
E. In the presence of lactose intolerance, use lactose-free dairy products such as Lactaid
F. Provide skin care (Lincoln & Roberts, 1989) by:
   1. Cleaning the skin thoroughly and gently
   2. Because water alone usually is not an adequate means of cleansing, using commercial spray cleaner (e.g., Peri Wash, Uni Wash, and Hollister Skin Cleanser, which contain substances that emulsify the stool and aid in its removal)
   3. If skin is intact, after cleansing apply a petrolatum-based protective ointmet to limit further contact of stool on the skin
   4. If skin is denuded, after cleansing apply a coat of protective powder such as Stomahesive and then apply a petrolatum-based protective ointment
G. For ambulatory persons:
   1. Use plastic squeeze bottle filled with warm water and spray cleaner to wash perianal area while sitting on toilet after each bowel movement
   2. Carry Tucks disposable wipes to cleanse perianal area when not home
   3. Wear absorbent "shields" to line un-

derwear and protect clothing to prevent embarrassment because of incontinence or staining by fecal liquid or
creams applied to perianal region; if
incontinence is severe, adult diaper
may be used
4. Assess client for orthostatic hypotension and teach gradual assumption of
upright position
H. For bed-bound patients with large-volume
or continuous diarrhea, a fecal incontinence pouch connected to gravity drainage can be used (Lincoln & Roberts, 1989)
I. Avoid anal intercourse or oral-anal sexual
activities
J. Encourage the use of antidiarrheal agents
on a scheduled basis, not an as-desired
(p.r.n.) basis

Referrals:

A. Dietitian
B. CNS in HIV disease or ostomy care
C. Visiting nurse

Evaluation:

The client will:

A. Identify factors that contribute to diarrhea
B. Plan a 24-hour menu of low-residue, high-
protein, high-caloric foods and adequate
hydration
C. Demonstrate the ability to provide proper
skin care after each bowel movement
D. Verbalize the need to avoid anal sexual
practices
E. Verbalize a decrease in the number of
bowel movements for a 24-hour period

SYMPTOM: *Dry and Painful Mouth*

Etiology:

A. Primary infection of HIV: diffuse infiltrative lymphocytosis syndrome (Itescu et al.,
1990)
B. Secondary infections caused by:
1. Bacteria (e.g., *Mycobacterium avium-intracellulare*)
2. Fungi (e.g., *Candida albicans, Cryptococcus neoformans, Histoplasma capsulatum*)
3. Viruses (e.g., herpes simplex virus, var-

icella-zoster virus, papillomavirus, Ep-
stein-Barr [causing oral hairy leuko-
plakia])
C. Malnutrition
D. Dehydration
E. Reaction to drug therapy or local radia-
tion therapy
F. Dentures that fit poorly because of weight
loss
G. Mouth breathing
H. Inadequate oral hygiene
I. Continued alcohol and tobacco use
J. Periodontal disease

Nursing Assessment:

A. Subjective data
1. History of symptoms
2. Associated symptoms
3. History of recent nutritional intake
4. History of oral hygiene habits
5. Use of alcohol and tobacco
6. Medical, surgical, and dental history
7. Current drug therapy
B. Objective data
1. Examination of the lips, tongue, buccal
mucosal surfaces, teeth, and dental appliances
2. Assessment for pain
C. Assessment tool: Oral Assessment Guide
(Eilers et al., 1988)

Nursing Diagnosis:

Altered oral mucous membrane

Goals:

After discussing the findings of assessment
and validating the nursing diagnosis, the
client and/or care partner and the nurse will
select interventions to:

A. Establish a routine oral hygiene regimen
B. Minimize the potential for or severity of
stomatitis

**Considerations for Nursing Care and
Health Teaching** (Greifzu et al., 1990;
Liebman, 1992):

A. Implement an oral hygiene regimen
1. Perform oral hygiene with a mirror
over the sink and with an emesis basin
in the bed

2. Remove dental appliances
3. Examine oral cavity with adequate lighting
4. Brush teeth with a small, soft toothbrush; avoid brushing mucosal surfaces
5. Use a foam swab or large cotton swab instead of a toothbrush if the platelet count falls to less than 50,000 mm³
6. Advise against commercial mouthwashes that contain alcohol or glycerin; substitute mouthwash with a solution of 1 quart warm water with one-half teaspoon each of salt and baking soda (change solution daily)
7. Rinse thoroughly with cool water
8. Floss between teeth and avoid flossing near gumline
9. When away from home and unable to perform detailed oral hygiene procedures, at least:
   a. Wipe surfaces of teeth with paper napkin after eating
   b. Rinse with a saltwater solution
10. Perform oral hygiene after meals and before going to sleep at night
11. If peroxide is used to remove tenacious secretions or crusted exudate, rinse well with normal saline solution and avoid overuse because it will interfere with healing

B. For profound fatigue or the client who is not capable of complying with a regimen of oral hygiene, consider:
   1. Using saline mouth rinses after meals, and wiping teeth with a paper napkin
   2. Consulting with the physician about ordering an oral pharmacologic rinse such as chlorhexidine (National Institutes of Health, 1990)
C. For oral pain:
   1. Provide straws
   2. Popsicles and ice cream can temporarily numb painful lesions
   3. Avoid very hot or spicy foods
   4. Apply topical agents to control pain before meals
   5. Evaluate the need for systemic analgesia

D. For xerostomia (dryness of mouth)
   1. Avoid tobacco, alcohol, spicy foods, very hot and very cold foods, citrus juices, commercial mouthwashes, coarse foods, and hard foods
   2. Use a salt-and-baking-soda rinse solution
   3. Take frequent sips of fluid; keep water at the bedside
   4. Use commercially prepared artificial saliva
   5. Suck on sugarless hard candies or chew sugarless gum
   6. Use lip balms to keep lips moist
E. Provide adequate nutrition; see "Weight Loss"

Referrals:

A. Dentist or dental hygienist
B. CNS in HIV disease
C. Visiting nurse

Evaluation:

The client will:

A. Demonstrate the ability to assess oral cavity before and after hygiene
B. Demonstrate the ability to perform an oral hygiene routine
C. Demonstrate moist, pink, intact mucosal surfaces
D. Verbalize a decrease in perceived symptoms

SYMPTOM: *Dry Skin and Skin Lesions*

Etiology:

A. Commonly seen skin conditions in HIV diseases (Berger, 1990)
   1. Herpes simplex
   2. Herpes zoster (shingles)
   3. *Candida albicans* infection
   4. *Mycobacterium avium-intracellulare* infection
   5. Staphylococcal folliculitis
   6. Bacillary angiomatosis
   7. Molluscum contagiosum
   8. Insect bite reactions
   9. Photosensitivity
   10. Eosinophilic folliculitis

11. Seborrheic dermatitis
12. Psoriasis or Reiter's syndrome
B. Dry skin caused by diaphoresis and febrile states associated with HIV disease
C. Anemia
D. Cutaneous invasion by Kaposi's sarcoma
E. Immobility
F. Malnutrition
G. Cutaneous reactions to drug therapy

Nursing Assessment:

A. Subjective data
  1. History of symptoms
  2. Usual patterns of bathing and skin care
  3. Bathing facilities in home
  4. Current nutritional history
  5. Past medical and surgical history
  6. Exercise and rest patterns
  7. Current drug therapy
  8. Continence patterns
  9. Client's and care partner's knowledge of risks and prevention strategies related to dry skin and skin lesions
B. Objective data
  1. Examine skin, paying particular attention to:
     a. Areas under skin folds
     b. Pressure points
     c. Sites of invasive procedures (e.g., incisions, biopsy sites, venipuncture sites)
     d. Genital, perineal, and perianal regions
  2. Palpate skin for temperature, texture, pain, turgor, moisture, circulation, and edema
  3. Observe skin for redness, scaling, cracking, flaking
  4. Perform motor and sensory examination and evaluate ability to transfer, change position, and ambulate
  5. Assess cerebral functions (ability to learn, follow instructions, and recall from memory)
C. Assessment tools
  1. To monitor and evaluate the client for dry skin, use the modified Skin Condition Data Form (SCDF) (Hardy, 1992)
  2. To monitor potential or actual development of pressure ulcers, use the Braden Scale or Norton Scale (Panel for the Prediction and Prevention of Ulcers in Adults, 1992)

Nursing Diagnosis:

High risk of impaired skin integrity

Goals:

After discussing and validating the findings of the assessment and the nursing diagnoses, the client and/or care partner and the nurse will select intervention to:

A. Add moisture to the skin through bathing
B. Maintain and improve tissue tolerance to pressure for prevention of injury
C. Protect the client's skin against the adverse effects of external mechanical forces: pressure, friction, and shear

Considerations for Nursing Care and Health Teaching:

A. Keep skin clean and well moisturized (Hardy, 1992, p. 46)
  1. Shower with a continuous spray over all body parts for 10 minutes (facilitated by the use of handheld showerhead)
  2. Maintain water temperature of 90° F to 105° F
  3. Use a superfatted soap for cleansing
  4. Pat the skin dry with a cotton towel rather than by rubbing
  5. Apply an emollient while skin is damp over all body parts (as an occlusive agent to keep moisture in skin)
  6. Maintain a humid environment
  7. Use clothing and linen that have been thoroughly rinsed of detergent, without antistatic rinses or dryer products
  8. Wear cotton clothing
B. Prevent dissemination of infection or development of secondary infection
  1. Avoid tub baths or sitz baths if skin lesions are present
  2. Avoid bar soap
  3. Use separate washcloth to bathe areas with infectious lesions

4. Explain dangers of scratching and extension of infection and lesions

C. Minimize the potential for skin breakdown and pressure ulcers in persons with mobility and activity deficits (Panel for the Prediction and Prevention of Ulcers in Adults, 1992)

1. Establish a prevention plan
   a. Inspect skin at least once a day
   b. Individualize bathing schedule
   c. Minimize environmental factors such as low humidity and cold air
   d. Avoid massage over bony prominences (Dyson, 1978; Ek et al., 1985)
   e. Use proper positioning, transferring, and turning techniques
   f. Use lubricants to reduce friction injuries
   g. Assess the need for physical therapy consultation to institute a plan for rehabilitation

2. Reduce the potential for injury
   a. For bed-bound individuals
      (1) Reposition at least every 2 hours
      (2) Use pillows or foam wedges to keep bony prominences from direct contact
      (3) Use devices that totally relieve pressure on the heels; do not use doughnut-shaped devices (more likely to cause pressure ulcers than to prevent them)
      (4) Avoid positioning directly on the trochanter
      (5) Elevate the head of the bed as little as possible and for as short a time as possible
      (6) Use lifting devices to move, rather than drag, individuals during transfers and position changes
      (7) Place at-risk individuals on pressure-reducing mattresses; do not use doughnut-shaped devices
   b. For chair-bound individuals
      (1) Reposition at least every hour
      (2) Have patient shift weight every 15 minutes if capable
      (3) Use pressure-reducing devices for seating surfaces; do not use doughnut-shaped devices
      (4) Consider postural alignment, distribution of weight, balance, and stability, and pressure relief when positioning individuals in chairs or wheelchairs

3. Minimize skin exposure to moisture caused by incontinence
   a. Cleanse skin at time of soiling
   b. Assess for treatment of urinary incontinence
   c. When moisture cannot be controlled, use underpads or briefs (or shields) that are absorbent and present a quick-drying surface to the skin

4. Identify related factors, such as nutritional deficits, especially in protein and calories; see "Weight Loss"

D. Memory deficits; see "Impaired Cognition"

E. Provide a written plan of care and instructions to the client and care partner, including:

1. The cause of and risk factors for pressure ulcers
2. Risk assessment tools and their application
3. Skin assessment
4. Selection and/or use of support devices
5. Development and implementation of an individualized program of skin care
6. Demonstration of positioning to decrease risk of tissue breakdown
7. Instruction on accurate documentation of pertinent data

NOTE WELL: "Occlusive dressings such as Stomahesive, Op-Site, and Duo-Derm are contraindicated for immunocompromised patients" (McDonnell & Sevedge, 1986, p. 572). For safe use of this type of dressing, the body's host defenses should be intact (Hotter, 1990). In vitro studies have shown that, in PWHIV, the body's chemotactic responses to bacterial substances are altered, interfering with monocyte-macrophage–mediated organisms (Crowe et al., 1990). In addition, *Candida al-*

bicans flourishes under occlusive dressings (Cuzzel, 1990). Hoffmann and associates (1992) demonstrated a significantly increased risk of catheter-tip infection with the use of transparent compared with gauze dressings used with either central or peripheral intravenous catheters.

Referrals:

A. Physical therapist
B. CNS in HIV disease, dermatologic disorders
C. Visiting nurse

Evaluation:

The client and/or caregiver will:

A. Verbalize causes and risk factors for skin breakdown and pressure ulcers
B. Demonstrate the ability to perform a skin and risk assessment, use support devices, and position properly
C. Show evidence that the plan of care is being followed
D. Maintain intact skin surfaces without evidence of redness, dryness, or infection

SYMPTOM: *Pain*

Etiology:

A. Localized pain in bone, nerve, and viscera caused by:
   1. Tumor invasion
   2. Opportunistic infection(s)
B. Generalized arthralgia and myalgia associated with chronic HIV disease
C. Autoimmune response to HIV disease, resulting in:
   1. Vasculitis
   2. Chronic demyelinating neuropathy
   3. Inflammatory myopathy
D. Related to therapy
   1. Acute postoperative pain
   2. Postradiotherapy pain
   3. Postchemotherapy pain
   4. Pain caused by diagnostic procedures

Nursing Assessment:

A. Subjective data (Acute Pain Management Guideline Panel, 1992)
   1. Significant previous and/or ongoing instances of pain and its effect on the patient
   2. Previously used methods of pain control that the patient has found either helpful or unhelpful
   3. The patient's attitude toward the use of opioid, anxiolytic, or other medications, including any history of substance abuse
   4. The patient's typical coping response to stress or pain, including more broadly the presence or absence of psychiatric disorders such as depression, anxiety, or psychosis
   5. Family expectations and beliefs concerning pain and stress
   6. Ways that the patient describes or shows pain
   7. The patient's knowledge of, expectations about, and preferences for pain management methods and for receiving information about pain management
   8. Self-report about pain including description, location, intensity/severity, and aggravating and relieving factors
B. Objective data
   1. Assess heart rate, blood pressure, and respiratory rate
   2. Observe the client's ability and willingness to participate in ADL.

NOTE WELL: The Acute Pain Management Guideline Panel (1992), in a review of the literature, concluded that (1) the single most reliable indicator of the existence and intensity of acute pain and any related discomfort or distress is the patient's self-report; (2) neither behavior nor vital signs can substitute for self-report; and (3) patients may be having excruciating pain even while smiling or using laughter as a coping mechanism.

C. Assessment tools (Acute Pain Management Guideline Panel, 1992)
   1. A numeric rating scale (NRS)
   2. A visual analog scale (VAS)
   3. An adjective rating scale (ARS)
   4. McGill (MPQ) Short Form (Melzack, 1987)

Nursing Diagnosis:

Pain

Goals:

After discussing and validating the findings of assessment and the nursing diagnosis, the client and/or care partner and the nurse will seek interventions to:

A. Reduce the incidence and severity of pain
B. Communicate effectively about pain experiences
C. Enhance comfort and satisfaction

Considerations for Nursing Care and Health Teaching (Acute Pain Management Guidelines Panel, 1992):

A. Identify activities of daily living that appear to increase the intensity and severity of the pain experience
B. Provide nonpharmacologic interventions to reduce pain and anxiety and control mild pain, but not as a substitute for the pharmacologic management of moderate to severe pain:
   1. Cognitive-behavioral interventions such as:
      a. Education and instruction in pain control
      b. Relaxation exercises
      c. Imagery
      d. Music distraction
      e. Biofeedback
   2. Physical agents such as:
      a. Application of heat or cold (e.g., warm soaks to painful muscles or joints, or a cold washcloth or ice bag for headaches)
      b. Massage (e.g., back rubs)
      c. Transcutaneous electrical nerve stimulation (TENS)
C. Provide additional comfort measures such as:
   1. Using egg crate mattress, air mattress, or other comfortable surface
   2. Positioning and supporting limbs comfortably when client is lying in bed or sitting up in chair
   3. Using a "pull sheet" to move patient and/or to help patient change position

D. When client is institutionalized, encourage family or significant other to bring in familiar objects such as:
   1. Pillows and blankets
   2. Favorite photographs
   3. Religious articles
   4. Personal clothing
   5. Cologne, makeup, face powder, and other cosmetic articles
E. Pharmacologic treatments should include consideration of:
   1. The efficacy of nonsteroidal antiinflammatory drugs in pain management as primary or adjunctive therapy in pain control
   2. Opioid analgesic requirements as an individual matter
   3. Orders for opioid analgesics, which should include "rescue" doses for instances when regularly scheduled doses are insufficient
   4. Orders for p.r.n. analgesics, which produce delays in administration and intervals of inadequate pain control
   5. Dosage frequency, which should be adjusted to prevent recurrence of pain once the duration of analgesic action is determined
   6. The possibility that the patient may wish to refuse an analgesic agent if not in pain or to forego it if asleep; however, an explanation should be provided that lower blood analgesia levels may result in resurgence of pain

Referrals:

A. Occupational/physical therapist
B. CNS in HIV disease, hospice care, or mental health
C. Pharmacist
D. Psychologist
E. Visiting nurse

Evaluation:

The client will:

A. Identify aggravating or precipitating factors related to the pain experienced
B. Identify measures to control pain
C. Verbalize a decrease in the amount and

type of pain experienced for a 24-hour period

SYMPTOM: *Dyspnea*

Etiology:

A. Infections of the respiratory system caused by:
1. Bacteria (e.g., *Mycobacterium tuberculosis*, atypical *Mycobacterium*)
2. Fungi (e.g., *Candida albicans*, *Histoplasma capsulatum*, *Coccidioides immitis*, *Cryptococcus neoformans*)
3. Protozoa (e.g., *Pneumocystis carinii*, *Cryptosporidium*)
4. Viruses (e.g., cytomegalovirus, herpes simplex virus)
B. Respiratory tract invasion by:
1. Kaposi's sarcoma
2. Lymphoma
C. Autoimmune manifestation of HIV infection
1. Lymphocytic interstitial pneumonitis
2. Diffuse infiltrative lymphocytosis syndrome (Itescu et al., 1990)
D. Anemia
E. Exercise intolerance

Nursing Assessment:

A. Subjective data
1. History of problem
2. Associated symptoms (e.g., fatigue, pain, suffocation, tightness, congestion, tingling, and loud heartbeat) (Janson-Bjerklie et al., 1986)
3. Identification of situational factors that may precipitate dyspnea (e.g., bad weather, wind, pollens in the air, crowds, smoke, living arrangements, social support, attitude, air pollution, life events, daily hassles) (Gift & Pugh, 1993)
4. Medical and surgical history
5. Current drug therapy
6. Self-evaluation by client of ability to dress, bathe, toilet, ambulate, and so forth
B. Objective data
1. Detailed respiratory assessment, including observation, palpation, and auscultation
2. Cardiovascular assessment, including blood pressure, pulse, and skin color
3. Evaluation of cardiovascular and respiratory system in relation to client's response to ADL
4. Situational assessment, including living arrangements, presence of significant other(s), and community and social support
5. Laboratory evaluation of arterial blood gases (especially with pneumonia)
C. Assessment tools
1. A visual analog scale (VAS) (Gift et al., 1986; Gift, 1989)
2. The Symptom Distress Scale (SDS) (McCorkle & Young, 1978)
3. American Thoracic Society's Breathlessness Scale (American Thoracic Society, 1978)
4. Borg Scale (Borg, 1982)

Nursing Diagnoses:

Activity intolerance; ineffective breathing pattern

Goals:

After discussing the findings of assessment and the nursing diagnosis, the client and/or care partner and the nurse will select interventions to:

A. Identify factors that may precipitate dyspnea
B. Identify strategies to prevent and control dyspnea
C. Develop a lifestyle that keeps the client involved in ADL, independent, and socially active

Considerations for Nursing Care and Health Teaching:

A. Physiologic therapies to control breathing patterns when dyspnea occurs
1. Teach pursed-lips breathing (Carrieri and Janson-Bjerklie, 1986)
   a. Inhaling deeply
   b. Exhaling slowly through lips that are pursed (similar to whistling)
2. Body positioning (Sharp et al., 1980)

a. Sitting upright
b. Leaning forward
c. Elevating and supporting arms

B. Psychologic therapies to control responses (Gift, 1993)
1. Coping with anxiety
    a. Use relaxation techniques either with instruction or a tape recording (Gift et al., 1992; Renfroe, 1988)
    b. Practice relaxation either on a daily basis or when an acute attack of dyspnea occurs
2. Preventing or controlling depression (Gift, 1993)
    a. Encourage regular exercise (Gift & Austin, 1992)
    b. Promote independence by encouraging patient to remain as active as possible
    c. Explore physically efficient ways to perform self-care ADL
    d. Participate in support groups
    e. Structured Life Review (Butler, 1963; 1974), although used primarily with older adults, may be of benefit in increasing life satisfaction and psychologic well-being in the HIV-infected individual
    f. Arrange for physical therapy consultation for upper body extremity exercise training (Carrieri-Kohlman & Janson-Bjerklie, 1993)
3. Coping with hostility when dyspnea occurs by understanding that hostility may occur when a sudden bout of dyspnea occurs, especially if it interferes with planned activities

C. Social therapies to minimize social restrictions and prevent dyspnea (Gift, 1993)
1. Teach pacing of activities, including:
    a. Developing a written daily/weekly plan of activities
    b. Performing activities at a slower pace
    c. Planning frequent rest periods
    d. Limiting the number of daily activities
2. See "Fatigue"
3. See "Sexual Dysfunction"

D. Cognitive therapies to restructure the patient's perception of dyspnea (Gift, 1993)

1. Changing the perception of symptom by:
    a. Treating the underlying cause of dyspnea (if known)
    b. Exploring the patient's perception of dyspnea and ability to cope with the symptom
2. Altering the interpretation of dyspnea through desensitization by having the patient exercise to the point of dyspnea and then teaching the patient to control the symptom
3. Recalling past experiences in which dyspnea was handled effectively

E. Minimizing of factors contributing to the client's perception of dyspnea
1. For smoking:
    a. Discuss the possibility of a smoking cessation program
    b. If client has a need to continue, discourage smoking before eating and before, during, and immediately after ADL are performed
    c. Discuss a daily schedule of reduction of cigarettes smoked
    d. Consider use of commercial filters to reduce the amount of tar, nicotine, and carbon monoxide inhaled (especially if client uses marijuana)
2. For inadequate pulmonary hygiene or immobility:
    a. Change position frequently
    b. For immobilized client, develop a regimen of frequent coughing and deep breathing exercises
    c. If necessary and not contraindicated, consider use of incentive spirometer and chest physical therapy
    d. Provide adequate hydration: 2 to 2.5 liters of fluid per day; monitor fluid intake and output
    e. If client has productive cough or copious secretions, see "Cough"
3. There is evidence that blowing of air on the face (using a fan) may have some beneficial effect in the reduction of dyspnea (Schwartzstein et al., 1987)

Referrals:

A. Physical therapist
B. Occupational therapist

C. CNS in HIV disease or respiratory disorders
D. Visiting nurse

Evaluation:

The client will:

A. Identify the contributing factors related to dyspnea
B. Develop a plan of self-care by pacing ADL
C. Verbalize a decrease in the number of times per day that dyspnea is experienced

SYMPTOM: *Cough*

Etiology:

A. See "Dyspnea"
B. Respiratory therapy or procedures

Nursing Assessment:

A. See "Dyspnea"
B. Observation of client with chronic coughing

Nursing Diagnosis:

Ineffective airway clearance

Goals:

After discussing and validating the findings of assessment and the nursing diagnosis, the client and/or care partner and the nurse will select interventions to:

A. Promote optimal respiratory function
B. Minimize the discomfort associated with chronic cough

Considerations for Nursing Care and Health Teaching:

A. Minimize discomfort associated with chronic nonrelieved cough
 1. Encourage client to take cough medications on a scheduled basis rather than p.r.n. and to schedule doses appropriately between, not with, meals
 2. Encourage use of cough drops and of tea with lemon and honey
 3. Consider warm saline gargle frequently to soothe sore throat
 4. Avoid oxygen administration without adequate humidification

B. Minimize factors that contribute to cough suppression
 1. If chest pain from chronic, nonrelieved cough is present, medicate on a scheduled basis rather than p.r.n.
 2. Demonstrate splinting techniques to minimize pain associated with coughing
C. Minimize cough related to viscous secretions
 1. Hydrate with 2 to 2.5 liters of fluid per day
 2. Assist client in controlled coughing exercise schedule

Referrals:

A. CNS in HIV disease or respiratory disorders
B. Visiting nurse

Evaluation:

The client will:

A. Identify effective cough remedies
B. Demonstrate the ability to cough effectively
C. Verbalize a decrease in the amount of cough experienced daily

SYMPTOM: *Impaired Cognition*

Etiology:

A. HIV induced (primary infection) such as:
 1. AIDS dementia complex (subacute encephalitis)
 2. Aseptic meningitis
B. Opportunistic infections (secondary infection of central nervous system) caused by:
 1. Bacteria (e.g., *Mycobacterium tuberculosis,* atypical mycobacteria)
 2. Fungi (e.g., *Cryptococcus neoformans, Histoplasma capsulatum, Coccidioides immitis*)
 3. Protozoa (e.g., *Toxoplasma gondii*)
 4. Viruses (e.g., cytomegalovirus, J.C. virus, herpes simplex virus)
C. Other central nervous system infections caused by:
 1. Varicella-zoster virus
 2. *Treponema pallidum*

D. Malignancy (e.g., lymphoma, Kaposi's sarcoma)
E. Cerebrovascular accidents resulting from:
   1. Infarction
   2. Hemorrhage
   3. Vasculitis
F. Complications of HIV therapy such as:
   1. Drug side effects
   2. Irradiation side effects
G. Psychiatric disorders (e.g., psychosis, depression, anxiety)
H. Other causes (e.g., anemia, hypoxia, adrenal insufficiency, renal or liver disease, nutritional deficiencies)

Nursing Assessment (McArthur, 1990; Rasin, 1990; Ungvarski, 1989):

A. Subjective data (obtained from client and significant other)
   1. History of symptoms
   2. Problems with memory, concentration, and conversation
   3. Problems with missing appointments or forgetting to do things
   4. Changes in leisure activities (e.g., loss of interest in reading printed materials or watching television)
   5. Withdrawal from social activity
   6. History of lifestyle, including occupation, recreation and leisure interests, sleep patterns
   7. Coping patterns, including substance abuse
   8. Availability of support systems
   9. Ability and interest in performing ADL
   10. History of a typical week of client's activities
   11. Self-assessment
   12. Changes in upper motor function, such as signature change, or lower motor function, such as walking
   13. Behavior changes noticed by significant other
   14. Medical and surgical history
   15. Psychiatric history
   16. Current drug therapy
   17. Nutritional history
B. Objective data
   1. General appearance, including grooming and dress

   2. Examination of cerebral functioning, including level of consciousness, orientation, and cognitive function testing of calculations, memory, attention, and/or distraction during the interview
   3. Behavior (e.g., apathetic, withdrawn, irritable)
   4. Affect (e.g., appropriate or flat)
   5. Cranial nerve examination
   6. Motor examination
   7. Sensory examination
   8. Cerebellar examination
   9. Reflexes
   10. Meningeal signs
C. Assessment tools
   1. Mental Status Questionnaire (MSQ) (Kahn et al., 1960)
   2. Short Portable Mental Status Questionnaire (SPMSQ) (Pfeiffer, 1975)
   3. Mini-Mental State Examination (MMSE) (Folstein et al., 1975)
   4. Cognitive Capacity Screening Examination (CCSE) (Jacobs et al., 1977)
   5. New tools being tested with HIV/AIDS patients:
      a. Neurobehavioral Rating Scale (Hilton et al., 1990; Sultzer et al., 1992)
      b. Mattis Dementia Rating Scale (Kovner et al., 1992)
      c. AIDS Dementia Complex Rating Scale (van Gorp et al., 1992)

NOTE WELL: According to Rasin (1990), "For nursing, the value of using bedside cognitive instruments is not in the computation of a score so that the patient can be categorized as cognitively impaired or nonimpaired; it is in the ability to identify specific deficits in cognitive functioning" (p. 13).

Nursing Diagnosis:

Altered thought processes; self-care deficits

Goals:

After discussing and validating the findings of assessment and the nursing diagnosis, the client and/or care partner and the nurse will select interventions to:

A. Promote independence

B. Identify factors that contribute to sensory-perceptual alteration
C. Provide meaningful and sufficient sensory input
D. Minimize disorientation
E. Provide for safety
F. Improve the individual's ability to cope with reality

Considerations for Nursing Care and Health Teaching (McArthur, 1990; Muwaswes, 1993; Rasin, 1990; Ungvarski, 1989):

A. Assess for causative factors
  1. In the acute care setting
    a. Sleep interruption because of hospital routines
    b. Auditory overload because of staff talking at night, alarms going off, and other voices
    c. New, unfamiliar staff providing care
    d. Social isolation because of infection control practices
    e. Restricted environment
    f. Lack of routine
    g. Lack of familiar visitors
    h. Fear, especially of loss of control
    i. Medication side effects
    j. Physiologic alterations
  2. In the community
    a. Lack of supervision or motivation
    b. Change in housing (e.g., being placed in a nursing home or AIDS residence)
    c. Lack of social support (e.g., visitors)
    d. Lack of psychologic support (e.g., nonparticipation in peer support groups)
    e. Lack of established routines
    f. Changes in home care staff
    g. Medication side effects
    h. Continued substance use
    i. Physiologic alterations
B. Reduce or eliminate causative factors
  1. Provide a written schedule of activities for client and encourage all involved in care to adhere to schedule as much as possible

  2. Provide a copy of the routines for client to follow
  3. Avoid staff assignment changes as much as possible
  4. Decrease noise input, especially at night
  5. Encourage regular visiting by friends
  6. When friends visit, encourage them to take client out; in acute care settings, take client for a walk even to another area or for coffee
  7. Encourage participation in weekly peer support groups
  8. When barrier precautions are necessary, put them on in front of client, explaining the purpose
  9. Discuss dangers of substance use with impaired cognition (especially to friends who bring substances to client, and significant others)
  10. When external auditory stimuli cannot be controlled, consider use of personal radio with earplugs
  11. Keep pictures of loved ones nearby
C. Promote cognitive stimulation and orientation
  1. Address client by name
  2. Always maintain face-to-face contact during interactions
  3. Identify self frequently (especially important with telephone conversations)
  4. Explain all care activities
  5. Engage client in areas of pleasure or interest such as board games, cards
  6. Encourage friends to watch television and read newspapers with client
  7. Keep calendar visible and cross off each day
  8. Have client wear wristwatch, and check time with client periodically
D. Promote independence and self-esteem
  1. Engage client in decision making
  2. Keep important telephone numbers next to telephone for client's use
  3. Pre-pour medications for client and supervise client's ability to self-medicate
  4. Encourage client to do as much as possible in ADL, including cleaning, shopping, and cooking
  5. Have client dress and groom daily; do

not allow client to sit around in night-clothes

6. Encourage client to verbalize fears and concerns

E. Promote exercise
 1. Include exercise as a part of each day's routine
 2. Plan purposeful exercise (e.g., shopping or visiting a friend)
 3. If client was previously engaged in exercise (e.g., aerobics), continue within physical limitations of client's capabilities

F. Provide for safety
 1. Assist with potentially dangerous activities, such as cooking and using appliances
 2. Assess with client, significant other, and physician the client's ability to continue to drive a motor vehicle
 3. If client smokes, monitor safety and attempt to prohibit smoking in bed
 4. Assess the home for hazards and make necessary changes such as removing scatter rugs and breakable objects
 5. Continually assess the need for assistive devices such as a cane, walker, or bath bar

G. Pharmacologic treatment should include the following considerations:
 1. HIV-infected persons may be more prone to severe extrapyramidal symptoms when high-potency neuroleptic agents are used (Breitbart et al., 1988; Hriso et al., 1991; Swensen et al., 1989)
 2. Benzodiazepines that may be prescribed may alter the pharmacokinetics of zidovudine, potentially increasing toxicity (Burger et al., 1993)

NOTE WELL: Because of the nature of cognitive impairment, it is extremely important to include the client's designated care partner in all planning and health teaching. Documentation on the client's record should reflect all instruction and concerns provided to both individuals.

Referrals:

A. CNS in HIV disease, neurologic disorders, or mental health
B. Physical therapist
C. Occupational therapist
D. Community-based AIDS organization for participation in a volunteer visitor program, support groups
E. Day care program for cognitively impaired individuals (if available)

Evaluation:

The client or significant other will:

A. Identify causative factors contributing to sensory-perceptual alterations
B. Demonstrate the reduction or elimination of identified factors
C. Provide a safe home environment

The client will:

A. Participate in decision making
B. Maintain or improve appearance
C. Participate in plan of care
D. Verbalize fears and concerns
E. Be free from injury

SYMPTOM: *Impaired Vision*

Etiology (Heinemann, 1992):

A. HIV infection of the eye
B. Ocular infection caused by:
 1. Bacteria (e.g., *Mycobacterium avium-intracellulare,* endogenous bacterial endophthalmitis)
 2. Fungi (e.g., *Cryptococcus neoformans, Histoplasma capsulatum, Candida albicans*)
 3. Protozoa (e.g., *Toxoplasma gondii, Pneumocystis carinii*
 4. Viruses (e.g., cytomegalovirus, herpes simplex virus, varicella-zoster virus)
C. AIDS-related microangiopathy (noninfectious retinopathy)
D. Malignancy (e.g., Kaposi's sarcoma, lymphoma)
E. Complications of central nervous system disease (e.g., primary lymphoma of the brain, infection of the brain with J.C. virus)
F. Side effects of medications

Nursing Assessment (Heinemann, 1992; Plona & Schremp, 1992):

A. Subjective data
 1. Previous health history related to vision

2. History of visual impairment, with progression of vision loss noted
3. Self-reported changes in visual acuity (e.g., blurred vision, floaters, or gaps in vision, unilateral or bilateral)
4. Description of visual impairment, limitations on ADL, especially noting:
   a. Housing
   b. Egress from home
   c. Assistance needed
   d. Ability to summon assistance
   e. Ability to feed, bathe, dress, toilet, and medicate self
5. Current drug therapy
6. Emotional response and concerns about vision loss

B. Objective data
   1. Examination of cranial nerves II (optic); III, IV, and VI (oculomotor, trochlear, and abducens); V (trigeminal)
   2. Evaluation of ability to:
      a. Negotiate immediate surroundings
      b. Feed self
      c. Bathe self
      d. Dress self
      e. Toilet self
      f. Medicate self
   3. Mental status examination
C. Assessment tools
   1. Snellen chart
   2. Ophthalmoscope
   3. Self-reporting diary (tape recording if unable to write)

NOTE WELL: Allen (1990) identified three phases of adjustment to visual impairment:

A. Preimpact—associated with an insidious loss of vision in which the individual does not realize that vision changes are occurring
B. Impact—the point at which the individual recognizes and acknowledges visual impairment (often at the time of diagnosis; may be accompanied by emotional responses such as anger, sadness, depression, insecurity, feelings of wanting to give up, or self-pity)
C. After impact—learning to live with the impairment, coming to terms with the vision loss, and adapting activities

Nursing Diagnoses:

High risk for injury; self-care deficit(s); impaired home maintenance management

Goals:

After discussing and validating the assessment and the nursing diagnoses, the client and/or care partner and the nurse will select interventions to:

A. Identify potential hazards in the environment and methods to avoid injury
B. Adjust to vision loss and maintain maximum independence in ADL

Considerations for Nursing Care and Health Teaching:

A. Provide for safety
   1. Orient client to unfamiliar surroundings
      a. Explain call system and assess client's ability to use it
      b. Keep bed in lowest position
      c. Assess frequently at night and keep a night light on at all times
      d. Encourage client to ask for assistance at night, especially when first adjusting to impaired vision
   2. Discuss general safety measures for the home
      a. Avoid changing furniture arrangements
      b. Remove hazards such as small, unsecured area rugs and exposed sharp objects
      c. Avoid smoking when alone or unsupervised
B. Accommodate client with unilateral visual loss by:
   1. Assigning client to a bed in which client's intact visual field is toward the door
   2. Placing overbed table, telephone, call light, and so forth on appropriate side of person's bed
C. Minimize sensitivity to light by:
   1. Encouraging the use of sunglasses
   2. Keeping the environment dimly lit
   3. Encouraging client to wear brimmed hat when out of doors
   4. Keeping television at low level of brightness

D. Promote independence and assist in re-learning ADL
  1. Feeding self
    a. Describe location of utensils when serving food
    b. Describe locations of food on a plate referring to clock (e.g., the potatoes are at 12 o'clock, meat at 6 o'clock)
    c. Use "finger foods" for snacks
    d. Use cups or mugs for liquids such as soups
  2. Bathing and grooming self
    a. Arrange equipment according to client's preference and replace in same location when finished with toileting
    b. Consider use of assistive devices such as bath bar or shower chair
    c. Provide supervision until client is comfortable performing alone
    d. Encourage short hair styles that require a minimum of care and grooming
    e. Encourage use of electric shaver
  3. Dressing self
    a. Assist client in planning location of clothing
    b. Place matching clothing on same hanger
  4. Toileting self
    a. If bedpan or urinal is necessary, keep accessible at all times
    b. If diarrhea is present, evaluate usefulness of bedside commode
    c. If confusion is present, consider use of external catheter with drainage bag on leg or use of adult diapers
  5. Medicating self
    a. Develop a plan for medication
    b. Frequently review side effects of drugs, such as narcotic analgesics, that may further increase the potential for injury and need to restrict activities
E. Utilize sensory support techniques for visually impaired persons (Daly, 1990):
  1. Visual (for color impairments and limited vision)
    a. Print medications and activity schedules in letter size, in accor-dance with visual acuity; a magnifying glass is extremely useful
    b. Use red marker (Hi Marks, manufactured by Kentucky Industries for the Blind) that leaves a red-raised dot on medication bottles and vials, indicating frequency of dosing
  2. Auditory
    a. Speak to patient in a soft tone; loud auditory stimuli with visual loss may result in sensory overload
    b. For complete vision loss, teaching and instructions should be recorded on audiotape
  3. Tactile: When orienting client, point out descriptively the temperature and texture of environmental furniture and surroundings

Referrals:

A. Occupational therapist
B. CNS in HIV disease or in neurologic or ophthalmic disorders
C. Visiting nurse
D. Local organizations for the blind
E. Community-based support groups for PWHIV

Evaluation:

The client will:

A. Identify potential hazards in the environment
B. Demonstrate the ability to move about the environment safely
C. Demonstrate the ability to feed, bathe, dress, and toilet self
D. Describe a plan for assistance with medication administration and other ADL
E. Identify coping strategies to assist in adjusting to vision loss

SYMPTOM: *Insomnia*

Etiology:

A. Organic mental disorders such as AIDS dementia complex (Snyder et al., 1990; Wiegard et al., 1990)
B. Psychologic factors such as stress, anxiety, and depression (Nisita et al., 1991; Tostes, 1990)

C. Side effects of medications (e.g., zidovudine, didanosine) (Langtry & Campoli-Richards, 1989; Yarchoan et al., 1989)
D. Environmental conditions that are not conducive to sleep (e.g., noise, lights, interruptions for care during hospitalization) (Jensen & Herr, 1993)
E. Drug or alcohol dependency or preexisting psychiatric problems (Cohen & Merritt, 1992)

Nursing Assessment (Cohen & Merritt, 1992; North American Nursing Diagnosis Association, 1992):

A. Subjective data
1. History of symptom
2. Associated symptoms such as anxiety, depression, restlessness, irritability, lethargy, disorientation, pain, fever, night sweats
3. Usual patterns of sleep
4. Diet history and daily food intake patterns
5. Use of drugs, alcohol, and tobacco
6. Current ability to perform ADL
7. Medical and psychiatric findings
8. Current drug therapy
B. Objective data
1. Mild, fleeting nystagmus
2. Slight hand tremor
3. Ptosis of eyelids
4. Expressionless face
5. Dark circles under eyes
6. Frequent yawning
7. Changes in posture
8. Thick speech, with mispronunciation and incorrect words
C. Assessment tools
1. Sleep Pattern Questionnaire (SPQ) (Baekeland & Hoy, 1971)
2. Bedtime Routine Questionnaire (BRQ) (Johnson, 1986)

Nursing Diagnosis:

Sleep pattern disturbance

Goals:

After discussing the findings of assessment and the nursing diagnosis, the client and/or care partner and the nurse will select intervention to:

A. Promote healthy sleep
B. Increase energy levels and participation in ADL

Considerations for Nursing Care and Health Teaching:

A. Nonpharmacologic interventions may include (Cohen & Merritt, 1992):
1. Establishing regular times for sleep
2. Avoidance close to bedtime of:
   a. Strenuous exercise
   b. Heavy meals (but avoid going to bed hungry)
   c. Spicy foods
   d. Caffeine-containing beverages, and alcohol
   e. Smoking or other use of tobacco
3. Drinking a warm liquid containing milk, such as cocoa, before bedtime
4. Engaging in restful activities near bedtime, such as reading; avoid stimulating, anxiety producing activities (e.g., watching the news on television)
5. Providing quiet, dark, comfortable environment
6. Teaching progressive muscular relaxation techniques to be used (use when first getting into bed)
7. If unable to sleep (after about 30 minutes), engaging in a restful activity and avoiding lying in bed and thinking about insomnia
8. Using bed for sleeping (avoid using it for such activities as working and eating); to maintain an association with a restful place, one should rest during the day in other places (e.g., couch or chair) (Cohen, 1988; Golden and James, 1988)
B. Interventions identified by patients and nurses in hospital setting include (Pulling, 1991; Reimer, 1987):
1. Providing medication for sleep or pain
2. Providing a back rub
3. Turning lights down
4. Reminding the patient to void before retiring
5. Leaving the patient alone for at least 90 minutes, without interruption, after falling asleep
6. Decreasing staff conversations

7. Assuring the patient that the nurse is available if needed
C. Pharmacologic treatment should include the following considerations:
   1. Benzodiazepines that may be prescribed for insomnia may alter the pharmacokinetics of zidovudine, potentially increasing toxicity (Burger et al., 1993)
   2. Clients should be evaluated for history of drug abuse or for dependence before pharmacologic agents are provided

Referrals:

A. CNS in HIV disease or mental health
B. Community-based support groups
C. Visiting nurse

Evaluation:

The client will:

A. Identify strategies to improve sleep and prevent insomnia
B. Demonstrate increased participation in activities of daily living
C. Verbalize an improvement in sleep patterns

SYMPTOM: *Sexual Dysfunction*

Etiology:

A. Chronic genital lesions (e.g., herpes simplex or Kaposi's sarcoma)
B. Chronic *Candida* vaginitis
C. Physical limitations (e.g., fatigue, shortness of breath, paralysis)
D. Medications
E. Partner unwilling, uninformed, or unavailable
F. Religious conflict
G. Lack of knowledge
H. Pain
I. Substance abuse
J. Fear of failure
K. Fear of transmitting or acquiring infection
L. Depression

Nursing Assessment:

A. Subjective data
   1. History of problem

   2. Desire for sexual experience
      a. Changing patterns: increase or decrease or fluctuations
      b. Concern about adequacy
   3. Concerns about body image and desire to have sex
   4. Current sexual interactions with partner
   5. Initiation of sexual activity
      a. Communication, both verbal and nonverbal
      b. Use of substances (drugs and alcohol)
      c. Use of enhancements (e.g., clothing, sexual devices, videotapes)
   6. Use of fantasy during sexual activities
   7. Sexual dislikes
   8. Sexual experiences with multiple or different partners
   9. Male-specific questions
      a. Erections (quality, failure); satisfaction with size of penis
      b. Orgasms (frequency, how achieved [by penetration, oral sex, masturbation]); concern over whether partner will reach climax
      c. Sexual experiences; degree of experimentation
   10. Female-specific questions
      a. Facility for vaginal lubrication, sufficient time for lubrication, and vaginal pain with penile penetration
      b. Orgasms (frequency and method [masturbation, manual and oral manipulation by partners])
      c. Situations that inhibit orgasms
   11. Presence, absence, or fear of pain
   12. Knowledge of safer sexual practices
   13. Fear of infection
   14. Comfort level with sexual orientation
   15. Sexually related fears (e.g., conflict with religious belief, concern about disease transmission)
   16. Medical and surgical history
   17. Current drug therapy

B. Objective data
   1. Unwillingness to acknowledge problem
   2. Avoidance behaviors when topic is mentioned

3. Presence of physical limitations (e.g., dyspnea, paralysis)

Nursing Diagnoses:

Altered sexuality pattern; sexual dysfunction

Goals:

After discussing and validating the assessment and nursing diagnoses, the client and/or sex partner and the nurse will select the interventions to:

A. Encourage free expression of concerns about sexual activities
B. Minimize fear of sexual experience in the presence of HIV disease

Considerations for Nursing Care and Health Teaching (Annon, 1976):

A. Permission: provide a milieu in which the client and significant other can freely discuss their sexual feelings and concerns
   1. Assure the client that sexuality is an expression of an individual's identity
   2. Assess the client for areas of concern and factors contributing to sexual problems, both physiologic and physical
   3. Particularly note the knowledge deficits about sexual practices that may place the client at risk for disease transmission (e.g., exchange of body fluids)
   4. Assess the client for the presence of conflicts in sexual practices and in the client's spiritual beliefs
B. Limited information: provide information relevant to the client's concerns; explain effects of HIV disease and client's symptoms, as well as medication effects, on sexual desires and performance
C. Specific suggestions: offer suggestions that can facilitate sexual functioning
   1. Concern about having sex with a partner in the presence of HIV disease
      a. Explain prevention of potential harm to client and others during sexual activity through discussion of specific sexual behaviors
      b. Provide resource information on local AIDS support groups and

events sponsored for HIV-infected persons
      c. If having sex with a partner is unacceptable to client, consider masturbation
   2. Concern about genital lesions or infection
      a. For men, use of colored condoms
      b. For women, use of female condoms
   3. Concern about sexual appeal related to weight loss or to lesions on legs, torso, or arms
      a. Wear garments that may stimulate sexual arousal in both client and partner (encourage client and significant other to identify garments that stimulate sexual arousal)
      b. Consider reducing lighting in room when engaging in sexual activities
   4. Concern about need to stimulate all senses and perceptions
      a. Use oils for body rubs and use colognes
      b. Consider use of sexually explicit and appealing videotapes
      c. Consider use of sexual devices such as vibrators and dildos
   5. Concern about shortness of breath; client should:
      a. Remain passive in relation to position changes during sexual activities
      b. Avoid lying flat
      c. Use oxygen during sex if needed
      d. Avoid sexual practices (e.g., fellatio) that may interfere with breathing
   6. Concern about fatigue
      a. Plan rest before sexual activity
      b. Client should remain passive in relation to positional changes
   7. Concern about pain
      a. Assist client in determining the best time for medication in relation to sexual activities (e.g., 30 to 60 minutes before)
      b. Encourage client to use a water-soluble lubricant for intercourse
      c. For localized painful lesions, encourage client to use anesthetic

creams or ointments before sexual activity

D. Intensive therapy: when indicated, assist client with referral for counseling and therapy

Referrals:

A. CNS in HIV disease, human sexuality, or mental health
B. Psychologist or psychiatrist
C. Support groups for persons with HIV disease

Evaluation:

The client will:

A. Discuss sexual concerns and feelings
B. Identify sexual activities that prevent transmission of bodily fluids during sex
C. Express concerns over changes in body image and identify strategies to cope with the changes
D. Discuss physiologic limitations to having sex and strategies to minimize their interference with sex
E. When appropriate, identify the need for further counseling and seek out assistance with referral

HIV-RELATED RESEARCH ON NURSING CARE

Summary of Research

As the numbers of people living with HIV disease/AIDS increases, so does the need for nursing research to describe empirically patient problems, nursing interventions, and patient outcomes (Holzemer, 1992). In 1988 the National Center for Nursing Research (NCNR) identified five priority areas for nursing research related to HIV infection, including (1) prevention of HIV infection, (2) physiologic aspects of care, (3) psychosocial aspects of nursing care, (4) delivery of nursing care, and (5) applied ethics (Larson & Ropka, 1991). In a review of the literature from May 1987 to June 1990, Larson and Ropka (1991) found only 20 of 54 nursing research articles addressing the priority areas established by the NCNR. There were no studies that related to identifying the patient problems and link-

ing them to nursing activities and patient outcomes (Holzemer, 1992).

The need to identify empirically the nursing care of PWHIV is self-evident. Holzemer and Henry (1991) examined four standardized nursing care plans for PWHIV from four agencies with extensive experience in the clinical care of this client population. Although the agencies were located within a 4-mile radius of each other in the San Francisco Bay area, the authors not only found minimal agreement about nursing care problems of PWHIV but also noted differences in language, conceptual clarity, and level of complexity related to problem identification. The authors concluded that nurses need to define the problems of PWHIV adequately for appropriate planning of their nursing care and improvement of patient outcomes.

Janson-Bjerklie and colleagues (1992) studied PWHIV hospitalized with a medical diagnosis of *Pneumocystis carinii* pneumonia to identify patients' perceptions of pulmonary problems, especially dyspnea, and the nursing interventions perceived by the patients as helpful. Contrary to the authors' expectations, they found that dyspnea was not ubiquitous in the sample and that nonpulmonary concerns were the predominant problems reported by patients. This finding underscores the need for nurse researchers to conduct studies of patient problem identification that include self-reporting by the subjects. Additionally, the authors found that when dyspnea was present in the sample, there were few nursing interventions that patients could identify. This finding is similar to that of a study of patients with dyspnea and lung cancer who reported that nurses had not taught them how to manage their dyspnea but that they had learned on their own (Brown et al., 1986).

Hurley and Ungvarski (1994) conducted a retrospective study to identify both the physiologic and psychologic signs and symptoms of persons with AIDS admitted to a home care agency in New York City. The most frequent physiologic signs and symptoms identified in greater than 15% of the subjects (N = 244) were dyspnea (57%), weakness (53%), fatigue and lethargy (46%), pain (42%), ataxia (37%), cough (36%), skin lesions (34%), nocturia (26%), visual impairment (23%), paraparesis (23%), oral lesions, including thrush (21%), weight loss (19%), and diarrhea (16%). Psychologic signs and symptoms included memory deficit (34%), depression (28%), anxiety (27%), impaired judgment (18%), substance abuse (18%), and insomnia (16%). The signs and symptoms described in this study were identified on admission by the patient or the nurse or both.

Newshan (1993) explored common pain characteristics in both drug-using and non-drug-using PWHIV. The two most frequently cited types of pain for both groups were abdominal pain and neuropathic pain. Differences noted were a higher incidence of pain caused by esophagitis and headache in drug users and more Kaposi's sarcoma–associated pain in nonusers. The author also noted that drug users often required more frequent use of opiates.

The use of nursing diagnosis as a tool for identifying problems in individuals with HIV/AIDS has also been studied. Smith (1991) reviewed the literature on the nursing care of hospitalized adults with AIDS to examine the commonalities of identified nursing diagnoses, tabulated according to frequency. The author found that five of the nine problems with the highest frequency were physiologic (altered nutrition: less than body requirements; respiratory problems; impaired skin integrity; diarrhea; potential for infection), and the other four problems were cognitive (altered thought processes), safety (potential for injury), social (social isolation), and a combination of physiologic and cognitive (pain).

Hurley and Ungvarski (1993) explored the use of nursing diagnosis as a means of identifying the home care needs of adults with AIDS. The highest number of common diagnoses, identified in greater than 70% of the sample (N = 244) were impaired home health maintenance (98%); high risk of ineffective individual coping (94%); impaired physical mobility (85%); altered nutrition (82%); self-care deficit (80%); fatigue (74%); and dressing/grooming self-care deficit (70%).

Research Needed

Zeller and colleagues (1993) made recommendations for clinical nursing research related to symptom management in PWHIV, including:

1. Respiratory symptoms
   a. Management of dyspnea associated with *Pneumocystis carinii* pneumonia
   b. Determination of whether interventions developed for other types of patients with dyspnea are effective for PWHIV
   c. Study of the effects of these interventions on survival
2. Malnutrition and gastrointestinal symptoms
   a. Development and testing of nursing interventions to manage reduced nutrient intake, malabsorption, altered taste sensations, dysphagia, odynophagia, nausea and vomiting, and diarrhea
   b. Evaluation of the efficacy of oral rehydration therapies used for pediatric diarrhea in adult PWHIV
   c. Comparison of the benefits of enteral versus parenteral therapies
3. Neurologic symptoms: evaluation of the efficacy of strategies developed to maximize cognitive functioning in patients with Alzheimer's disease for PWHIV
4. Opportunistic and nosocomial infections
   a. Strategies to prevent opportunistic infections (e.g., *Candida* or *Cryptosporidium* infection)
   b. Treatment protocols for managing venous access devices and urinary catheters
   c. Studies of health care workers' handwashing techniques and skin cleansing agents
   d. Evaluation of the efficacy of low microbial diets in preventing infection
5. Pain
   a. Efficacy of nonpharmacologic nursing interventions (e.g., therapeutic touch, relaxation, and hypnosis)
   b. Comparative studies of delivery of prescribed analgesia (e.g., controlled-released analgesia vs traditional)

O'Brien and Pheifer (1993) recommended the study of physical and psychologic aspects of nursing care, including:

1. Examination of cultural variables associated with coping with HIV
2. Longitudinal research on continuing survival of HIV
3. Studies to test specific nursing therapeutic interventions in various settings such as hospital, home, and clinic
4. Descriptive research on the impact of HIV and AIDS on the family, including their functioning and adaptation

Additional considerations for future nursing research include:

1. Assessment
   a. Descriptive studies identifying the most frequent physiologic and psychologic responses encountered by PWHIV
   b. Congruency studies to determine the similarities to and differences in problems identified by clients in comparison with those identified by clinicians
   c. Identification of the comorbidity of symptoms in PWHIV
   d. Identification of problem differences in the different populations with HIV disease (e.g., gay men, drug users), as well as culturally related concerns
   e. Development, testing, and validation of assessment tools that are practical and user friendly for nurses performing patient assessment
2. Nursing treatments
   a. Development and testing of treatments for symptoms identified in PWHIV
   b. Identification and testing of nursing treatments that can be utilized in the presence of comorbid symptoms
3. Evaluation
   a. Evaluation of nursing treatments on the basis of patient preferences and outcomes
   b. Comparison of costs of nursing treatments

According to Holzemer (1992), research on the nursing care needs of the acute and chronically ill HIV-infected person should include a nursing framework that encompasses patient problems (inputs), nursing activities (processes), and patient responses (outcomes). Additionally, in the current climate of health care reform and cost containment, nurse researchers must begin routinely to include the economic impact of nursing services.

SUMMARY

Planning nursing care for clients with or at risk of having HIV disease begins with a knowledge of behaviors and activities that place individuals at risk. The findings of this risk assessment serve as the basis for assisting the client with making choices that protect the individual's health by reducing the potential for acquiring HIV. For HIV-infected individuals, nursing care focuses on providing information and options to change behavior for the purpose of maintaining and improving health. Because HIV disease has no cure, emphasis is placed on reducing symptoms through nursing interventions throughout the spectrum of illness (McMahon & Coyne, 1989). Nursing interventions should be based on research findings, and evaluation or their efficacy should be based on client outcomes and cost-effectiveness.

REFERENCES

Abbey, J.C., Andrews, C., Avigliano, K., et al. (1973). A pilot study: The control of shivering during hypothermia by a clinical nursing measure. *Journal of Neuroscience Nursing, 5*(2), 78–88.

Abrams, B., Duncan, D., Hertz-Piccotto, I. (1993). A prospective study of dietary intake and acquired immune deficiency syndrome in HIV-seropositive homosexual men. *Journal of Acquired Immune Deficiency Syndromes, 6*(8), 949–958.

Abramson, J.H. (1966). The Cornell Medical Index as an epidemiological tool. *American Journal of Public Health, 56*(2), 287–298.

Abramson, J.H., Terespolsky, L., Brook, J.G., et al. (1965). Cornell Medical Index as a health measure in epidemiological studies. *British Journal of Preventive Social Medicine, 19*(3), 103–110.

Acute Pain Management Guideline Panel (1992, February). *Acute pain management: Operative or medical procedures and trauma—clinical practice guideline.* (AHCPR Pub. No. 92-0032). Rockville, MD: Agency for Health Care Policy and Research, Public Health Service, U.S. Department of Health and Human Services.

AIDS Institute (1992, December). HIV medical evaluation and preventive care. In *Protocols for the medical care* of HIV infection (2nd ed.). Albany, NY: New York State Department of Health.

Allen, M. (1990). Adjusting to visual impairment. *Journal of Ophthalmic Nursing & Technology, 9*(2), 47–51.

American Thoracic Society (1978). Recommended respiratory disease questionnaire for use with adults and children in epidemiological research. *American Review of Respiratory Disease, 118,* 16.

Andrist, L.C. (1988). Taking a sexual history and educating clients about safe sex. *Nursing Clinics of North America, 23*(4), 959–973.

Annon, J.S. (1976). The PLISS and model: A proposed conceptual scheme for the behavioral treatment of sexual problems. *Journal of Sex Education and Therapy, 2*(1), 211–215.

Armistead, H.S. (1992). Aspirin and indomethacin may be potent immunomodulators in HIV disease. *International Conference on AIDS* [abstract No. 7016], *8*(3), 51.

Baekeland, F., Hoy, P. (1971). Reported versus recorded sleep characteristics. *Archives of General Psychiatry, 24*(6), 548–555.

Barnes, P.F., Bloch, A.B., Davidson, P.T., et al. (1991). Tuberculosis in patients with human immunodeficiency virus infection. *New England Journal of Medicine, 324*(23), 1644–1650.

Barringer, F. (1993, April 1). Viral sexual diseases are found in 1 of 5 in U.S. *The New York Times,* pA-1.

Bartlett, J.G. (1993). Routine laboratory testing in asymptomatic infection. *PAAC Notes: The Newsjournal of the Physicians in AIDS Care, 5*(5), 192–197.

Berger, T.G. (1990). Dermatologic care in the AIDS patient. In M.A. Sande & P.A. Volberding (Eds.), *The medical management of AIDS* (2nd ed.) (pp. 114–130). Philadelphia, PA: W.B. Saunders.

Blake, R.L., Vandiver, T.A. (1986). The reliability and validity of a ten-item measure of functional status. *Journal of Family Practice, 23*(5), 455–459.

Blum, J. (1987). *When you face the chemically dependent patient: A practical guide for nurses.* St. Louis: Ishiyaku Euro-America, Inc.

Borg, G. (1982). Psychophysical bases of perceived exertion. *Medicine and Science in Sports and Exercise, 14,* 337–381.

Bradley-Springer, L. (1991). Nutrition and support in HIV infection: A multilevel analysis. *Image: Journal of Nursing Scholarship, 23*(3), 155–159.

Breitbart, W., Marotta, R.F., Call, P. (1988). AIDS and neuroleptic malignant syndrome [letter]. *Lancet, 2*(8626-8627), 1488–1489.

Briscoe, K. (1989). Optimal management of nausea and vomiting in clinical oncology. *Oncology, 3*(suppl 8), 11–15.

Brown, M.L., Carrieri, V., Janson-Bjerklie, S., Dodd, M.J. (1986). Lung cancer and dyspnea: The patient's perception. *Oncology Nursing Forum, 13*(5), 19–24.

Burger, D.M., Meenhorst, P.L., Koks, C.H., et al. (1993). Drug interactions with zidovudine, *AIDS, 7*(4), 445–460.

Burish, T.G., Carey, M.P. (1984). Conditioned responses to cancer chemotherapy: Etiology and treatment. In B.H. Fox & B.H. Newberry (Eds.), *Impact of psychoendocrine systems in cancer and community* (p. 147). Lewiston, NY: C.J. Hogrefe.

Butler, R.N. (1963). The life review: An interpretation of reminiscence in the aged. *Psychiatry, 256,* 65–76.

Butler, R.N. (1974). Successful aging and the role of the life review. *Journal of the American Geriatric Society, 22*(12), 529–535.

Carrieri, V.K., Janson-Bjerklie, S. (1986). Strategies patients use to manage the sensation of dyspnea. *Western Journal of Nursing Research, 8*(3), 284–305.

Carrieri-Kohlman, V., Janson-Bjerklie, S. (1993). Dyspnea. In V. Carrieri-Kohlman, A.M. Lindsey, & C.M. West (Eds.), *Pathophysiological phenomena in nursing human responses to illness* (2nd ed.) (pp. 247–278). Philadelphia, PA: W.B. Saunders.

Caruso, C.C., Hadley, B.J., Shukla, R., et al. (1992). Cooling effects and comfort of four cooling blanket temperatures in humans with fever. *Nursing Research, 41*(2), 68–72.

Centers for Disease Control (1986). Diagnosis and management of mycobacterial infection and disease in persons with human T-lymphotropic virus type-III, lymphadenopathy-associated virus infection. *Morbidity and Mortality Weekly Report, 35*(28), 448–452.

Centers for Disease Control and Prevention (1990a). Risk for cervical disease in HIV-infected women—New York City. *Morbidity and Mortality Weekly Report, 39*(47), 846–849.

Centers for Disease Control and Prevention (1990b). *Health information for international travel.* (HHS Pub. No. CDC 90–8280.) Washington, DC: U.S. Government Printing Office.

Centers for Disease Control and Prevention (1991a). Purified protein derivative (PPD) – tuberculin anergy and HIV infection: Guidelines for anergy testing and management of anergic persons at risk of tuberculosis. *Morbidity and Mortality Weekly Report, 40*(RR-5), 27–33.

Centers for Disease Control and Prevention (1991b). Update on adult immunization practices advisory committee (ACIP). *Morbidity and Mortality Weekly Report, 40*(RR-12), 1–94.

Centers for Disease Control and Prevention (1992a). 1993 Revised classification system for HIV infection and expanded surveillance case definition for AIDS among adolescents and adults. *Morbidity and Mortality Weekly Report, 41*(RR-17), 1–19.

Centers for Disease Control and Prevention (1992b). Guidelines for the performance of CD4+ T-cell determinations in persons with human immunodeficiency virus infection. *Morbidity and Mortality Weekly Report, 41*(RR-8), 1–17.

Centers for Disease Control and Prevention (1992c). Recommendations for prophylaxis against *Pneumocystis carinii* pneumonia for adults and adolescents infected with human immunodeficiency virus. *Morbidity and Mortality Weekly Report, 41*(RR-4), 1–11.

Centers for Disease Control and Prevention (1993, October). *HIV AIDS Surveillance Report, 5*(3), 1–19.

Centers for Disease Control and Prevention (1993a). Update: Mortality attributable to HIV infection/AIDS among persons aged 25-44 years—United States, 1990 and 1991. *Morbidity and Mortality Weekly Report, 42*(25), 481–486.

Centers for Disease Control and Prevention (1993b). Recommendations of the advisory committee on immunization practices (ACIP): Use of vaccines and immune globulins in persons with altered immunocompetence. *Morbidity and Mortality Weekly Report, 42*(RR-4), 1–18.

Centers for Disease Control and Prevention (1993c). Recommendations on prophylaxis and therapy for disseminated *Mycobacterium avium* complex for adults and adolescents infected with human immunodeficiency virus. *Morbidity and Mortality Weekly Report, 42*(RR-9), 17–20.

Cheeseman, S.H. (1992). Cytomegalovirus. In S.L. Gorbach, J.G. Bartlett, & N.R. Blacklow (Eds.), *Infectious diseases* (pp. 1715–1720). Philadelphia, PA: W.B. Saunders.

Choi, S., Lagakos, S.W., Schooley, R.T. (1993). CD4$^+$ lymphocytes are an incomplete surrogate marker for clinical progression in persons with asymptomatic HIV infection. *Annals of Internal Medicine, 118*(9), 674–680.

Cockerell, C.J. (1991). Noninfectious inflammatory skin diseases in HIV-infected individuals. *Dermatologic Clinics, 9*(3), 531–541.

Cohen, F.L. (1988). Narocolepsy: A review of a common, life-long sleep disorder. *Journal of Advanced Nursing, 13*(5), 546–556.

Cohen, F.L., Merritt, S.L. (1992). Sleep promotion. In G.M. Bulechek & J.C. McCloskey (Eds.), *Nursing Interventions* (2nd ed.) (pp. 109–119). Philadelphia, PA: W.B. Saunders.

Cotton, D.J. (1993). Reports from Berlin: Disappointing assessment of current antiretrovirals. *AIDS Clinical Care, 5*(7), 52–53, 54, 58.

Crowe, S., Mills, J., McGrath, M.S. (1990). Monocyte/macrophage. In P.T. Cohen, M.A. Sande, & P.A. Volberding (Eds.), *The AIDS knowledge base* (pp. 324.1–324.2). Waltham, MA: Medical Publishing Group.

Culhane, B. (1984). Diarrhea. In J.M. Yasko (Ed.), *Nursing management of symptoms associated with chemotherapy* (pp. 41–47). Reston, VA: Reston Publishing.

Cuzzel, J.Z. (1990). Clues: Itching burning in skin folds. *American Journal of Nursing, 90*(1), 23–24.

Daly, M.R. (1990). Sensory supports for the visually impaired. *Journal of Ophthalmic Nursing & Technology, 9*(6), 243–244.

Dismukes, W.E. (1988). Cryptococcal meningitis in patients with AIDS. *Journal of Infectious Diseases, 157*(4), 624–628.

Dressler, D.K., Smejkal, C., Ruffolo, M.L. (1983). A comparison of oral and rectal temperature measurement on patients receiving oxygen by mask. *Nursing Research, 32*(6), 373–375.

Duigon, A. (1986). Anticipatory nausea and vomiting associated with cancer chemotherapy. *Oncology Nursing Forum, 13*(1), 35–40.

Dyson, R. (1978). Bed sores—the injuries hospital staff inflict on patients. *Nursing Mirror, 146*(24), 30–32.

Eilers, J., Berger, A.M., Petersen, M.C. (1988). Development, testing, and application of the oral assessment guide. *Oncology Nursing Forum, 15*(3), 325–330.

Ek, A.C., Gustavsson, G., Lewis, D.H. (1985). The local skin blood flow in areas at risk for pressure sores treated with massage. *Scandinavian Journal of Rehabilitation Medicine, 17*(2), 81–86.

Erickson, R. (1980). Oral temperature differences in relation to thermometer and technique. *Nursing Research, 29*(3), 157–164.

Fauci, A. (1993). CD4$^+$ T-lymphocytopenia with HIV infection—no lights, no camera, just facts [editorial]. *New England Journal of Medicine, 328*(6), 429–431.

Ferguson, K.J., Stapleton, J.T., Helms, C.M. (1991). Physicians' effectiveness in assessing risk for human immunodeficiency virus infection. *Archives of Internal Medicine, 151*(3), 561–564.

Filice, G.A., Pomeroy, C. (1991). Preventing secondary infections among HIV-positive persons. *Public Health Report, 106*(5), 503–517.

Fillit, H., Fruchtman, M.D., Sell, L., et al. (1990). AIDS in the elderly: A case and its implications. *AIDS Patients Care, 4*(1), 8–12.

Fischl, M.A., Uttamchandani, R.B., Daikos, G.L., et al. (1992). An outbreak of tuberculosis caused by multiple-drug–resistant tubercle bacilli among patients with HIV infection. *Annals of Internal Medicine, 117*(3), 177–183.

Fogel, C.I. (1990). Sexual health promotion. In C.I. Fogel & D. Lauver (Eds.), *Sexual health promotion* (pp. 1–18). Philadelphia, PA: W.B. Saunders.

Folstein, M.F., Folstein, S.E., McHugh, P.R. (1975). "Minimental state": A practical method for grading the cognitive state of patients for the clinician. *Journal of Psychiatric Research, 12*(3), 189–198.

Freud, M. (1923). The graphic rating scale. *Journal of Educational Psychology, 14*, 83.

Galgiani, J.N., Ampel, N.M. (1990). Coccidioidomycosis in human immunodeficiency virus–infected patients. *Journal of Infectious Diseases, 162*(5), 1165–1169.

Gemson, D.H., Colombotos, J., Elinson, J., et al. (1991). Acquired immunodeficiency syndrome prevention: Knowledge, attitudes, and practices of primary care physicians. *Archives of Internal Medicine, 151*(6), 1102–1108.

Giardino, E.R., Wolf, Z.R. (1993). Symptoms: Evidence and experience. *Holistic Nurse Practice, 7*(2), 1–12.

Gift, A.G. (1989). Visual analogue scales: Measurement of subjective phenomena. *Nursing Research, 38*(5), 286–288.

Gift, A. (1993). Therapies for dyspnea relief. *Holistic Nurse Practice, 7*(2), 57–63.

Gift, A.G., Austin, D.J. (1992). The effects of a program of systematic movement of COPD patients. *Rehabilitation Nursing, 17*(1), 6–10, 25.

Gift, A.G., Moore, T., Soeken, K. (1992). Relaxation to reduce dyspnea and anxiety in COPD patients. *Nursing Research, 41*(4), 242–246.

Gift, A.G., Plaut, S.M., Jacox, A.K. (1986). Psychologic and physiologic factors related to dyspnea in subjects with chronic obstructive pulmonary disease. *Heart & Lung, 15*(6), 595–601.

Gift, A.G., Pugh, L.C. (1993). Dyspnea and fatigue. *Nursing Clinics of North America, 28*(2), 373–384.

Golden, R.N., James, S.P. (1988). Insomnia. *Postgraduate Medicine, 83*(4), 251–258.

Goodman, E.L., Knochel, J.P. (1991). Heat stroke and other forms of hyperthermia. In P.A. Mackowiak (Ed.), *Fever: Basic mechanisms and management* (pp. 267–287). New York: Raven Press.

Grant, M. (1987). Nausea, vomiting, and anorexia. *Seminars in Oncology Nursing, 3*(4), 277–286.

Greifzu, S., Radjeski, D., Winnick, B. (1990). Oral care is part of cancer care. *RN, 53*(6), 9–10.

Grunfeld, C. (1992). Metabolic disturbances, anorexia, and wasting in HIV/AIDS. In G. Nary (Ed.), *Nutrition & HIV/AIDS* (vol. 1) (pp. 9–15). Chicago: PAAC Publishing.

Hardy, M.A. (1992). Dry skin care. In G.M. Bulechek & J.A. McCloskey (Eds.), *Nursing interventions: Essential nursing treatments* (2nd ed.) (pp. 34–47). Philadelphia: PA: W.B. Saunders.

Hargreaves, M.R., Fuller, G.N., Gazzard, B.G. (1988). Occult AIDS: *Pneumocystis carinii* pneumonia in elderly people. *British Medical Journal, 297*(6650), 721–722.

Hart, L.K., Freel, M.I., Milde, F.K. (1990). Fatigue. *Nursing Clinics of North America, 25*(4), 967–976.

Hecht, F.M., Soloway, B. (1993a). Identifying patients at risk for HIV infection. In D.J. Cotton & G.H. Friedland (Eds.), *HIV infection: A primary care approach* (rev. ed.) (pp. 3–7). Waltham, MA: Massachusetts Medical Society.

Hecht, F.M., Soloway, B. (1993b). Laboratory tests for monitoring HIV infection. In D.J. Cotton & G.H. Friedland (Eds.), *HIV infection: A primary care approach* (rev. ed.) (pp. 16–18). Waltham, MA: Massachusetts Medical Society.

Hecht, F.M., Soloway, B. (1993c). Immunizations in HIV-infected patients. In D.J. Cotton & G.H. Friedland (Eds.), *HIV infection: A primary care approach* (rev. ed.) (pp. 39–41). Waltham, MA: Massachusetts Medical Society.

Heinemann, M. (1992). Ophthalmic problems. *The Medical Clinics of North America, 76*(1), 83–97.

Hernandez, S.R. (1990). History and physical exam of HIV infected patients. In P.T. Cohen, M.A. Sande, & P.A. Volberding (Eds.), *The AIDS knowledge base* (pp. 421.1–421.7). Waltham, MA: Medical Publishing Group.

Henry, K., Sullivan, C., Campbell, S. (1993). Deficits in AIDS/HIV knowledge among physicians and nurses at a Minnesota public teaching hospital. *Minneosta Medicine, 76*(2), 23–27.

Hibberd, P.L., Rubin, R.H. (1991). Fever in the immunocompromised host. In P.A. Mackowick (Ed.), *Fever: Basic mechanisms and management* (pp. 197–218). New York: Raven Press.

Hilton, G., Sisson, R., Freeman, E. (1990). The Neurobehavioral Rating Scale: An interrator reliability study in the HIV seropositive population. *Journal of Neuroscience Nursing, 22*(1), 36–42.

Hinkle, K. (1991). A literature review: HIV seropositivity in the elderly. *Journal of Gerontological Nursing, 7*(10), 12–17.

Hoffmann, K.K., Weber, D.J., Samsa, P. (1992). Transparent polyurethane film as an intravenous catheter dressing: A meta-analysis of the infection risks. *Journal of the American Medical Association, 267*(15), 2072–2076.

Hogan, R. (1980). *Human sexuality: A nursing perspective.* New York: Appleton-Century-Crofts.

Holtzclaw, B.J. (1990a). Effects of extremity wraps to control drug induced shivering: A pilot study. *Nursing Research, 39*(5), 280–283.

Holtzclaw, B.J. (1990b). Control of febrile shivering during amphotericin B therapy. *Oncology Nursing Forum, 17*(4), 521–524.

Holtzclaw, B.J. (1992). The febrile response in critical care: State of the science. *Heart & Lung, 21*(5), 482–501.

Holzemer, W.L. (1992). Nursing effectivness research and patient outcomes. *Critical Care Nursing Clinics of North America, 4*(3), 429–435.

Holzemer, W.L., Henry, S.B. (1991). Nursing care plans for people with HIV-AIDS: Confusion or consensus? *Journal of Advanced Nursing, 16*(3), 257–261.

Hotter, A.N. (1990). Wound healing and immunocompromise. *Nursing Clinics of North America, 25*(1), 193–203.

Hriso, E., Kuhn, T., Masdey, J.C., et al. (1991). Extrapyramidal symptoms due to dopamine-blocking agents in patients with AIDS encephalopathy. *American Journal of Psychiatry, 148*(11), 1558–1561.

Hurley, P.M., Ungvarski, P.J. (1993, October). *Nursing care needs of adults with HIV disease/AIDS in homecare.* Paper presented at the First International Conference on Home Health Care for AIDS Patients, Lyon, France.

Hurley, P.M., Ungvarski, P.J. (1994). Home health care needs of adults living with HIV disease/AIDS in New York City. *Journal of the Association of Nurses in AIDS Care, 5*(2), 33–40.

Ilsley, A.H., Rutten, A.J., Runciman, W.B. (1983). An evaluation of body temperature measurement. *Anesthesia Intensive Care, 11*(1), 31–39.

Itescu, S., Brancato, L.J., Burnbaum, J., et al. (1990). A diffuse infiltrative CD8 lymphocytosis syndrome in human immunodeficiency virus (HIV) infection: A host immune response associated with HLA-DR5. *Annals of Internal Medicine, 112*(1), 3–10.

Jablonski, R.S. (1993). Nausea: The forgotten symptom. *Holistic Nursing Practice, 7*(2), 64–72.

Jacobs, J.W., Bernhard, M.K., Delgado, A., et al. (1977). Screening for organic mental syndromes in the medically ill. *Annals of Internal Medicine, 86*(1), 40–46.

Janson-Bjerklie, S., Carrieri, V.K., Hudes, M. (1986). The sensations of pulmonary dyspnea. *Nursing Research, 35*(3), 154–159.

Janson-Bjerklie, S., Holzemer, W., Henry, H.B. (1992). Patient's perceptions of pulmonary problems and nursing interventions during hospitalization for *Pneumocystis carinii* pneumonia. *American Journal of Critical Care, 1*(1), 114–121.

Jensen, D.P., Herr, K.A. (1993). Sleeplessness. *Nursing Clinics of North America, 28*(2), 385–405.

Jewitt, J.F., Hecht, F.M. (1993). Preventive health care for adults with HIV infection. *Journal of the American Medical Association, 269*(9), 1144–1153.

Johnson, J. (1986). Sleep and bedtime routines in non-institutionalized aged women. *Journal of Community Health Nursing, 3*(3), 117–125.

Kahn, R.L., Goldfarb, A.L., Polack, M., et al. (1960). Brief objective measures for the determination of mental status in the aged. *American Journal of Psychiatry, 117*, 326–328.

Kelly, P.J., Holman, S. (1993). The new face of AIDS. *American Journal of Nursing, 93*(3), 26–34.

Kelly, R.B., Zyanski, S.J., Alemagno, S.A. (1991). Prediction of motivation and behavior change following health promotion: Role of health beliefs, social support, and self-efficacy. *Social Science Medicine, 32*(3), 311–320.

King, A.B. (1990). Malnutrition in HIV infection: Prevalence, etiology and management. *PAACNOTES, 2*(3), 122–129.

Kotler, D.P. (1992). Causes and consequences of malnutrition in HIV/AIDS. In G. Nary (Ed.), *Nutrition and HIV/AIDS* (vol. 1) (pp. 5–8). Chicago: PAAC Publishing.

Kotler, D.P., Tierney, A.R., Wang, J., et al. (1989). Magnitude of body-cell-mass depletion and timing of death from wasting in AIDS. *American Journal of Clinical Nutrition, 50*(3), 444–437.

Kovner, R., Lazar, J.W., Lesser, M., et al. (1992). Use of the Dementia Rating Scale as a test for neuropsychological dysfunction in HIV-positive i.v. drug users. *Journal of Substance Abuse Treatment, 9*(2), 133–137.

Langtry, H.D., Campoli-Richards, D.M. (1989). Zidovudine: A review of its pharmacodynamic and pharacokinetic properties, and therapeutic efficacy. *Drugs, 37*(4), 408–450.

Larson, E., Ropka, M.E. (1991). An update on nursing research and HIV infection. *Image: Journal of Nursing Scholarship, 23*(1), 4–12.

Lee, K.A., Hicks, G., Nino-Murcia, C. (1991). Validity and reliability of a scale to assess fatigue. *Psychiatry Research, 36*(3), 291–298.

Liebman, M.C. (1992). Practice corner: Oral care. *Oncology Nursing Forum, 19*(6), 939–941.

Life Sciences Research Office, Federation of American Societies for Experimental Biology (1990, November). *Nutrition and HIV infection.* Washington, D.C.: Center for Food Safety and Applied Nutrition, Food and Drug Administration, U.S. Department of Health and Human Services.

Lincoln, R., Roberts, R. (1989). Continence issues in acute care. *Nursing Clinics of North America, 24*(3), 741–754.

Lindsey, A.M. (1993). Cancer cachexia. In V. Carrieri-Kohlman, A.M. Lindsey, & C.M. West (Eds.), *Pathophysiological phenomena in nursing human responses to illness* (2nd ed.) (pp. 133–152). Philadelphia, PA: W.B. Saunders.

Lyles, J.N., Burish, T.G., Krozely, M.G., et al. (1982). Efficacy of relaxation training and guided imagery in reducing the aversiveness of cancer chemotherapy. *Journal of Consulting and Clinical Psychology, 50*(4), 509–524.

Macilwain, C. (1993). Aspirin on trial as HIV treatment. *Nature, 364*(6436), 369.

MacVicar, A.G., Winningham, M.L. (1986). Promoting functional capacity of cancer patients. *Cancer Bulletin, 38,* 235–239.

Mahoudi, A., Iseman, M.D. (1993). Pitfalls in the care of patients with tuberculosis: Common errors and their association with the acquisition of drug resistance. *Journal of the American Medical Association, 270*(1), 65–68.

Mackowiak, P.A., Wasserman, S.S., Levine, M.M. (1993). A critical appraisal of 98.6 degrees F, the upper limit of the normal body temperature, and other legacies of Carl Reinhold August Wunderlich. *Journal of the American Medical Association, 268*(12), 1578–1580.

Malone, J.L., Simms, T.E., Gray, G.C., et al. (1990). Sources of variability in repeated T-helper lymphocyte counts from human immunodeficiency virus type 1–infected patients: Total lymphocyte count of fluctuations and diurnal cycle are important. *Journal of Acquired Immune Deficiency Syndromes, 3*(2), 144–151.

Mann, J., Tarantola, D.J., Netter, T.W. (1992). *A global report: AIDS in the world.* Cambridge, MA: Harvard University Press.

McArthur, J. (1990). AIDS dementia: Your assessment can make all the difference. *RN, 53*(3), 36–42.

McCarthy, P.L. (1991). Fever in infants and children. In P.A. Mackowiak (Ed.), *Fever: Basic mechanisms and management* (pp. 219–231). New York: Raven Press.

McCorkle, R., Young, K. (1978). Development of a symptom distress scale. *Cancer Nursing, 1*(5), 373–378.

McDonnell, M., Sevedge, K. (1986). Acquired immune deficiency syndrome (AIDS). In M.H. Brown, M.E. Kiss, E.M. Outlaw, & C.M. Viamontes (Eds.), *Standards of oncology practice* (pp. 565–594). New York: John Wiley & Sons.

McMahon, K.M., Coyne, N. (1989). Symptom management in patients with AIDS. *Seminars in Oncology Nursing, 5*(4), 288–301.

Melzack, R. (1987). The short form McGill Pain Questionnaire. *Pain, 30*(2), 191–197.

Morgan, S.P. (1990). A comparison of three methods of managing fever in the neurologic patient. *Journal of Neuroscience Nursing, 22*(1), 19–24.

Morrow, G.R. (1984). Methodology in behavioral and psychosocial cancer research: The assessment of nausea and vomiting—past problems, current issues and suggestions for future research. *Cancer, 53*(10 suppl), 2267–2280.

Murphy, R., Chmiel, J. (1992). Prognostic value of the CD4 count and other surrogate markers. *HIV: Advances in Research and Therapy, 2*(2), 25–29.

Muwaswes, M. (1993). Alterations in consciousness. In V. Carrieri-Kohlman, A.M. Lindsey, & C.M. West (Eds.), *Pathophysiological phenomena in nursing human responses to illness* (2nd ed.) (pp. 195–220). Philadelphia: W.B. Saunders.

National Institute of Allergy and Infectious Diseases (1993, summer). Preliminary guidelines take more patient-tailored approach to HIV therapy. *NIAID AIDS Agenda,* p. 1, 11.

National Institutes of Health (1990). Oral complications of cancer therapies: Diagnosis, prevention and treatment. *Clinical Courier, 8*(3), 1–8.

Newman, C.F. (1992). The role of nutritional assessments and nutritional plans in the management of HIV/AIDS. In G. Nary (Ed.), *Nutrition and HIV/AIDS* (vol. 1) (pp. 57–106). Chicago: PAAC Publishing.

Newman, J. (1985). Evaluation of sponging to reduce body temperature in febrile children. *Canadian Medical Association Journal, 132*(6), 641–642.

Newshan, G.T. (1993). Pain characteristics and their management in persons with AIDS. *Journal of the Association of Nurses in AIDS Care, 4*(2), 53–59.

Nisita, C., Perretta, P., Gallic, L., et al. (1991). Symptomatological aspects of anxiety and depression in a cohort of HIV-positive patients and their relationship with the phase of infection and the belonging to a group at risk. *International Conference on AIDS* [abstract No. M.B. 2107], *7*(1), 208.

North American Nursing Diagnosis Association (1992). *NANDA Nursing diagnoses: Definitions and Classification 1992.* St. Louis: The Association.

O'Brien, M.E., Pheifer, W.G. (1993). Physical and psychological nursing care for patients with HIV infection. *Nursing Clinics of North America, 28*(2), 303–316.

O'Brien, W.A., Ovcak, S., Kalhor, H., et al. (1993). HIV-1 replication can be increased in blood from seropositive patients following influenza immunization. *International Conference on AIDS* [abstract No. PO-A12-0209], *9*(1), 169.

Onorato, I.M., Markowitz, L.E., Oxtoby, M.J. (1988). Childhood immunization, vaccine-preventable diseases and infection with human immunodeficiency virus. *Pediatric Infectious Disease, 7*(8), 588–595.

Palmes, E.D., Park, C.R. (1965). The regulation of body temperature during fever. *Archives of Environmental Health, 11*(6), 749–759.

Panel for the Prediction and Prevention of Ulcers in Adults (1992, May). *Pressure ulcers in adults: prediction and prevention. Clinical practice guideline, No. 3* (AHCPR Pub. No. 92-0047). Rockville, MD: Agency for Health Care Policy and Research, Public Health Service, U.S. Department of Health and Human Services.

Pape, J.W., Johnson, W.D. (1989). HIV-1 infection and AIDS in Haiti. In R.A. Kaslow & D.P. Francis (Eds.), *The epidemiology of AIDS* (pp. 194–221). New York: Oxford University Press.

Pardue, N.H. (1984). Energy expenditure and subjective fatigue of chronic obstructive pulmonary disease patients before and after a pulmonary rehabilitation. [doctoral dissertation]. Washington, D.C.: Catholic University.

Parkerson, G.R., Broadhead, W.E., Tse C.-K.J. (1990). The Duke health profile: A 17-item measure of health and dysfunction. *Medical Care, 28*(11), 1056–1069.

Parkerson, G.R., Gehlbach, S.H., Wagner, E.H., et al. (1981). The Duke-UNC health profile: an adult health status instrument for primary care. *Medical Care,* 19(8), 806–823.

Passannante, M.R., French, J., Louria, D.B. (1993). How much do health care providers know about AIDS? *American Journal of Preventive Medicine, 9*(1), 62–64.

Pearson, R.G., Byars, G.E., Jr. (1956). *The development and validation of a checklist for measuring subjective fatigue.* [report No. 56–115]. Randolph AFB, TX: USAF School of Aviation Medicine.

Pearson, M.L., Jereb, J.A., Frieden, T.R., et al. (1992). Nosocomial transmission of multidrug-resistant *Mycobacterium tuberculosis.* A risk to patients and health care workers. *Annals of Internal Medicine, 117*(30) 191–196.

Pfeiffer, E. (1975). A short portable mental status questionnaire for the assessment of organic brain deficit in elderly patients. *Journal of the American Geriatric Society, 23*(10), 433–441.

Piper, B. (1993). Fatigue. In V. Carrieri-Kohlman, A.M. Lindsey, & C.M. West (Eds.), *Pathophysiological phenomena in nursing human responses to illness* (2nd ed.) (pp. 279–302). Philadelphia: W.B. Saunders.

Piper, B.F., Rieger, P.T., Brophy, L., et al. (1989). Recent advances in the management of biotherapy-related side effects: Fatigue. *Oncology Nursing Forum, 16*(suppl 6), 27–34.

Plasse, T.F., Gorter, R.W., Krasnow, S.H., et al. (1991). Recent clinical experience with dronabinol. *Pharmacology, Biochemistry and Behavior, 40*(3), 695–700.

Plona, R.P., Schremp, P.S. (1992). Nursing care of patients with ocular manifestations of human immunodeficiency virus infection. *Nursing Clinics of North America, 27*(3), 793–805.

Porter, S., Sande, M.A. (1992). Toxoplasmosis of the central nervous system in the acquired immunodeficiency syndrome. *New England Journal of Medicine, 327*(23), 1643–1648.

Pratt, A., Lazar, R.M., Penman, D., et al. (1984). Psychological parameters of chemotherapy-induced nausea and vomiting: A review. *Cancer Nursing, 7*(12), 483–490.

Pulling, C.A. (1991). The relationship between critical care nurses' knowledge about sleep, and the initiation of sleep-promoting nursing interventions. *Axone, 13*(2), 57–62.

Rasin, J.H. (1990). Confusion. *Nursing Clinics of North America, 25*(4), 909–918.

Redd, W.H. (1984). Control of nausea and vomiting in chemotherapy patients: Four effective behavior methods. *Postgraduate Medicine, 75*(5), 105–107.

Redland, A.R., Stuifbergen, A.K. (1993). Strategies for maintenance of health-promoting behaviors. *Nursing Clinics of North America, 28*(2), 427–442.

Reimer, M. (1987). Sleep pattern disturbance: Nursing interventions perceived by patients and their nurses as facilitating nocturnal sleep in hospital. *Classification of Nursing diagnoses: Proceedings of the Seventh Conference of the North American Nursing Diagnosis Association* (pp.

372–376). St. Louis: North American Nursing Diagnosis Association.

Renfroe, K.L. (1988). Effect of progressive relaxation on dyspnea and state anxiety in patients with chronic obstructive pulmonary disease. *Heart & Lung 17*(4), 408–413.

Rhodes, V.A. (1990). Nausea, vomiting and retching. *Nursing Clinics of North America, 25*(4), 885–900.

Rhodes, V.A., Watson, P.M., Johnson, M.H. (1986). Association of chemotherapy-related nausea and vomiting with pretreatment and posttreatment anxiety. *Oncology Nursing Forum, 13*(4), 41–47.

Rhodes, V.A., Watson, P.M. (1987). Symptom distress: The concept, past and present. *Seminars in Oncology Nursing, 3*(4), 242–247.

Roberts, M.F. (1993). Diarrhea: A symptom. *Holistic Nurse Practice, 7*(2), 73–80.

Rodrigues, L., Moreno, C.G. (1991). HIV transmission to women in stable relationships [letter]. *New England Journal of Medicine, 325*(13), 966.

Rowbottom, J. (1993). STDs and the overseas traveller. *Australian Family Physician, 22*(2), 125–131.

Sattler, F.R., Ko, R., Antoniskis, D., et al. (1991). Acetaminophen does not impair clearance of zidovudine. *Annals of Internal Medicine, 114*(11), 937–940.

Schuchat, A., Broome, C.V., Hightower, A., et al. (1991). Use of surveillance for invasive pneumococcal disease to estimate the size of the immunosuppressed HIV-infected population. *Journal of the American Medical Association, 265*(24), 3275–3279.

Schwartzstein, R.M., Lahive, K., Pope, A., et al. (1987). Cold facial stimulation reduces breathlessness induced in normal subjects. *American Review of Respiratory Disease, 136*(1), 58–61.

Sharp, J.T., Drutz, W.S., Moisan, T., et al. (1980). Postural relief of dyspnea in severe chronic obstructive pulmonary disease. *American Review of Respiratory Disease, 122*(2), 201–211.

Shriner, K., Goetz, M.B. (1992). Severe hepatotoxicity in a patient receiving both acetaminophen and zidovudine. *American Journal of Medicine, 93*(1), 94–96.

Smeltzer, S.C., Whipple, B. (1991). Women and HIV infection. *Image, 23*(4), 249–256.

Smith, A.R. (1991). Examination of nursing diagnoses for adults hospitalized with acquired immunodeficiency syndrome, 1982–1990. *Nursing Diagnosis, 2*(3), 111 118.

Snyder, S., Strain, J.J., Fulop, G. (1990). Evaluation and treatment of mental disorders in patients with AIDS. *Comprehensive Therapy, 16*(8), 34–41.

Sprauer, M.A., Markowitz, L.E., Nicholson, J.K., et al. (1993). Response of human immunodeficiency virus–infected adults to measles-rubella vaccination. *Journal of Acquired Immune Deficiency Syndromes, 6*(9), 1013–1016.

Staff (1993). Clinical topic: NIAID issues preliminary recommendations on antiretrovirals. *AIDS Clinical Care, 6*(8), 64–65.

Steffe, E.M., King, J.H., Inciardi, J.F., et al. (1990). The effect of acetaminophen on zidovudine metabolism in HIV-infected patients. *Journal of Acquired Immune Deficiency Syndromes, 3*(7), 691–694.

Stein, D.S., Korvick, J.A., Vermund, S.H. (1992). $CD4^+$ lymphocyte cell enumeration for prediction of clinical course of human immunodeficiency virus disease: A review. *Journal of Infectious Diseases, 165*(2), 352–363.

Steinhart, R., Reingold, A.L., Taylor, F., et al. (1992). Invasive *Haemophilus influenzae* infections in men with

HIV infection. *Journal of the American Medical Association, 268*(23), 3350–3352.

Stephenson, B.J., Rowe, B.H., Haynes, R.B. (1993). Is this patient taking their treatment as prescribed? *Journal of the American Medical Association, 269*(21), 2779–2781.

Sultzer, D.L., Levin, H.S., Mahler, M.E., et al. (1992). Assessment of cognitive, psychiatric, and behavioral disturbances in patients with dementia: The neurobehavioral rating scale. *Journal of the American Geriatric Society, 40*(6), 549–555.

Swensen, J.R., Erman, M., Labelle, J., et al. (1989). Extrapyramidal reactions: Neuropsychiatric mimics in patients with AIDS. *General Hospital Psychiatry, 11*(4), 248–253.

Task Force on Nutrition Support in AIDS (1989). Guidelines for nutrition support in AIDS. *Nutrition, 5*(1), 39–45.

Temple, M.T., Leigh, B.C., Schafer, J. (1993). Unsafe sexual behavior and alcohol use at the event level: Results of a national survey. *Journal of Acquired Immunodeficiency Syndromes, 6*(4), 393–401.

Thayer, R.E. (1987). Energy, tiredness and tension effects of a sugar snack versus moderate exercise. *Journal of Personality and Social Psychology, 52*(1), 119–125.

Tichy, A.M., Talashek, M.L. (1992). Older women: Sexually transmitted diseases and acquired immunodeficiency syndrome. *Nursing Clinics of North America, 27*(4), 937–949.

Tostes, M.A. (1990). Psychiatric emergencies in HIV disease and AIDS. *International Conference on AIDS* [abstract No. S.B. 397], *6*(3), 185.

Ungvarski, P.J. (1989). AIDS dementia complex: Considerations for nursing. *Journal of the Association of Nurses in AIDS Care, 1*(1), 10–12.

U.S. Preventive Services Task Force (1989a). Screening for chlamydial infections. In M. Fisher (Ed.), *Guide to clinical prevention services: An assessment of the effectiveness of 169 interventions* (pp. 147–150). Baltimore: Williams & Wilkins.

U.S. Preventive Services Task Force (1989b). Screening for gonorrhea. In M. Fisher (Ed.), *Guide to clinical prevention services: An assessment of the effectiveness of 169 interventions* (pp. 135–138). Baltimore: Williams & Wilkins.

van Gorp, W.G., Mandelkern, M.A., Gee, M., et al. (1992). Cerebral metabolic dysfunction in AIDS: Findings in a sample with and without dementia. *Journal of Neuropsychiatry and Clinical Neuroscience, 4*(3), 280–287.

van Servellen, G.M., Lewis, C.E., Leake, B. (1988). Nurses' responses to the AIDS crisis: Implications for continuing education programs. *The Journal of Continuing Education in Nursing, 19*(1), 4–8.

Wallace, J.I., Paauw, D.S., Spack, D.H. (1993). HIV infection in older patients: When to suspect the unexpected. *Geriatrics, 48*(6), 69–70.

Weiler, P.G., Mungas, D., Pomerantz, S. (1988). AIDS: A cause of dementia in the elderly. *Journal of the American Geriatric Society, 36*(2), 139–141.

Weiner, A., Wallace, J.I., Steinberg, A., et al. (1992). Intravenous drug use, inconsistent condom use, and fellatio in relationship to crack smoking are risk behaviors for acquiring AIDS in streetwalkers. *International Conference on AIDS* [abstract No. PoC 4560], *8*(2), C338.

Weisman, A.D. (1979). A model for psychological phasing in cancer. *General Hospital Psychiatry, 1*(1), 187–195.

Weitzel, E.A. (1992). Medication management. In G.M. Bulechek & J.C. McCloskey (Eds.), *Nursing interventions: Essential nursing treatments* (2nd ed.) (pp. 213–220). Philadelphia: W.B. Saunders.

Wheat, L.J., Connolly-Stringfield, P., Williams, B., et al (1992). Diagnosis of histoplasmosis in patients with the acquired immunodeficiency syndrome by detection of *Histoplasma capsulatum* polysaccharide antigen in bronchoalveolar lavage fluid. *American Review of Respiratory Disease, 145*(6), 1421–1424.

Wiegard, M., Moller, A.A., Schreiber, W., et al. (1991). Alterations of nocturnal sleep in patients with HIV infection. *Acta Neurologica Scandinavia, 83*(2), 141–142.

Yarchoan, R., Mitsuya, H., Thomas, R.V. (1989). In vivo activity against HIV and favorable toxicity profile of 2′,3′-dideoxyinosine. *Science, 245*(4916), 412–415.

Yerly, S., Wyler, C.A., Kaiser, L., et al. (1993). Antigenic stimulation by immunization does not increase HIV viral load. *International Conference on AIDS* [abstract No. PO-B22-1929], *9*(1), 457.

Zeller, J.M., Swanson, B., Cohen, F.L. (1993) Suggestions for clinical nursing research: Symptom management in AIDS patients. *Journal of the Association of Nurses in AIDS Care, 4*(3), 13–17.

Nursing Care of the Child

Mary G. Boland and Lynn Czarniecki

As the decade of the 1990s continues, the HIV epidemic is spreading with particular rapidity among infants and children. In the United States the Centers for Disease Control and Prevention (CDC) has recorded more than 4,000 cases of pediatric AIDS, and experts predict as many as 1.2 million HIV-infected infants and children in the world by 1995 (Mann et al., 1992). Although in the mid-1980s the cases of pediatric AIDS in the United States were concentrated in urban centers in New York, New Jersey, and Florida, today the pediatric HIV epidemic reaches into rural areas and the country's heartland (Wasser et al., 1993).

Many of the earliest cases of pediatric AIDS in the United States resulted from the use of infected blood in transfusions and in blood products administered to people with hemophilia. Since the screening of blood and the treatment of blood products began in 1985, however, the vast majority of pediatric HIV infection in the United States has been a result of perinatal transmission. This is most often related to the intravenous use of illicit drugs by the infant's mother or heterosexual transmission of HIV to the mother from a sexual partner who has injected drugs. Several cases of HIV infection have also been traced to transmission through breast-feeding. In addition, a small proportion of the cases of HIV infection among children have resulted from sexual abuse.

Until recently the prognosis for infected children was generally poor; without medical intervention, most perinatally infected children had symptoms of HIV infection within a year, and most with HIV-related conditions survived for less than 3 years. In a far smaller proportion of children, disease manifestations did not become evident for as long as 9 years.

That symptoms of HIV infection generally develop so much more rapidly in infants than in adults may be attributed to the infant's immature immune systems. However, there are growing indications that early intervention and prophylaxis for infected infants and children can allow their more normal development, forestalling the onset and lessening the effects of life-threatening conditions (Pizzo, 1989). Zidovudine (ZDV; azidothymidine [AZT]) has been approved for use in children, and clinical trials of other drugs with immunomodulating and prophylactic effects have increasingly included children. Clinical care and research have become more closely intertwined as the medical community searches for a definitive treatment for HIV infection.

The identification of HIV-infected infants is complicated by the fact that infants receive maternal antibodies to HIV transplacentally and retain them for up to 15 months. Because tests currently available in clinical settings detect HIV antibodies rather than the virus itself, virtually all infants born to infected mothers initially have positive HIV test results. However, evidence suggests that HIV infection will develop in only about 15% to 25% of these infants. The remainder will have seroconversion, eventually showing no signs of HIV antibody or HIV infection. The stages of pregnancy or delivery at which infants can become infected are not yet known because the virus is capable of interacting with the fetal immune system at various stages of development (Delfraissy et al., 1992). There are several ways to obtain information about which infants are infected and would benefit from early intervention to slow the progression of HIV disease. Knowledge of the HIV status of all pregnant women would help health care professionals know which infants are at risk of acquiring HIV. For this reason many public health officials have recommended that testing be offered routinely, particularly to women whose histories indicate a risk of exposure to HIV. For other women of childbearing age, knowledge of their serostatus could have an important influence on their decision of whether to become pregnant. In general, HIV symptoms in infants and children are different from those in adults. Among the HIV-related symptoms often seen in children are recurrent fever, serious bacterial infections, failure to thrive, developmental delay, and loss of developmental milestones. Health care workers who know how HIV infection manifests itself among children can conduct regular medical checkups to look for those manifestations. Such checkups also allow health professionals to monitor growth and development, provide appropriate immunizations, and perform laboratory evaluations of immune function.

CARE DELIVERY

Results of recently published retrospective studies and analysis of pediatric AIDS case reports in the United States and Europe provide strong evidence that HIV disease can take two forms in infants. Between 10% and 15% of infants will have severe immunodeficiency with clinical symptoms before 1 year of age. Such infants are extremely sick and do not respond well to intervention; the result is high morbidity and mortality rates (Delfraissy et al., 1992). For the remainder of infected children, the risk of having symptoms and progression to AIDS is similar to that for adults. Studies from France show that 60% of children with HIV are more than 6 years of age and 49.5% are 9 years of age or older (Duliege et al., 1992). These older children have more chronic multiorgan complications such as chronic lung disease and gastrointestinal manifestations such as diarrhea, anorexia, and wasting (Grubman & Oleske, 1993). They are also more prone to acquiring opportunistic infections not seen as frequently in noninfected infants and younger children, such as toxoplasmosis, cryptococ-

cosis, and infection with *Myobacterium avium* complex.

The care of this population becomes increasingly complex as the disease progresses. Children can be receiving many potent medications and high-technology care in the home. Stresses on the child and family can be overwhelming. Constructing a home care plan often requires an enormous amount of time, ingenuity, and coordination. Services from multiple agencies may be needed and must be orchestrated in such a way as to provide optimal care without redundancy. Skilled case managers are essential. Patients and families need to be helped to decide which therapies they can manage at home. Allowing older school-aged children and adolescents to participate in the decision making and planning is crucial so that the child will adhere to the medical regimen. The child's lifestyle and desire for normalcy must be factored into the plan. Quality-of-life issues need to be constantly weighed against prolonged longevity.

HIV-infected children have a better quality of life when as much of their care as possible is administered at home or in community-based settings. As noted previously, however, a majority of infected children in the United States are from families in which one or both parents are infected. As both a cause and a consequence of injection drug use, these families are often disorganized and have poor access to health care (including prenatal care), substandard housing, inadequate nutrition, and little money. Moreover, one or both parents may already have HIV-related illnesses, rendering them psychologically unwilling or physically unable to care for their children. In such cases, foster care may be necessary and is often available from members of the extended family. In contrast, some infected mothers dedicate themselves to the care of their ailing children and neglect their own need for services (Abrams & Nicholas, 1990). All these factors complicate the delivery of care to HIV-infected children. The development of comprehensive networks of community-based, family-centered, multidisciplinary services can help deliver care to both infected children and their mothers.

ROLE OF NURSES

Nurses have played a central role in building and staffing networks for HIV-infected infants, children, and their families. The range of services needed by infected families is broad and may include home care, hospice care, counseling, nutrition, housing, transportation, financial and legal assistance, many forms of outpatient care and therapy, and inpatient care. Hospital and community-based nurses can contribute to the success of patient outcomes by functioning as case managers who quickly link children and their families with the services they need. Nurses can also provide the support and educational services that help make adult family members (whether natural, foster, or extended) part of the child's primary caregiving team, promoting the normal growth and development of both infected children and their siblings.

Progress in the development of antiretroviral and prophylactic drugs for infected children will increase their life spans substantially. Longer survival will create a demand for health and social services for extended periods and in an increasing variety of settings, including long-term care facilities, day care centers, and schools. To protect infected children against prejudice and discrimination, and to protect themselves against infection, workers in these settings will need accurate information about HIV transmission and must be comfortable in working with infected children. Nurses can play an important role in providing authoritative information and reshaping the attitudes of others who work with infected children. In addition, nurses will continue to be a key source of support in providing critical services and comfort to this newest population of chronically ill children.

PERINATAL TRANSMISSION OF HIV

HIV infection in infants and children is primarily due to perinatal transmission from the mother of the fetus or neonate. Although much remains to be learned regarding transmission and infection, there is increasing evidence that transmission occurs not only in utero and through breast milk but also in the peripartum period (Wara et al., 1993). The risk factors for perinatal transmission, its timing, and the early diagnosis of HIV-infected infants are being widely investigated throughout the world. Different modes of transmission have been described, but the relative risk of each is unknown, as is its potential influence on the course of infection in the infant.

Several factors probably contribute to the rate of transmission. These include stage of maternal infection, maternal immune response, infant's gestational age, mode of delivery, and breast-feeding. Although some studies indicate that women with symptoms and low CD4$^+$ cell counts (less than 200/mm^3) are more likely to transmit virus to their infants, other researchers have found no association. Our knowledge in this area is limited but can be expected to increase with time.

Preliminary results of clinical trials of the use of zidovudine in pregnant women, have revealed a transmission rate of 8.3% when both mothers and their newborn babies received zidovudine, in comparison with a transmission rate of 25.5% among those receiving a placebo (National Institute of Allergy and Infectious Disease, 1994). Because the long-term effects of therapy remains unknown, researchers will monitor the growth and development and any unusual illnesses of the infants.

HIV has been detected in breast milk and colostrum both by culture and polymerase chain reaction (PCR). Whereas proving direct transmission of a pathogen by breast milk is difficult, it is known that cytomegalovirus (CMV) and the retrovirus human T-cell leukemia virus (HTLV-1) are transmitted by breast-feeding. Several case reports have described transmission of HIV by breast milk from an infected mother to her infant; however, the risk of transmission has not been quantified (Goldfarb, 1993). Several studies have attempted to compare rates of transmission in breast-feeding and in formula-feeding infants of chronically HIV-infected women. The studies have been clinically based and hampered by the lack of an early diagnostic test for infection in the infant. The conflicting results indicate clearly that transmission does occur, but it is impossible to definitively implicate breast-feeding as the sole factor.

Breast milk is the ideal food for infants. The nutritional and psychologic benefits to both mother and infant are unquestionable. The early recommendation to use formula feeding in the United States because of the potential benefit of preventing infection remains valid. Women must be provided with adequate and accurate information when making the decision regarding feeding their infant.

DIAGNOSIS OF HIV IN INFANTS

The diagnosis of HIV in children older than 18 months is based on detection of anti-HIV antibodies in serum by means of enzyme-linked immunosorbent assay (ELISA) and the Western blot test. HIV-exposed infants can be identified at birth if pregnant women are tested. For this reason, public health officials increasingly recommend voluntary confidential testing of all pregnant women and those contemplating pregnancy, particularly if they have a history of risk activity. Such testing should always be accompanied by culturally sensitive counseling, both before tests are conducted and when the results are given. At a minimum, pretest counseling should clarify the purpose of the test, the relation of HIV infection to AIDS, the reason that the test is desirable, and the possible outcomes and consequences of the test. Techniques to prevent HIV transmission can also be discussed at counseling sessions. Before an infant is tested, the consent of a parent or guardian (or a child protective agency, when appropriate) should be obtained. Test results should be given only in person to the test subject (in the case of infants, to the caregiver), and the implications should be carefully explored.

Early intervention can be of substantial benefit to HIV-infected infants. Because of the toxicities associated with antiviral treatments, however, only truly infected infants, not all HIV-exposed infants, should be treated. Because infants retain maternal HIV antibodies for as long as 15 months after birth, the standard ELISA and Western blot test used to diagnose HIV infection in older children and adults yield indeterminate results for infants. Consequently, a variety of other diagnostic tools are used to detect HIV infection in infants. These are often employed in combination with nonspecific laboratory measures. Among the diagnostic tools currently in use or development are detection of HIV antigen, viral culture, and PCR.

Antigen Testing

One approach to diagnosing HIV infection in infants is to look for the presence of a specific HIV antigen (p24) in blood or tissue specimens. The level of this antigen, however, varies with the amount of virus in the subject, making it particularly difficult to detect in the early, asymptomatic phase of HIV infection. High levels of maternal antibody, passively acquired by the newborn, may interfere with this assay. When acid washing is used to disrupt antigen-antibody complexes in serum, the sensitivity can be increased. A positive antigen test result may indicate HIV infection, especially when there are other positive test results or clinical signs of immunocompromise.

Viral Culture

Another approach to testing infants is co-culturing of peripheral blood mononuclear cells with uninfected mononuclear cells that can support HIV growth. HIV presence in such samples can be determined through measurement of p24 antigen or reverse transcriptase activity. Viral cultures have yielded positive results in more than 90% of infected adults regardless of their stage of infection. However, because this method has failed to detect infection in almost 10% of infected adult subjects, cultures negative for HIV in infants do not definitively rule out HIV infection.

Polymerase Chain Reaction

PCR amplifies specific nucleic acid sequences, such as HIV proviral DNA, facilitating their detection. This technique's sen-

Table 6–1. Indicators of Pediatric HIV Infection

MEDICAL HISTORY	PHYSICAL EXAMINATION	LABORATORY RESULTS
Recurrent fever	Failure to maintain percentiles or gain weight	Anemia
Serious bacterial infections		Thrombocytopenia
Recurrent otitis media	Failure to grow in length or head circumference	Leukopenia
Recurrent sinusitis		Liver function elevations
Recurrent or chronic oral thrush	Loss of developmental milestones	Hypergammaglobulinemia
Recurrent or chronic diarrhea	Diaper dermatitis or condyloma	p24 antigen
Failure to thrive	*Candida* or seborrhea	Reactive HIV culture
Poor feeding	Otitis media, rhinitis, parotitis	Reactive HIV PCR
Developmental delay	Generalized lymphadenopathy (>0.5 cm), cervical, axillary, or inguinal	Low $CD4^+$ cell count for age
	Hepatomegaly	
	Splenomegaly	
	Clubbing	

sitivity in diagnosing HIV has been greater in adults than in infants, especially those in whom AIDS does not develop in the first year of life. Moreover, viral levels in the months immediately after birth are often below the current limits of detection of the PCR assay. As with HIV culture, sensitivity increases with age. With these techniques, approximately 50% of infants can be identified soon after birth and greater than 95% by 3 to 6 months of age.

Combinations of these investigational tests, along with nonspecific laboratory tests for immunoglobulin levels and T cells, are often used to detect HIV infection in infants. The nonspecific tests can be ordered by pediatricians and performed at many local laboratories; experimental tests and HIV culture may be available only at referral centers.

Seropositive infants who do not have a definite diagnosis of HIV infection should continue to be tested every 3 months, until 18 months of age, by ELISA and Western blot test, with final testing at 24 months of age (Pizzo & Wilfert, 1993).

Other Indicators

In addition to depressed CD4 levels, nonspecific clinical findings that suggest an HIV diagnosis include hepatomegaly, splenomegaly, or lymphadenopathy; hypergammaglobulinemia; nonspecific pulmonary infiltrates; and opportunistic infections in the absence of other causes of immunodeficiency (Husson et al., 1990). Table 6–1 lists conditions suggestive of HIV infection that can be detected through medical history, physical examination, and laboratory tests. Many of these conditions may have causes other than HIV infection, but their presence should raise the index of suspicion that a young child is infected, especially when other indicators of infection are present. The prolonged indeterminate HIV status of an infant is a source of stress for the family and caregivers, even when the infant eventually becomes seronegative. Nurses should thus be aware of the need for strong medical and social support systems to help families cope with the immediate and the long-term implications of an HIV diagnosis.

CLASSIFICATION OF PEDIATRIC HIV

The CDC has issued several classification schemes for pediatric HIV infection. The system currently in use, issued in 1987, was developed for epidemiologic purposes. It classifies pediatric infection according to the presentation of symptoms, and it does not necessarily correlate with stage of illness. Efforts are under way to develop schemes that are both clinically relevant and helpful in predicting the course of infection. The majority of clinical settings describe disease status in children as indeterminate, asymptomatic, symptomatic, and AIDS. These correspond roughly to the CDC scheme of P-0, P-1, P-2, and P-2 AIDS. This chapter will use this scheme to describe the management and treatment of illness and the corresponding nursing care needs.

CARE OF THE SYMPTOM-FREE CHILD WITH INDETERMINATE TEST RESULTS

Immunization

Infants whose mothers had positive test results prenatally and infants with HIV antibody by ELISA and Western blot test in the newborn period should be watched closely for the signs of immunocompromise listed in Table 6–1. If an infant is well and has no physical symptoms or laboratory findings associated with HIV infection, it is impossible to know whether infection is present. Viral cultures and other immunologic studies should be performed during the first few months of life, and, depending on the results, ELISA, immunoblot test, and CD4$^+$ cell counts, as well as experimental tests, should be performed every 3 to 6 months until the children are 2 years old. Because HIV-infected children are particularly susceptible to disease, all at-risk children should be immunized against childhood diseases according to the CDC schedule, with inactivated polio vaccine (Salk) substituted for oral vaccine (Sabin). Recommendations for the immunization of HIV-infected children are shown in Table 6–2.

HIV-infected children who have been exposed to such diseases as measles should be immunized within 72 hours of exposure, even if they have not yet reached the normal age for immunization. The increased mortality and morbidity rates for measles have led to the recommendation that children in high-prevalence measles areas in whom protective antibody fails to develop after two measles-mumps-rubella immunizations should receive regular intravenous infusion of immune globulin.

Parents should report varicella (chickenpox) exposure immediately, and HIV-in-

Table 6–2. Recommendations for Routine Immunization of HIV-Infected Children in the United States

VACCINE	KNOWN ASYMPTOMATIC HIV INFECTION	SYMPTOMATIC HIV INFECTION/AIDS
DTP	Yes	Yes
OPV	No	No
IPV	Yes	Yes
MMR	Yes	Yes
Hib	Yes	Yes
Hepatitis B	Yes	Yes
Pneumococcal	Yes	Yes
Influenza	Should be considered	Yes

DTP, Diphtheria and tetanus toxoids and pertussis vaccine; *OPV*, oral poliovirus vaccine; *IPV*, inactivated poliovirus vaccine; *MMR*, live-virus measles-mumps-rubella vaccine; *Hib*, *H. influenzae* type b vaccine.
From Recommendations of the Advisory Committee on Immunization Practices (ACIP). Use of vaccines and immune globulins for persons with altered immunocompetence. *Morbidity and Mortality Weekly Reports, 42* RR-4, April 9, 1993.

fected children should receive varicella-zoster immune golublin (VZIG) within 96 hours of exposure to prevent or modify infection. Nurses must be aware that VZIG prolongs the incubation period to 10 to 28 days. Normally, varicella virus is controlled by cell-mediated immune mechanisms and is a self-limited illness. In children with immune system impairment however, it can cause prolonged and disseminated morbidity, with complications including neurologic encephalitis and pneumonia. Its symptoms include pruritic vesicular rash on the face, scalp, and trunk; these may be preceded by systemic symptoms including fever, chills, myalgia, and arthralgia. Treatment is intravenous administration of acyclovir, 10 mg/kg administered every 8 hours for 5 to 7 days or until lesions dry. This decreases pain and hastens healing. Immunocompromised children who have had varicella are at risk for its reactivation as herpes zoster (shingles), which can be severe and disseminated. Zoster in children is treated with intravenous infusion of acyclovir, 10 mg/kg every 8 hours for 5 to 7 days or until lesions dry. Side effects of acyclovir include renal toxic effects and an increase in the serum creatinine level.

Symptom-free, immunocompetent children would be expected to produce protective antibody in response to immunization. Some care providers document such antibody by obtaining postvaccination titers. Children with symptomatic infection and/or documented humoral or antibody deficiencies may have a poor immunologic response, resulting in lack of protective antibody. Such children, when exposed to a vaccine-preventable disease such as measles, should be considered susceptible regardless of the history of vaccination.

Home Care

Illnesses contracted by children with indeterminate HIV status and those with asymptomatic HIV infection rarely require hospitalization; most of their care can be given on an outpatient basis. The major goal of care for children with asymptomatic HIV infection is to prevent infections and opportunistic illnesses, through both supportive care and prophylaxis. Educating parents or other caregivers about supportive care is basic and important. Topics covered should include hand washing; bathing children regularly (daily or every other day); keeping the children's skin clean and dry, especially in the diaper area; moisturizing the skin in other areas to prevent cracking and itching and thus preventing fungal infections and impetigo; changing diapers; and cleaning bottles. Nurses can be instrumental in providing this education and can also sensitize caregivers to the signs and symptoms of infection that should lead them to seek medical attention.

Prophylaxis

Prophylaxis is intended to prevent primary or recurrent infection in children known to be infected with HIV. Although studies of prophylaxis against *Pneumocystis carinii* pneumonia (PCP) have not yet been conducted on children, results in adults have shown aerosolized pentamidine and trimethoprim-sulfamethoxazole (TMP-SMX; Bactrim, Septra) to be effective in both preventing the onset of PCP and reducing morbidity and mortality rates. TMP-SMX can also prevent recurrent otitis media and other infections in children.

Because PCP may be the initial illness associated with AIDS, HIV-exposed and HIV-infected infants must be identified as early as possible so that primary prophylaxis can begin. Prophylaxis is recommended for infants under 1 year of age born to infected mothers with CD4$^+$ T-lymphocyte counts less than 1500 cells/mm^3, for seropositive children between 1 and 2 years of age with CD4$^+$ cell counts less than 750 cells/mm^3, and for infected children more than 2 years of age with CD4$^+$ cell counts less than 500 cells/mm^3 (Connor et al., 1991). Some observers recommend prophylaxis for all seropositive infants more than 1 month of age, regardless of their ultimate serostatus (Leibovitz et al., 1990). Dapsone is recommended as the oral drug alternative to TMP-SMX at any age. The recommended dose is 1 mg/kg given orally once daily (not to exceed 100 mg per dose) to minimize toxic effects. As with TMP-SMX, monthly complete blood cell counts, with differential cell and platelet counts, should be done to monitor the patient for hematologic toxic effects. TMP-SMX, dapsone, and other sulfa drugs may be more likely to cause hematologic anemia in patients with glucose-6 phosphate dehydrogenase deficiency. Other prophylactic and antiviral therapies for use in children are discussed later in the chapter.

CARE AND DISEASE PREVENTION IN CHILDREN WITH SYMPTOMS

Immune Function, Nutrition, and Infection

A child's immune function interacts with his or her nutrition and infection status: if one is impaired, the others tend to worsen as well. For example, malnutrition impairs immune function (even in a healthy child), and an immunodeficiency (an inability to produce functioning antibody) increases the risk of infection. Infections in immunocompromised children have more rapid onset and greater severity than in normal children; they also typically involve more than one infectious agent.

Age and Symptoms

Symptoms and their presentation vary by age among HIV-infected children. Infants frequently have recurrent infections of bacterial, fungal, or protozoal origin. In early childhood most infections are bacterial and not life threatening; they should generally be handled in the same way as for young children who are not immunocompromised.

Hospitalization

When infected children are hospitalized, the risk of acquiring nosocomially transmitted infections should be recognized. Following universal precautions in the handling of blood and body fluids from these patients is critical. Hand washing by caregivers between patients is the single most effective way of preventing the spread of disease. An HIV-infected child admitted to the hospital with a diagnosis of possible infection should be given a private room for 24 to 48 hours or until a definitive cause or agent has been ruled out. HIV-infected children who are hospitalized with a noninfectious process or who are completing treatment for an infectious disease do not need a private room. However, most institutions still place such children by themselves or in a room with other HIV-infected children.

Acute Treatment

For acute treatment of children thought to have infectious conditions, diagnosis is often the most challenging problem. Many times such children run a fever but no infectious agent can be identified. It is appropriate to treat these children with empiric therapy and broad-spectrum antibiotics for 3 to 5 days pending the results of bacterial cultures. Pending diagnosis, treatment should cover organisms associated with B-cell defects, such as *Staphylococcus aureus*, *Streptococcus pneumoneia*, and *Haemophilus influenzae*. However, infectious viral and fungal organisms can rarely be eradicated in an immunocompromised child; once treatment is halted, the organism reappears. If an agent is identified for which there is no definitive treatment, supportive or symptomatic treatment can be given.

Continuing Care

Once an agent of opportunistic infection has been identified, lifelong treatment will be required. For some opportunistic infections, no treatment is currently available; for others, existing experimental treatments often have side effects. Decisions about what course to follow should be discussed between the physician and the parents or other caregivers. Factors to be taken into account include the child's overall medical condition, the accessibility of treatment, the ability of parents or caregivers to administer necessary treatment, the stage of the child's illness, the family's ability to obtain needed services, the financial impact of treatment decisions on the family, and the impact of these decisions on the quality of the child's life. The nurse can play an important role in working with the family to provide information and validate the impact of treatment. Because nurses often understand better than physicians how treatment will affect the lives of the child and the family, they should be actively involved in decision making.

As a child's degree of immunocompromise increases, more frequent hospitalizations will be required. In children with less severe symptoms, most conditions can be treated on an outpatient basis. However, once AIDS has developed, it is not unusual for a child to be hospitalized as many as three times in a year for the treatment of acute illnesses. Each hospitalization forces families to confront anew the uncertain outcome of the illness.

INFECTIOUS COMPLICATIONS

Bacterial Infections

Bacterial and fungal skin infections have been noted at many sites in HIV-infected children. The most recent (1987) CDC definition of AIDS-related conditions among children less than 13 years of age includes at least two multiple or recurrent bacterial infections within 2 years, excluding skin and otitis media. Because of secondary impaired humoral response, HIV-infected children are susceptible to both gram-positive and gram-negative bacterial infections, and these can become acute if treatment is absent or incomplete. Bacterial infections affect a variety of organ systems, including the skin, respiratory system, gastrointestinal tract, and blood.

Common skin infections include cellulitis and abscess caused by staphylococcus and streptococcus; the latter is the bacterial pathogen most frequently identified in children with HIV disease and is often implicated in pneumonia and bacteremia (Hauger & Powell, 1990). Skin infections may follow bites, eczema, or the insertion of catheters. Sinopulmonary complications include chronic otitis media, sinusitis, and pneumonia; chronic recurrent pneumonia predisposes some children to chronic lung diseases such as bronchiectasis. In the gastrointestinal tract, diarrhea is the most common symptom, and infectious agents are usually opportunistic, including CMV, *Salmonella, Cryptosporidium, Mycobacterium avium-intracellulare* and *Giardia.* In the blood, any bacterial agent (e.g., *H. influenzae*) can cause sepsis. Blood infections often occur secondarily in children hospitalized for acute infections. Like other bacterial infections, they are appropriately treated with antibiotics administered for the maximum "normal" time with follow-up to ensure that the infection has been resolved. When care is given at home, nurses can teach parents or other caregivers to administer required medication.

Treatment with intravenous immune globulin (IVIG) has been shown to reduce bacterial infections and hospitalizations in some HIV-infected children (National Institute of Child Health and Human Development, 1991). The drug did not appear to benefit children receiving TMP-SMX for PCP prophylaxis or those with severe immunocompromise and less than 200 $CD4^+$ cells/mm^3. IVIG is used in the treatment of those HIV-infected infants and children with hypogammaglobulinemia, poor functional antibody, or recurrent bacterial infections including chronic sinusitis and bronchiectasis. Infusions of 400 mg/kg every 21 to 28 days can be given in the ambulatory care or home settings.

Tuberculosis

In 1987, rates of tuberculosis (TB) began to increase and by 1991 more than 26,000 cases had been reported in the United States. These cases, primarily in young adults, represent an increasing risk of exposure to children. Between 1985 and 1991, cases of TB in children aged 14 years or younger increased by 24%. Presently there are few reported studies regarding TB in HIV-infected children, although clinicians around the country are reporting increasing cases of TB in HIV-infected children.

Active TB is diagnosed in more than 1,000 children annually in the United States. TB infection without disease is the preclinical stage of infection with *Mycobacterium tuberculosis.* The tuberculin skin test reaction is positive, but the chest radiograph is normal and the child is free of signs or symptoms. TB occurs when clinical manifestations or pulmonary or extrapulmonary TB become apparent, either by chest radiograph or by clinical signs and symptoms. In adults, there is a clear time distinction of weeks or years between asymptomatic infection and clinical disease. However, in young children, the two stages are less distinct (Starke et al., 1992). Younger children (less than 4 years of age), children whose exposure occurs within a household, and those with immunocompromise are considered at greatest risk for progression to the disease. Some experience suggests that HIV-infected children who acquire TB may also have worsened pulmonary disease, more rapid progression, and possibly increased rates of extrapulmonary disease (Gutman, 1993).

The clinical presentation of TB in HIV-infected children is not well described, and the diagnosis may be hampered by cutaneous anergy and difficulty in obtaining adequate sputum samples for culture. The two factors that determine the chance that TB will develop are (1) environmental, that is, the potential for exposure to an infectious person, and (2) host related, that is, the ability of the immune system to control the infection. Children with HIV infection are placed at risk through exposure in households with HIV-infected adults coinfected with TB and by the potential inability of the children's immune system to control the infection. It is recommended that HIV-infected children who are household contacts of adults with diagnosed

Table 6–3. Positive Mantoux Tuberculin Reactions (Stratification by Immunologic Function, Exposure Characteristics, and Reaction Size)*

PATIENT IMMUNOLOGIC STATUS	REACTION SIZE		
	5 MM	**>10 MM**	**>15 MM**
Normal cell-mediated immune function	Contacts of cases Abnormal chest radiograph	Children aged <4 years Children or contacts of persons considered at high risk for TB	No risk factors identified
	2–5 MM	**>5 MM**	
Comprised cell-mediated immune function	Contacts or suspected contacts of cases Abnormal chest radiograph	All others, including children with no known risk factors	

From Gutman, L. (1993). Recent developments in the intersection of the epidemics of tuberculosis and HIV in children. *Pediatric HIV Forum, 1*(1):3.

*Failure of a Mantoux test to produce a reaction which meets these definitions of "positive" is not necessarily evidence that the child is free of TB exposure, infection, or disease.

TB receive preventive therapy regardless of the results of intradermal skin testing or radiography of the chest.

Children whose intradermal tuberculin skin test result is "positive" are presumed to be infected. In the child with documented immunocompromise, a "negative" skin test result does not rule out infection. Presently, clinicians consider test results of an erythematous area 2 to 10 mm in diameter to be positive in certain children (Table 6–3).

Standardized regimens for treatment of TB have been complicated by the emergence of strains resistant to therapy. The role of such strains in the infection of children is not yet known. Choice of drug for treatment can be guided by the sensitivity patterns of the infecting strain. When the treatment is "preventive" or the strain is not known, treatment should include at least three drugs initially and be continued for at least 9 months (Committee on Infectious Diseases, Academy of Pediatrics, 1992).

Treatment adherence is critical to prevention of complications in the HIV-infected child receiving treatment for TB. Noncompliance can be anticipated because of the long-term nature of treatment. The nurse should provide anticipatory guidance regarding administration of medications and development of a dosing schedule and routine. It is critical to assess the ability of family members to obtain medication, their understanding of what is expected of them, and their recognition that therapy must be completed. Missed appointments must receive follow-up. Directly observed therapy, if available within the community, should be considered if the child's parent is ill or the family situation unstable.

OPPORTUNISTIC INFECTIONS

Infectious agents that present no threat to people with healthy immune systems can cause serious damage in immunocompromised individuals. Some of the common sources of opportunistic infection in infants and children with HIV disease and typical therapeutic responses are found in Table 6–4. Primary and secondary prophylaxis may be offered to children in particular situations. A more detailed discussion of several of these infections follows.

Pneumocystis carinii Pneumonia

The protozoan that causes PCP is commonly found in air, water, and soil (although some geographic variation exists) and is carried by many domestic animals and people. Most children are exposed to the protozoan by the age of 4 years and form specific anti-

Table 6–4. Opportunistic Infections in Infants and Children with HIV Disease

OPPORTUNISTIC INFECTION	THERAPY	COMMENTS
Pneumocystis carinii pneumonia	Trimethoprim-sulfamethoxazole Pentamidine Dapsone	Prophylaxis indicated in children with immunocompromise Postinfection prophylaxis indicated Diagnosis established by bronchoalveolar lavage or open lung biopsy
Candida esophagitis (thrush)	Nystatin Clotrimazole troches Ketoconazole Fluconazole Amphotericin B	Recalcitrant oral thrush may require treatment for esophagitis Appropriate prophylaxis regimen not established, but prolonged use of nystatin relatively safe
CMV	Ganciclovir Foscarnet*	No established treatment HIV-infected infants who have no CMV antibodies should receive CMV-negative blood
MAI	No therapy effective Amikacin sulfate* Clarithromycin* Ethambutol* Rifabutin*	*Mycobacterium tuberculosis hominis* may become more prevalent in pediatric HIV infection, with unusual manifestations
Cryptococcus meningitis (and other systemic infections)	Amphotericin B 5-Fluorocytosine Fluconozole	After initial daily treatment for 4–6 weeks, lifelong daily treatment with fluconazole; CSF and serum cryptococcal antigen should be serially measured
CNS toxoplasmosis	Sulfadiazine and pyrimethamine Folic acid Clindamycin*	Biopsy of CNS lesion may be needed to differentiate from CNS lymphoma Lifelong treatment necessary
Cryptosporidiosis	No therapy effective Azithromycin* Bovine colostrum*	MAI of GI tract and cryptosporidiosis potentiate malnutrition, intermittent ileus

CMV, Cytomegalovirus; *MAI, Mycobacterium avium-intracellulare; CSF,* cerebrospinal fluid; *CNS,* central nervous system; *GI,* gastrointestinal.
Adapted from Boland, M. (1991). The child with HIV infection. In J. Durham & F. Cohen (Eds.), *The person with AIDS: Nursing perspectives* (2nd ed.) (pp. 324–326). New York: Springer.
*Denotes investigational use.

bodies to it. However, illness from PCP has occurred in more than 25% of the pediatric AIDS cases reported to the CDC. Before the use of prophylaxis, both adults and children had a high mortality rate from PCP, with about half of the deaths among children occurring during the first episode and a large proportion of the rest occurring during the second. With prophylaxis the prognosis has improved substantially, although PCP remains the most serious opportunistic infection in children and is often observed in conjunc-

tion with a failure to thrive, encephalopathy, and renal disease. Its onset is quicker and its progression more fulminant than in adults (Hauger & Powell, 1990). Correlates of death from PCP in children include young age, depleted CD4+ cell counts, and associated clinical manifestations, including failure to thrive, oral or esophageal candidiasis, and encephalopathy. Survival times for children with PCP are shorter than those for adults.

The primary site of PCP infection is the lungs, although disseminated infection is also found in the spleen, lymphatic system, and blood. Clinical symptoms of disease include acute tachypnea, dyspnea, fever, dry cough, hypoxemia, and bilateral pulmonary infiltrates. Definitive diagnosis can be made through lung biopsy or bronchofibroscopy performed with brochoalveolar lavage. The most prominent laboratory finding is a large alveolar-arterial oxygen gradient, denoting hypoxemia. The roentgenographic pattern is similar to that seen in diffuse interstitial lung disease; PCP should be suspected when hypoxemia is out of proportion. Isomorphic elevation of lactate dehydrogenase levels is sensitive to PCP but not specific. However, given the high mortality rates associated with untreated PCP, a presumptive diagnosis based on clinical symptoms is preferable to waiting for a definitive diagnosis.

Treatment is generally with TMP-SMX. The recommended dosages are intravenous infusions of TMP, 20 mg/kg, and SMX, 100 mg/kg given daily, divided into four doses, for 21 days (Hauger & Powell, 1990). TMP-SMX appears to be better tolerated in children than in adults. Adverse reactions to TMP-SMX include rash, fever, leukopenia, acute hypoglycemia, and a drop in blood pressure. For children whose condition fails to improve within a few days or who cannot tolerate TMP-SMX, an alternative treatment is intravenous infusion of pentamidine, 4 mg/kg, given for 21 days, although this regimen has been associated with a high incidence of side effects, including renal insufficiency. Coadministration of corticosteroids to adults with PCP has helped to improve outcomes, but no information about their effectiveness in children is available. Aerosolized pentamidine, used for prophylaxis, is an ineffective treatment for acute PCP, and in children its use has still not been standardized. Side effects of aerosol treatment include bronchospasm and hypoglycemia as well as a strong metallic taste. These can be offset by preceding treatment with a bronchodilator, ventilating the room well, and offering hard candy or mints.

PCP is generally recurrent, necessitating prophylactic use of TMP-SMX, pentamidine, or dapsone. Recommended drugs, used in the past in children with leukemia, are TMP, 75 mg/m², and SMX, 375 mg/m², respectively, administered orally every 12 hours on 3 consecutive days a week (Connor et al., 1991).

Candidiasis

Candidiasis is a fungal (yeast) infection often encountered in children. Before the HIV epidemic, *Candida* infection was seen in infants less than 2 months of age, particularly in the mouth and diaper areas. In all children this organism also inhabits the oropharynx, vagina, large intestine, and skin but rarely causes disease unless the child is immunocompromised. *Candida* infection is most commonly localized but can be disseminated. Its symptoms vary with the site. Along with herpes simplex virus and CMV, it is among the causes of dysphagia (difficulty in swallowing) and odynophagia (pain in swallowing), both of which adversely affect infant feeding behaviors.

Treatment of *Candida* infection is site specific. When it occurs on the skin, mucous membranes, or diaper area, it calls for an antifungal cream. Oral thrush is generally treated with an antifungal agent such as nystatin or clotrimazole (Mycelex) troches; parents need to be instructed about cleaning bottles. If no improvement occurs, short courses of ketoconazole can be given. *Candida* infection in the esophagus or trachea (diagnosed through a barium-swallow x-ray examination) is treated with systemic doses of amphotericin B. As in adults, amphotericin B can produce severe reactions. Thus the child must be monitored closely and may require premedication with diphenhydramine (Benadryl) or corticosteroid or both. Complaints such as fever and abdominal pain must be reported promptly to a physician. Disseminated *Candida* infection has recently been treated with fluconazole administered daily. Because fungal infection in children tends to be a recurrent problem, prophylactic treatment may be indicated. For oral thrush, nystatin can be administered prophylactically once or twice daily; in the dipaer area, antifungal cream should be used.

Nontuberculous Mycobacterial Disease

Nontuberculous mycobacterial disease occurs in 6% to 11% of children with AIDS and is usually extra pulmonary, most often affecting the gastrointestinal tract. Infection with *M. avium-intracellulare* (MAI) is responsible for more than 85% of cases (Horsburgh et al., 1993). Because MAI is resistant to many antimicrobial agents, the outcome is generally poor. In addition to the gastrointestinal tract, sites include the blood, bone marrow, liver, spleen, adrenal glands, lungs, brain, and skin. The clinical presentation is often nonspecific, involving recurrent fever, chills, abdominal pain, failure to gain or maintain weight, hepatosplenomegaly, anemia, and diarrhea. Definitive diagnosis can be made by cultures of blood, sputum, bone marrow, or stool or through tissue biopsy. No curative therapy is available, and treatment decisions should be based on the child's condition; comfort and nutrition are the main issues to consider (Hoyt et al., 1992). Although MAI is not communicable, enteric precautions should be followed.

Cryptosporidiosis

Cryptosporidium is an enteric protozoan that causes acute, self-limited disease in immunocompetent children but severe and persistent enteritis in those with HIV/AIDS. Because it is communicable, only toilet-trained children with symptoms should be permitted in group settings. Symptoms of cryptosporidiosis include fever, frequent and voluminous watery diarrhea, cramps and abdominal pain, weight loss and dehydration, and lactose intolerance. This condition is not life threatening, but early manifestations should be treated symptomatically. Total parenteral hyperalimentation is beneficial and may be decreased or terminated once the child is able to eat. Definitive diagnosis can be made from stool samples. No definitive treatment is available.

Herpes

Children with HIV/AIDS can have recurrent herpes zoster and herpes simplex. Varicella in an immunocompromised host can be life threatening if not treated early. Recurrent herpes infections can also cause increased pain and discomfort. Both herpes zoster and herpes simplex type 1 are treated with acyclovir, 10/mg/kg per dose every 8 hours intravenously. Acyclovir is also given daily for prophylaxis in children with recurrent herpes infections.

MALIGNANCIES

Kaposi's Sarcoma

Malignancies occur less frequently in HIV-infected children than in infected adults, although this discrepancy may not necessarily continue as survival times for children with HIV increase. Kaposi's sarcoma (KS), which is far more common in homosexual men than in other adults with HIV, is relatively rare in children, with few cases among the first 500 children with AIDS reported to the CDC (McClain & Rosenblatt, 1990). KS has occurred mostly among children with Haitian-born parents from the Miami area (Falloon et al., 1989). A variety of chemotherapeutic agents in combination—vincristine with bleomycin or methotrexate—have yielded response rates from 40% to 80%, as in adults with KS. However, a biologic response modifier, interferon alfa, has been effective in 20% to 50% of adults treated early and does not have the immunosuppressive effects of chemotherapy. For this reason it may prove more appropriate than chemotherapy for children with KS. Eight children with HIV have been identified with leiomyosarcoma. This tumor, rarely seen in healthy children, has become the most common disseminated solid tumor in HIV-infected children.

Lymphomas

Some evidence of B- and T-cell lymphomas in children has been found; these were present in 7 of 300 HIV-infected children in one study and 3% to 4% in a larger sample (Wiznia & Nicholas, 1990; McClain & Rosenblatt, 1990). HIV-associated lymphomas are uncommon in childhood, however, and B-cell lymphomas in HIV-infected children may be hard to recognize as HIV related because they are similar to those found in about 25% of all children with lymphomas (Falloon et al., 1989; McClain & Rosenblatt, 1990). Symptoms of lymphoma in children include fever, weight loss, diffuse adenopathy, jaundice, hepatomegaly, abdominal distention, and pain. Early institution of intravenous chemotherapy with combinations of cyclophosphamide, vincristine, doxorubicin, methotrexate, cytarabine, and prednisone may extend life for these children (McClain & Rosenblatt, 1990). However, the course of lymphomas in some children is so rapid and severe that chemotherapy and radiation therapy may be precluded.

ORGAN SYSTEM INVOLVEMENT IN HIV INFECTION

Oral Manifestations

HIV infection in children causes many oral and dental problems. There is a high rate of dental caries, especially in the primary teeth (Howell et al., 1992). Primary dental care with frequent dental visits and fluoride therapy are important to prevent serious complications.

Oral candidiasis is also very common. Even when treatment has been completed and the oropharynx appears clear, *Candida* colonies can be found in the vestibules. Nystatin, which is commonly used to treat *Candida* infection, has a high sucrose content that may contribute to dental caries. Clotrimazole (Mycelex) troches or antifungal creams such as miconazole (Monistat) can be used orally.

Herpes lesions are common and frequently painful and can lead to decreased intake of food and fluid, weight loss, and dehydration. The current treatment is acyclovir. Topical anesthetics such as dyclonine (mixed with diphenhydramine [Benadryl] suspension) or Oratec gel may be helpful.

Children with HIV also experience HIV-associated periodontal disease and HIV-associated gingivitis. These problems have been reported in adults, but less is known about them in children. The initial presentation of gingivitis is gingival inflammation with minimal amounts of plaque; conventional treatment—plaque removal—is not effective. In one study 37% of 67 children were found to have HIV gingivitis. Periodontitis, which progresses rapidly, manifests as intense erythema, moderate to extensive generalized bone loss, pain, and gingival bleeding. The incidence of periodontitis is about 4% to 5%. Treatment includes extraction of teeth or, if failing health precludes extraction, administration of amoxicillin or of amoxicillin plus clavulanate (Augmentin). In severe cases, clindamycin is recommended.

The numerous oral problems associated with HIV in children requires that nurses caring for HIV-infected children provide careful oral assessment and care. In the ambulatory setting the nurse can assess the oral cavity at each visit, teach good oral hygiene to the child and family, prescribe fluoride if the water is not fluoridated, and refer the child to dental services. The sick hospitalized child must also receive scrupulous oral assessment and care. Special attention needs to be paid to children who are on a "nothing by mouth" regimen or are receiving broad-spectrum antibiotics. The nurse should suspect oral problems if a patient's appetite decreases suddenly. The best intervention for these oral problems is prevention coupled with early identification and treatment.

Gastrointestinal Tract Disorders

Diarrhea in HIV-infected children has both common and uncommon causes. When it is preceded by vomiting but the stool does not contain blood or mucus, viral (e.g., rotavirus) gastroenteritis should be the presumptive diagnosis. Diarrhea along with fever and abdominal pain may result from CMV infection, which can be diagnosed by endoscopic biopsy. Although no standard therapy for CMV infection has been established, ganciclovir is believed to be effective in the treatment of adult enterocolitis. *Escherichia coli,* another cause of enterocolitis, responds to antibiotic therapy. *Yersinia* enterocolitis is also seen and responds to TMP-SMX and other broad-spectrum antibiotics. *Salmonella, Shigella,* and *Campylobacter* can also cause acute bacterial gastroenteritis (Hauger & Powell, 1990).

In addition to the loss of nutrients from diarrhea, children with HIV also show evidence of malabsorption even in the absence of diarrhea (Miller et al., 1991). Abnormal d-xylose results are frequently associated with enteric infections (Miller et al., 1991). Patients may also have decreased intake of nutrients because of esophagitis, difficulty in chewing and swallowing as a result of neurologic problems, nausea, oral lesions, dental caries, anorexia caused by certain medications, abdominal pain, and depression (Winter & Chang, 1993). Frequent infections, fevers, and alterations in metabolic function can also increase nutrient requirements.

The assessment and management of nutritional problems need to be multidimensional. Nutrition counseling and intervention should be part of the routine care of children with HIV. Close monitoring of weight, height, and lean body mass as measured by triceps skin-fold thickness and arm circumference can help detect changes in nutritional status early. A complete diet history should be obtained at intervals to assess the quantity and nutritional value of food being eaten. Counseling regarding dietary changes must take into account the child's preferences, the family culture, and the family's financial ability to provide necessary supplements. For children with decreased intake, a multivitamin and mineral supplement that provides the U.S. recommended daily amount of each nutrient is advisable. Commercially prepared supplements can be offered but need to be tailored to the child's preferences, which often change with time. Families can be taught how to increase the nutritional value of their regularly prepared foods.

When weight can no longer be maintained or gained by oral feedings, it may be necessary to attempt feeding through either a nasogastric tube or a gastrostomy tube. These methods allow for the use of high-calorie, high-protein, nutritionally complete formulas to be given either by bolus feedings or by continuous drip for a number of hours, usually during the night. The correct formula and total volume need to be determined to avoid increased diarrhea, abdominal distention, and vomiting. Parents can be taught how to administer these feedings at home, and older children can be taught how to pass their own tubes and set up the equipment.

When the enteral route fails completely for whatever reason, parenteral nutrition can be an option. This intervention requires the surgical insertion of a central catheter (preferably a double-lumen tube whenever possible) and a great deal of caregiver education. The risks of infection and bleeding need to be weighed against the potential nutritional benefits. The patient's overall health status and prognosis need to be examined carefully. An assessment of the home and of the family's ability and willingness to undertake this responsibility must be conducted. If the decision is made to begin total parenteral nutrition (TPN), then the patient and family must be thoroughly educated about all aspects of its administration and the care of the central line. When the primary caregiver is the mother who is also infected or an elderly grandparent, it is good to educate a backup person as well. Referrals to home care agencies for assistance and support in the home must be in place before discharge whenever possible. The vendor supplying the TPN and equipment must be available for emergencies 24 hours a day and preferably will have nursing and pharmacy services with whom you can form a working relationship. TPN has increased weight and improved the quality of life for children with HIV for a while and is therefore worth considering for a patient who is nutritionally failing as evidenced by loss of weight.

Pulmonary Disease

Pulmonary examinations of HIV-infected children should include roentgenography of the chest, quantification of blood oxygenation (arterial blood gases or transcutaneous pulse oximetry), and in selected cases a computed tomography scan of the chest. Lymphoid interstitial pneumonitis (LIP) is the most frequently occurring pulmonary disease among HIV-infected children. Other pulmonary complications include bacterial pneumonia, lower respiratory tract viral infection, bronchiectasis, and reactive airway disease.

LIP is sometimes associated with hyperplasia of bronchus-associated lymphoid tissue (pulmonary lymphoid hyperplasia [PLH]). A slowly progressive disease with presentation in the second or third year of life, LIP-PLH causes chronic, nonproductive cough and exertional dyspnea, leading to dyspnea and finally hypoxemia at rest (Pitt, 1991). Chronic hypoxemia causes digital clubbing, mild lactate dehydrogenase elevation, and a widened alveolar-arterial oxygen gradient. A roentgenogram of the chest may be helpful in diagnosis, although definitive diagnosis is based on lung biopsy. Signs of infection include worsening cough, increased respiratory rate, dyspnea, color changes, distress in feeding, and fatigue. LIP is often accompanied by wheezing, marked lymphadenopathy and hepatosplenomegaly, sharply elevated serum gamma globulin levels, and occasional parotitis. The progression of LIP is insidious; fever is usually absent, and short-term effects are far less serious than those of PCP. LIP-PLH responds to corticosteroid therapy, but this therapy should be withheld until there is evidence of significant hypoxemia. Then treatment should begin with prednisone, 2 mg/kg per day for 2 to 4 weeks, tapered to 0.5 to 0.75 mg/kg on alternate days.

The long-term management of LIP, when there is bronchiectasis or multiple episodes of bacterial pneumonia, includes admission of the patient to the hospital every 3 months to receive intravenous infusion of antibiotics, frequent bronchodilator treatments, and frequent chest physiotherapy for 10 to 14 days. This regimen is similar to that offered to patients with cystic fibrosis.

In HIV-infected children, bacterial pneumonia is generally manifested as an acute febrile illness with fever, malaise, and cough; most often the infectious agent is *Streptococcus*, *H. influenzae*, or *Staphylococcus*. Lower respiratory tract viral infection also occurs frequently, often as a result of respiratory syncytial virus. This is treated with aerosolized ribavirin, 6 gm in 300 ml sterile water nebulized over 12 hours for a maximum of 5 days. Intermittent adenovirus infection occurs also, with a course similar to that in immunocompetent infants.

Central Nervous System Disorders

Encephalitis is the central nervous system infection of greatest concern in HIV-infected children. Primary infection with HIV is the most common cause, although other viruses (CMV, herpes simplex, varicella-zoster, Epstein-Barr) can cause encephalitis as well as meningitis or retinitis. *Toxoplasma gondii* infection is relatively uncommon in young HIV-infected children, although it does occur in older, school-age children and adolescents. Children with HIV infection can also have CMV retinitis, which frequently progresses despite therapy with ganciclovir.

Developmental delay is a key symptom of HIV infection, and it may be compounded in children born to mothers who injected recreational drugs during pregnancy. Other signs of involvement of the central nervous system include acquired microcephaly, cognitive impairment, loss of milestones, seizures, ataxia, abnormal tonicity, and spasticity. Encephalopathy can be static or progressive. Cerebrospinal fluid may be normal or may reveal mild pleocytosis and elevated protein levels. Corticospinal tract degeneration is frequently seen in HIV-infected children. Therefore children with HIV infection require regular neurodevelopmental evaluations. Intervention can be of benefit for mild delays. Children with severe neurologic involvement require therapy to maximize ability and manage abnormal tone and spasticity.

Hematologic Disease

Hematologic disease may result directly from HIV or appear as a secondary consequence of immune system dysfunction. Moderate anemia is present in nearly all perinatally infected infants by their fifth month, and severe anemia requiring aggressive intervention occurs in some children. Anemia is a side effect of ZDV, and some children require repeated blood transfusions while receiving ZDV therapy. Thrombocytopenia occurs in 10% to 15% of HIV-infected children, in whom it is often the initial symptom of HIV infection. Most hematologic disease in infected children results from an increased rate of platelet destruction; drug therapy should be considered if the platelet count is consistently fewer than 40,000/mm. The count may rise spontaneously; therapy with IVIG (1 g/kg for 3 days, with additional infusions every 2 to 4 weeks) frequently results in a significant but transient increase in the platelet count. The use of corticosteroid is also beneficial but may result in further immunosuppression. Splenectomy has had limited success in older infected children but carries the risk of sepsis. Growth factors (granulocyte-macrophage and granulocyte colony-stimulating factors, erythropoietin) have had some success in the treatment of secondary neutropenia and anemia in HIV-infected children, but their definitive role has not yet been established in controlled studies.

Renal Complications

HIV-associated nephropathy has been described in about 30% of children with perinatally transmitted HIV infection and only rarely in those who acquired HIV through infected blood or blood products. Renal complications of HIV infection include parenchymal disease, B- and T-cell lymphomas infiltrating the kidney, electrolyte abnormalities (often a result of other organ system involvement), hyponatremia, hypokalemia and hyperkalemia, and metabolic acidosis. Especially if nephrotoxic drugs such as pentamidine are used, renal function tests should be performed regularly on HIV-infected children. The cause of renal involvement is unclear and treatment is symptomatic. Unlike adults, children with renal disease only rarely progress to renal failure. In children with acute and chronic renal failure, use of hemodialysis or peritoneal dialysis requires that the ethical, financial, and legal aspects of intervention be addressed (Strauss et al., 1992).

Cardiomyopathy

Because HIV-infected children have multiorgan involvement, cardiac involvement must be assessed in relation to other complications. Autopsy reveals evidence of cardiomyopathy in a majority of children with HIV, but whether this is primarily or secondarily related to HIV infection is unknown. Decreased left ventricular contractility and dilation develop in some children and result in congestive heart failure with pulmonary edema, tachycardia, tachypnea, hepatomegaly, and decreased peripheral pulses. The optimal management of cardiac disease in HIV-infected children is unclear. Baseline evaluation should include a thorough physical examination, electrocardiography, radiography of the chest, and echocardiography. As with other organ system dysfunction, treatment is directed toward the symptoms presenting difficulty to the child. Long-term treatment may be required for some children, including the use of cardiotropic drugs and diuretics (Vogel, 1992).

INVESTIGATIONAL AND ANTIVIRAL THERAPIES

Strategies to prevent serious illness in HIV-infected children include attempts to block the action of specific infectious agents, to block replication of HIV, and to strengthen the immune system. For many of the conditions affecting HIV-infected children, investigational therapies offer the only hope for curative treatment. HIV damages multiple body systems. Therapy must reach diverse sites, and because proviral sequences are integrated into target cells, treatment may have to continue as long as the child lives (Pizzo & Wilfert, 1991). Probably no one drug will be effective for the long term. Therapy will require multiple agents used in combination to minimize side effects or toxic effects while providing benefit. Investigational drugs are available through the AIDS Clinical Trials Group (1-800-TRIALS-A) and the Pediatric Branch, National Cancer Institute (301-402-0696).

Antiviral drugs are now available to treat HIV infection in children. Therapeutic intervention should be evaluated for all children with an established diagnosis of HIV infection, although therapy may not be indicated for all children. Presently, antiviral therapy is recommended for children with evidence of significant immunodeficiency or HIV-associated symptoms (National Pediatric HIV Re-

Table 6–5. CD4⁺ Lymphocyte Values for the Initiation of Antiretroviral Therapy and PCP Prophylaxis

	CRITERIA FOR ANTIRETROVIRAL THERAPY	CRITERIA FOR PCP PROPHYLAXIS
CD4 (%)		
<1 year	<30	<20
1–2 year	<25	<20
>2 years	<20	<20
CD4 (cells/mm³)		
<1 year	<1,750	<1,500
1–2 year	<1,000	<750
2–6 years	<750	<500
>6 years	<500	<200

Reprinted with permission from National Pediatric HIV Resource Center (1993). Antiretroviral therapy and medical management of the human immunodeficiency virus infected child. *Pediatric Infectious Disease Journal, 12,* 513–522. © 1993.

source Center, 1993). Routine therapy is not recommended for HIV-infected children who are free of symptoms and have normal immune status, including those with lymphadenopathy, hepatomegaly, or hypergammaglobulinemia.

As with adults, return to function and/or prolongation of life should be the goal of effective therapy. Besides these clinical end points, surrogate markers such as CD4 and p24 antigen levels are used to indicate response to treatment. Although shortcomings are recognized, use of these markers is the standard approach in the absence of clinical change. CD4⁺ lymphocyte counts are used as the primary criterion for a diagnosis of immunodeficiency, with recognition of the changes that occur with age. Criteria for instituting antiretroviral therapy are found in Table 6–5.

The U.S. Food and Drug Administration approved use of the antiviral drug ZDV for children in the late spring of 1990, more than 3 years after its use in adults had become widespread. ZDV is now officially recommended for use as initial therapy in children. Early studies of ZDV in children consistently showed improvements such as weight gain, improved neurologic function, and decreased levels of serum immunoglobulin. However, the effects were only temporary and did not reverse disease progression.

As in adults, ZDV has bone marrow toxicity, necessitating regular monitoring of patients for anemia and neutropenia. The recommended dosage for children 4 weeks to 13 years of age is 180 mg/m² orally every 6 hours. Because this was the dosage used in the initial studies in children, clinicians have been reluctant to decrease the recommended dosage to adult levels. Toxic effects may occur at any time during treatment and is related to ZDV dose and the stage of disease at which treatment is begun. Complete blood cell counts should be obtained monthly.

ZDV failure or intolerance are indications for changing antiviral therapy. Intolerance is defined as persistent or severe adverse reactions to therapeutic doses of ZDV. Failure is defined as progression of HIV disease while the patient is adherent to therapy (National Pediatric HIV Resource Center, 1993). The primary indications are growth failure and/or progressive central nervous system disease. Didanosine (dideoxyinosine [ddI]) is the only approved second-line therapy for children and is suggested for children with ZDV intolerance or failure. Although ddI does not suppress bone marrow function, pancreatitis and peripheral retinal depigmentation have occurred in 5% of children taking the drug. The recommended dosage is 90 to 135 mg/m² orally every 12 hours.

Zalcitabine (dideoxycytidine [ddC]) is available for use in combination therapy and can be used as an alternative to ZDV or in combination with it or ddI. Clinical trials of these therapeutic agents are ongoing. Table 6–6 lists medications commonly prescribed to treat HIV- and AIDS-related disorders in children.

CHRONICITY OF DISEASE AND DELIVERY OF CARE

Both psychosocial issues (discussed in more detail later in the chapter) and the progressive nature of HIV disease complicate the management of HIV infection as a chronic childhood illness. Nevertheless, it is critical for the child that the process begin early: if the signs and symptoms of HIV infection are recognized at the outset, the effects of the illness can be minimized through supportive and antiretroviral therapies. More widespread HIV testing and greater awareness of early signs of pediatric HIV infection by health care workers will result in more diagnoses before the appearance of symptoms. Early diagnosis will require that pediatric health professionals deal with issues not typically encountered in pediatric practice in the past, including substance abuse, sexuality, reproductive rights, early death, and bereavement.

In general, persons who provide care for chronically ill children should strive to minimize the disruption made by the disease process and treatment regimen in the family unit and in the development of the children. In recent years the focus of pediatrics has shifted from an exclusive concern with medical care toward psychosocial problem solving with an awareness of the contributions other disciplines can make to long-term care. This shift has contributed to the development of care models that promote a normal life for the chronically ill child. In the case of HIV-infected children, health care and psychosocial needs are particularly complex and demand coordination. Most of these needs can be met by community-based providers, but regional tertiary care centers should be available to treat the children for severe infection or illness and to provide periodic evaluation and antiviral treatment. Acute care hospitalization is seldom needed before symptomatic AIDS develops.

Challenges of Home Care

The ideal locus for the management of chronic childhood illnesses is the home. Often the parents of a chronically ill child are the only consistent link in the care system; they know the most about the child's symptoms, treatments, and responses (Boland & Czarniecki, 1991). Even in the best of circumstances, however, managing a chronic illness introduces stresses into the family (Jessop & Stein, 1989): it must reorient its existence around the child's constant need for care and deal with the concomitant financial, social, and emotional strains. In the case of HIV-infected children, however, family stability may already have been compromised by drug addiction and a host of other social problems, such as poverty, substandard housing, inad-

equate support networks, and poor access to community resources, including medical care. Moreover, parents frequently discover that they are HIV infected only when HIV symptoms are diagnosed in their newborn child. This discovery, which may be the first concrete evidence of one partner's drug use or bisexuality, invariably transforms the relationship, often further destabilizing family life. The first reaction may be a denial of the child's diagnosis.

HIV-infected children and their families require services from many helping professions. In addition to nurses, these may include physicians, social workers, psychologists, dietitians, teachers, clergy, and occupational, physical, and recreational therapists. Care from these many sources can be coordinated through case management, which can prevent the two extremes of a failure to meet needs and the duplication of services. Indeed, families of HIV-infected children have testified that the constant availability of a single identified person to link them with services is the key factor that has enabled them to care for their children at home (McGonigel, 1988). Outpatient care can be made particularly accessible and effective if it is offered in special clinics that provide comprehensive care for both children and adults. In all care settings the special needs of children, such as the need to play, should be acknowledged and accommodated. In addition, health care professionals must be culturally sensitive and nonjudgmental. By adopting positive attitudes, these professionals can promote such attitudes in families, which bear the brunt of care.

A formal assessment of the family members is important to determine their willingness and ability to provide care for the HIV-infected child (Boland & Harris, 1992). Home care workers need to know how the family regards the diagnosis and who in the family is aware of it (Boland et al., 1989). The limited capacity of the medical profession to provide help for HIV-infected children may have shattered trust in the profession, and this trust will have to be rebuilt (Thorne & Robinson, 1989). Trust may be an issue particularly when the source of infection was blood products provided by medical authorities for a family member with hemophilia (Tiblier et al.,

Text continued on page 210

Table 6–6. Medications Commonly Prescribed for Children with HIV

MEDICATION	INDICATION	DOSE
A. Therapy Aimed at Combating HIV Infection		
Zidovudine (ZDV; azidothymidine [AZT]; Retrovir)	Proven HIV infection with CD4$^+$ cell count inadequate for age. HIV encephalopathy or other symptoms of disease.	By mouth: <12 yr 180 mg/m^2 q6hr; >12 yr 100 mg.po 5× daily **IV:** 480 mg/m^2 daily continuously or 120 mg/m^2 infused over 1 hour q6hr. When drug unable to be delivered by mouth or in children with progressive encephalopathy not responsive to oral AZT
Didanosine (dideoxyinosine [ddI], Videx)	Same	90–150 mg/m^2 bid given po
Zalcitabine (dideoxycytidine [ddC], HIVID)	Same	0.005 mg/kg or 0.01 mg/kg po q8hr Recommended for use only in alternating or combination schedules with ZDV to alleviate toxic effects and limit emergence of drug resistant strains
B. Prevention and Treatment of Concurrent Infections		
Trimethoprim-sulfamethoxazole (TMP-SMX; Septra, Bactrim)	Treatment of *Pneumocystis carinii* pneumonia (PCP) Prophylaxis of PCP in the child with inadequate CD4$^+$ cell counts, in any child with a history of previous PCP infection or in the seropositive infant <1 yr of age with presence of HIV-related symptoms	Trimethoprim, 5 mg/kg q6hr IV or po 75 mg/m^2 bid on Monday, Tuesday, and Wednesday only

SIDE EFFECTS, TOXIC EFFECTS, COMMENTS	NURSING INTERVENTIONS
Neutropenia, anemia Increased mean corpuscular volume Myopathy, particularly in lower extremities Hyperactivity Short serum half-life Drug is acid labile	Carefully follow complete blood cell count with differential cell count. Assist as monitor of compliance. Monitor serum levels of muscle enzymes; observe gait; monitor for signs of muscle weakness, tenderness, wasting. Elicit history of sleep difficulties, distractibility, change in school performance; may need further evaluation and referral. Families must be educated concerning need for drug administration q6hr and assisted with identifying a schedule allowing ease of compliance; especially during the school day and night sleep.
Drug is suspended in magnesia and alumina Peripheral neuropathy correlated with administration of ddI in adults Pancreatitis associated with high doses (540 mg/m²/day) or concurrent use of pentamidine Variable absorption of drug even when taken under optimal circumstances, especially in children with gastrointestinal symptoms	Instruct family to administer drug to child one-half hour after meals. Suspension may cause diarrhea and require taking alumina hydroxide before each dose. Discuss potential with family, observe child for signs of pain, changes in gait, complaints of numbness, pain, or tingling in hands or feet or signs of constipation. Monitor serum amylase, lipase, and triglycerides before initiation of drug and routinely throughout therapy. Teach family to immediately report abdominal pain, nausea, or vomiting; avoid caffeine, carbonated drinks, and chocolate, all of which can cause gastrointestinal symptoms. Careful monitoring of clinical response by history taking, physical examination, neurodevelopmental assessment, and laboratory evaluation. Participation in therapeutic drug monitoring.
Ulcers in oral cavity and on tongue and lips	Inform family of potential. Inspection of oral cavity. Teach concerning oral hygiene to prevent infection. Monitor oral intake/hydration status.
Erythematous maculopapular rash on trunk and extremities, including palms Reports of peripheral neuropathy in adults	Inform family of potential. Observe for symptoms, including change in gait, refusal to walk, jaw pain; complaints of numbness, pain, tingling; and complaints of constipation.
Anemia, neutropenia, thrombocytopenia, rash, fever, Stevens-Johnson syndrome	Monitor complete blood cell count and differential cell count. Educate caregivers concerning potential for side effects; impress need for visit to medical care provider if fever and/or rash occurs for assessment. Inform caregivers of devastating impact of PCP on infants and discourage discontinuation of prophylaxis without consulting an HIV specialist.
Interstitial nephritis	Monitor renal function.

Continued on following page

Table 6–6. Medications Commonly Prescribed for Children with HIV *Continued*

MEDICATION	INDICATION	DOSE
Pentamidine (Pentam 300)	Treatment of PCP Prophylaxis of PCP (when child hypersensitive to TMP-SMX or bone marrow suppression interfering with antiretroviral therapy)	4 mg/kg IV q24hr 4 mg/kg IV once a month 300 mg via aerosol once a month
Dapsone	Prophylaxis of PCP when unable to give TMP-SMX (Bactrim) because of allergy or severe neutropenia.	1 mg/kg dose per day
Intravenous immune globulin	Prevention of serious bacterial infections in children with $CD4^+$ cell count greater than 200/ mm^3	400 mg/kg monthly intravenously
Nystatin (Mycostatin)	Mild mucocutaneous candidiasis Candidal diaper dermatitis	1–6 ml po each cheek 4 or 5 times daily after feeding for oral lesions. Apply cream in thin film to diaper area after thorough cleansing 4 or 5 times daily for diaper dermatitis.
Fluconozole	Systemic fungal infection Esophagitis Severe oral candidiasis Maintenance for cryptococcal disease	6 mg/kg once a day po or IV
Terconazole (Terazol) vaginal cream	Oral candidiasis	Apply orally bid to qid

SIDE EFFECTS, TOXIC EFFECTS, COMMENTS	NURSING INTERVENTIONS
Hypotension related to rate of infusion	Administer for 60 to 90 min with monitoring of blood pressure throughout infusion.
Hypoglycemia with long-term use	Use reagent strip (Dextrostix) 45 min into and after infusion.
Bronchospasm related to aerosol administration	Monitor for effects especially when used with other drugs (ddI, ddC) with pancreatic toxicity.
Necessitates cooperation of child for effective delivery of medication via aerosol	Assess for history of prior bronchospasm during therapy.
Burning in back of throat, metallic taste in mouth during inhalation	Administered by a respiratory therapist using a Respirgard II jet nebulizer, with frequent pulmonary assessment. Medication and equipment available for treatment of acute respiratory distress. Premedication may be necessary.
No data concerning efficacy of aerosol or intravenous pentamidine in children as prophylaxis	Room used for administration must be ventilated according to Occupational Safety and Health Administration standards.
	Careful assessment of child's developmental and emotional ability to cooperate with a lengthy and somewhat unpleasant procedure.
	Allow careful use of hard candies, flavored drinks during treatment.
	Inform parents. Emphasize need to report immediately fever, shortness of breath, rapid respirations, and cough to a health professional aware of the child's HIV status.
Exfoliative dermatitis	Not absorbed in alkaline pH. Give 2 hours before or after ddI.
Convulsions (rare)	
Methemoglobinemia (rare)	Monitor complete blood cell count, liver studies, renal status.
Potential for adverse events including pyrogenic reactions, systemic reactions, cardiovascular manifestations, or hypersensitivity	Have epinephrine immediately available.
	Administer with an escalating-rate regimen, monitoring patient throughout and assessing vital sign before rate escalation.
	Patient may require premedication with hydrocortisone.
Interferes with immunogenicity of measles, mumps, rubella vaccine	Plan administration of measles-mumps-rubella vaccine 3 months after last IVIG dose. Readminister vaccine if immune globulin is administered within 14 days after immunization.
Consider home administration in appropriate families under constant supervision of registered nurse	
Prolonged use safe, but may cause problems with dentition in older children related to sugar content of suspension	Instruct family in oral hygiene measures.
Frequency of administration difficult to comply with, and families often cease therapy when plaques not visible	Instruct family of need to continue therapy beyond resolution of visible lesions.
	Assist family in identifying a schedule to optimize compliance.
Candidal diaper dermatitis frequently occurs coincidentally with oral disease	Assess diaper area.
	Anticipate occurrence of diaper area lesions and provide therapy.
Skin rash	
Allergic reaction (adults)	
	Coat oral membranes

Continued on following page

MEDICATION	INDICATION	DOSE
Ketoconazole	Severe or recalcitrant mucotaneous esophageal candidiasis Candidal diaper dermatitis	3.3–6.6 mg/kg in one daily dose by mouth for mucotaneous lesion Apply cream in thin film to diaper area once daily after thorough cleansing
Amphotericin B	Invasive or disseminated candidiasis Cryptococcal disease	Assess febrile/hemodynamic response with test dose 0.1 mg/kg/day. After 1 week of therapy, may give double the daily dose on alternative days; duration of therapy dependent on type and extent of infection
Clarithromycin	*Mycobacterium avium* complex (MAC)	15 mg/kg/day, bid po
Ethambutol	MAC	15 mg/kg/day, po
Rifabutin	MAC	10–20 mg/kg/day, po
Amikacin	MAC	10 mg/kg/day IV

C. Drugs Used to Mediate Toxic Effects of Therapy

Granulocyte colony-stimulating factor (G-CSF; filgrastim [Neupogen])	Neutropenia related to antiretroviral therapy or HIV infection itself	1–10 mg/kg subcutaneously daily and titrated to maintain absolute neutrophil count between 2000 and 6000 cells/mm^3
Erythropoietin (EPO; epoetin [Eprex])	Long-term transfusion-dependent anemia related to drug therapy or HIV-related autoimmune phenomena	50–100 IU/kg IV or sq three times weekly; dose reduced when hemoglobin level reaches 10–11.5 gm/dl

Adapted from Boland, M., Santacroce, S. (in press). Nursing Care of the Child. In P. Pizzo & C. Wilfert (Eds.), *Pediatric HIV/AIDS* 2nd ed. © Williams & Wilkins, Baltimore.

SIDE EFFECTS, TOXIC EFFECTS, COMMENTS	NURSING INTERVENTIONS
Potential hepatotoxic effects	Evaluate liver function before and during course of therapy.
Should *not* be taken with antacids; best absorbed when taken after a fatty meal or with milk products	Assist families in determining optimum dosing schedule, especially those whose children also receive ddI.
Potential for rash, pruritus	Inform family, monitor child, prevent skin injury.
Fever with shaking chills	Premedication with acetaminophen and hydrocortisone may reduce systemic reactions. Give meperidine (Demerol) by intravenous push for shaking chills. Monitor platelet count.
Abnormal renal function (hypokalemia, elevated serum creatinine and blood urea nitrogen, hypomagnesemia)	Monitor and replace electrolytes. Monitor renal function.
Consider outpatient and home infusion for appropriate children and families after resolution of acute illness	Refer to experienced home health agency for teaching and at-home supervision as well as laboratory evaluation.
Hepatotoxic effects	Monitor liver studies.
Thrombocytopenia	Monitor liver studies. Monitor complete blood cell count.
Hepatotoxic effects	Monitor liver studies.
Hepatotoxic reaction Renal toxic reaction Ototoxic reaction Agranulocytosis Thrombocytopenia Leukopenia Eosinophilia Anemia	Monitor complete blood cell count and differential cell count, liver function, and hearing status.
Mild fever, arthralgia, myalgia, headache and nausea, rash, and swelling at injection site	Assess child for symptoms, teaching regarding symptom management.
Medication administered subcutaneously	Assess family's ability and willingness to administer injections to child. Educate family and backup caregiver concerning home injection therapy.
Doses titrated in response to blood chemistry values	Make appropriate home health referrals for monitoring of injection administration, support, and potential administration of drug. Arrange for home or community laboratory evaluation and reporting to prescribing physician.
May cause hypertension in children with renal disease related to increased blood viscosity	Monitor blood pressure. Obtain laboratory evaluation.
Adequate iron stores; ferritin necessary for optimum response	Assess family for ability and willingness to administer injections to child.
Drug given intravenously or subcutaneously	Educate family and backup caregiver regarding medication administration.
Doses titrated in response to blood chemistry values	Make appropriate home health referrals for monitoring, support, and medication administration.
Mild skin rash possible	Arrange for home/community laboratory evaluation and reporting to prescribing physician. Inform family.

1989). Families may also have a general suspicion of authorities if injecting drug use was the route of infection. Even without these complicating factors, caretakers often do not understand the meaning of HIV testing or the complexities of immune system functioning. They may be overwhelmed with the amount of information provided them and many have difficulty remembering what was said. Education for parents or guardians should be provided at the many occasions on which they encounter health professionals, and it should be reinforced with printed and video materials. Parents of infected children have requested particular assistance in getting information about HIV disease and its treatment and in disclosing the diagnosis to family and friends (Falloon et al., 1989). Some parental concerns can be addressed in the context of support groups. Although many parents of infected children shy away from formal support group meetings, organized group social activities often spawn informal support systems (Mayers & Spiegel 1992).

Planning Care

The caregiving team should meet regularly to plan and coordinate patient and family care and to make referrals concerning such issues as child care, foster care, child custody, school arrangements, home health care, finances, and substance use. Initial assessments of seropositive infants should include information about maternal drug withdrawal and sexually transmitted diseases, for which infants should be given appropriate treatment (Mendez, 1990). Ongoing outpatient care of the seropositive infant should include HIV antibody testing at regular intervals until the infant is 2 years of age. Growth (height, weight, head circumference) and development should be monitored at regular intervals with a growth chart and the Denver Developmental Screening Test or the Bayley or McCarthy scales. Regular immunizations with vaccines such as measles-mumps-rubella, influenza, and pneumococcus vaccines should be administered.

The need for preventive therapy should be reviewed early in the course of a child's illness and should include consideration of prophylaxis against PCP, the potential benefits of intravenous administration of gamma globulin, and the timing of ZDV dosing. For school-age children the development of treatment protocols and drug regimens should take into account school schedules; late afternoon or evening clinic visits and adjusted medication schedules best accommodate the needs of these children (Abrams & Nicholas, 1990). As noted previously, ongoing information and education should be provided for parents or guardians. Infected parents should be encouraged to obtain regular health care, and health care workers should look for signs of parental compromise that could affect the care of the child, such as fatigue, weight loss, forgetfulness, or an inability to follow through with treatment.

The Role of the Home Care Nurse

The home care nurse can act as a liaison between the family and the child's medical team and can serve as an advocate for the family in dealing with other providers. Because of the impairment in humoral and cell-mediated immunity, HIV-infected children are susceptible to bacterial, viral, and fungal infections. The nurse must have a good working knowledge of HIV disease processes, how they affect children at various stages of infection, and appropriate phamacologic and non-pharmacologic interventions. The home care nurse should also know how well the child and caregivers understand diagnosis and treatment, sites of infection, respiratory status, growth and development, thought processes, physical mobility, nutritional status, skin integrity, level of comfort, and compliance with medical regimens (Lincoln & Hanley, 1991). The most common nursing diagnoses in immunocompromised children include increased susceptibility to infection, fever, increased pain, opportunistic infection, alteration in gas exchange, alteration in cognitive and motor function, alteration in nutrition, potential for bleeding, alteration in fluid-and-electrolyte balance, potential impairment of skin integrity, and potential fatigue and exhaustion of caregivers (Boland et al., 1989).

Ambulatory Care

Even with well-coordinated home care, infected children are likely to make periodic visits to the hospital emergency department. Parents or guardians should be instructed to tell staff there about the child's HIV sero-status (Mendez, 1990). As symptoms develop, the frequency of outpatient visits will increase and hospitalizations will begin. This will make denial of the diagnosis more difficult, and parents will often ask for detailed information as they experience a loss of control and as treatment regimens become more complicated. These regimens may include intravenous and high-technology therapies that can be safely administered in the home. Nurses should be aware, however, that when denial does not interfere with medical care, it serves as a protective measure, decreasing stress and allowing caregivers to function.

Pain Management

It has been reported in studies of adults with HIV/AIDS that pain is a frequently reported symptom during all stages of the disease, but most significantly during the terminal stage (O'Neill & Sherrard, 1993). Types of pain reported include headaches, mouth and throat pain, chest pain, myalgia, peripheral neuritis, arthralgia, and the pain associated with medical procedures (O'Neill & Sherrard, 1993; Lebovitz et al., 1989; Singer et al., 1993).

Pain in children with HIV infection has been studied less. Retrospective studies document that children also have similar types of pain related to their disease and its diagnosis, course, and treatment. One retrospective chart audit of 149 children with HIV infection showed that 88% of patients had at least one HIV-related complication (i.e., thrush, herpes, stomatitis, esophagitis, sinusitis, otitis, opportunistic infections, or multiple organ problems) that could be reasonably expected to cause pain (Czarniecki and Oleske, 1993). In this same group only 24% had reports of pain documented in the chart. Episodes of pain included headache, abdominal pain, oral cavity pain, neuromuscular pain, peripheral neuropathy, chest pain, earache, odynophagia, myalgia, and arthralgia.

Pain in children with HIV poses several unique problems. As the survival of children with perinatally acquired HIV infection lengthens, the potential that multiple complications will create pain increases. Children who are nonverbal because of age or neurologic complications cannot self-report their pain. Parents and health care professionals may deny a child's pain because it represents progression of disease. Families who have a history of substance abuse may be very resistant to the use of opioid analgesics for fear of addiction.

For effective management of pain in children with HIV infection, it must first be recognized. This can occur only if pain is consistently assessed. Reports of pain should be taken at face value. Pain should be treated while a cause is being determined and even if a cause is not identified. It is frequently found that patients with HIV have pain of unknown cause. If there is a reason to suspect pain, but the patient cannot tell you about it, it is within reasonable treatment guidelines to begin a trial of pain management to see how the patient responds. Frequently children's chronic pain will manifest itself by depressed affect, lack of activity, or anorexia, rather than by crying or grimacing.

The backbone of good pain management should be appropriate use of analgesics with a pain ladder: *mild pain*, nonsteroidal antiinflammatory drugs (NSAIDs), acetaminophen; *moderate pain*, continue NSAIDs or acetaminophen and add a mild opioid such as codeine; and *severe pain*, continue NSAIDs or acetaminophen and add a strong opioid, morphine being the first choice. There is no ceiling on the dose of opioids to achieve pain relief, and doses can go very high. Longer-acting opioids such as liquid methadone or time-released morphine can be used once the correct dose is determined by using short-acting morphine. Families must be educated about the difference between physical dependence and addiction. Side effects of opioids should be treated aggressively.

In addition to analgesics, other nonpharmacologic measures such as distraction, hypnosis, application of heat or cold, massage, relaxation, and music therapy can be tried. Many of these methods have been found to help children cope with painful procedures.

Terminal Care

As it becomes evident that a child with HIV infection is nearing the end of life, attention must be paid to helping the child and family move through this time with the least amount of suffering and the most support and dignity possible. For this to happen, all the people involved—child, family, and health care professionals—must be communicating as openly as possible about what is happening. Physicians and nurses must speak clearly and explain the child's condition to parents so that they can make informed decisions about their child's care and final days. Euphemisms can be confusing and can send double messages. Most parents do not want professionals to "give up" on their child, but if it is explained that, rather than giving up, there is simply no more that can be done, parents will understand the difference and begin to make decisions.

Discussions about "do not resuscitate" orders need to take place before a crisis arises. This discussion is a process in which families are helped to understand their child's medical condition, the treatment options that still remain, and the most likely consequences of those treatments. For example, a child with end-stage cardiomyopathy might live awhile longer with intravenous infusions of cardiac inotropic medications and mechanical ventilation, but it is not likely that the child would ever be weaned from those therapies and would die slowly while connected to a machine in the intensive care unit. In this instance a parent could also be given the option of foregoing the inotropes and ventilator and have the child die peacefully at home. These discussions are never easy, and families and health care professionals can have ambiguous feelings and go back and forth with the decision. The most important thing to do is to keep communication open at all times.

If a decision has been made to cease any further treatment of the disease and to focus only on comfort and quality of life, then certain interventions can be very helpful to patients and families. First, the family can decide to have the child die at home or in the hospital. If at home, referrals to hospice programs or home health agencies can be made. Hospice programs offer a wide array of services including nursing care, volunteers, spiritual support, support groups, and expertise in symptom management. If the family opts for in-hospital care, then every effort should be made to provide hospicelike services. Nurses can make sure that the child is kept clean and smelling as good as possible, that no needless tests are performed, that parents are involved in their child's care as much as they desire, and that the child is as pain-free as possible, with other symptoms optimally controlled. Helping families prepare in advance for the death, including teaching them how their child might look and act, can decrease their fear of the unknown. Talking openly with the child about what is happening to him or her, reading stories about death, and talking with the child about his or her feelings and beliefs about death can reduce the child's fears and sense of isolation. Families may now want certain spiritual rituals performed that they could not endure earlier. Decisions about autopsy and funeral arrangements can be made in advance, thereby decreasing stress at the time of death. Older children often want to help plan their funeral.

When death occurs, parents and other family members need adequate time to say good-bye, which may involve bathing the child's body or fixing the child's hair. Although such time is seldom provided in busy hospital settings, these hours are invaluable to parents. The family cannot be rushed; nurses who provide such support can assist the family in beginning the mourning process.

Financial constraints on home care and the safety of personnel if the home is in a high-crime area are often provider concerns in the terminal stage of illness. Parents who have provided excellent home care may wish to place a child in the hospital as death approaches; some may refuse home-based hospice care because they do not want new people introduced into their lives. Rehospitalization should remain an option for terminally ill children. When all treatments have failed, and death is the sure outcome, there is still much to be done for the child with HIV infection and the family.

MANAGEMENT OF CHRONIC ILLNESS BY FAMILY

It was noted earlier that a majority of HIV-infected children in the United States have one or both parents infected and that the parents' infections are frequently a consequence of injection drug use. A mother's illness or addiction may interfere with her ability to care for an infected child, both physically and psychologically. She may be fearful of sharing her diagnosis with her significant other because of the possibility of rejection, abandonment, withdrawal of economic support, or even physical violence. Similar fears may isolate her and her partner from the network of friends or family to whom they would normally turn for support. The diagnosis may also precipitate arguments between a couple about who is to blame, or it may reactivate previously buried family issues. In addition to the disruption of the relationship with the partner, an infected mother may be burdened by guilt over her child's condition. Moreover, although a diagnosis of HIV infection should be the occasion for adopting safer sexual behaviors, cultural or religious beliefs often make it difficult for a woman to initiate changes in sexual behaviors with her partner.

The mother's responses to HIV infection are further complicated when she has a history of substance use. She may continue to use drugs as an escape, and this may prevent her from coping with the child's infection or providing needed care and treatment (Boland & Harris, 1992). Addicted parents may be skilled at manipulating medical staff members and turning them against one another. There is also the risk that addicted parents may inappropriately use pain medications prescribed for their children; health care workers should monitor the children for adequacy of pain medication. Health care professionals can be helpful in making parents with substance use problems aware of the benefit of seeking treatment for these problems. When treatment is not an option and the parents' actions are disruptive, professionals experienced in dealing with substance use must be consulted. Nursing and medical staff members must be consistent and clear about their expectations of parents and the plan of care. A concrete plan and frequent communication among care providers can minimize splitting and manipulation of the staff by family members. Health care workers can help parents overcome guilt for their past actions by refocusing them on the good they can do for their infected children in the present.

Surrogate Caregivers

In some circumstances, surrogate caregivers are needed for infected children. Often they can be found within the extended family; in many black or Hispanic families the pattern of care involves extended family members such as grandmothers or aunts (Boyd-Franklin & Aleman, 1990). However, these caregivers may be impeded by struggles related to the lifestyles, illnesses, or deaths of their own children. If they are advanced in age, they may lack the physical strength and stamina to provide care for young children at a time in their lives when they themselves might reasonably expect to receive care. Although extended family members in some places are reimbursed for the foster care of a relative, services available to other caregivers, such as respite care, may not be available to them.

Early in the pediatric HIV epidemic there were periodic horror stories in the press about infected children who lived their entire lives as "boarder babies" in acute care hospitals. By 1990 the situation had changed markedly. Most states had improved their resources for recruiting and training foster care families; transitional care facilities for children awaiting foster care placements had been developed in many localities (Abrams & Nicholas, 1990). Foster parents of HIV-infected children have some of the same fears of rejection and isolation as do natural parents, but they face some additional challenges. They may lack the legal authority to participate in decision making about a child's medical treatment. In addition, they may be unrealistic in their expectations about what will be involved in caregiving. Their involvement may grow out of spiritual beliefs, a sense of higher calling, a strong sense of advocacy, or a belief that love will heal. Proper training for foster parents, conducted in hospitals and transitional care facilities, will help prepare them for the realities of caring for chronically ill children (Groth, 1993).

Dealing With Stress

The manner in which a biologic, extended, or foster family copes with an HIV diagnosis in a child is related to its previously established ways of dealing with crises and stresses. A diagnosis of HIV can magnify feelings of hopelessness and precipitate suicidal ideation in adults; in some cultural contexts, adults may view illnesses as a moral judgment or punishment for past behavior. Similar feelings are involved when a child has HIV infection. A parent's guilt may manifest itself in overprotective or permissive behavior toward the child, possibly interfering with the child's development (Jessop & Stein, 1989). If the family fears the stigma often attached to an HIV diagnosis, they may be secretive and may isolate themselves. This may confuse older siblings, who frequently become involved in caring for an ailing child and parents. These children may face the prospect of requiring a new home without understanding the illness that is the cause of their relocation (Abrams & Nicholas, 1990). Families often need assistance in dealing with issues of confidentiality and disclosure, that is, thinking through whom to tell, when, and how. Because of difficulty in adjusting to the diagnosis, the family may have only intermittent contact with clinics at crisis or decision points and may otherwise be unavailable. This intermittent contact may also be an outgrowth of a family's perception of outside agencies as intrusive, which may be more common in minority families with multiple socioeconomic problems who are most in need of help (Boyd-Franklin & Aleman, 1990).

Families with HIV-infected children may have to deal with the illness for many years and are likely to encounter practical problems that have no easy solutions. Most families with infected children are totally dependent on public health care programs, such as Medicaid, that are often inadequately funded. Even adequately insured families may have difficulty in getting complete coverage for HIV-related conditions in children. Other financial stressors include the loss of work time when a child must be supervised constantly, lost opportunities for career advancement, and the expenses involved in transporting the child to the clinic and other social service appointments (Jessop & Stein, 1989). Chronic illnesses such as HIV can also be more draining emotionally than acute illnesses. Parents of chronically ill children often fluctuate among a variety of reactions—shock, denial, sadness, and anger—between periods of relative acceptance and equilibrium. Their feelings of guilt or inadequacy are brought to the fore repeatedly as they are confronted by the child's difference from healthy peers, especially at critical developmental stages such as starting day care or school (Jessop & Stein, 1989). Most of the literature on chronic illness has focused on children in middle-class families, so there is little understanding of how deprived and chaotic families may deal with a chronic illness such as HIV over the long run. In addition, families with an HIV-infected child typically have more than one chronically ill member. Early results from one study of biologic, extended, and foster parents of children indicate similarities in coping styles of the three types of family units (Sherwen et al., 1993).

Once AIDS is diagnosed, the prognosis is generally poor. Most children die within 2 years of diagnosis. Most often the AIDS diagnosis results from a progression of existing symptoms such as failure to thrive, encephalopathy, or untreatable opportunistic infection. High levels of service and intervention are required, and these greatly increase the potential for parent-provider conflict as the involved parties grapple with the risks and benefits of aggressive, intrusive, and investigational therapies. An AIDS diagnosis is often accompanied by an immediate family crisis, manifested in guilt, shock, shame, and confusion. Families often need assistance in clarifying issues and getting support for decision making. Disadvantaged families especially may assume that the physician is always right and may not realize how actively they can participate in making decisions. The family should be encouraged to discuss feelings about the child's prognosis, including the desire for pain management, use of life support mechanisms, and confidentiality. Often at a time when the medical staff has come to accept the child's impending death, parents favor heroic lifesaving measures. Conversely, some parents perceive and accept impending death before the medical team does. The different expectations of parent and provider must be recognized and addressed. The nurse can initiate discussion and facilitate recognition of differing perceptions.

Maintaining Family Autonomy

As noted earlier, health care professionals treating a chronic childhood illness should try to prevent both the illness and the treatment regimen from disrupting the child's development and the family unit. Typically the medical establishment reinforces the role of passive, dependent parents. This is particularly inappropriate in the management of a chronic illness such as HIV. Furthermore, forcing parents into a dependent role is counterproductive in families that are determined to maintain control over the child; enforced dependence makes the lives of the adults, as well as that of the child, feel out of control. Health care workers should attempt to establish a partnership with the family (Boland et al., 1989). This may be challenging in the case of families unaccustomed to dealing with the health care system. To them, monthly appointments may appear time-consuming, cost prohibitive, and unnecessary if they result in no prescription, procedure, or treatment. In addition, where case management and coordinated care systems have not been developed, the variety of sources and providers with whom the family must deal may include medical subspecialists with conflicting demands. This situation sets the stage for clashes between the values of middle-class professionals who provide services and those of poor families struggling to survive. Because responsibility for day-to-day supervision falls to family members, respecting their autonomy and providing a flexible system of care are important. The family of the HIV-infected child should be able to maintain its independence, autonomy, and self-determination without undue supervision and paternalism (Jessop & Stein, 1989). Health care workers must convince families that the services they offer are necessary if they expect parents to make use of these services. In addition, the workers sometimes have to deal with their own feelings of anger and blame toward parents if fantasies of rescuing children from "evil" parents are to be avoided.

A complex interaction occurs among chronic illness, the family's response, and the child's developmental status. Changes in all three occur simultaneously: the child develops, the chronic condition changes as its course continues, and the family changes throughout its life cycle and as its adaptation to the child's condition unfolds (Jessop & Stein, 1989). The care of most HIV-infected children requires lifelong treatment involving multiple drug regimens with oral and intravenous treatments and complex medical interventions. As care proceeds, both medical professionals and caregivers need to be sensitive to changes in the child, the child's medical condition, and the family situation.

PSYCHOSOCIAL ISSUES

Infected children are children first, with typical wishes for acceptance and understanding. HIV infection compromises their development, and societal reactions to the illness—such as fear and rejection—impede their struggles for normal life experiences. These children may have lived with several caretakers and lacked a consistent parental figure; this lack of a consistent family structure may inhibit their ability to deal with the diagnosis. Medical care is also stressful for them; they can expect to undergo repeated anxiety-producing, painful, and intrusive procedures throughout their treatment. Their ability to assimilate information is limited, and they may misunderstand what is told them. Young children often believe that their chronic illness is a result of magic or of their own action or inaction. As they grow older and more aware of their peers, they may worry about their differences from others, and these differences could become a primary mode of identification. Concealing their condition from others—however warranted it may be—may lead them to believe that their illness is something to be ashamed of (Perrin & Gerrity, 1984). Thus children with chronic conditions appear to have a greater incidence of psychosocial problems than others (Pless, 1984).

Disclosure of the Diagnosis

Parents and caregivers of chronically ill older children and adolescents often struggle over whether to tell them the nature of their illness, what to tell them, when is the best time, and who should do the telling. The truth is less threatening to children than fear of the unknown, but the information given to a child has to be geared to the child's developmental level. Psychologists can figure critically in the decision-making process, helping to frame the information given to the child and helping the child to survive the aftermath of the disclosure. Before a disclosure is made, the child's and parents' understanding of illness causality should be assessed. Awareness of the family's level of health knowledge and of their beliefs about health and illness is also important in determining how to help them integrate the necessary medical information. Often families need assistance in finding words that they can say comfortably and that the child will understand (Pollock & Boland, 1990). Because HIV-infected children with neurologic involvement may not be functioning at normal age levels, developmental evaluation may be helpful in determining how to communicate with them. It may be necessary to relate the information more than once. Developmentally appropriate language is needed when medical procedures and treatments are explained to children; play therapy and discussion may be helpful. The stigma and shame

that often accompany an HIV diagnosis must be addressed therapeutically as well. Disclosure should be considered an ongoing process, especially as the survival of children increases.

Overcoming Isolation

Some families of infected children isolate themselves in an attempt to maintain control over the child and the situation; their isolation may be a result of disapproval or fear of contagion by family members and friends. Caregivers may feel that they and their children are contaminated, and they may be angry with the medical profession and depressed over the many losses and potential losses they face. Counseling and psychologic support may be indicated to help caregivers—including mothers, grandmothers, and foster parents—and siblings deal with denial and feelings of shame or fear. Families that have dealt with racism, poverty, and the intrusive scrutiny of entitlement programs may have strict rules about the privacy of family-related matters that have to be overcome (Boyd-Franklin & Aleman, 1990). Still, it is important for children to have contact with their peers, particularly in school settings.

Grief and Bereavement

Often the mental health needs of HIV-infected children are neglected. The death of friends from the clinic may heighten the child's fear of death; a variety of approaches, including behavior therapy, play therapy, and medication, may be salutary. Therapy can be offered at the clinic, during hospitalizations, or at home. Offering children access to one another in play or support groups may also help them grieve. Children who survive the death of a parent, whether the children are infected or not, may need emotional support that is not available from their caregivers. Signs of their distress may include disruptive behavior at home and in school, increased aggression, and substance use (Boyd-Franklin & Aleman, 1990). Again, these cases require therapeutic intervention.

The stigma associated with HIV disease and the resultant secrecy complicate the grieving process. Health and social service professionals should respect the family's need to maintain secrecy about the diagnosis. People vary greatly in the ways they handle their grief—what they feel, how deeply and intensely they feel, how they respond, and what coping mechanisms produce relief. Options for support include counseling, support groups, telephone calls, contact with other bereaved families, home visits, and the use of volunteers or others who have established a close relationship with the family. Spiritual beliefs and connections with others in church communities may also be important coping mechanisms. A postdeath conference scheduled with the medical care providers can give parents an opportunity to ask about the events leading to the death and can help provide closure for both the providers and the parents.

NURSING RESEARCH

So that nurses can further influence the care of children with HIV infection, these children must become a focus of concern for clinical nursing research (Boland & Santacroce, in press). With increased survival comes the necessity to expand concerns to the broader sphere of the child's life—to the psychosocial aspects of living with HIV, as well as the psychologic and medical aspects. As with children with other chronic illnesses, research must increasingly be directed toward the psychologic, social and cultural dimensions (Sherwen & Boland, in press).

Particular priorities are the development of innovative programs for drug users and the management of acute, procedural, and chronic pain; supportive care needs of children; methods of case management; maintenance of adequate nutrition; models for providing hospice care; and models for accessing natural social support systems as part of the continuum of care. Investigation in these priority areas will assist in the development of theory for pediatric HIV infection nursing practice.

SUMMARY

As the techniques for identifying HIV infection in infants and treating infected children with antiretroviral and prophylactic therapies improve, so does the prognosis for HIV-infected children. Already the management of HIV illness has shifted to a chronic illness model. As the life expectancy of infected children increases, the quality of their lives assumes greater importance. Many infected children will be able to participate in the normal growth processes and activities of childhood. Thoughtfully designed systems of care delivery and competently administered care will help HIV-infected children to live for many years.

REFERENCES

Abrams, E.J., Nicholas, S.W. (1990). Pediatric HIV infection. *Pediatric Annals, 19,* 482–487.

Andiman, W.A., Simpson, B.J., Olson, B., et al. (1990). Rate of transmission of human immunodeficiency virus type 1 infection from mother to child and short-term outcome of neonatal function. *American Journal of Disease in Children, 144,* 758–768.

Blanche, S., Rouzioux, C., Moscato, M.L.G., et al. (1989). A prospective study of infants born to women sero positive for human immunodeficiency virus type 1. *New England Journal of Medicine, 320,* 1643–1648.

Boland, M.G. (1990). HIV infection in children. *NAACOG's Clinical Issues in Perinatal and Women's Health Nursing, 1,* 53–59.

Boland, M., Czarniecki, L. (1991). Starting life with HIV. *RN 54*(1), 54–58.

Boland, M., Harris, D. (1992). Living with HIV infection. In E. Connor & R. Yogev (Eds.), *The child with HIV infection* (pp. 533–550). Chicago: Year Book Medical Publishers.

Boland, M.G., Mahan-Rudolph, P., Evans, P. (1989). Special issues in the care of the child with HIV infection/AIDS. In B. Martin (Ed.), *Pediatric hospice care: What helps* (pp. 116–144). Los Angeles: Los Angeles Children's Hospital.

Boland, M.G., Santacroce, S. (in press). Nursing care of the child. In P.A. Pizzo & C. Wilfert (Eds.), *Pediatric HIV/AIDS* (2nd ed.). Baltimore: Williams & Wilkins.

Borkowsky, W., Steel, C.J., Grubman, S., et al. (1987). Antibody responses to bacterial toxoids in children infected with human immunodeficiency virus. *The Journal of Pediatrics, 110*(4), 563–566.

Boyd-Franklin, N., Aleman, J. (1990). Black, inner-city families and multigenerational issues: The impact of AIDS. *Psychologist, 40*(3), 14–17.

Bremer, J.W., Holtinger, F.B. (1990). Pediatric HIV infection and AIDS: Diagnostic tests. *Seminars in Pediatric Infectious Diseases, 1*(1), 27–30.

Burns, D. (1992). The neuropathology of pediatric acquired immunodeficiency syndrome. *Journal of Child Neurology, 7,* 332–346.

Centers for Disease Control (1987). Classification system for human immunodeficiency virus (HIV) infection in children under 13 years of age. *Morbidity and Mortality Weekly Report, 36,* 225–230.

Committee on Infectious Diseases, Academy of Pediatrics (1992). Chemotherapy for tuberculosis in infants and children. *Pediatrics, 89,* 161–165.

Connor, E., Bagarzzi, M., McSherry, G., et al. (1991). Clinical and laboratory correlates of *Pneumocystis carinii* pneumonia in children infected with HIV. *Journal of the American Medical Association 265,* 1693–1697.

Czarniecki, L., Oleske, J. (1993). Pain in children with HIV infection (p. 74). Presented at an International Conference on AIDS, Berlin, June 1993 (W.S.B. 31–33).

Delfraissy, J.F., Blanche, S., Rouzioux, C., Mayaux, M.J. (1992). Perinatal HIV transmission facts and controversies. *Immunodeficiency Reviews, 3,* 305–327.

Duliege, A., Messiah, A., Blanche, S., et al. (1992). Natural history of human immunodeficiency virus type 1 infection in children: Prognostic value of laboratory tests on the bimodal progression of the disease. *Pediatric Infectious Diseases, 11,* 630–635.

Eaton, A.P., Coury, D.L., Kern, R.A. (1989). The roles of professionals and institutions. In R. Stein, (Ed.), *Caring for children with chronic illness* (pp. 75–86). New York: Springer.

Falloon, J., Eddy, J., Wiener, L., Pizzo, P. (1989). Human immunodeficiency virus infection in children. *Journal of Pediatrics, 115,* 1–30.

Goldfarb, J. (1993). Breastfeeding AIDS and other infectious diseases. *Clinics in Perinatology, 20,* 225–243.

Gonik, B., Hammill, H.A. (1990). AIDS in pregnancy. *Seminars in Pediatric Infectious Diseases, 1*(1), 82–88.

Groth, B. (1993). Resource availability versus need: Perceptions of foster parents of HIV positive children. *Pediatric AIDS & HIV Infection: Fetus to Adolescent, 4,* 367–372.

Grubman, S., Oleske, J. (1993). The maturation of an epidemic: Update on pediatric HIV infection. *AIDS 1993, 7*(suppl 1), 5225–5234.

Gutman, L.T. (1993). Recent developments in the intersection of the epidemics of tuberculosis and HIV in children. *Pediatric HIV Forum, 1*(1), 1–5.

Hauger, S.B., Powell, K.R. (1990). Infectious complications in children with HIV infection. *Pediatric Annals, 19,* 421–436.

Horsburgh, C.R., Caldwell, M.D., Simonds, R.J. (1993). Epidemiology of disseminated nontuberculous mycobacterial disease in children with acquired immunodeficiency syndrome. *Pediatric Infectious Disease Journal, 12,* 219–221.

Hoyt, L., Oleske, J., Holland, B., Connor, E. (1992). Nontuberculous mycobacteria in children with acquired immunodeficiency syndrome. *Pediatric Infectious Disease Journal, 11,* 354–360.

Howell, R., Jandinski, J., Palumbo, P., et al. (1992). Dental caries in HIV-infected children. *Pediatric Dentistry, 14,* 370–371.

Husson, R.N., Corneau, A.M., Hoff, R. (1990). Diagnosis of human immunodeficiency virus infection in infants and children. *Pediatrics 86*(1), 1–10.

Jessop, D.J., Stein, R.E.K. (1989). Meeting the needs of individuals and families. In R. Stein, (Ed.), *Caring for children with chronic illness* (pp. 63–74). New York: Springer.

Krivine, A., Firtion, G., Cao, L., et al. (1992). HIV replication during the first weeks of life. *Lancet, 339,* 1187–1189.

Lebovitz, A., Lefkowitz, M., McCarthy, D., et al. (1989). The prevalence and management of pain in patients with AIDS: A review of 134 cases. *Clinical Journal of Pain, 5,* 245–248.

Leibovitz, E., Rigaud, M., Pollack, H., et al. (1990). *Pneumocystis carinii* pneumonia in infants infected with the human immunodeficiency virus with more than 450 CD4 lymphocytes per cubic millimeter. *New England Journal of Medicine, 323*(8), 531–533.

Lincoln, P., Hanely, E. (1991). Pediatric HIV infection: Clinical and social management issues. *Journal of Home Health Care Practice 3*(3), 24–33.

Mann, J., Tarantola, D.J., Netter, T.W. (1992). *AIDS in the world.* Boston: Harvard University Press.

Mayers, A., Spiegel, L. (1992). A parental support group in a pediatric AIDS clinic: Its usefulness and limitations. *Health and Social Work, 17,* 184–191.

McClain, K.L., Rosenblatt, H. (1990). Pediatric HIV infection and AIDS: Clinical expression of malignancy. *Seminars in Pediatric Infectious Diseases, 1*(1), 124–129.

McGonigel, M. (1988). *Family meeting on pediatric AIDS.* Washington, DC: Association for the Care of Children's Health.

Mendez, H. (1990). Ambulatory care of infants and children born to HIV-infected mothers. *Pediatric Annals, 17,* 439–447.

Miller, T., Orav, E.J., Martin, S., et al. (1991). Malnutrition and carbohydrate malabsorption in children with vertically transmitted human immunodeficiency virus-1 infection. *Gastroenterology, 100,* 1296–1302.

National Institute of Allergy and Infectious Disease (1994, February 21). AZT reduces rate of maternal transmission of HIV. *NIAID News.* Bethesda, MD: National Institutes of Health, U.S. Public Health Service.

National Institute of Child Health and Human Development (1991). Intravenous immune globulin for the prevention of bacterial infections in children with symptomatic human immunodeficiency virus infection. *New England Journal of Medicine, 325,* 73–80.

National Pediatric HIV Resource Center (1993). Antiretroviral therapy and medical management of the human immunodeficiency virus–infected child. *Pediatric Infectious Disease Journal, 12,* 513–522.

O'Neill, W., Sherrard, J. (1993). Pain in human immunodeficiency disease: A review. *Pain, 54,* 3–14.

Perrin, E.C., Gerrity, P.S. (1984). Development of children wth a chronic illness. *Pediatric Clinics of North America, 31,* 19–31.

Pitt, J. (1991). Lymphocytic interstitial pneumonia. *Pediatric Clinics of North America, 38*(1), 89–96.

Pizzo, P.A. (1989). Emerging concepts in the treatment of HIV infection in children. *Journal of the American Medical Association, 262,* 1989–1992.

Pizzo, P.A., Wilfert, C. (1991). Treatment considerations for children with HIV infection. In P. Pizzo, C. Wilfert, (Eds.), *Pediatric AIDS: The challenge of HIV infection in infants, children, and adolescents* (pp. 478–494). Baltimore: Williams & Wilkins.

Pless, I.B. (1984). Clinical assessment: Physical and psychological functioning. *Pediatric Clinics of North America, 31,* 33–45.

Pollock, S., Boland, M. (1990). Children and HIV infection. *Psychologist, 40,* 17–21.

Prober, C., Gershon, A. (1991). Medical management of newborns and infants born to seropositive mothers. In P. Pizzo, C. Wilfert, (Eds.), *Pediatric AIDS: The challenge of HIV infection in infants, children, and adolescents* (pp. 516–530). Baltimore: Williams & Wilkins.

Rosenblatt, H.M., Englund, J.A., Shearer, W.T. (1990). Immunotherapeutic approaches to pediatric HIV infection. *Seminars in Pediatric Infectious Diseases, 1*(1), 140–149.

Sherwen, L., Boland, M., Gilchrist, M. (1993). Stress, coping and perception of child vulnerability in female caretakers of HIV-infected children: A preliminary report. *Pediatric AIDS and HIV Infection: Fetus to Adolescent, (4)*, 358–366.

Sherwen, L., Boland, M.G., (in press). Overview of psychosocial research concerning pediatric HIV infection.

Singer, E., Zorella, C., Fahy-Chandon, B., et al. (1993). Painful symptoms reported by ambulatory HIV-infected men in a longitudinal study. *Pain, 54*, 15–19.

Starke, J.R., Jacobs, R.F., Jereb, J. (1992). Resurgence of tuberculosis in children. *The Journal of Pediatrics, 120*, 839–855.

Steiner, G.L. (1990). Children, families and AIDS: Psychosocial and psychotherapeutic aspects. *N.J. Psychologist, 40*(3), 11–14.

Strauss, J., Abitol, C., Zilleruelo, G., et al. (1990). Renal disease in children with the acquired immunodeficiency syndrome. *New England Journal of Medicine, 321*(10), 625–630.

Strauss, J., Zilleruelo, G., Abitbol, C., Montane, B. (1992). Pediatric AIDS and renal genitourinary changes. In R.

Yogev & E. Connor (Eds.), *Management of HIV infection in infants and children* (pp. 389–405). St. Louis: Mosby–Year Book.

Tasker, M. (1992). *How can I tell you?* Bethesda, MD: Association for the Care of Children's Health.

Thorne, S.E., Robinson, C.A. (1989). Guarded alliance: Health care relationships in chronic illness. *Image: Journal of Nursing Scholarship, 21*, 153–157.

Tiblier, K.B., Walker, G., Rolland, J.S. (1989). Therapeutic issues when working with families of persons with AIDS. In J. Macklin (Ed.), *AIDS and families* (pp. 81–128). New York: Harrington Park Press.

Vogel, L. (1992). Cardiac manifestations of pediatric AIDS. In R. Yogev & E. Connor (Eds.), *The child with HIV infection* (pp. 357–369). Chicago: Year Book Medical Publishers.

Wara, D., Luzuriaga, K., Martin, N., et al. (1993). Maternal transmission and diagnosis of human immunodeficiency virus during pregnancy. *Annals of the New York Academy of Sciences, 693*, 14–19.

Wasser, S., Gwinn, M., Fleming, P. (1993). Urban-nonurban distribution of HIV infection in childbearing women in the United States. *Journal of Acquired Immunodeficiency Syndromes, 6*(9) 1035–1041.

Winter, H., Chang, T. (1993). Nutrition in children with HIV infection. *Pediatric HIV Forum Focus on Nutrition, 1*(2), 1–5.

Wiznia, A., Nichols, S. (1990). Organ system involvement in HIV-infected children. *Pediatric Annals, 19*, 475–476, 479–481.

Nursing Care of the Adolescent

Martha W. Moon

Adolescents are the next wave of persons to be affected by the HIV epidemic. Because of the 7- to 9-year latency period between HIV infection and the onset of AIDS-defining illnesses, many adolescents who are infected with HIV will not have AIDS until they are adults (Persaud et al., 1992; Weiss, 1993). Thus they will not be accounted for in AIDS surveillance data, with the result that adolescent issues will be underrepresented in AIDS policy and funding discussions. The fact that many HIV-infected adolescents are unaware of their HIV status or appear to be in good health makes it difficult to conduct effective education, treatment, and research. It is important that nurses understand adolescent risks of having HIV infection, methods of prevention, and how to care for adolescents who have HIV or AIDS. This chapter will review the epidemiology of HIV in adolescents, pertinent growth and developmental issues, risk factors, prevention and education strategies, care of HIV-infected youth, and nursing research to date and the gaps therein.

ADOLESCENTS AND HIV EPIDEMIOLOGY

The Centers for Disease Control and Prevention (CDC) reports adolescent patients with AIDS from 13 to 19 years of age (CDC, 1993). This age category has been criticized by several experts in the field of AIDS in adolescents, who recommend the period from 13 to 21 years of age because they believe that 13- to 19-year-olds are unable to appreciate HIV transmission, inasmuch as few adolescents actually have AIDS by age 19 years (Kunins et al., 1993). How adolescence is defined

is an important issue for service delivery, particularly in regard to legal and consent issues. This chapter will define adolescence as the period from 13 to 19 years of age unless otherwise noted.

Diagnosed AIDS Cases

As of June 30, 1993, there were 1,301 reported cases of AIDS in the 13- to 19-year age range (CDC, 1993). Although this number may appear small, the concern is that because of the latency period between HIV infection and the onset of AIDS (at which time the infection is reported), many adolescents are currently infected but not included in AIDS surveillance data. It may be 7 to 9 years before AIDS develops in an adolescent with HIV infection; thus it is important to look at the number of reported cases of AIDS in the 20- to 24-year age category, which may more accurately reflect the prevalence of HIV in the adolescent population. In the 20- to 24-year age range, there were 11,840 reported cases of AIDS as of June 30, 1993 (CDC, 1993). Comparing the exposure categories for these two age groups is useful in determining the risk factors for HIV infection in adolescents. Table 7–1 provides the transmission route by age and gender of the diagnosed AIDS cases in the 13- to 19-year and the 20- to 24-year age ranges.

As in adults, sexual activity and injection drug use are the two risk activities that lead to AIDS in adolescents. Also noteworthy from the surveillance data is the lower ratio of male to female cases among adolescents (4:1), in comparison with that among adults (9:1). Fifty-three percent of male adolescents and young adults aged 13 to 24 years who have

Table 7–1. Cumulative Totals of AIDS Cases in Adolescents and Young Adults Under Age 25 Years, by Gender and Exposure Category Through June 1993, in the United States

	ADOLESCENTS AGED 13–19 YEARS CUMULATIVE TOTAL		YOUNG ADULTS AGED 20–24 YEARS CUMULATIVE TOTAL	
	NO.	(%)	NO.	(%)
Male exposure category				
Men who have sex with men	299	(33)	6,116	(65)
Injecting drug use	61	(7)	1,166	(12)
Men who have sex with men and inject drugs	42	(5)	995	(11)
Hemophilia/coagulation disorder	409	(45)	352	(4)
Heterosexual contact	28	(3)	330	(3)
Receipt of blood transfusion	36	(4)	78	(1)
Risk not identified	38	(4)	409	(4)
Male subtotal	913	(100)	9,446	(100)
Female exposure category				
Injecting drug use	82	(21)	847	(35)
Hemophilia/coagulation disorder	4	(0)	8	(0)
Heterosexual contact	208	(54)	1,193	(50)
Receipt of blood transfusion	36	(9)	79	(3)
Risk not identified	58	(15)	267	(11)
Female subtotal	388	(100)	2,394	(100)
Total	1,301		11,840	

Data from Centers for Disease Control and Prevention (1993). *HIV/AIDS Surveillance Report* 5(2), 1–19.

AIDS are black, Latino, Asian, or American Indian, and 75% of female adolescents and young adults with AIDS are from these racial/ethnic groups. In adults, these proportions are 44% and 74%, respectively. As with adults, AIDS disproportionately affects nonwhite adolescents.

Figures 7–1 and 7–2 show the exposure categories for male and female patients with AIDS by age group. Note that by age 20 to 24 years, homosexual-bisexual transmission is the predominant category of risk for young men with AIDS, which mirrors that of adult men with AIDS. It is thought that the majority of the 20- to 24-year-old patients were exposed to HIV when they were younger adolescents. Note in Figure 7–2 that heterosexual transmission is the largest category of risk for adolescent girls, even more so than for adult women, who are at risk primarily because of injection drug use.

HIV Seroprevalence

The number of AIDS cases shown in column 1 of Table 7–1 reflects only those cases in which individuals have been infected with HIV early enough to have AIDS as adolescents, or before age 19 years. To date, no seroprevalence study has described HIV infection among a random sample of adolescents (Kunins et al., 1993), and few HIV seroprevalence studies have included adolescents. Thus there is currently no way to determine seroprevalence among adolescents as a group. A few studies have been conducted on special populations of adolescents, including applicants to the U.S. military services, Job Corps applicants, and adolescent clients at selected runaway and homeless shelters.

HIV seroprevalence was 34 per 100,000 among 1,141,164 youths less than 20 years of age applying for military service between October 1985 and March 1989 (Burke et al.,

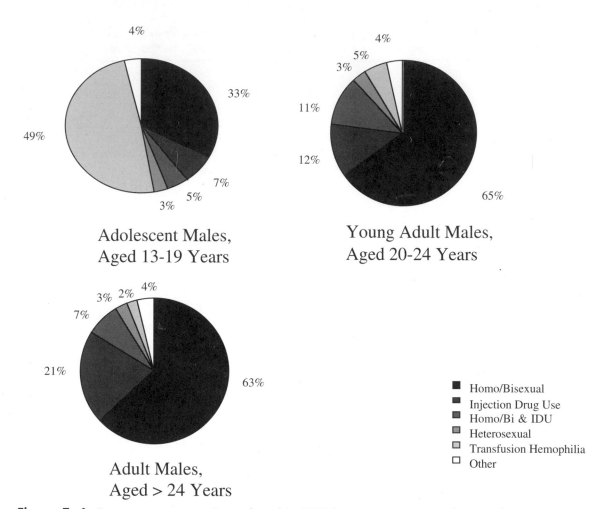

Figure 7–1. Exposure categories for males with AIDS by age group. (Data from Centers for Disease Control and Prevention (1993). *HIV/AIDS Surveillance Report, 5*(2), 1–19.)

1990). The prevalence among black adolescent applicants (106 per 100,000) was greater than among white (18 per 100,000) or Hispanic applicants (31 per 100,000) (Burke et al., 1990). HIV prevalences among adolescent applicants to military service were greater among those who were nonwhite, who lived in densely populated counties, and who lived in metropolitan areas with high incidences of reported cases of AIDS (Burke et al., 1990). The HIV prevalences drawn from this study are lower than those from other studies (see below). One explanation is that male adolescents at highest risk for HIV may be underrepresented in the population of military applicants because of self-exclusion as a result of same-gender sexual activities.

HIV seroprevalence was 360 per 100,000 among all 137,209 Job Corps applicants aged 16 to 21 years who were screened from October 1987 through February 1990 (St. Louis et al., 1991). Seroprevalence in Job Corps applicants increased with the age of applicants and with the size of the statistical metropolitan area in which they lived. By age 21 years, the HIV seroprevalence was 890 per 100,000. Seroprevalence varied by ethnicity; the rate of increase for black applicants was 210 per 100,000 per year, for Hispanic applicants, 150 per 100,000 per year, and for white applicants, 70 per 100,000 per year. For black and Hispanic 21-year-old applicants from large Northeastern cities, seroprevalence reached 2,480 per 100,000 (2.48%), or 1 in 40 (St.

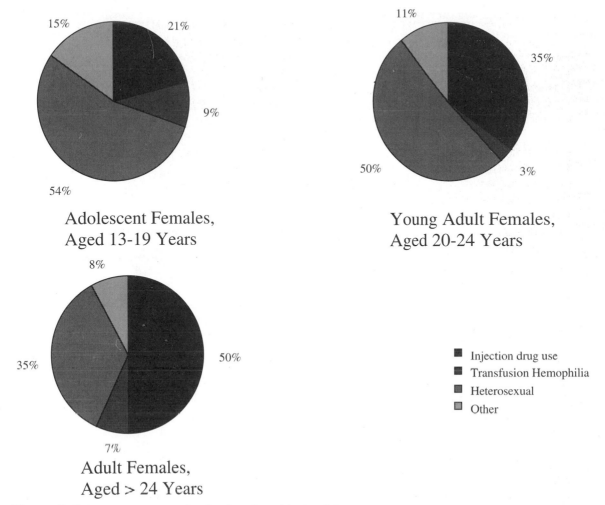

15%   21%

9%

54%

Adolescent Females,
Aged 13-19 Years

11%

35%

50%   3%

Young Adult Females,
Aged 20-24 Years

8%

35%   50%

7%

Adult Females,
Aged > 24 Years

■ Injection drug use
■ Transfusion Hemophilia
■ Heterosexual
□ Other

Figure 7–2. Exposure categories for females with AIDS by age group. (Data from Centers for Disease Control and Prevention (1993). *HIV/AIDS Surveillance Report*, 5(2), 1–19.)

Louis et al., 1991). The HIV seroprevalence in Job Corps and U.S. military applicants is low, however, compared with that in street youth.

A study of 2,667 homeless and street youth conducted in a shelter in New York City found that 5,300 per 100,000 overall had HIV antibodies. By age, the seroprevalence went from 2.2% of 15- to 16-year-olds to 8.6% of 20-year-olds tested (Stricof et al., 1991). By gender, 4.2% of female clients and 6.0% of male clients had HIV antibodies. HIV testing was conducted on all clients of the shelter who underwent an initial medical evaluation between Oct. 1, 1987, and Dec. 31, 1989; thus this study sample was fairly representative of homeless and runaway youth seeking care at shelters in New York City at the time. Street youth are more likely than other at-risk adolescents to inject drugs and to have unprotected sexual activities in exchange for food, shelter, and drugs, which may account for this dramatically higher rate of HIV prevalence than in the military applicants or the Job Corps applicants (Stricof et al., 1991; St. Louis et al., 1991).

In seroprevalence surveys conducted in 1993 among youth attending clinics at homeless youth centers in San Francisco, HIV seroprevalence was 26% among men who have sex with men, 50% among men who have sex with men and who are injection drug users (IDUs), 0% among heterosexual male IDUs, 2.8% among heterosexual female clients, 0.7% among male heterosexual clients who are not IDUs, and 0.8% among female heterosexual clients who are not IDUs (Givertz & Katz, 1993).

The increasing incidence of AIDS and the high rates of HIV infection among young persons in their early and mid twenties lends urgency to the need for effective HIV prevention programs for adolescents. Adolescents may not yet have established their sexual habits, and if safer behaviors can become their norm, then there is an opportunity to limit infection in the next generation (Mann et al., 1992).

ADOLESCENT DEVELOPMENT

The unique developmental stages of adolescence add complexity to issues surrounding HIV risk and infection among teenagers. Risk taking is normal during adolescence (Irwin, 1993) but may have deadly consequences in the context of the HIV epidemic.

Identity Formation and Limits

Tremendous confusion and risk taking occurs during this stage as adolescents acquire a sense of identity. Erikson's psychosocial theory of human development describes adolescents' struggles with personal identity versus identity confusion (Erikson, 1963). Subsumed under this task are sexual identity and orientation, choices about types and frequency of sexual activity, and use of recreational drugs (Janke, 1989).

Peer group and family are important in the development of adolescent behavior and behavior related to the acquisition of HIV. Havighurst's learning theory emphasizes society's influence on behavior and personal development. He believed that human behavior is learned behavior (Havighurst, 1972).

Living in the Present

There is tendency for adolescents to think about the present without thought of future consequences. This may translate into a sense of immunity from HIV in adolescents. Piaget's theory of cognitive development emphasizes the importance of continuous interaction between individuals and their environment. Adolescents are struggling with formal operational thought, which involves the transition from concrete thinking to abstract thinking (Piaget, 1969). Because of the inability to think abstractly, many adolescents cannot correlate the risk of infection today with the consequence of having AIDS in the future.

The Role of the Environment

The Panel on High-Risk Youth of the National Research Council (1993), which recently released its findings regarding adolescent risk taking, concluded that the environments, or settings, in which adolescents live are the most important factors determining risk behaviors, with family income being the most critical factor in determining in which setting an adolescent lives. Financial status determines the location or neighborhood in which an adolescent is raised, the presence or absence of a parent from the home, whether there is enough food to eat, the school the adolescent attends, and whether the adolescent even attends school. Understanding the implications of violence, crime, poverty, abuse, malnutrition, drugs, and the juvenile justice and welfare systems for the lives and behaviors of adolescents is the challenge of many researchers today (Bell & Bell, 1993; Garbarino et al., 1992; Panel on High-Risk Youth, 1993). The interaction between the environment and development is critical in defining subsequent risk behaviors in adolescents.

SPECIFIC RISK FACTORS FOR HIV IN ADOLESCENTS

Risk factors can be understood from an ecologic framework, that is, by looking at the environment of the developing adolescent in conjunction with the developmental stage, historical factors, and predisposing biologic factors. Hemophilia is considered to be a predisposing biologic factor that put persons at risk for HIV infection before 1985. The other factors reviewed are not biologic but are important determinants of risk taking.

Hemophilia

As of 1993, 45% of male adolescents with AIDS diagnosed between the ages of 13 and 19 years and 6% of young men with AIDS diagnosed between the ages of 20 and 24 years were exposed to HIV because of hemophilia or a coagulation disorder (CDC, 1993). Only 12 adolescent girls and young adult women with hemophilia (aged 13 to 24 years) had AIDS as of this time. Before the screening of blood products for HIV antibodies in 1985, many persons with hemophilia were exposed to HIV through transfusions of HIV-infected blood products. The CDC reports that about 70% of persons with hemophilia A (factor VIII deficiency) and 35% of persons with hemophilia B (factor IX deficiency) were HIV seropositive (CDC, 1987). Without new breakthroughs in AIDS treatments, it is assumed that these persons will eventually have AIDS. The current risk to those with hemophilia for HIV infection is small because of the screening of blood products for HIV. Thus the number of adolescents with hemophilia who are infected with HIV because of blood transfusions should decrease with time as this risk factor diminishes.

Sexual Behaviors

HIV infection can be transmitted from one person to another through sexual activities in which blood and body fluids are shared. Sexual activities can be consensual, both persons agreeing to participate, or nonconsensual, one person not agreeing to participate without coercion or threat. Unprotected or unsafe sexual activities that can lead to HIV infection occur in both categories.

Nonconsensual Sexual Behaviors
Sexual Abuse. The transmission of HIV to children and adolescents through sexual abuse is well documented, but its frequency is unknown (Gellert et al., 1993). Although the incidence of HIV infection is small relative to other exposure categories, it may explain some of the reported cases of AIDS in young adolescents who were not infected perinatally or through blood transfusions. Not only is sexual abuse a direct means of contracting HIV infection (from an HIV-infected perpetrator), but a history of sexual abuse can affect subsequent behaviors of the survivor. Researchers concur that the sexually abused adolescent is at heightened risk for HIV infection (Allers et al., 1993). Two factors contributing to this increased risk include (1) the abused adolescents' focus on present survival, which outweighs any concerns for future health, and (2) the adolescent survivors' depression, passive suicidal behaviors, and the view that exposure to HIV is a way to end their worries (Allers et al., 1993).

Adolescents who were sexually abused as children are more likely than others to engage in high-risk sexual activity such as prostitution or sex with multiple partners without contraception or condom use (Friedrich, 1993). Such behavior will, in turn, increase their risk for contracting HIV or other sexually transmitted diseases (STDs). Several studies reviewed below have documented the relation between a history of sexual abuse and subsequent sexual acting out, drug use, and risk taking.

One study of HIV transmission in heterosexual adults found that approximately half of the women and one fifth of the men reported a history of rape during childhood or adulthood (Zierler et al., 1991). Twenty-eight percent of the women and 15% of the men recalled that they had been sexually abused during childhood or adolescence. Survivors of childhood sexual abuse, both men and women, were four times more likely to report having worked as prostitutes at some time than were those who reported no history of abuse. In adults with no history of injection drug use, survivors of sexual abuse had 70% and 80% greater rates of tranquilizer and heavy alcohol use, respectively, than persons reporting no sexual abuse (Zierler et al., 1991). In a study of 34 HIV-infected adolescents and young adults (aged 12 to 20 years), 41% admitted to a history of sexual abuse by their caretaker (Dekker et al., 1990). The authors point out that sexual abuse may be the sentinel event in the lives of HIV-infected adolescents and young adults.

Polit and colleagues (1990), in a study of 177 adolescent women who were part of the public child welfare system, found that victims of sexual abuse were more likely to have engaged in voluntary sexual intercourse than those who had not been sexually abused. Burgess and associates (1987) found a link between childhood sexual abuse and later drug abuse, juvenile delinquency, and criminal behavior in 34 adolescents. Cunningham and associates (1991) also found a significant relationship between previous sexual abuse and HIV infection in a cohort of randomly sampled adolescents (n = 602) from public health clinics in 10 U.S. cities.

Adolescents who are living on the street are at particular risk for HIV infection. Pennbridge and colleagues (1990) estimated that 36% of street youth run from physical or sexual abuse, 44% leave because of other severe long-term problems such as substance-abusing parents, and 20% leave because of temporary or less severe crises such as divorce, sickness, and school problems. Up to 73% of female runaways may have experienced some form of sexual abuse (McCormack et al., 1986). Comparing the extent of sexual abuse among runaways with that among all teenagers is difficult, because two thirds of all cases are not reported to the proper authorities (American Humane Association, 1984). Some studies estimate that as many as 20% of all adolescents experience incestuous sexual abuse (Kercher & McShane, 1984); estimates of any form of sexual abuse range from 20% (Kercher & McShane, 1984) to 38% (Russell, 1984). In a study by Janus and associates (1987), 38.2% of the 89 adolescent male runaways interviewed had been sexually abused.

A study of a small sample of hospitalized adolescent psychiatric patients identified cutting behavior, defined as self-mutilation with sharp instruments without conscious suicidal intent, as a previously unreported risk behavior for HIV infection. The study found that a high proportion of adolescents in this sample shared cutting implements with other adolescents, thereby increasing the risk of HIV infection. A significant association was identified between adolescents who reported sexual abuse and those reporting cutting behavior in this sample (DiClemente et al., 1991).

Sexual abuse may lead to HIV infection directly, through exchange of body fluids, or indirectly, through survivors' increased risk activities. The risk of HIV infection is especially great for runaway or homeless adolescents who lack physical, emotional, and economic support.

Economically Coerced Sexual Activities. Adolescent prostitutes are at particular risk for HIV infection, especially if they are street youth and are dependent on trading sex for money in order to live. Several studies of special populations suggest a connection between child sexual abuse and later prostitution (Browne & Finkelhor, 1986). Seng (1989) found, in a review of literature on male and female prostitutes, that early childhood sexual abuse and incest were a recurring characteristic in this population. Prevalence of this characteristic varied in the literature between 28.5% and 65% for female prostitutes and between 10% and 85.5% for male prostitutes (Seng, 1989). Silbert and Pines (1982) found that 60% of the female subjects that they studied who were involved in prostitution had been sexually abused, and James and Meyerding (1977) found that 86% of their sample of male prostitutes in Boston had a history of sexual abuse. Yates and colleagues (1991) found that 56% of the runaway adolescents in their study in Los Angeles who were involved in prostitution had a history of sexual abuse, compared with 17% of those who were not involved in prostitution. The early experience with sex is thought to condition children to view sex as a means of communication with adults while retaining a level of control as prostitutes that was lacking in their earlier victim-abuser relationships (Rickel & Hendren, 1993). Additionally, the low self-esteem characteristic of sexually abused children aids the pimp and the prostitute in keeping the latter in this self-abusing profession (Rickel & Hendren, 1993).

Runaway adolescents must cope with the dangers and stress of living on the street. Fewer than 10% are ready to live independently (Pennbridge et al., 1990). Few of them have marketable job skills for legitimate occupations, and many turn to illicit activities, including prostitution and selling drugs as a means of survival (Yates et al., 1991). Both male and female adolescents engage in prostitution. Estimates of runaways who engage in prostitution range from 54% (U.S. Public Health Service, 1991) to 63% (Schram & Giovengo, 1991). As with female adolescents, most adolescent male prostitutes are runaways (Rickel & Hendren, 1993). Male runaways quickly find that prostitution is an easy way to make money, and they may find themselves in this lifestyle with no prior intention of selling themselves for sex (Rickel & Hendren, 1993). Adolescent male prostitutes may be heterosexually or homosexually identified. Young prostitutes are at the mercy of those who pay for their services. Many prostitutes are paid extra for sex without a condom. To many adolescents who cannot think past the present, this may seem a small price to pay for needed cash.

Unprotected Recreational/Comfort Sexual Activities. Recreational sexual activities are those which are consensual and are engaged in for pleasure. Comfort sexual activities are engaged in by persons who are lonely in an attempt to gain a sense of security or reassurance through intimacy. Approximately half of American teenagers have had sexual intercourse by age 18 years (Castro, 1990). One large national study has documented an overall increase in women aged 15 to 19 years who reported having had premarital sexual intercourse from 28.6% in 1970 to 51.5% in 1988 (CDC, 1991).

In a 1988 analysis of data from the National Survey of Family Growth (n = 8,450 women 15 to 44 years of age), the investigators found that 25.6% of 15-year-old, 31.8% of 16-year-old, 51.0% of 17-year-old, 69.5% of 18-year-old, and 75.3% of 19-year-old adolescent women reported having had premarital sexual intercourse (CDC, 1991). In the recent National Survey of Adolescent Males, 20% of black male adolescents said that their first intercourse took place before age 13 years, compared with only 3% of white and 4% of Hispanic male adolescents. Stated differently, black male adolescents are about 2 years

ahead of white and Hispanic male adolescents in the proportion who report having had sexual intercourse by a given age (Miller et al., 1993). In the National Youth Risk Behavior Survey, which collected data from 11,631 students in grades 9 to 12, 48% of female students of all races and 60.8% of male students of all races reported having had sexual intercourse (CDC, 1992). These data also showed that more black male and female adolescents reported a history of sexual intercourse (60.0% black female and 87.8% black male adolescents) than did their white or Hispanic counterparts (47.0% white female and 56.4% white male adolescents; 45.0% Hispanic female and 63.0% Hispanic male adolescents) (CDC, 1992).

Many studies show that despite the facts that AIDS education messages consistently include information about condom use, and that adolescents are able to state that condoms are effective in helping to prevent HIV infection and other STDs, they are not using them (Barling, 1990; Kegeles et al., 1988; DiClemente et al., 1988; Keller et al., 1991; Rickert et al., 1989; Nader et al., 1989). In the most recent wave of the National Survey of Adolescent Males (n = 1,676), the proportion of young male subjects using condoms at last intercourse fell by 12 percentage points, from 56% in 1988 to 44% in 1991 (Ku et al., 1993). In a San Francisco sample of homeless youth, only 39.3% of those who reported engaging in vaginal sex had used a condom during their last sex act (U.S. Public Health Service, 1991).

It is estimated that 17% to 37% of male adolescents participate in homosexual activity to orgasm on at least one occasion (Remafedi, 1988). Ten percent of all adults are homosexual, and homosexual identity may surface during adolescence (Janke, 1989). Studies differ on the age of homosexual identity formation for males, varying from age 14 years (Remafedi, 1987) to 19 to 21 years (Troiden, 1988). Savin-Williams and Rodriguez (1993) believe that it is easier today for youths to identify as gay because of the visibility of homosexuality in our culture. They argue that the media, AIDS, and local and state ordinances establishing gay rights have all made homosexuality more of a public issue than previously. They believe that this means that homosexually inclined youth are "coming out" at younger ages than ever before (Savin-Williams & Rodriguez, 1993). For those who do not deny their sexual preference and come out during adolescence, a different type of denial may occur. Because young gay men see AIDS only in older gay men, because of the long latency period of HIV infection, they falsely conclude that only older men are affected (Feldman, 1989). This denial can lead to the belief that sex with men their own age, or with those who look healthy, is free of HIV risk.

In a study of HIV risk-taking behavior among young gay men (n = 99) in three medium-sized West Coast communities, 43% reported having engaged in unprotected anal intercourse during the previous 6 months (Hays et al., 1990). Male adolescents who engaged in unprotected anal intercourse reported greater enjoyment of unprotected anal intercourse, perceived less risk of unprotected anal intercourse, labeled themselves as more at risk for AIDS, reported poorer communication skills with sexual partners, and were more likely to have a boyfriend/lover than men who had not engaged in high-risk sex. In addition, respondents perceived the likelihood of acquiring HIV from unprotected anal intercourse with young gay men to be significantly lower than with older gay men (Hays et al., 1990).

Young gay men are not allowed in gay bars and may not have access to gay newspapers, where much of the information about safe sex and HIV is disseminated. Therefore it cannot be assumed that they, as a group, are as informed about AIDS as the adult gay male community. Coates and colleagues (1989) discuss the vulnerability of the adolescent who is just beginning to explore homosexual feelings and activities. A runaway adolescent may act on feelings that otherwise would be restrained by parental control or monitoring, or by peer control.

Few HIV seroprevalence studies have been conducted on lesbians. In a study of 498 lesbians and bisexual women 17 years of age and older conducted in 1993 in San Francisco and Berkeley, California, 1.2% of lesbians and bisexual women were infected with HIV (San Francisco Department of Public Health, 1993). This study found no clear evidence of woman-to-woman transmission among the six HIV-infected women in the survey. All six infected women reported a history of either injection drug use or anal or vaginal sex with men. Only 3.8% of the survey participants were in the age range of 17 to 19 years, and none were infected at this time. Lesbians are susceptible to HIV infection through the same routes as other women—injection drug use, cutting, and unprotected penetrative sex with men. Prevention and education programs that frankly discuss women's risks of having HIV infection, regardless of whether they identify as lesbians, bisexuals, or heterosexuals, are needed.

Drug Use

Hein (1989) reported that there has been a decline in drug use, including marijuana, alcohol, and tobacco, among high school students since the early 1980s. The percentage of high school seniors using cocaine has decreased in the past 5 years. However, in the areas with high HIV prevalence, the high school dropout rate can be as high as 40%. In adolescents at highest risk of HIV acquisition, drug use patterns may be different from those of adolescents enrolled in schools. Kipke and associates (1993) found, in a study of 1,121 homeless and nonhomeless youth in Los Angeles, that homeless youth were significantly more likely to report the use of alcohol and illicit drugs, including involvement in injection drug use, than nonhomeless youth. These findings suggest that drug use may be higher in youth seen at community primary health clinics than in youth currently enrolled in schools.

In addition to injection drug use with needle sharing, which is a very high risk activity for HIV transmission, using drugs orally is associated with riskier sexual behaviors (Castro, 1990). An adolescent who is high on drugs, whether injected, smoked, or swallowed, may engage in high-risk activities not normally engaged in because of a decrease in

Table 7–2. Percentages of Female and Male Adolescents' Responses Regarding Why They Used Alcohol and Drugs Around Sexual Activities

RESPONSE	% FEMALES WHO USED ALCOHOL (n = 528)	% FEMALES WHO USED ILLEGAL SUBSTANCES (n = 387)	% MALES WHO USED ALCOHOL (n = 158)	% MALES WHO USED ILLEGAL SUBSTANCES (n = 113)
Easier to have sex	77	50	76	45
Enjoyed sex more	77	57	82	60
Worried less about birth control	49	38	65	61

Data from Moscicki, A., Millstein, S.G., Broering, J., Irwin, C.E., Jr. (1993). Risks of human immunodeficiency virus infection among adolescents attending three diverse clinics. *The Journal of Pediatrics, 122,* 813–820.

inhibitions. Adolescents who inject anabolic steroids, used for body building and strengthening, may also place themselves at risk of acquiring HIV infection if they share contaminated injection equipment (Blanken, 1993).

In a study of HIV risks among adolescents attending three clinics (n = 671 female and 207 male adolescents), 29% of female and 33% of male subjects used alcohol and drugs around sexual activity (Moscicki et al., 1993). Adolescents often use substances to enhance enjoyment of sex and to forget about their worries, thereby greatly increasing their risk of HIV infection (Table 7–2).

In another study that assessed the relation between alcohol and drug use during sexual activity and HIV risk–associated behavior in 108 inner-city black male adolescents, the investigators found that adolescents who reported a greater number of days on which they had sex while "high" reported more unprotected intercourse, a greater number of risky partners, and more frequent insertive anal intercourse than did those who reported fewer days on which they had sex while high (Jemmott & Jemmott, 1993).

Crack use and unprotected sex are also closely associated. In a study of 222 self-identified black adolescent crack users that looked at the relation between high-risk activities and the transmission of HIV and other STDs, investigators found that 73% of the respondents reported having engaged in at least one HIV risk activity. Half of the respondents combined sex with crack use, and only 26% of the male and 18% of the female adolescents had

used a condom in their last sexual encounter (Fullilove et al., 1990). One respondent in four reported having been involved in an exchange of sexual favors for money and/or drugs.

PREVENTION OF HIV RISK BEHAVIORS

During the early years of the HIV epidemic, policy makers paid little attention to adolescents as a susceptible population. Policy was focused on gay men, persons with hemophilia, IDUs, and infants born to HIV-infected mothers (Wilcox, 1990). Part of this lack of attention resulted from denial regarding adolescent sexuality, particularly homosexuality, coupled with a lack of understanding about the latency of HIV infection. A dearth of advocates to speak on behalf of adolescents played a critical role in the delay of initiatives aimed at this population. The role of vocal advocacy is well illustrated by the organization of the gay community early in the epidemic, which is credited with stemming the spread of HIV in that population (Shilts, 1987). With no organized interest group, adolescents, particularly disenfranchised adolescents such as incarcerated or runaway adolescents, were among the last vulnerable groups to be represented in the discussions about how money for HIV prevention and care should be spent. In the past few years, however, many programs have been developed and implemented for education and prevention of HIV in adolescent populations, both school-based and out-of-school youth.

It has been demonstrated consistently that adolescent HIV knowledge is a necessary but not a sufficient condition for adolescents to adopt preventive practices (Fisher & Fisher, 1992). Nevertheless, the vast majority of HIV risk reduction interventions for adolescents have focused and continue to focus on providing adolescents with HIV information (Fisher et al., 1992). Bandura (1992) argued that knowledge alone is insufficient for behavior change—that translating health knowledge into effective self-protection action against HIV infection requires social and self-regulative skills and a sense of personal power to exercise control over sexual situations. Teaching people safer sexual guidelines is easy; what is difficult is equipping them with skills that enable them to put the guidelines consistently into practice in the face of counteracting influences (Bandura, 1992). Perceived self-efficacy is concerned with individuals' belief that they can exert control over their motivation, behavior, and social environment. The weaker the perceived self-efficacy, the more that social and affective factors can increase the likelihood of risky behavior (Bandura, 1992). People must believe that they can control and change their own behavior. Behavior change must be modeled and reinforced before it can be incorporated into their behavior. The interventions by Walter and Vaughan (1993) and Kelly et al. (1989), discussed below, used Bandura's ideas about self-efficacy and modeling with some success in changing behaviors.

School-based Prevention and Education Models

Walter and Vaughan (1993) discussed a school-based AIDS risk reduction curriculum which they used in a sample of 1,316 New York City high school students. The curriculum focused on conveying facts about AIDS, fostering theoretically derived beliefs favorable to AIDS prevention, and teaching skills necessary for the successful performance of AIDS-preventive behaviors. Results included modest but significant effects in knowledge, beliefs, self-efficacy, and risk behavior scores for the students.

Catania and associates (1990) proposed a three-stage theoretical model that applies to a person's efforts to change sexual behaviors related to HIV transmission. The AIDS Risk Reduction Model (ARRM) focuses on social and psychologic factors that are hypothesized to influence (1) labeling of high-risk behaviors as problematic, (2) making a commitment to changing high-risk behaviors, and (3) seeking and enacting solutions directed at reducing high-risk activities. ARRM emphasizes the goal of understanding why people fail to progress over the change process. Factors identified as important include the following:

1. Knowledge of the risks associated with various sexual practices and ways of incorporating low-risk sexual activities into one's sexual relationships in a satisfying manner
2. Perceptions of susceptibility to contracting HIV
3. Perceived costs and benefits associated with reducing high-risk and increasing low-risk sexual activities
4. Self-efficacy beliefs
5. Emotional states
6. Social factors, including verbal communication skills, reference group norms, help-seeking processes, and social support

Boyer and Kegeles (1991) adapted the ARRM to the adolescent population and recommend that prevention programs for adolescents emphasize cognitive and behavioral skills training as well as education. They state that schools are the logical location for these prevention programs and that adolescents who are not in school (dropouts, runaways, street youth) are at increased risk of acquiring HIV and will have to be reached through other strategies. Data from and evaluation of these interventions are forthcoming.

Lewis et al. (1990) reviewed several school-based primary prevention programs. They believe that adolescent problem behavior is due to poor socialization in the family, which subsequently leads to early emotional and conduct problems in school, which leads to decreased learning and poor academic performance. Poor academic performance is linked to delinquency and drug use. Problems in school lead to disillusionment with schooling, withdrawal of effort, and rebelliousness, which contribute to further academic failure (Lewis et al., 1990). The authors suggested that there are seven characteristics of an effective school-based prevention program:

1. Prevention programs should be clearly derived from theories that recognize the multidimensionality of risk behaviors,
2. School-based prevention programs should be directed at influencing the general social milieu of the school, not as a separate entity, but as an integral part of school life,
3. Programs that promote positive influences on social development may be more effective than programs that attempt to counteract negative social norms,
4. Because socialization is a continuous process, prevention programs should also be comprehensive and long lasting,
5. School-based prevention programs should be incorporated into the overall mission of the school, rather than being introduced as independent units, to produce a widespread and enduring effect,
6. Prevention programs must be implemented early enough to precede the emergence of the problem behavior. Because it is harder to change established attitudes and behaviors than to prevent their initial formation, programs must be initiated so that they are preventive and not remedial,
7. Prevention programs must be monitored and evaluated carefully to ensure that they are being implemented as planned.

Many school districts have wrestled with the issue of condom distribution to their students. The evaluation of one program in which condoms are distributed in conjunction with HIV information under the supervision of the school nurses by faculty members indicates that more students would utilize the program if condoms were available from other students (peers) or from vending machines (U.S. Conference of Mayors, 1992).

Prevention and Education Programs for Street Youth

Many of the major cities that attract runaway adolescents have established outreach programs for these youth through public or private agencies. Several of these will be reviewed below.

Houston. Covenant House Texas (CHT) is a crisis shelter for runaway, homeless, and "throwaway" youth less than the age of 21 years located in the Inner Loop area of central Houston (U.S. Conference of Mayors, 1993). CHT assists youths by trying to reunite them with their families, helping them find jobs, helping them complete their education, and teaching them the skills needed to become independent and productive citizens while improving their self-esteem. CHT implemented the Teen Health Teaching Modules (THTM) curriculum, designed by the Rocky Mountain Center for Health Promotion, in Lakewood, Colorado. In addition to covering basic health issues, two AIDS-related modules were added. The curriculum was modified for their population and was tailored to meet the needs of different subsets of the population, including older adolescents, younger adolescents, and pregnant and parenting women.

New York City. At a homeless shelter in New York City, an AIDS education intervention was offered to 78 adolescent clients, and outcomes were compared with those for 67 runaways at another shelter (Rotheram-Borus et al., 1991). The intervention included general knowledge about HIV/AIDS, coping skills, access to health care and other resources, and individual barriers to safer sex. The outcomes measured were consistent condom use, high-risk patterns of sexual behavior, and sexual abstinence for 3 months. The investigators found that as the number of intervention sessions increased, runaways' reports of consistent condom use increased significantly, and their reports of engaging in high-risk patterns of sexual behavior decreased significantly. Abstinence did not change. In a previous study, Rotheram-Borus and Koopman (1991) found that 126 runaways demonstrated moderately high AIDS knowledge and beliefs endorsing AIDS prevention and that condom use and abstinence were directly related to beliefs about preventing AIDS.

San Francisco. At Larkin Street Youth Center, in San Francisco, California, outreach teams go out on the streets in the evenings to talk with adolescents, to distribute condoms and bleach, to give out HIV information, and to encourage them to stop by the clinic for health care. Once the street youth are in the clinic, the nurse practitioner can assess them individually for HIV-related risk behaviors and psychologic status, to determine whether the topic of HIV testing should be raised. The HIV antibody test is performed after two sessions of pretest counseling are given and informed consent is obtained. The pretest and posttest counseling sessions are used to give HIV information and to answer questions that the adolescent may have about HIV or risk behaviors (Goulart & Madover, 1991).

Seattle. The city of Seattle, Washington, offers services for street youth that include drop-in centers, shelters, drug treatment, and health care. A report addressing the needs of Seattle's homeless youth (Smart, 1991) points out that Seattle has made significant progress in addressing the needs but that gaps still exist in service provision to street youth. The Threshold Project is a residential treatment program designed to work with homeless and alienated young women who are approaching 18 years of age but lack the skills, values, and attitudes necessary to care for themselves and to assume the responsibilities of adulthood (Schram & Giovengo, 1991). The project offers a series of progressively more independent living experiences to young women who have a history of sexual, physical, or emotional abuse or neglect, and who had been or are at high risk of being involved in prostitution. In the initial 2 years of the project, 24 female clients were served. An evaluation of follow-up data on these adolescents showed that 42% of them lived in stable situations, were employed and/or attending school, were not misusing or abusing drugs, and were not involved in prostitution or other criminal activity.

Community-based Models of HIV Prevention

The two models reviewed below are not based in schools or shelters, but in community settings. They both offer content beyond education alone and may prove to be useful for prevention of HIV in the adolescent population.

Peer-counseled AIDS Education Program. Rickert and colleagues (1991) described a study in which they compared peer-led versus adult-led AIDS education programs on the knowledge, attitudes, and satisfaction of 82 adolescents with their education. The intervention consisted of one session in which adolescents received didactic information and viewed a videotape about AIDS transmission and prevention. The results showed that both adult and peer counselors were equally effective in promoting knowledge gains and appropriate attitude changes, but that more questions were asked of the peer counselors. The authors suggested that when education is presented by peer counselors, adolescents may be more likely to see AIDS as a personal danger and that peer counselors should be considered when comprehensive AIDS education programs are designed. The adolescents were recruited from local community and church organizations. This intervention has not been used with street youth, but given its brevity, it might prove effective for this transient population.

DiClemente (1993) believes that the use of peer educators as behavior-change agents is the most underutilized prevention strategy for adolescents. Trained peer educators may be a more credible source of information, they communicate in a language that is more likely to be understood, and they can serve as positive role models to dispel the misconception that most adolescents are engaging in high-risk behaviors.

Skills-Training Model. Kelly and associates (1989), in research on gay men, showed that there are psychologic factors that predict AIDS high-risk behaviors. These investigators developed a skills-training group model that has been effective in achieving long-range behavioral changes in gay male adults regarding HIV risk behaviors. The intervention consisted of twelve 75- to 90-minute weekly group sessions led by two clinical psychologists and two project assistants. Session content focused on AIDS risk education (two sessions), behavioral self-management skills training (three sessions), assertion training (three sessions), and relationship skills and social support development (three sessions). In the final session, participants identified the risk reduction changes they had made and the strategies they had used to make them. Their findings were that perceived peer norms concerning the acceptability of safer sex practices, AIDS health locus-of-control scores, knowledge of risk behaviors, age, and accuracy of personal risk estimation, but not personal HIV serostatus knowledge, were associated with change in high-risk and precaution-taking behavior. In a study with 104 gay men, Kelly and associates (1989) concluded that men changed their behaviors and had maintained these changes at the 8-month follow-up, as measured by self-reported sexual behaviors. This intervention has not been used with adolescents. The intervention as described requires a time commitment and a group setting, which may be difficult to implement in a population of street youth but may be successful as a school-based intervention.

HIV COUNSELING AND TESTING

The developmental stage of the adolescent must be taken into account during counseling for HIV testing. By establishing rapport and engaging in conversation with the adolescent, the counselor can determine the developmental level of the adolescent and then tailor the counseling to the adolescent's developmental needs. For example, the adolescent may be thinking concretely, be a magical thinker, be in denial, or be feeling invulnerable.

Many sites require more than one pretest counseling session because of the multiplicity of issues that need to be covered, coupled with the developmental issues of the adolescent. Adolescents need to understand the social, medical, psychologic, and legal consequences of learning their HIV antibody status (negative vs positive) (Table 7–3). The benefits of knowing one's HIV serostatus through HIV

Table 7–3. Elements of Pretest HIV Counseling for Adolescents

- Establish rapport
- Ensure confidentiality
- Assess developmental stage
- Conduct risk assessment
- Discuss methods of risk reduction
- Discuss the meaning and implications of the HIV test
- Conduct a risk/benefit analysis
- Investigate adolescent's coping history and develop future strategies
- Forecast and role-play possible reactions to a positive test result
- Forecast and role-play possible reactions to a negative test result
- Discuss the waiting period
- Investigate and help develop adolescent's support systems
- Discuss notifying partners
- Discuss confidentiality and determine capacity to consent
- Assist in reading and signing consent form

Data from Kunins, H., Hein, K., Futterman, D., Tapley, F., Elliot, A.S. (1993). Guide to adolescent HIV/AIDS program development. *Journal of Adolescent Health, 14,* 1S–140S.

antibody testing include potential access to medical treatments and services. These benefits must be weighed against the potential harm of knowing, including discrimination and negative psychologic outcomes, particularly in adolescents (Kunins et al., 1993). There is no evidence that knowledge of serostatus alone affects sexual or drug use behaviors (Kunins et al., 1993), so testing should not be used as a sole method of prevention. Testing should be voluntary, not mandatory, and the adolescent should decide whether it is to be confidential or anonymous.

Counseling adolescents for HIV antibody testing requires specialized training in some states because of the myriad of issues involved, many of which differ from those of adults. Nurses are advised to contact their local or state health department for protocols and policies regarding testing and counseling in adolescents. Suggestions for further information and protocols for HIV antibody testing in adolescents were given by Kunins and associates (1993) and by Tighe (1993).

CARE OF THE ADOLESCENT WITH HIV INFECTION

In many locations, there are no adolescent specialist providers, so adolescents receive care from childhood pediatricians or family practitioners. Regardless of the type of provider, the care of HIV-infected youth should be conducted in an adolescent-friendly environment. Adolescents should have access to providers whom they can trust not to disclose intimate information to their parents. Laws vary from state to state regarding consent and confidentiality, but in many states, HIV and STD treatment, pregnancy, and family planning care do not require parental consent (English, 1992).

Health histories for adolescents should include social, psychologic, sexual, drug use, and family histories, including direct questions about physical and sexual abuse (see Chapter 5). It is important to use concrete language, nonmedical jargon, and open-ended questions when one is talking with adolescents. Providers should make no assumptions about an adolescent's sexual identity, orientation, or activities. It is also important to elicit accurate information about drug use, including route, frequency, quantity, and sharing habits. The physical examination is similar to that in adults. Providers should include a sexual maturity rating, such as the one developed by Tanner (1962), which allows for concise description of the stage of development of secondary sexual characteristics.

Adolescents with HIV should be given their age-specified immunizations as recommended by the CDC, including pneumococcal vaccine, influenza vaccine (yearly), tetanus and diphtheria (Td) toxoids, and measles-mumps-rubella (MMR) vaccine. Hepatitis B vaccine is also recommended for those adolescents who do not have immunity (Kunins et al., 1993). Medically, treatment is based on adult guidelines (or pediatric guidelines if the adolescent is very small in stature) because of the lack of adolescent-specific guidelines. Because of the rapid changes in medical treatment for HIV and related illnesses, always consult the latest guidelines first. (See resource list at end of chapter.)

Special sensitivity is required because of developmental issues in adolescents. Many adolescents with HIV cope by denying their infection and resisting treatment regimens. Like many adults, these adolescents may wait until the last minute to seek care because of their denial. Providers should be aware of this and encourage regular visits even when the adolescents are well.

Adolescents may need special assistance in integrating their medications into their daily routine, as well as remembering their appointments and getting to referral sites. Providers can try problem solving with adolescents to determine which obstacles they need to overcome. Do they have bus money? Have they lost their pills? Are they not taking their pills at home because they do not want their families to know their diagnosis? Who is paying for their care and their medications? Are they on their parents' insurance plan or are they without assistance? With good case management, most low-income, runaway, or homeless adolescents can qualify for Medicaid and other forms of public assistance. Adolescents who are recently infected may not develop HIV-related illnesses for many years. It is important to ensure that infected adolescents understand how to prevent transmission of HIV and how to take care of themselves by preventing and recognizing the onset of opportunistic infections.

Primary care providers, including nurse practitioners, should be comfortable caring for HIV-infected adolescents, but may want backup from a specialist on occasion. In many urban areas in the United States, specialized adolescent HIV centers have been developed. AIDS-indicator diseases, such as *Pneumocystis carinii* pneumonia, wasting syndrome, and candidiasis are the same for adolescents as for adults. See Chapters 4 and 5 for more about these diseases and their clinical management guidelines.

ETHICAL AND LEGAL CONSIDERATIONS FOR ADOLESCENTS

Access to HIV treatment and research for adolescents raises many ethical and legal concerns because of their age and level of maturity. These include questions regarding adolescents' ability to give true informed consent, concerns about confidentiality and disclosure of HIV test results, and potential conflicts between research and service delivery. For many adolescents, as well as adults, with HIV, enrollment in clinical trials may provide the only access to quality care.

Access to Clinical Trials

Access to clinical trials is a complex issue. For a patient to gain access, he or she must have (1) a provider who is knowledgeable about HIV and the available trials, and who is willing to refer the patient to the trial and (2) access to the clinical trial site, meaning time off work or school to meet appointments, transportation to and from the site, and the ability to negotiate the building after arrival at the site. Some urban areas are fortunate to have active community-based research programs, but many locations in the United States are limited to the federally funded ACTG (AIDS Clinical Trials Group). This system, sponsored by the National Institute of Allergy and Infectious Diseases (NIAID), includes 41 research institutions or AIDS Clinical Trial Units (ACTUs) across the country (Levine et al., 1991). The inclusion criteria for trials in the ACTG system are strictly defined to make the population as homogeneous as possible; as a result, many people are ineligible (Levine et al., 1991). Until recently a person had to be at least 18 years of age or be a child born with HIV infection in order to enroll in these clinical trials.

Pediatric trials began a few years ago, with the purpose of examining transmission from mother to infant *in utero*. Adolescents are excluded. They are too old for the pediatric trials and too young for the adult trials, the majority of which still have a minimum age of 18 years. As results of trials began to be disseminated, health care providers were left with no data specific to adolescents. Do providers prescribe zidovudine for adolescents on a pediatric schedule or on an adult schedule? How do adolescents respond to zidovudine? Answers to these questions are still unknown

because of the almost complete absence of adolescents in clinical trials.

In 1991, NIAID agreed to fund six sites throughout the United States for enrollment of adolescents in the existing ACTU studies. No other funding for including adolescents in preexisting trials and no other clinical trials specifically for adolescents are known to exist at this time. Whereas clinical trials have been well accepted in the adult gay community as a means of access to care, as well as a means of altruism, the recent initiative to recruit adolescents into trials has not been as successful. The reasons are currently being investigated.

Under the regulations promulgated by the federal government governing human subjects research (U.S. Department of Health and Human Services Rules and Regulations 45 CFR 46), parents must give permission (distinguished from *consent*) before their children may participate in research, but in most instances minors retain the power of *assent*, which is essentially a veto power (Melton, 1989). This divided authority is based on the assumption that parents will act in the best interests of their children. How does this apply to an adolescent who has run away from an abusive relationship with the parents? Are abusive parents acting in the "best interest of the child"? Fortunately, the federal regulations provide that minors may consent to research in situations in which they would be able to consent to treatment, as well as stating that parental permission may be waived "if the IRB [institutional review board] determines that a research protocol is designed for conditions or for a subject population for which parental or guardian permission is not a reasonable requirement to protect the subjects (for example, neglected or abused children)" (Levine, 1986, p. 412).

Access to Clinical Care

The legal issues surrounding adolescents' rights are ambiguous. Melton (1989) states that the trends in children's law are toward ever-increasing recognition of liberty and privacy for youth, recognition of privacy for families, and coercive intervention in the lives of children, youth, and families. He also describes a rise in the "new paternalism" in America, which is a reconceptualization in recent years of social problems as problems of public health and a corresponding willingness to regulate unhealthy behavior, especially that of adolescents (Melton, 1989).

The provisions for minors' independent consent to treatment vary from state to state and are often unclear. Even if a provision for independent consent to treatment is clearly available, such a provision cannot be presumed by itself to create a right to consent to related research under *state* law. The federal regulations providing for research without parental consent do not resolve the matter (Melton, 1989).

Criteria for legal emancipation of minors also vary from state to state. The consequences of emancipation generally include termination of parents' obligation of support and authorization for emancipated minors to establish their own residence and to enter into binding contracts (English, 1990). In addition, many states have statutes regarding "medically emancipated minors," which include minors who are older than a specified age, pregnant minors, minor parents, minors who have run away from home, and minors who are living apart from their parents and managing their own financial affairs, even if they are not considered fully emancipated (English, 1990). States differ on how medically emancipated minors are defined, but services for which these minors are most commonly permitted to give their own consent are pregnancy-related care and family planning services, including contraception; diagnosis and treatment of sexually transmitted or contagious diseases, including HIV infection; treatment of substance abuse problems; and outpatient mental health counseling. These statutes reflect a public policy of encouraging adolescents to seek care for problems that, if left untreated, not only would jeopardize their own health and welfare but also would create public health hazards and significant social burdens (Capron, 1982). Nurses should be aware of the laws regarding care for adolescents with HIV infection in the state in which they practice.

In a hospital setting, who has the right and responsibility to tell the adolescent the truth about medical diagnosis and prognosis? The nurse or nurse practitioner spends more time with the patient than does the physician, particularly in the clinic or hospital setting. If the nurse establishes a good rapport with the patient, most likely the nurse will be the one who gains the adolescent's trust. The nurse should make every effort to be present when the physician is discussing treatment plans with the patient, but, if not, the nurse can ask the patient what the physician said and then clarify or elaborate for the patient (Farrell, 1987). The nurse can act as liaison between physician and patient. Remember that the adolescent may not be able to understand abstract concepts, so it is important to speak in terms as concrete as possible without changing the content of the subject.

What if the family does not believe that the adolescent should know his or her diagnosis or prognosis? The nurse can assist in the decision making regarding whether the patient is able to understand and cope with the truth and can speak with the family and the physician about the ramifications of withholding this information. As part of the nursing assessment, the nurse should assess the adolescent's psychologic functioning and be aware that suicide is always a potential in this population (Low & Andrews, 1990), not only because of the stress of adolescence, but because of the stress of being infected with HIV (Farrell, 1987). Mental health consultation should be established immediately if this seems to be a present danger.

REVIEW OF NURSING RESEARCH ON ADOLESCENTS AND HIV

Nurses have been actively conducting research and writing on several topics related to adolescents and HIV infection. These topics include knowledge, attitudes, beliefs, and practices; gay youth and AIDS; and mental health issues. A brief review of these recent articles will follow.

Knowledge, Attitudes, Beliefs, and Practices Research

In the area of knowledge, attitudes, beliefs, and practices (KABP), nurses are conducting research on providers, adolescents, students, and student nurses. A nurse investigator has conducted research with black male and female adolescents, and has measured the intention to use condoms after an AIDS-related intervention with young black women (Jemmott, 1993; Jemmott & Jemmott, 1992). The investigators found that women scored higher in the intention to use condoms, AIDS knowledge, outcome expectancies regarding condom use, and self-efficacy to use condoms after the intervention than before the intervention. Robb and colleagues (1991) conducted a telephone survey among university students to assess knowledge of AIDS transmission, prevalence, and infectivity. They concluded that students are in need of education that stresses the ways that AIDS is *not* transmitted.

DuRant and associates (1992) looked at AIDS knowledge and perceived risk of HIV infection in eleventh- and twelfth-grade students and found that many adolescents incorrectly answered questions on the survey. Walker (1992) surveyed high school students for knowledge of and risk behaviors for HIV infection and found that the students had the knowledge but were still engaging in risky behaviors. Tyden and colleagues (1991) conducted a survey of adolescents in secondary school in Sweden to assess their sexual behaviors. The students had a low rate of condom usage. In another study of the evaluation of a school-based AIDS education program, the investigators found that the program was effective in affecting adolescents' knowledge, attitudes, and beliefs (Alteneder et al. 1992). DiIorio and associates (1992) developed an instrument to measure use of safe sex practices among adolescents. The results established construct validity for the Safe Sex Behavior Questionnaire, which they designed.

Stierborg (1992) assessed nursing students' knowledge about HIV in Sydney. The investigator found that nursing students with AIDS care experience had significantly more positive attitudes than those who had no such experience, and concluded that training programs should include experiential learning to address fear, discomfort, and anxiety about HIV. Campbell and colleagues (1991) studied knowledge, attitudes, and behavior in relation to AIDS among registered nurses who practiced in a hospital setting. They found a considerable level of misinformation, mistrust, and fear regarding AIDS among registered nurses practicing in the hospital setting.

Research on Special Needs of Gay Youth

Taylor and Remafedi (1993) discussed the special needs of gay youth and suggested resources to help school nurses reach out to these underserved youth. Remafedi (1993) surveyed professionals who had been given training on adolescent homosexuality and HIV and a control group that had not received the training and found that those who had special training were most knowledgeable and most able to assist gay adolescents to find needed resources. Treadway and Yoakam (1992) described their experiences in working with the Youth and AIDS Project, a primary prevention program for gay and bisexual male youth aged 14 to 21 years. They discussed the youths' behaviors and coping strategies, and the role of school professionals in assisting these youth. Gay youth are often overlooked in research studies related to HIV.

Research on Mental Health Issues

Van Servellen and colleagues (1993) studied depression and hopelessness in persons with AIDS and found that stress-resistant resources are important in promoting health in persons with AIDS. Graham and Cates (1992) discussed the need for HIV education in the severely mentally ill population and suggested that effective programs can be developed by following community health nursing principles. The relation between mental health problems during adolescence and high-risk behaviors has been well documented (Stiffman et al., 1992). These mental health problems include conduct disorder, depression, anxiety, suicidality, and posttraumatic stress. Scharer and associates (1990) described the development and implementation of a health promotion and primary mental health prevention program for junior high students. Both cognitive and affective learning strategies were used in the program.

AREAS IN WHICH MORE NURSING RESEARCH IS NEEDED

More effective methods of affecting knowledge, attitudes, beliefs, and practices of adolescents regading HIV are urgently needed. The measurement of these variables seems clear; the difficulty lies in designing interventions that change these variables. The purely cognitive approach to HIV education has not proved to be effective in adolescents. Researchers are in a race against time to develop methods that will effectively change risky behaviors in adolescents and thus save this generation from AIDS. More research is necessary to determine the best method for each different subgroup of adolescents, including runaways, gay male adolescents, lesbians, drug users, ethnic and racial groups, and urban, rural, suburban, school-based, homeless, military, affluent, poor, and middle-class groups. How can safer sexual and drug-using practices be normalized in this population? The answers are not yet clear.

How is behavior change sustained in adolescents? The research shows a drop in the use of condoms during the past few years in this population. What must be done to make barrier protection the norm and not the exception for all sexual activities in our society?

Understanding the link between adolescents' risk behaviors and HIV and their histories of sexual and physical abuse through well-designed research studies should be a priority for the next few years in AIDS research. More nursing research is needed to understand gay youths' behaviors, attitudes, knowledge, beliefs, and need for intervention.

Research on intervention to decrease nurses' attitudes on homophobia and AIDS fear should be encouraged. What will help nurses overcome their fear, discomfort, and anxieties about caring for persons with HIV infection? What are the most effective training methods to dispel misconceptions? Creating environments in clinical settings that have high standards for quality care and a low tolerance for prejudice and bigotry should be a priority.

There is a great need for nursing research on female adolescents regarding sexual behaviors, knowledge, attitudes, beliefs, and effective interventions for prevention. Nurses interested in women's health will find a wealth of untapped research opportunities to investigate by interviewing and working with adolescent women who attend STD clinics, family planning clinics, or prenatal clinics; attend schools; or are involved in the social services or juvenile justice system.

Mental health issues are critical when dealing with adolescents and HIV. How does an HIV diagnosis affect an adolescent's sexual identity formation? How do adolescents with HIV infection compare with non-HIV infected youths in rates of depression or suicide? Why are adolescents not joining clinical trials? Why should they be interested? Which are the best ways of looking at this issue?

With the advent of health care reform, nurses' voices must be heard regarding policy on the role of nursing care in the HIV epidemic, the ethics of care, and nurses as advocates for adolescents. These voices will be stronger if backed by rigorous research on these issues.

Are there differences between adolescents and adults in the clinical manifestations of HIV infection? Do adolescents differ from adults in their responses, both psychologic and physiologic, to HIV? What are the most appropriate service models for adolescents with HIV?

SUMMARY

Adolescents are being infected by HIV at an alarming rate. Unless effective prevention and education interventions are implemented in the adolescent population, significant portions of this generation—including disproportionate numbers of nonwhite adolescents—will be devastated by HIV. Adolescents are infected with HIV through the same transmission routes as adults—through the exchange of blood and body fluids. The interplay of historical risk factors, such as sexual abuse and poverty, with adolescent development tasks may predispose an adolescent to engage in risk activities that can lead to HIV infection. These activities include unprotected sexual activity and drug use.

Education and prevention programs should include a social skills–building component, not just a cognitive approach. Adolescents must be instructed on and allowed to practice negotiating safe risk taking. HIV counseling and testing should be done in an adolescent-friendly setting and should take as much time as the adolescent needs to feel comfortable with the decision to test.

The main legal and ethical issues regarding adolescents and HIV involve informed consent for treatment and research, confidentiality, and access to care. Health care for HIV-infected youths is similar to that for adults, although the absence of adolescents in clinical trials has left many questions unanswered. Nurses should stay alert to new developments and changes in treatment regimens for HIV infection that may affect care of the adolescent. Nurses have been active in HIV-related research on adolescents. More research is needed in this area.

Acknowledgment: Thanks to Judy Heiman for her support, encouragement, and editorial skills.

REFERENCES

Allers, C.T., Benjack, K.J., White, J., Rousey, J.T. (1993). HIV vulnerability and the adult survivor of childhood sexual abuse. *Child Abuse & Neglect, 17,* 291–298.

Alteneder, R.R., Price, J.H., Telljohann, S.K., Didion, J., Locher, A. (1992). Using the PRECEDE model to determine junior high school students' knowledge, attitudes, and beliefs about AIDS. *Journal of School Health, 62,* 464–470.

American Humane Association (1984). *Trends in child abuse and neglect: A national perspective.* Denver: The Association.

Bandura, A. (1992). A social cognitive approach to the exercise of control over AIDS infection. In R.J. DiClemente (Ed.), *Adolescents and AIDS: A generation in jeopardy* (pp. 89–116). Newbury Park, CA: Sage.

Barling, N.R. (1990). Adolescents' attitudes towards AIDS precautions and intention to use condoms. *Psychological Reports, 67,* 883–890.

Bell, N.J., Bell, R.W. (Eds.) (1993). *Adolescent risk taking.* Newbury Park, CA: Sage.

Blanken, A.J. (1993). Measuring use of alcohol and other drugs among adolescents. *Public Health Reports, 108* (suppl 1), 25–30.

Boyer, C.B., Kegeles, S.M. (1991). AIDS risk and prevention among adolescents. *Social Science and Medicine, 33*(1), 11–23.

Browne, A., Finkelhor, D. (1986). Impact of child sexual abuse: A review of the research. *Psychological Bulletin, 99,* 66–77.

Burgess, A.W., Hartman, C.R., McCormack, A. (1987). Abused to abuser: Antecedents of socially deviant behaviors. *American Journal of Psychiatry, 144,* 1431–1436.

Burke, D.S., Brundage, J.F., Goldenbaum, M., Gardner, L.I., Peterson, M., Visintine, R., Redfield, R.R., and the Walter Reed Retrovirus Research Group (1990). Human immunodeficiency virus infections in teenagers: Seroprevalence among applicants for U.S. military service. *Journal of the American Medical Association, 263,* 2074–2077.

Campbell, S., Maki, M., Willenbring, K., Henry, K. (1991). AIDS-related knowledge, attitudes, and behaviors among 629 registered nurses at a Minnesota hospital: A descriptive study. *Journal of the Association of Nurses in AIDS Care, 2,* 15–23.

Capron, A.M. (1982). The competence of children as self-deciders in biomedical interventions. In W. Gaylin & R. Macklin (Eds.), *Who speaks for the child: The problems of proxy consent* (pp. 57–114). New York: Plenum Press.

Castro, O.C.R. (1990). Adolescents and AIDS: A special population. *NAACOG's Clinical Issues in Perinatal and Women's Health Nursing, 1,* 99–109.

Catania, J.A., Kegeles, S.M., Coates, T.J. (1990). Towards an understanding of risk behavior: An AIDS risk reduction model (ARRM). *Health Education Quarterly, 17*(1), 53–72.

Centers for Disease Control (1987). Human immunodeficiency virus infection in the United States: A review of current knowledge. *Morbidity and Mortality Weekly Report, 36*(S-6), 1–48.

Centers for Disease Control (1991). Premarital sexual experience among adolescent women—United States, 1970–1988. *Morbidity and Mortality Weekly Report, 39* (51, 52), 929–932.

Centers for Disease Control (1992). Sexual behavior among high school students—United States, 1990. *Morbidity and Mortality Weekly Report, 40*(51, 52), 885–888.

Centers for Disease Control and Prevention (1993). *HIV/ AIDS Surveillance Report, 5*(2), 1–19.

Coates, T.J., Stall, R., Catania, J.A., Dolcini, M.M., Hoff, C.C. (1989). Priorities for AIDS risk reduction: Research and programmatic direction. *AIDS Clinical Review,* 29–52.

Cunningham, R.M., Stiffman, A., Earls, F., Dore, P. (1991). Abused adolescents at risk for AIDS: Implications for public health. Abstract presented at the VIIth International Conference on AIDS, Florence, Italy, June 16–21, 1991. Abstract Book, p. 424.

Dekker, A.H., Earl, D.T., McKeigue, J.T., Aguila-Manalo, M., Torres, H., Ahart, S. (1990). The incidence of sexual abuse in HIV-infected adolescents and young adults [abstract]. *Journal of Adolescent Health Care, 11*(3), 282.

DiClemente, R.J. (1993). Preventing HIV/AIDS among adolescents: Schools as agents of behavior change. *Journal of the American Medical Association, 270,* 760–762.

DiClemente, R.J., Boyer, C.B., Morales, E.S. (1988). Minorities and AIDS: Knowledge, attitudes, and misconceptions among black and Latino adolescents. *American Journal of Public Health, 78,* 55–57.

DiClemente, R.J., Ponton, L.E., Hartley, D. (1991). Prevalence and correlates of cutting behavior: Risk for HIV transmission. *Journal of the American Academy of Child Adolescent Psychiatry, 30,* 735–738.

DiIorio, C., Parsons, M., Lehr, S., Adame, D., Carlone, J. (1992). Measurement of safe sex behavior in adolescents and young adults. *Nursing Research, 41,* 203–208.

DuRant, R.H., Ashworth, C.S., Newman, C., Gaillard, G. (1992). High school students' knowledge of HIV/AIDS and perceived risk of currently having AIDS. *Journal of School Health, 62,* 59–63.

English, A. (1990). Treating adolescents: Legal and ethical considerations. *Medical Clinics of North America, 74,* 1097–1109.

English, A. (1992). Expanding access to HIV services for adolescents: Legal and ethical issues. In R.J. DiClemente (Ed.), *Adolescents and AIDS: A generation in jeopardy* (pp. 262–283). Newbury Park, CA: Sage.

Erikson, E.H. (1963). *Childhood and society* (2nd ed.). New York: W.W. Norton.

Farrell, B. (1987). AIDS patients: Values in conflict. *Critical Care Nursing Quarterly, 10*(2), 74–85.

Feldman, D.A. (1989). Gay youth and AIDS. *Journal of Homosexuality, 17*(1/2), 185–193.

Fisher, J.D., Fisher, W.A. (1992). A general social psychological model for changing HIV risk behavior. *Psychological Bulletin, 111,* 455–474.

Fisher, J.D., Misovich, S.J., Fisher, W.A. (1992). Impact of perceived social norms on adolescents' AIDS-risk behavior and prevention. In R.J. DiClemente (Ed.), *Adolescents and AIDS: A generation in jeopardy* (pp. 117–136). Newbury Park, CA: Sage.

Friedrich, W.N. (1993). Sexual victimization and sexual behavior in children: A review of recent literature. *Child Abuse and Neglect, 17,* 59–66.

Fullilove, R.E., Fullilove, M.T., Bowser, B.P., Gross, S.A. (1990). Risk of sexually transmitted disease among black adolescent crack users in Oakland and San Francisco, Calif. *Journal of the American Medical Association, 263,* 851–855.

Garbarino, J., Dubrow, N., Kostelny, K., Pardo, C. (1992). *Children in danger: Coping with the consequences of community violence.* San Francisco: Jossey-Bass.

Gellert, G.A., Berkowitz, C.D., Gellert, M.J., Durfee, M.J. (1993). Testing the sexually abused child for the HIV antibody: Issues for the social worker. *Social Work, 38,* 389–394.

Givertz, D., Katz, M. (1993). *Youth and HIV Disease in San Francisco.* San Francisco: Department of Public Health AIDS Office and Special Programs for Youth.

Goulart, M., Madover, S. (1991). An AIDS prevention program for homeless youth. *Journal of Adolescent Health, 12,* 573–575.

Graham, L.L., Cates, J.A. (1992). How to reduce the risk of HIV infection for the seriously mentally ill. *Journal of Psychosocial Nursing and Mental Health Services, 30*(6), 9–13.

Havighurst, R.J. (1972). *Developmental tasks and education* (3rd ed.). New York: David McKay.

Hays, R.B., Kegeles, S.M., Coates, T.J. (1990). High HIV risk-taking among young gay men. *AIDS, 4,* 901–907.

Hein, K. (1989). AIDS in adolescence: Exploring the challenge. *Journal of Adolescent Health Care, 10,* 10S–35S.

Irwin, C.E., Jr. (1993). Adolescence and risk taking: How are they related? In N.J. Bell & R.W. Bell (Eds.), *Adolescent risk taking* (pp. 7–28). Newbury Park, CA: Sage.

James, J., Meyerding, J. (1977). Early sexual experience and prostitution. *American Journal of Psychiatry, 134,* 1381–1385.

Janke, J. (1989). Dealing with AIDS and the adolescent population. *Nurse Practitioner, 14*(11), 35, 36, 38, 41.

Janus, M., Burgess, A.W., McCormack, A. (1987). Histories of sexual abuse in adolescent male runaways. *Adolescence, 32*(86), 405–417.

Jemmott, J.B., III, Jemmott, L.S. (1993). Alcohol and drug use during sexual activity: Predicting the HIV-risk–related behaviors of inner-city black male adolescents. *Journal of Adolescent Research, 8,* 41–57.

Jemmott, L.S. (1993). AIDS risk among black male adolescents: Implications for nursing interventions. *Journal of Pediatric Health Care, 7,* 3–11.

Jemmott, L.S., Jemmott, J.B., III (1992). Increasing condom-use intentions among sexually active black adolescent women. *Nursing Research, 41,* 273–279.

Kegeles, S.M., Adler, N.E., Irwin, C.E., Jr. (1988). Sexually active adolescents and condoms: Changes over one year in knowledge, attitudes and use. *American Journal of Public Health, 78,* 460–461.

Keller, S.E., Bartlett, J.A., Schleifer, S.J., Johnson, R.L., Pinner, E., Delaney, B. (1991). HIV-relevant sexual behavior among a healthy inner-city heterosexual adolescent population in an endemic area of HIV. *Journal of Adolescent Health, 12,* 44–48.

Kelly, J.A., St. Lawrence, J.S., Hood, H.V., Brasfield, T.L. (1989). Behavioral intervention to reduce AIDS risk activities. *Journal of Consulting and Clinical Psychology, 57*(1), 60–67.

Kercher, G.A., McShane, M. (1984). The prevalence of child sexual victimization in an adult sample of Texas residents. *Child Abuse & Neglect, 8,* 495–501.

Kipke, M.D., Montgomery, S., MacKenzie, R.G. (1993). Substance use among youth seen at a community-based health clinic. *Journal of Adolescent Health, 14,* 289–294.

Ku, L., Sonenstein, F.L., Pleck, J.H. (1993). Young men's risk behaviors for HIV infection and sexually transmitted diseases, 1988 through 1991. *American Journal of Public Health, 83,* 1609–1615.

Kunins, H., Hein, K., Futterman, D., Tapley, E., Elliot, A.S. (1993). Guide to adolescent HIV/AIDS program development. *Journal of Adolescent Health, 14,* 1S–140S.

Levine, C., Dubler, N.N., Levine, R.J. (1991). Building a new consensus: Ethical principles and policies for clinical research on HIV/AIDS. *IRB: A Review of Human Subjects Research, 13*(1-2), 1–17.

Levine, R.J. (1986). *Ethics and Regulation of Clinical Research* (2nd ed.). Baltimore: Urban & Schwarzenberg.

Lewis, C., Battistich, V., Schaps, E. (1990). School-based primary prevention: What is an effective program? *New Directions for Child Development, 50,* 35–59.

Low, B.P., Andrews, S.F. (1990). Adolescent suicide. *Medical Clinics of North America, 74,* 1251–1274.

Mann, J.M., Tarantola, D.J.M., Netter, T.W. (1992). *AIDS in the world.* Cambridge, MA: Harvard University Press.

McCormack, A., Janus, M.D., Burgess, A.W. (1986). Runaway youths and sexual victimization: Gender differences in an adolescent runaway population. *Child Abuse & Neglect, 10,* 387–395.

Melton, G.B. (1989). Ethical and legal issues in research and intervention. *Journal of Adolescent Health Care, 10,* 36S–44S.

Miller, B.C., Christopherson, C.R., King, P.K. (1993). Sexual behavior in adolescence. In T.P. Gullotta, G.R. Adams, & R. Montemayor (Eds.), *Adolescent sexuality* (pp. 57–76). Newbury Park, CA: Sage.

Moscicki, A., Millstein, S.G., Broering, J., Irwin, C.E., Jr. (1993). Risks of human immunodeficiency virus infection among adolescents attending three diverse clinics. *Journal of Pediatrics, 122,* 813–820.

Nader, P.R., Wexler, D.B., Patterson, T.L., McKusick, L., Coates, T. (1989). Comparison of beliefs about AIDS among urban, suburban, incarcerated, and gay adolescents. *Journal of Adolescent Health Care, 10,* 413–418.

Panel on High-Risk Youth, Commission on Behavioral and Social Sciences and Education, National Research Council (1993). *Losing generations: Adolescents in high-risk settings.* Washington, DC: National Academy Press.

Pennbridge, J.N., Yates, G.L., David, T.G., Mackenzie, R.G. (1990). Runaway and homeless youth in Los Angeles County, California. *Journal of Adolescent Health Care, 11,* 159–165.

Persaud, D., Chandwani, S., Rigaud, M., Leibovitz, E., Kaul, A., Lawrence, R., Pollack, H., DiJohn, D., Krasinski, K., Borkowsky, W. (1992). Delayed recognition of human immunodeficiency virus infection in pre-adolescent children. *Pediatrics, 90*(5), 688–691.

Piaget, J. (1969). The intellectual development of the adolescent. In G. Caplan & S. Lebovici (Eds.), *Adolescence: Psychosocial perspective.* New York: Basic Books.

Polit, D.F., White, C.M., Morton, T.D. (1990). Child sexual abuse and premarital intercourse among high-risk adolescents. *Journal of Adolescent Health Care, 11,* 231–234.

Remafedi, G. (1987). Male homosexuality: The adolescent's perspective. *Pediatrics, 79,* 326–330.

Remafedi, G.J. (1988). Preventing the sexual transmission of AIDS during adolescence. *Journal of Adolescent Health Care, 9,* 139–143.

Remafedi, G. (1993). The impact of training on school professionals' knowledge, beliefs, and behaviors regarding HIV/AIDS and adolescent homosexuality. *Journal of School Health, 63,* 153–157.

Rickel, A.U., Hendren, M.C. (1993). Aberrant sexual experiences in adolescence. In T.P. Gullotta, G.R. Adams, & R. Montemayor (Eds.), *Adolescent sexuality* (pp. 141–160). Newbury Park, CA: Sage.

Rickert, V.I., Jay, S., Gottlieb, A. (1991). Effects of a peer-counseled AIDS education program on knowledge, attitudes, and satisfaction of adolescents. *Journal of Adolescent Health, 12,* 38–43.

Rickert, V.I., Jay, M.S., Gottlieb, A., Bridges, C. (1989). Adolescents and AIDS: Female attitudes and behaviors toward condom purchase and use. *Journal of Adolescent Health Care, 10,* 313–316.

Robb, H., Beltran, E.D., Katz, D., Foxman, B. (1991). Sociodemographic factors associated with AIDS knowledge in a random sample of university students. *Public Health Nursing, 8,* 113–118.

Rotheram-Borus, M.J., Koopman, C. (1991). Sexual risk behaviors, AIDS knowledge, and beliefs about AIDS among runaways. *American Journal of Public Health, 81,* 206–208.

Rotheram-Borus, M.J., Koopman, C., Haignere, C., Davies, M. (1991). Reducing HIV sexual risk behaviors among runaway adolescents. *Journal of the American Medical Association, 266,* 1237–1241.

Russell, D.E.H. (1984). The prevalence and seriousness of incestuous abuse: Stepfathers vs. biological fathers. *Child Abuse & Neglect, 8,* 15–22.

San Francisco Department of Public Health (1993). *HIV seroprevalence and risk behaviors among lesbians and bisexual women: The 1993 San Francisco/Berkeley women's survey, October 19, 1993.* San Francisco: Surveillance Branch, AIDS Office, Department of Public Health.

Savin-Williams, R.C., Rodriguez, R.G. (1993). A developmental, clinical perspective on lesbian, gay male, and bisexual youths. In T.P. Gullotta, G.R. Adams, & R. Montemayor (Eds.), *Adolescent sexuality* (pp. 77–101). Newbury Park, CA: Sage.

Scharer, K., Challberg, C., Rearick, T. (1990). Young people and AIDS: Mental health promotion in action. *Journal of Child and Adolescent Psychiatric Mental Health Nursing, 3*(2), 41–45.

Schram, D.D., Giovengo, M.A. (1991). Evaluation of threshold: An independent living program for homeless adolescents. *Journal of Adolescent Health, 12,* 567–572.

Seng, M.J. (1989). Child sexual abuse and adolescent prostitution: A comparative analysis. *Adolescence, 24,* 665–675.

Shilts, R. (1987). *And the band played on: Politics, people and the AIDS epidemic.* New York: St. Martin's Press.

Silbert, M., Pines, A. (1982). Entrance into prostitution. *Youth and Society, 13,* 471–500.

Smart, D.H. (1991). Homeless youth in Seattle: Planning and policy-making at the local government level. *Journal of Adolescent Health, 12,* 519–527.

Stierborg, M. (1992). Knowledge about, and attitudes to, HIV/AIDS among students in a Sydney nursing college. *Nurse Education Today, 12,* 207–214.

Stiffman, A.R., Dore, P., Earls, F., Cunningham, R. (1992). The influence of mental health problems on AIDS-related risk behaviors in young adults. *Journal of Nervous and Mental Disorders, 180,* 314–320.

St. Louis, M.E., Conway, G.A., Hayman, C.R., Miller, C., Petersen, L.R., Dondero, T.J. (1991). Human immunodeficiency virus infection in disadvantaged adolescents: Findings from the U.S. Job Corps. *Journal of the American Medical Association, 266,* 2387–2391.

Stricof, R.L., Kennedy, J.T., Nattell, T.C., Weisfuse, I.B., Novick, L.F. (1991). HIV seroprevalence in a facility for runaway and homeless adolescents. *American Journal of Public Health, 81*(suppl), 50–53.

Tanner, J.M. (1962). *Growth at adolescence* (2nd ed.). Oxford: Blackwell Scientific.

Taylor, B.A., Remafedi, G. (1993). Youth coping with sexual orientation issues. *Journal of School Nursing, 9*(2), 26–27, 30–39.

Tighe, J. (1993). Young people & HIV. *HIV Counselor Perspectives, 3*(3), 1–8. [San Francisco: UCSF AIDS Health Project.]

Treadway, L., Yoakam, J. (1992). Creating a safer school environment for lesbian and gay students. *Journal of School Health, 62,* 352–357.

Troiden, R.R. (1988). Homosexual identity development. *Journal of Adolescent Health Care, 9,* 105–113.

Tyden, T., Norden, L., Ruusuvaara, L. (1991). Swedish adolescents' knowledge of sexually transmitted diseases and their attitudes to the condom. *Midwifery, 7*(1), 25–30.

U.S. Conference of Mayors (1992). Condom availability in high school: A local response. *AIDS Information Exchange, 9*(3), 1–12.

U.S. Conference of Mayors (1993). HIV/AIDS education and prevention for homeless youth: The CHT experience. *HIV Education Case Studies, 7*(July), 1–19.

U.S. Public Health Service (1991). *Homeless and runaway youth: Public health issues and the need for action.* San Francisco, CA: U.S. Public Health Service, Region XI.

Van Servellen, G., Padilla, G., Brecht, M.L., Knoll, L. (1993). The relationship of stressful life events, health status and stress-resistance resources in persons with AIDS. *Journal of the Association of Nurses in AIDS Care, 4,* 11–22.

Walker, S.H. (1992). Teenagers' knowledge of the acquired immunodeficiency syndrome and associated risk behaviors. *Journal of Pediatric Nursing, 7,* 246–250.

Walter, H.J., Vaughan, R.D. (1993). AIDS risk reduction among a multiethnic sample of urban high school students. *Journal of the American Medical Association, 270,* 725–730.

Weiss, R.A. (1993). How does HIV cause AIDS? *Science, 260,* 1273–1279.

Wilcox, B.L. (1990). Federal policy and adolescent AIDS. *New Directions for Child Development, 50,* 61–70.

Yates, G.L., Mackenzie, R.G., Pennbridge, J., Swofford, A. (1991). A risk profile comparison of homeless youth involved in prostitution and homeless youth not involved. *Journal of Adolescent Health, 12,* 545–548.

Zierler, S., Feingold, L., Laufer, D., Velentgas, P., Kantrowitz-Gordon, I., Mayer, K. (1991). Adult survivors of childhood sexual abuse and subsequent risk of HIV infection. *American Journal of Public Health, 81,* 572–575.

RESOURCES FOR FURTHER READING

Bell, N.J., Bell, R.W. (Eds.) (1993). *Adolescent risk taking.* Newbury Park, CA: Sage.

DiClemente, R.J. (Ed.) (1992). *Adolescents and AIDS: A generation in jeopardy.* Newbury Park, CA: Sage.

El-Sadr, W., Oleske, J.M., Agins, B.D., et al. (1994). *Evaluation and management of early HIV infection: Clinical practice guideline No. 7.* Publication No. 94–0572. Rockville, MD: Agency for Health Care Policy and Research, Public Health Service, U.S. Department of Health and Human Services. (For free copies, call 1-800-342-AIDS.)

English, A. (1988). *Adolescent health care: A manual of California law* (3rd ed.). San Francisco: Adolescent Health Care Project of the National Center for Youth Law.

Grady, C., Vogel, S. (1993). Laboratory methods for diagnosing and monitoring HIV infection. *Journal of the Association of Nurses in AIDS Care, 4*(2), 11–21.

Gullotta, T.P., Adams, G.R., Montemayor, R. (Eds.) (1993). *Adolescent sexuality.* Newbury Park, CA: Sage.

Kunins, H., Hein, K., Futterman, D., Tapley, E., Elliot, A.S. (1993). Guide to adolescent HIV/AIDS program development. *Journal of Adolescent Health, 14,* 1S–140S.

Panel on High-Risk Youth, Commission on Behavioral and Social Sciences and Education, National Research Council (1993). *Losing generations: Adolescents in high-risk settings.* Washington, DC: National Academy Press.

Sanford, N.D. (1989). Providing sensitive health care to gay and lesbian youth. *Nurse Practitioner, 14*(5), 30, 32, 35–37, 42, 47.

Nursing Care of Women

Kathleen M. Nokes

Since HIV infection was first identified in gay men, much of the focus has been on how the disease manifests itself in men. In the United States, HIV/AIDS is now among the 10 leading causes of death in women of reproductive age, and the death rate for HIV/AIDS continues to rise (Chu et al., 1990; Selik et al., 1993). AIDS is the leading cause of death among women aged 25 to 34 years in New York City (Allen, 1990; Selik et al., 1993). Among Latinas, these same statistics apply (Maldonado, 1991) but among African American women in New York and New Jersey, the statistics are more startling. AIDS is the leading cause of death in African American women aged 15 to 44 years in these two states (Alexander, 1991). The estimated rate per 1,000 women of HIV seroprevalence, as determined by blinded samples of blood obtained from newborn infants, is 6.0, 0.5, 1.6, and 0.5 for the Northeast, Midwest, South, and West regions of the United States, respectively. However, when HIV seroprevalence rates were compared between black and white women in nearly every state, the highest rates were among black women in urban areas, followed by black women in nonurban areas, followed by white women in urban areas, with the lowest rates among nonurban white women (Wasser et al., 1993).

The sociodemographic characteristics of women likely to be infected with HIV differ vastly from those of men in that the women are often poor, use public facilities, are suspicious of institutions or agencies, and are crisis oriented in their health-seeking behaviors (Alexander, 1991; Maldonado, 1991; Mitchell et al., 1992). Women are often perceived as vectors of HIV infection—transmitters of the virus to their sexual partners and their unborn children (Mitchell, 1988). This perspective negates the role of women as competent adults, contributes to feelings of helplessness, and limits their access to treatment (Shayne & Kaplan, 1991).

INJECTION DRUG USE

At present, most AIDS cases among women of childbearing age are related to injection drug use—either directly or indirectly through sexual contact with an injection drug user (Gayle et al., 1990). A plethora of problems accompanies drug use among women. Female drug users usually have drug-using sexual partners. Chemically dependent women generally have low self-esteem, are not independent and autonomous, and are often in traditional roles in their relationships with men (Mitchell, 1990). They have more obstacles to overcome in protecting themselves from HIV infection. Alcohol and other drugs may relax inhibitions and result in unsafe needle-sharing and sexual practices (Karan, 1989). Cocaine use is associated with the acquisition of both HIV and syphilis because women may trade sex for drugs. Additionally, women using cocaine may fail to use prenatal services (Minkoff et al., 1990a, 1990b). Finally, drug users are more susceptible to rape and physical abuse than are women who do not use drugs.

Female drug users often have irregular menses, which they may incorrectly interpret to mean that they are not fertile. These women often come from dysfunctional, abusive families. Their children often experience the effects of their mothers' drug use *in utero* and after birth may be hyperirritable and sickly. Their condition heightens the difficulty in achieving adequate parenting skills and bonding between mother and baby. Women in the African American and Latino communities who use injection drugs are different from women in these cultural groups who do not use drugs. Chapter 9 addresses the problems and treatments for injection drug users in detail, and Chapter 15 discusses culture and ethnicity.

SEXUAL PRACTICES

Sexually active women (aged 15 to 44 years) report that they have changed their sexual practices in response to fear of becoming infected, with HIV and other sexually transmitted pathogens. These changes include using condoms, having sexual relations with fewer partners, reducing the frequency of sexual intercourse, changing specific sexual activities, and avoiding sex with unknown men, bisexual men, and injection drug users (Campbell & Baldwin, 1991). A group of drug-using HIV-infected (n = 38) and uninfected (n = 37) women reported marked prevalence of problems in sexual functioning in all major phases of the sexual-response cycle (desire, sexual arousal, and orgasmic functioning) and in vaginismus and vaginal pain (Meyer-Bahlburg et al., 1993). HIV-infected women reported significantly worse sexual problems even relatively early in the course of their HIV disease. The high rate of vaginal pain was associated with lack of vaginal lubrication, which may lead to injury and increased transmission of HIV during unprotected sex. In another study, advanced age (more than 45 years) of the uninfected female sexual partner was associated with increased risk of HIV transmission. The investigators suggested that this may have been due to increased fragility of the genital mucosa in perimenopausal women (European Study Group, 1992). Health care providers need to make an assessment of potential sexual dysfunction and instruct women about the availability of water-soluble lubricants and contraceptive creams and foams that may increase lubrication and reduce vaginal pain.

PREVENTION

To effect behavior change in the community, educational and prevention programs must be culturally relevant and competent to the community served (Flaskerud & Rush, 1989). Women with HIV infection are a diverse group. Many are poor but others are not; many are African American or Latina but others are from various cultural groups; most are heterosexual but some are lesbians; urban living is common but HIV infection is growing in rural areas. The nurse should avoid generalizations regarding women with HIV infection and should evaluate whether intervention is appropriate for particular clients.

Condoms

Women in preexisting relationships are particularly resistant to introducing condom use, even when a partner is known to be infected (Saracco et al., 1993). In heterosexual, monogamous women reporting irregular condom use, HIV seroconversion was associated with partners who had symptoms, with a low $CD4^+$ cell count (less than $400/mm^3$), or with detectable p24 antigen (Saracco et al., 1993). Similarly, women in a long-term, monogamous relationship with HIV-infected men with hemophilia reported that condom use was not significantly related to frequency of intercourse, knowledge about HIV and risk reduction, or other variables (Mayes et al., 1992).

Condoms for many individuals are symbols of sexual activity outside the relationship (Worth, 1989). A woman who does not use drugs and has one steady partner may not believe that she is at risk. This belief may be erroneous. Although the woman may be monogamous, her male sexual partner may live according to a different standard. A sample of sexually active married Americans was asked in 1990 about their sexual activity with a person other than their spouse. Of the men (n = 400), 1.8% reported having had sexual partners other then their spouse during the previous 30-day period; of the women (n = 481), .06% reported the same. These propor-

Table 8–1. Resistance to Condom Use in Heterosexual Relationships

Cultural	Belief that condoms are a symbol of promiscuity
	Passive role of women in sexual decision making
	Embarrassment associated with obtaining condoms
Economic	Fear of loss of financial support from sexual partner for self and children
	Expense involved in buying condoms, contraceptives
Mechanical	Feelings of vaginal and urinary irritation, both from condom and from nonoxynol 9
	Artificial barrier created during intimate behaviors
	Condom failure caused by (1) improper application, (2) breakage, and (3) slipping off as penis is removed
Psychologic	Denial of risk because not aware of behaviors of sexual partner
	Reluctance to introduce with steady partners because of implication of mistrust
	Feelings of powerlessness when partner refuses to use
	Uncertainty about whether condom will truly protect against HIV transmission

tions increased to 4.4% of the men (n = 405) and 2.9% of the women (n = 495) during the previous 12-month period; and 8.5% (n = 356) of the men and 4.3% of the women (n = 426) during the previous 5-year period (Leigh et al., 1993).

A woman trying to introduce condom use may be physically abused or abandoned. Even though the man's behavior may place the dyad at risk for HIV infection, he may blame her for infecting him if she is the first person to receive the diagnosis. Contact notification of partners is an important way of slowing HIV transmission. Table 8–1 outlines some of the problems and resistance women may experience related to the use of condoms.

Little attention has been given to barriers to HIV transmission that depend on the woman for their use (Stein, 1990). Some possibilities of barrier protection methods applied by the woman are the female condom, dental or latex dams, and topical agents inserted into the vagina.

Female Condoms

The female condom (Fig. 8–1) was approved by the U.S. Food and Drug Administration (FDA) in May 1993. It consists of a soft polyurethane sheath with two flexible rings. The ring at the closed end is inserted into the vagina and anchored under the pubic bone—similar to the diaphragm. The ring at the other end is much bigger and covers the labia and the base of the partner's penis (Rispin, 1989). Although the female condom was met with surprising disfavor by the popular press (Stein, 1993), African American women who participated in one of three focus groups that discussed the female condom positively endorsed it. The women liked the fact that it gives them control over its use, and the group members who particularly liked the female condom were women who had friends or family members who were dying or had died of AIDS (Shervington, 1993).

Latex Dams

Dental or latex dams are flat squares of latex, often 6 inches by 6 inches, that come in different colors and may have fruit or candy flavors. These squares are held in place over the external genitalia during oral sex by either partner. Some consumer groups have advocated the use of nonmicrowavable plastic wrap such as Saran Wrap during oral sex (New York City Department of Health, 1989), but the pores in the plastic wrap may allow passage of HIV. If dental dams are unavailable and the use of Saran Wrap is perceived as too uncertain, the nurse can advise the woman either to cut the fingers off a glove or to split a condom and cover the woman's external genitalia. The nurse should also advise the person to mark the barrier in some way so that the side with the vaginal secretions is replaced correctly should it slip. If this precaution is not taken, the partially used barrier can

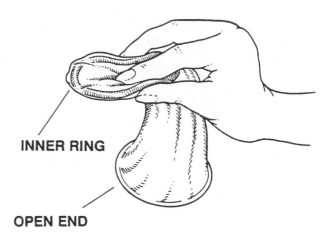

INNER RING

OPEN END

Figure 8–1. Insertion of the Reality vaginal pouch. (Courtesy Wisconsin Pharmacal Company, Chicago, Ill.)

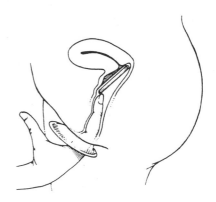

be replaced incorrectly and the partner could come in contact with vaginal secretions. Both the female condom and the latex dam require at least implicit consent from the sexual partner because the external genitalia are covered.

Topical Agents

Spermicides or topical creams and foams that are inserted into the vagina are usually available at the drugstore and do not necessarily require the consent of the woman's sexual partner. Barriers that depend exclusively on the woman may not be as efficacious as condoms but may be better than no barrier at all. Some contraceptive creams and foams contain nonoxynol 9, which is known to be effective in killing HIV. The barrier and/or the spermicide can be irritating to the penis or vagina, especially if one partner is allergic to the substance being used (Schaaf et al., 1990). Local sensitivity may be affected by the

vehicle, the stage in the woman's menstrual cycle, the presence of low-grade infections, and the woman's age and nutritional status (Stein, 1993). Questions have been raised about whether the use of spermicides may facilitate HIV transmission because of irritation to the vaginal mucosa.

No *in vivo* research findings are available at present regarding the effectiveness of using a contraceptive vaginal cream or foam with nonoxynol 9 versus no protection. *In vitro* research has demonstrated that nonoxynol 9 kills the virus and therefore may be considered effective on its own. Research is needed to address the question of the effectiveness of a vaginally inserted spermicide containing nonoxynol 9 used with a condom versus used without any other barrier. Questions also persist about the effectiveness of diaphragms and cervical caps in reducing HIV transmission from an HIV-infected woman to her uninfected partner (Stein, 1993).

Pregnancy

HIV-discordant couples (seropositive husband and seronegative wife) may be interested in having children. Several studies are in process that may affect childbearing in these couples. Since theoretically the spermatozoa could proceed to the cervical os without being surrounded by infected seminal fluid, a virucide that would be inserted into the vagina has been proposed (Stein, 1990). The virucide would kill HIV without killing the sperm, thus allowing the possibility of pregnancy while preventing transmission of HIV. No vaginal virucide currently exists, and whether development of one is planned is not known.

Artificial insemination is one option for achieving pregnancy. However, transmission of HIV through artificial insemination has been documented (Centers for Disease Control [CDC], 1990a) and is a source of infection in women. In one case a woman was inseminated three times with semen from her HIV-seropositive hemophiliac husband. His semen had been treated to remove HIV. No other risk behavior existed in this case because the couple reported protected sex and did not engage in oral or anal intercourse. However, the woman became HIV seropositive. There is no procedure that reliably eliminates HIV from semen, and the CDC advises against artificial insemination when the donor is infected with HIV (CDC, 1990a, p. 255). More recently, a research team in Milan, Italy, treated semen from HIV-infected men by using a "swim up" method before the semen was implanted in the HIV-negative spouses. The treated implanted semen resulted in 17 pregnancies and 10 births, and all the women and offspring remained uninfected (Semprini et al., 1992). The Milan study has elicited great interest from HIV-discordant couples who want to conceive, but that method of treating semen is not available currently in the United States (Connett, 1993).

HIV-infected women may want to use oral contraceptives to prevent pregnancy. Current information is insufficient to contraindicate the use of oral contraceptives in women with HIV disease as long as there are no other contraindications to hormone therapy and barrier methods are used to prevent HIV transmission (New York State Department of Health, 1992). Although it is not known whether there are any drug interactions between antiretroviral medications and oral contraceptives, a number of other drugs, such as rifampin, do interact with oral contraceptives. Anergy may be increased in women who are taking oral contraceptives, and thus an anergy study should be performed before oral contraceptives are prescribed (Denenberg, 1993a).

Prevention Among Lesbians

Female-female sexual transmission of HIV is the least efficient means of transmission among any of the possible sexual pairings. HIV infection among women as a result of female-female sexual contact is extremely low. However, lesbians with HIV are a virtually unstudied subpopulation affected by the AIDS epidemic (Cole & Cooper, 1991; Stevens, 1993). Lesbians who are bisexuals and/or who inject drugs run the same risks of infection with HIV as do any other persons. Lesbians who are sexual partners of bisexual lesbians or of women who inject drugs should take several precautions to reduce risk. Lesbians are particularly at risk of acquiring HIV infection during oral sex if one woman is menstruating. Barrier protection is recommended for all oral sex and for unprotected contact of hand or fingers to the vagina or anus if cuts are present on the hand. Lesbians should be instructed to use barriers such as gloves to prevent the exchange of vaginal secretions, urine, feces, menstrual blood, or breast milk (Cole & Cooper, 1991; Women's AIDS Network, 1988). Lesbians may also be at risk as a result of artificial insemination. Furthermore, lesbians who use drugs and share needles should take the same precautions as other injection drug users. Lesbians who are bisexual should practice the same sexual precautions during female-male contacts as do other female-male sexual pairings (see Chapters 2 and 9).

Household Precautions

Because HIV is transmitted by blood, infected women should be counseled about safely disposing of their menstrual products and using bleach solutions to remove blood from their underpants. Like men, they should be advised to keep their toothbrushes and razors separate from those of other family members and reassured that HIV is not spread through casual contact.

The issues surrounding prevention of HIV in women are not simple. Nurses need to be clear about their personal beliefs and open to hearing about the situation from the woman's perspective. This can be challenging when the woman is acting in ways that the nurse believes are irresponsible. Judging the behaviors of others and giving advice are easy, but it is much more difficult to truly respect the client by helping her make realistic changes within her existing constraints. The nurse does not have to agree with the woman's choice but, rather, should create an environment in which the woman can feel safe to explore alternatives.

CLINICAL MANIFESTATIONS IN WOMEN

Recognition of early HIV infection in women is particularly lacking, as illustrated by the findings of an emergency department chart review (Schoenbaum & Webber, 1993). In this study, HIV was completely unrecognized among all adolescent, young adult, and older women (25 years of age or less and 45 years or more) who were treated in this inner-city emergency department. The New York State Department of Health (1992) clinical standards for women with HIV disease are outlined in Table 8–2.

Assessment

Nurses need to become more comfortable in assessing sexual behaviors and teaching safer sex strategies that will decrease the risk of infection among women (Whipple, 1992). When taking a sexual history, the nurse must consider different attitudes, cultural and religious influences, developmental levels, and cognitive skills (Nolte et al., 1993). Irrespective of the skill of the assesser, up to half of the women in one group who had acquired HIV heterosexually did not know that they

Table 8–2. Comprehensive Gynecologic Evaluation for HIV-infected Women

History
Menstrual history
Obstetric history
Contraceptive use
History of sexual practices
Previous diagnosis of sexually transmitted diseases
Vulvovaginal and pelvic infections
Previous Pap smear results
Surgical procedures
Current abdominal and pelvic symptoms

Physical Examination
Clinical breast examination
Inspection of external genitalia: vaginal canal, cervix, perianal area
Rectal and bimanual examination

Laboratory and Other Diagnostic Procedures
Urinalysis
Syphilis serologic screening
Gonorrhea testing
Chlamydia testing
Pap smears (every 6 to 12 months)
Mammography (according to recommendations of American Cancer Society)
Pregnancy test

From New York State Department of Health. (1992). *Gynecologic services for women with HIV infection.* New York: The Department.

had been exposed to HIV even when closely questioned (Wofsy, 1992). To assess an HIV-infected woman's illness cognition (picture of her illness), the nurse must determine how the woman contracted the virus, her role in the transmission of the disease with past and current sexual partners and her children, and her role as a parent (Regan-Kubinski & Sharts-Engel, 1992).

Clinical Signs and Symptoms

The interactions among the neurologic, endocrine, and immune systems are complex (Denenberg, 1993a). As an example, menstrual disorders may occur in greater frequency in HIV-infected women. These disorders include amenorrhea and between-periods bleeding, but other factors such as continued use of recreational drugs or use of medications for HIV infection may be found to be the cause. In addition, the HIV infection itself, as well as the loss of weight and body fat, can disrupt menstruation. In the case of missed or late periods, pregnancy should always be considered (Kelly & Holman, 1993). Blood loss from heavy periods can predispose a woman to anemia or exacerbate it (Denenberg, 1993a). Premature menopause appears frequently in women with HIV illness, and ovarian failure should promote a consideration of hormone replacement, especially if the woman has menopausal symptoms (Denenberg, 1993a).

Comorbidity

Women with other sexually transmitted diseases (STDs) should be considered at risk of acquiring HIV infection and should be presented with the issues surrounding a decision to take the HIV antibody test. Evidence suggests that genital ulcer diseases such as genital herpes, chancroid, genital warts, syphilis, and possibly *Chlamydia* infection and gonorrhea increase the risk of HIV transmission during sexual activity (New Jersey Women & AIDS Network, 1990; Stein, 1993). HIV infection should be considered as a differential diagnosis in women with *Candida* vaginitis, severe pelvic inflammatory disease (PID), infection with herpes simplex virus (HSV) or human papillomavirus, or neoplasia. When any one of these conditions is characterized by unusual severity, resistance to treatment, or frequent recurrence, a concurrent HIV infection is a possibility.

Vaginal yeast infections may be another sign of HIV infection. In June 1992 the FDA approved nonprescription sale of creams and suppositories for the treatment of vaginal candidiasis. More recently, the FDA required that the manufacturers add an additional warning: "In women with frequently recurrent vaginal yeast infections, especially infections that do not clear up easily with proper treatment, the vaginal yeast infections may also be the result of serious medical conditions, including infection with HIV, that can damage the body's normal defenses against infection" (Clardy, 1993). To raise awareness about this issue and because clients have variable levels of reading competency and understanding of English,

nurses must highlight this warning as they care for any woman.

Table 8–3 presents common vaginal infections, but despite these symptoms some clinicians fail to make a diagnosis of HIV (Schaaf et al., 1990). HIV infection should be considered a possibility in all women with recurrent or persistent vaginal candidiasis. Vaginal candidiasis is especially prevalent in HIV-infected women. It usually responds well to topical antifungal agents such as clotrimazole (Gyne-Lotrimin) (Wofsy, 1992). For more refractory cases, ketoconazole (400 mg/day for 14 days, followed by 5-day courses each month for 6 months, with monitoring by means of liver function tests) or fluconazole is also extremely effective but expensive (Wofsy, 1992). Vaginal candidiasis may precede oral thrush. Table 8–4 presents assessment and intervention strategies for women with *Candida* vaginitis.

PID includes endometritis, salpingitis, tuboovarian abscess, and pelvic peritonitis. Symptoms of PID include (1) bilateral sharp, cramping pain in the lower abdominal quadrants, (2) fever, (3) chills, (4) purulent vaginal discharge, (5) irregular menstrual bleeding, (6) malaise, and (7) nausea and vomiting. In some cases the woman may have normal laboratory findings and no symptoms (Schober, 1986). Many cases of PID are associated with *Neisseria gonorrhoeae* infections but chlamydia should also be considered. PID is confirmed by laparoscopy but since this diagnostic procedure is often unavailable, women are frequently treated empirically with antibiotics. Depending on the severity of the case, women should be advised that hospitalization with parenteral antibiotics is the strategy of choice especially if the woman is interested in future pregnancies. However, some providers are reluctant to treat PID aggressively in HIV seropositive women. A common sequela to untreated PID is sterility and the health care provider may perceive this as a desirable outcome in the HIV-positive women. Since intrauterine devices increase the risk of PID, they should be avoided in HIV infected women (Smeltzer & Whipple, 1991).

Recurrent or persistent HSV infection is associated with an increased risk of HIV infection. HIV-infected women with herpes infection might shed virus more frequently than

Table 8–3. Common Vaginal Infections

PROBLEM	SYMPTOMS	LABORATORY FINDINGS
Yeast *(Candida albicans)*	Vaginal pruritus White, clumped discharge Vaginal wall inflammation	Microscopic yeast Discharge with pH of 4.5 or lower
Trichomonas	Profuse, often malodorous yellow discharge of low viscosity Vaginal wall inflammation	Discharge with pH higher than 5.0 Microscopic leukocytes and trichomonads
Bacterial vaginosis	Gray-white, malodorous discharge with thin, homogeneous consistency	Discharge pH of 4.5 or higher Amine or fishy odor when potassium hydroxide is applied to the discharge Clue cells on microscopic examination

women not infected with HIV and thereby pose an increased risk of HIV transmission to sexual partners (Minkoff & DeHovitz, 1991). Higher doses of acyclovir may be needed to control the infection and achieve remission. Symptoms often recur when the medication is discontinued and the drug may not be effective when it is resumed. Suppressive therapy may be necessary for chronic HSV infections.

Different types of human papillomavirus are associated with benign condylomata acuminata (genital warts), vulvar intraepithelial neoplasia, and most invasive cancers of the cervix (Wright & Ferenczy, 1993). Condylomata acuminata appear as white or gray fleshy clusters that resemble cauliflower. They are often treated with local applications of trichloroacetic or bichloroacetic acid (50% to 85%); podophyllum resin is not usually recommended as the first line of treatment (Denenberg, 1993b).

Laboratory Findings

HIV-infected women have a high prevalence of cervical and vaginal cytologic abnormalities (CDC, 1990b; Schrager et al., 1989). In one study, fivefold to eightfold increased rates of abnormal smears in HIV-infected women were observed, and these abnormalities increased as the HIV-infected women's CD4+ cells decreased (Marte et al., 1992). HIV-infected women often have mild, chronic cervicitis (Allen, 1990). They are at significant risk of having cervical cancer be-

cause they have a high prevalence of cervical intraepithelial neoplasia and infection with human papillomavirus (McCann, 1990). Since 1993, cervical cancer has been included as an AIDS-defining diagnosis in HIV-infected women. Nursing issues for HIV-infected women with cervical cancer are discussed further in Chapter 5.

Papanicolaou (Pap) smears are used to diagnose cervical cancer. Preparation for a Pap smear should include instructing the woman that the best smears are obtained in mid cycle, that smears cannot be obtained when there is any vaginal bleeding, and that douching, use of tampons, and vaginal intercourse should be avoided for 48 hours before the smear (Denenberg, 1993b). If sampling is adequate and cytologic findings are normal, Pap smears should be obtained every 6 to 12 months. If any atypia is noted or sampling is inadequate, additional smears should be obtained after treatment. The frequency of subsequent Pap smears depends on the woman's history of cervical dysplasia (or neoplasia) and colposcopic examination findings (New York State Department of Health, 1992). Women often react to an abnormal Pap smear with concern, so the nurse should be prepared to give information and should leave time for emotional support.

Treatment and Nursing Care

The survival time of HIV-infected women and heterosexual men is similar. Issues affecting treatment with medications include

Table 8–4. *Candida* Vaginitis

Medical diagnosis: *Candida* vaginitis
Nursing diagnosis: Alteration in comfort related to recurrent vaginal *Candida* infections

Assessment
1. Assess for the presence of symptoms.
2. Determine prior response to treatment.
3. Determine $CD4^+/CD8^+$ T-cell counts and ratio.
4. Assess whether other risk factors are present, such as the use of birth control pills or antibiotics, pregnancy, or diabetes.
5. Determine whether symptoms are related to menstrual cycle, especially menstrual period.
6. Determine whether partner also has symptoms, because treatment of both will then be indicated.

Planning and Intervention
1. Provide safe environment in which woman can describe her symptoms.
2. Obtain vaginal discharge for culture.
3. Discuss self-help strategies such as:
   a. Wearing cotton underpants
   b. Avoiding tight-fitting clothing
   c. Avoiding spreading anal secretions to vaginal area both during sex and after bowel movement
   d. Avoiding douching and feminine hygiene products
   e. Minimizing sugar, sweets, and refined foods in diet
   f. Killing yeast on underpants by boiling, bleaching, ironing, or, if damp, microwaving for 5 minutes (Hackney, 1990)
   g. Eating 8 ounces of yogurt containing *Lactobacillus acidophilus* each day (Hilton et al., 1992)
4. Determine whether woman wants to use alternative therapies such as:
   a. Vinegar rinse
   b. Garlic vaginal suppositories
   c. Acidophilus vaginal suppositories or two acidophilus tablets daily for 1 week, starting after the course of antibiotics is completed
   d. Yogurt tablets inserted into vagina, or plain, unsweetened yogurt inserted with applicator into vagina
   e. Golden seal and myrrh douche (Gardner, 1989)
5. Discuss prescriptive therapies with physician, such as:
   a. Miconazole intravaginal cream 2% or suppository (100 mg) every day for 7 days
   b. Mystatin intravaginal cream or tablet (100,000 units) twice a day for 7 days
   c. Clotrimazole intravaginal cream (1%) or tablet (100 mg) every day for 7 days
   d. Ketaconazole (200 mg) orally twice a day for 5 to 7 days (Bartlett, 1990)
   e. Fluconazole
6. Teach woman how to insert suppository or applicator and make sure that she understands technique.

Evaluation
1. Woman shares feedback about the effectiveness of different strategies.
2. Sexual partner does not reinfect the woman.
3. Barriers are used during sexual activity to prevent transmission of HIV and other organisms.

lower mean body weight in women, lower mean hemoglobin level, and the absence of established controls for $CD4^+$ cell counts in men versus women (Wofsy, 1992). Kaposi's sarcoma in women is probably related to infection through sexual activity with bisexual partners. Kaposi's sarcoma is four times more common in women with bisexual partners than in women with partners in other HIV risk groups (Beral et al., 1990). This evidence lends support to the proposal that Kaposi's sarcoma may be caused by a sexually transmitted infectious agent. AIDS-indicator diseases occur with similar frequency in men and women (Farizo et al., 1992).

Nurses also need to serve as advocates for HIV-infected women to ensure that their multiple social and health care needs are met. In one study, HIV-infected women had more unmet needs for services in the areas of mental health, drug treatment, housing, home care, transportation, and entitlements than HIV-infected men (Piette et al., 1993). Specific assistance in planning for the care and guardianship of children and in settling financial affairs may be needed (Hanley & Lincoln, 1992). Women are now included, unlike in the early years of the epidemic, in most clinical trials of medications to treat HIV and related problems (Murphy, 1991). The FDA published a guideline that outlines the expectation that women will be included in clinical trials and revised the 1977 guideline that excluded women of childbearing potential from participating in early studies of most drugs (Nightingale, 1993). Nurses need to know how to assist women in gaining access to clinical trials and how to act as advocates for transportation and child-care as services offered to subjects in clinical trials. Support groups for women, such as the one described by Haynes (1993), may be one way to assist HIV-infected women to cope with HIV disease.

HIV INFECTION AND PREGNANCY

To date, there has been a disproportionate focus on pregnancy in the study of HIV disease and women (Hankins & Handley, 1992). Pregnancy may be associated with a decrease in cell-mediated immunity (Nanda & Minkoff, 1989). Research has demonstrated a significant decrease in the relative and absolute numbers of helper T lymphocytes (CD4$^+$ cells) during pregnancy, with a return to normal levels by the fifth postpartum month (Nanda & Minkoff, 1989). HIV also decreases the number of helper T cells, and therefore it was initially believed that pregnancy would adversely affect the health of an HIV-infected woman (Minkoff, 1987). Other studies did not support the claim that HIV infection progresses more rapidly during pregnancy (Coyne & Landers, 1990). However, recent research suggests that there is a trend toward earlier manifestation of HIV-related symptoms in pregnant women and a higher maternal mortality rate in seropositive than seronegative women (Deschamps et al., 1993; Mmiro et al., 1993).

Perinatal Transmission

The process of vertical transmission or transmission of HIV from the mother to the fetus is still unclear (Touchette, 1993). During the course of gestation, the embryo/fetus could, in theory, become infected with HIV at any number of times and places. Infection could occur as a result of gametic infection, during development and transport of the embryo in the oviduct and uterus, during the periimplantation period, or via the placenta during the remainder of gestation (Douglas & King, 1992). That only 14% to 30% of the infants are actually infected with HIV has generated a number of research studies. Serum and amniotic fluid from 13 HIV-seropositive women and their fetuses before elective termination of pregnancy (mean gestational age was 18.8 weeks) were examined (Viscarello et al., 1992). HIV antibody was detected in maternal serum, amniotic fluid, and fetal serum from all subjects. The p24 antigen was found in maternal serum and amniotic fluid from 38% (n = 5) of the women and in serum from 23% (n = 3) of the fetuses.

A carefully designed study in Zaire suggested some factors associated with vertical transmission. In this study of 324 HIV-seropositive women and 253 uninfected women, prolonged fever during pregnancy, a CD4$^+$ lymphocyte count less than 24%, a CD8$^+$ lymphocyte count greater than 1.80 cells × 100, maternal p24 antigenemia, and placental membrane inflammation were all significantly and independently related to HIV infection of the offspring (St. Louis et al., 1993). Maternal anemia was also associated with vertical transmission, but the anemia was probably secondary to advanced maternal HIV disease rather than to an independent predictor of vertical transmission. As opposed to industrialized countries, where labor is induced when the woman continues past term, late gestational age (longer than 42 weeks after term) was also a predictor of vertical transmission by women delivering in a developing country (St. Louis et al., 1993). These researchers suggested that interventions to prevent vertical transmission will vary according to the stage of maternal HIV infection. Antiretroviral therapy may be more effective both very early and late in the course of maternal HIV infection, and antimicrobial prophylaxis for chorioamnionitis might be considered as a potential strategy to decrease placental inflammation.

In another study with women in Baltimore, vertical transmission was associated with clinical chorioamnionitis, STDs during pregnancy, and continued illicit drug use (Nair et al., 1993). Both the importance of avoiding illicit drugs and reinforcement of the use of barrier protection should be emphasized when HIV-infected pregnant women are taught how to decrease HIV transmission to the fetus.

Many women seek confirmation and treatment from the health care system when they suspect that they are pregnant. The CDC recommends HIV testing of women who are at risk of infection through injection drug use or unprotected sexual contact with an HIV-infected partner. Nonspecific symptoms such as fatigue, anorexia, and weight loss are common in both pregnancy and HIV infection. A woman may not know that her sexual partner has engaged in behaviors that place her at risk. The impact of learning of HIV infection during pregnancy is unique and overwhelming (Beevor & Catalan, 1993). The health care provider needs to be sensitive to the issues that are important to the client.

Abortion

Health care providers should be aware of their own values about continuing or terminating pregnancy in HIV-seropositive women and of how these values may influence their relationship with the client. When a pregnant woman learns early in the pregnancy that she is infected with HIV, she may choose to terminate the pregnancy. Because many women with HIV are poor and only 12 states in the United States provide Medicaid (MediCal) funds to poor women seeking abortions, this option may be severely limited (Mitchell, 1988).

Other factors also influence the decision to continue a pregnancy. Sixty-four uninfected and HIV-infected women with a history of injection drug use were asked about their decision to continue or terminate pregnancy (Selwyn et al., 1989). Half of the women infected with HIV (n = 28) chose to have an abortion. Neither the perceived personal risk of becoming sicker nor concern about AIDS was associated with termination of pregnancy. In another study, drug users did not vary significantly from nonusers in their decision to abort, whether they were seropositive or seronegative (Sunderland et al., 1992). Decisions about continuing or aborting the pregnancy were highly individual, and some women were psychologically unable to make a decision. Culture, ethnicity, and religion also may influence the decision to have an abortion. In some cultures, procreation and children are valued to the extent that the fear of disease may not override these values (Lifshitz, 1991; Maldonado, 1991).

To make informed decisions about pregnancy, HIV-infected pregnant women need to be told that the chances are approximately 3 in 10 that their offspring will actually be infected with HIV. In one study of poor HIV-infected pregnant women, 59% believed that all their babies would have AIDS (Kass et al., 1992). This same group of women were very knowledgeable about other routes of HIV transmission, leading the investigators to question whether health care providers were being clear in their communication about the incidence of vertical transmission.

Timing is crucial in the decision to terminate a pregnancy. In one study, 27 of 82 pregnant HIV-infected women learned their test results early enough in pregnancy to consider abortion (Holman et al., 1989). All were counseled about the issues surrounding HIV and pregnancy. Four of these women chose to abort, citing concern about their health and/or reluctance to risk having an infected child. One of these four women was unable to secure an abortion. She wanted the abortion performed on an outpatient basis, but available facilities had policies against doing outpatient abortions on women who were taking methadone. In another study conducted for a 4-year period, 20% of the pregnant women who had received extensive counseling chose to terminate pregnancy (Lindsay, 1993). Table 8–5 presents some of the issues generated by pregnancy in the HIV-infected woman.

Table 8–5. Pregnancy in Women Infected With HIV

ASSESSMENT	FACTORS TO CONSIDER
Whether pregnancy is wanted	1. Sociocultural values 2. Social support, especially from father of child or current sexual partner 3. Presence of other children who are well
Knowledge of HIV and pregnancy	1. Stage of HIV infection 2. Feelings about baby possibly being infected 3. Access to prenatal care 4. Willingness to adopt positive health behaviors 5. Concerns over personal health
Decision about continuation or termination of pregnancy	1. Stage of pregnancy 2. Religious beliefs 3. Economic resources 4. Access to abortion services 5. Abortion history 6. Feelings about transmitting HIV infection to unborn baby

Treatment

Health care for a pregnant HIV-infected woman depends on her stage of HIV infection. For the most part, management of the woman with no symptoms or mild symptoms does not differ from standard prenatal care (Connor et al., 1989). The standard approach to the symptom-free individual, including laboratory tests, skin tests, and vaccinations, need not be altered because of pregnancy (Minkoff & DeHovitz, 1991). Case finding for other sexually infectious and blood-borne diseases should be done because of similar routes of transmission. To prevent congenital syphilis, some providers suggest that pregnant HIV-infected women with syphilis be hospitalized for 10 to 14 days of intravenous penicillin therapy instead of the recommended 3-week regimen of 2.4 million units of benzathine penicillin G (Bicillin) (Mitchell et al., 1992). Infection with *Mycobacterium tuberculosis* should always be considered in an HIV-infected person. Because pregnancy may depress immune function, reactivation of latent infections can be a problem. In at least one case, a placental lymphoma (non-Hodgkins lymphoma) led to the diagnosis of AIDS (Pollack et al., 1993).

Medications are limited during pregnancy because of potential adverse effects on the fetus. Many of the common medications used to treat persons with HIV disease (acyclovir, clotrimazole troches, dapsone, fluconazole, inhaled pentamidine, trimethoprim-sulfamethoxazole [TMP-SMX], and zidovudine) are in FDA pregnancy category C; that is, animal studies have demonstrated fetal risk but there are no human trials, or neither human nor animal studies are available. Use of zidovudine (AZT) by 43 pregnant HIV-infected women failed to show any pattern of adverse outcomes of pregnancy that could be attributed directly to maternal zidovudine therapy (Sperling et al., 1992). In another study, AZT caused only limited toxic effects among the infants, and the authors suggest that its administration to large numbers of mothers in treatment trials should be considered relatively safe for both mother and child (Ferrazin et al., 1993).

It was recently reported that vertical transmission of HIV from infected mothers to their infants has been significantly reduced by the use of AZT by the mother during the pregnancy and labor and by the newborn for the first 6 weeks of life (CDC, 1993–1994). On February 21, 1994, the NIH's National Institute of Allergy and Infectious Diseases (NIAID) and National Institute of Child Health and Human Development (NICHD) announced preliminary results from a randomized multicenter, double-blinded clinical trial (AIDS Clinical Trials Group Protocol 076 [ACTG 076]) of AZT to prevent HIV transmission from mothers to their infants (CDC, April 29, 1994). Based on the analysis of data for 364 births through December 1993, AZT therapy was associated with a 67.5% reduction in the risk for HIV transmission. The ACTG protocol 076 included:

1. Oral administration of 100 mg of AZT five times daily initiated at 14 to 34 weeks' gestation and continued for the remainder of the pregnancy.
2. During labor, intravenous administration of AZT in a loading dose of 2 mg per kg of body weight given over 1 hour, followed by continuous infusion of 1 mg per kg of body weight per hour until delivery.
3. Oral administration of AZT to the newborn (AZT syrup at 2 mg per kg body weight per dose given every 6 hours) for the first 6 weeks of life, beginning 8–12 hours after birth.

Based on the findings of ACTG protocol 076, the Public Health Service (PHS) provided the following interim recommendations:

1. All health care workers providing care to pregnant women and women of childbearing age should be informed of the results of ACTG protocol 076.
2. HIV-infected pregnant women meeting the protocol eligibility criteria should be informed of the potential benefits but unknown long-term risks of AZT therapy as administered in ACTG protocol 076, and decisions to use AZT for prevention of perinatal transmission should be made in consultation with their health-care providers.
3. Health care providers should inform their patients that this AZT regimen substantially reduced, but did not eliminate, the risk for HIV infection among the infants; and

4. Until the potential risk for teratogenicity and other complications from AZT therapy given in the first trimester can be assessed, AZT therapy only for the purpose of reducing the risk for perinatal transmission should not be instituted earlier than the 14th week of gestation.

PHS is developing further recommendations for the uses of AZT for HIV-infected pregnant women whose clinical indications differ from the ACTG protocol 076 eligibility criteria and for counseling and HIV-antibody testing for women of childbearing age (CDC, April 29, 1994).

Immunotherapy in the mother also may interrupt vertical transmission of virus to the fetus. One of the HIV envelope proteins is gp120, and within gp120 is a hypervariable region known as the V3 loop. The absence of maternal antibody to the V3 loop correlates with vertical transmission. Passive immunization of pregnant, HIV-infected women with antibody preparations containing high titers against gp120, harvested from HIV-infected volunteers, is currently under study in clinical trials (Toltzis, 1993). This research is highly uncertain because in another study, mothers of infants who acquired HIV-1 infections did not differ significantly from the mothers of uninfected infants in the prevalence or concentration of antibodies to gp120 (Halsey et al., 1992). The nurse, acting in an advocacy role, will need to ensure that informed consent is carefully obtained and that the pregnant woman understands the extent of uncertainty related to vaccine clinical trials during pregnancy.

Finally, prophylaxis against *Pneumocystis carinii* pneumonia (PCP) during pregnancy may decrease the risk of hypoxic damage to the fetus (Landesman, 1989), but the use of teratogenic drugs such as trimethoprim and most antiviral agents should be avoided unless the mother has PCP (Wofsy, 1992). For the treatment of PCP, TMP-SMX is the most attractive therapeutic option, whereas intravenous pentamidine therapy should be avoided and dapsone held in reserve (Wofsy, 1992). Monitoring the woman's medication blood levels during pregnancy is essential because the physiologic changes of pregnancy alter the excretion and sometimes the metabolism of drugs (Mitchell, 1990).

Obstetric Complications

There have been no major obstetric complications related directly to HIV infection of the mother (Ukwu et al., 1992). A risk-benefit analysis should be carefully weighed before antepartum practices, such as an amniocentesis, are used that could theoretically increase the risk of perinatal HIV infection (DeFerrari et al., 1993). Monitoring the fetus during labor will be more difficult, because it is advisable to avoid the use of internal scalp electrodes and scalp pH so that the integrity of the fetus' scalp can be maintained as a barrier to infected vaginal secretions. External fetal monitoring devices should be used when feasible (Minkoff, 1987). Forceps delivery should be avoided (DeFerrari et al., 1993). Table 8–5 presents a summary of some of the issues surrounding HIV infection and pregnancy.

Another focus during the delivery period should be avoidance of occupational exposure to health care workers. Suction devices that use mouth suction to clear the neonate's airway, such as the DeLee suction device, should be replaced by mechanisms that use wall or bulb suction. Quality care should be delivered in a manner that protects both the client and the provider. Chapter 10 provides a detailed description of infection control practices for health care workers, including those in the delivery room.

Finally, new mothers should be cautioned about breast-feeding. Breast milk has been implicated as a mode of transmission of HIV. In the United States, where other sources of infant food are readily available, women should be counseled to avoid breast-feeding. In pattern II countries, such as those in Africa, other sources of food are not available and therefore breast-feeding is still encouraged; otherwise, the baby will starve to death long before the development of HIV disease.

NURSING RESEARCH IN THE CARE OF WOMEN

Flaskerud and colleagues conducted early research on the knowledge, attitudes, and practices of different groups of women with respect to HIV transmission and infection (Flaskerud and Nyamathi, 1989, 1990; Flaskerud & Rush, 1989). These studies contributed greatly to an understanding of the factors that need to be considered in planning primary and secondary intervention strategies. Other nurses have served as coinvestigators in studies that examined clinical issues related to HIV, such as the relation between human papillomavirus and the development of cervical cancer. Several clinical articles on health care of women with HIV have been published (DeFerrari et al., 1993; Hanley & Lincoln, 1992; Haynes, 1993; Kelly & Homan, 1993; Smeltzer & Whipple, 1991; Whipple, 1992; Williams, 1991). A body of knowledge is being generated by research that is examining the health care experiences of the HIV-infected woman (Regan-Kubinski & Sharts-Engel, 1992; Torres & Gallison, 1993), as well as her relationship with her children (Andrews et al., 1993) and with other family members (Sowell et al., 1993).

A number of questions persist that nurses could study in relation to women and HIV disease. Primary prevention questions that remain include the impact of the woman's social class and socioeconomic status on primary prevention strategies. Another area of questioning might involve barrier protection. For instance, would use of supplemental lubricants decrease vaginal irritation and increase acceptability of condoms and spermicides? Secondary prevention questions include the following: How does HIV disease manifest itself in older women, and what are their unique issues? How can health care delivery systems adapt themselves to be more responsive to women with children and multiple responsibilities? Do medications used to treat HIV disease manifest toxic effects differently in women from men (with control for the woman's body surface area)? Finally, how can women combine alternative therapies with medical models of treatment for HIV disease?

Tertiary prevention issues should address responses of women with AIDS to guardianship issues and advance directives and should assist terminally ill women with AIDS in planning for the future care of their infected and uninfected children.

SUMMARY

Although much has been learned about HIV disease in women, many questions persist. This chapter briefly addressed the epidemiology of HIV/AIDS in women in the United States, examined injection drug use and sexual practices that heighten the risk of infection, identified issues related to HIV primary and secondary prevention, discussed the unique clinical manifestations of HIV disease in women, and presented the current thinking about pregnancy and HIV-infected women. Although the clinical picture of HIV disease in women is clearer, vertical transmission remains confusing. A clearer understanding about vertical transmission should assist in clarifying the pathogenicity of HIV infection. Nursing research related to the care of women with HIV disease is needed. Areas of research in primary, secondary, and tertiary care were identified in this chapter.

REFERENCES

Alexander, V. (1991). Black women and HIV/AIDS. *SIECUS Report, 19*(2), 8–10.

Allen, M. (1990). Primary care of women infected with the HIV. *Obstetrics & Gynecology Clinics of North America, 17*(3), 557–569.

Andrews, S., Williams, A., Neil, K. (1993). The mother-child relationship in the HIV-1–positive family. *Image, Journal of Nursing Scholarship, 25*(3), 193–198.

Bartlett, J. (1990). *Pocketbook of infectious disease therapy.* Baltimore: Williams & Wilkins.

Beevor, A.S., Catalan, J. (1993). Women's experience of HIV testing: The views of HIV positive and HIV negative women. *AIDS Care, 5*(2), 177–186.

Beral, V., Peterman, T., Berkelman, R., et al. (1990). Kaposi's sarcoma among persons with AIDS: A sexually transmitted infection? *Lancet, 335*(8682), 123–128.

Campbell, A., Baldwin, W. (1991). The response of American women to the threat of AIDS and other sexually transmitted diseases. *Journal of Acquired Immune Deficiency Syndromes, 4*(11), 1133–1140.

Centers for Disease Control (1990a). HIV-1 infection and artificial insemination with processed semen. *Morbidity and Mortality Weekly Report, 249,* 255–256.

Centers for Disease Control (1990b). Risk for cervical disease in HIV-infected women—New York City. *Morbidity and Mortality Weekly Report, 39*(47), 846–849.

Centers for Disease Control and Prevention (Winter/Spring, 1993–1994). AZT found to reduce rate of maternal HIV transmission. *HIV/AIDS Prevention,* US DHHS, PHS, *4*(4), 3.

Centers for Disease Control and Prevention (April 29, 1994). Zidovudine for the prevention of HIV transmission from mother to infant. *Morbidity and Mortality Weekly Report, 43*(16), 285–287.

Chu, S., Buehler, J., Berkelman, R. (1990). Impact of the HIV epidemic on mortality in women of reproductive age, United States. *Journal of the American Medical Association, 264*(2), 225–229.

Clardy, T. (1993). Women and HIV/AIDS. *PI Perspective.* San Francisco, CA: Project Inform, 10.

Cole, R., Cooper, S. (1991). Lesbian exclusion from HIV/AIDS education. *SIECUS Report, 19*(2), 18–21.

Connett, S. (Ed.) (1993). Sperm washing study encouraging but U.S. researcher leery of risks. *AIDS Alert, 8*(4), 53, 55–56.

Connor, E., Bardeguez, A., Apuzzio, J. (1989). The intrapartum management of the HIV infected mother and her infant. *Clinics in Perinatology, 16*(4), 899–908.

Coyne, B., Landers, D. (1990). The immunology of HIV disease and pregnancy and possible interactions. *Obstetrics and Gynecology Clinics of North America, 17*(3), 595–606.

DeFerrari, E., Gegor, E., Gummers, L., et al. (1993). Nurse-midwifery management of women with HIV disease. *Journal of Nurse-Midwifery, 38*(2), 86–96.

Denenberg, R. (1993a). Female sex hormones and HIV. *AIDS Clinical Care, 5*(9), 69–71, 76.

Denenberg, R. (1993b). *Gynecological care manual for HIV positive women.* Durant, OK: Essential Medical Information Systems, Inc.

Deschamps, M., Pape, M.J.W., Desvarieux, M., et al. (1993). A prospective study of HIV seropositive asymptomatic women of childbearing age in a developing country. *Journal of Acquired Immune Deficiency Syndromes, 6*(5), 446–451.

Douglas, G., King, B. (1992). Maternal-fetal transmission of HIV: A review of possible routes and cellular mechanisms of infection. *Clinical Infectious Diseases, 15*(4), 678–691.

European Study Group on Heterosexual Transmission of HIV (1992). Comparison of female to male and male to female transmission of HIV in 563 stable couples. *British Medical Journal, 304,* 809–812.

Farizo, K., Buehler, J., Chamberland, M., et al. (1992). Spectrum of disease in persons with HIV infection in the United States. *Journal of the American Medical Association, 267*(13), 1798–1805.

Ferrazin, A., DeMaria, A., Gotta, C., et al. (1993). Zidovudine therapy of HIV-1 infection during pregnancy: Assessment of the effect on the newborns. *Journal of Acquired Immune Deficiency Syndromes, 6*(4), 376–379.

Flaskerud, J., Nyamathi, A. (1989). Black and Latina womens' AIDS-related knowledge, attitudes, and practices. *Research in Nursing and Health, 12*(6), 339–346.

Flaskerud, J., Nyamathi, A. (1990). Effects of an AIDS education program on the knowledge, attitudes and practices of low income black and Latina women. *Research in Nursing and Health, 15*(6), 343–354.

Flaskerud, J., Rush, C. (1989). AIDS and traditional health beliefs and practices of black women. *Nursing Research, 3*(4), 210–215.

Gardner, J. (1989). *The new healing yourself.* Freedom, California: The Crossing Press.

Gayle, J., Selik, R., Chu, S. (1990). Surveillance for AIDS and HIV infection among black and Hispanic children and women of childbearing age, 1981–1989. *Morbidity and Mortality Weekly Report, 39 (SS-3)*, 23–30.

Hackney, A. (1990). Women's health section. *American Journal of Nursing, 90*(9), 17.

Halsey, N., Markham, R., Wahren, B., et al. (1992). Lack of association between maternal antibodies to V3 loop peptides and maternal-infant HIV-1 transmission. *Journal of Acquired Immune Deficiency Syndromes, 5*(2), 153–157.

Hankins, C., Handley, M. (1992). HIV disease and AIDS in women: Current knowledge and a research agenda. *Journal of Acquired Immune Deficiency Syndromes, 5*(10), 957–971.

Hanley, E., Lincoln, P. (1992). HIV infection in women: Implications for nursing practice. *Nursing Clinics of North America, 27*(4), 925–926.

Haynes, Y. (1993). A women's issue: HIV/AIDS. *Perspectives in Psychiatric Care, 29*(1), 23–25.

Hilton, E., Isenberg, H., Alperstein, P., et al. (1992). Ingestion of yogurt containing *Lactobacillus acidophilus* as prophylaxis for candidal vaginitis. *Annals of Internal Medicine, 116*(5), 353–357.

Holman, S., Berthaud, M., Sunderland, A., et al. (1989). Women infected with HIV: Counseling and testing during pregnancy. *Seminars in Perinatology, 13*(1), 7–15.

Karan, L. (1989). AIDS prevention & chemical dependence treatment needs of women and their children. *Journal of Psychoactive Drugs, 21*(4), 395–399.

Kass, N., Faden, R., Gielen, A., O'Campo, P. (1992). Pregnant women's knowledge of the HIV: Implications for education and counseling. *Women's Health Issues, 2*(1), 17–25.

Kelly, P., Holman, S. (1993). The new face of AIDS. *American Journal of Nursing, 9*(3), 26–34.

Landesman, S. (1989). HIV in women: An overview. *Seminars in Perinatology, 13*(1), 2–6.

Leigh, B., Temple, M., Trocki, K. (1993). The sexual behavior of U.S. adults: Results from a national survey. *American Journal of Public Health, 83*(10), 1400–1408.

Lifshitz, A. (1991). Critical cultural barriers that bar meeting the needs of Latinas, *SIECUS Report, 19*(2), 16–17.

Lindsay, M. (1993). A protocol for routine voluntary antepartum HIV antibody screening. *American Journal of Obstetrics & Gynecology, 168*(2), 476–479.

Maldonado, M. (1991). Latinas and HIV/AIDS. *SIECUS Report, 19*(2), 11–15.

Marte, C., Kelly, P., Cohen, M., et al. (1992). Papanicolaou smear abnormalities in ambulatory care sites in women infected with the HIV. *American Journal of Obstetrics & Gynecology, 166*(4), 1232–1237.

Mayes, S., Elsesser, V., Schaefer, J., et al. (1992). Sexual practices and AIDS knowledge among women partners of HIV-infected hemophiliacs. *Public Health Reports, 107*(5), 504–514.

McCann, J. (1990). Anal, cervical cancers increasing in HIV infected. *Oncology & Biotechnology News, 4*(8), 16.

Meyer-Bahlburg, H., Nostlinger, C., Exner, T., et al. (1993). Sexual functioning in HIV⁺ and HIV⁻ injecting drug-using women. *Journal of Sex and Marital Therapy, 19*(1), 56–68.

Minkoff, H. (1987). Care of pregnant women infected with HIV. *Journal of the American Medical Association, 258*(19), 2714–2717.

Minkoff, H., DeHovitz, J. (1991). Care of women infected with the HIV. *Journal of the American Medical Association, 266*(16), 2253–2258.

Minkoff, H., McCalla, S., Delke, I., et al. (1990b). The relationship of cocaine use to syphilis and HIV infection among inner city parturient women. *American Journal of Obstetrics and Gynecology, 163*(2), 521–526.

Minkoff, K., Willoughby, A., Mendez, H., et al. (1990a). Serious infections during pregnancy among women with advanced HIV infection. *American Journal of Obstetrics and Gynecology, 162*(1), 30–34.

Mitchell, J. (1988). Women, AIDS, and public policy. *AIDS and Public Policy Journal, 3*(1), 50–51.

Mitchell, J. (1990). Treating HIV-infected women in chemical dependency programs. *AIDS Patient Care, 4*(4), 36–37.

Mitchell, J., Tucker, J., Loftman, P., et al. (1992). HIV and women: Current controversies and clinical relevance. *Journal of Women's Health, 1*(1), 35–39.

Mmiro, F., Ndugwa, C., Guay, L., et al. (1993). Effect of human immunodeficiency virus-1 infection on the outcome of pregnancy in Ugandan women. *Pediatrics AIDS HIV Infection in Fetus and Adolescent, 4*(2), 67–73.

Murphy, T. (1991). Women and drug users: The changing faces of HIV clinical drug trials. *Quality Review Bulletin, 17*(1), 26–32.

Nair, P., Alger, L., Hines, S., et al. (1993). Maternal and neonatal characteristics associated with HIV infection in infants of seropositive women. *Journal of Acquired Immune Deficiency Syndromes, 6*(3), 298–302.

Nanda, D., Minkoff, H. (1989). HIV in pregnancy: Transmission and immune effects. *Clinical Obstetrics & Gynecology, 32*(3), 456–466.

New Jersey Women & AIDS Network (1990). *Me first! Medical manifestations of HIV in women.* The Network, 5 Elm Row, New Brunswick, NJ, 08901.

New York City Department of Health (1989). *A woman's guide to AIDS.* New York: The Department.

New York State Department of Health (1992). *Gynecologic services for women with HIV infection.* New York: The Department.

Nightingale, S. (1993). FDA guidelines on women in clinical trials. *Journal of the American Medical Association, 270*(11), 1290.

Nolte, S., Sohn, M., Koons, B. (1993). Prevention of HIV infection in women. *Journal of Obstetrics, Gynecologic and Neonatal Nursing, 22*(2), 128–134.

Piette, J., Fleishman, J., Stein, M., et al. (1993). Perceived needs and unmet needs for formal services among people with HIV disease. *Journal of Community Health, 18*(1), 11–23.

Pollack, R., Sklarin, N., Rao, S., et al. (1993). Metastatic placental lymphoma associated with maternal HIV infection. *Obstetrics & Gynecology, 81*(5[Pt 2]), 856–857.

Regan-Kubinski, M., Sharts-Engel, N. (1992). HIV-infected women: Illness cognition assessment. *Journal of Psychosocial Nursing, 30*(2), 11–15.

Rispin, P. (1989, June 8). Female condom rates high in trials. *Dimensions, Vth International Conference on AIDS*, p. 3.

Saracco, A., Musicco, M., Nicolosi, A., et al. (1993). Man-to-woman sexual transmission of HIV: Longitudinal study of 343 steady partners of infected men. *Journal of Acquired Immune Deficiency Syndromes, 6*(5), 497–502.

Schaaf, V., Perez-Stable, E., Borchardt, K. (1990). The limited value of symptoms and signs in the diagnosis of vaginal infections. *Archives of Internal Medicine, 150*(9), 1929–1933.

Schober, M. (1986). Gynecologic and urinary problems. In J. Griffith-Kenney (Ed.), *Contemporary women's health* (pp. 588–602). Menlo, CA: Addison-Wesley.

Schoenbaum, E., Webber, M. (1993). The underrecognition of HIV infection in women in an inner-city emergency room. *American Journal of Public Health, 83*(3), 363–368.

Schrager, L., Friedland, G., Maude, D., et al. (1989). Cervical and vaginal squamous cell abnormalities in women infected with HIV. *Journal of Acquired Immune Deficiency Syndromes, 2*(6), 570–575.

Selik, R.M., Chu, S.Y., Buehler, J.W. (1993). HIV infection as a leading cause of death among young adults in U.S. cities and states. *Journal of the American Medical Association, 269*(23), 2991.

Selwyn, P., Carter, R., Schoenbaum, E., et al. (1989). Knowledge of HIV antibody status and decisions to continue or terminate pregnancy among IVDU. *Journal of the American Medical Association, 262*(24), 3567–3571.

Semprini, A., Levi-Setti, P., Bozzo, M., et al. (1992). Insemination of HIV negative women with processed semen of HIV positive partners. *Lancet, 340*(8831), 1317–1319.

Shayne, V.T., Kaplan, B.J. (1991). Double victims: Poor women and AIDS. *Women and Health, 17*, 21–37.

Shervington, D. (1993). The acceptability of the female condom among low-income African-American women. *Journal of the National Medical Association, 85*(5), 341–347.

Smeltzer, S., Whipple, B. (1991). Women and HIV infection. *Image: Journal of Nursing Scholarship, 23*(4), 249–255.

Sowell, R., Demi, A., Moneyham, L., et al. (1993). Effect of AIDS/HIV infection in families in Georgia. *Reflections, 19*(3), 33.

Sperling, R., Stratton, P., O'Sullivan, M., et al. (1992). A survey of zidovudine use in pregnant women with HIV infection. *New England Journal of Medicine, 326*(13), 857–861.

St. Louis, M., Munkolenkole, K., Brown, C., et al. (1993). Risk for perinatal HIV-1 transmission according to maternal immunologic, virologic, and placental factors. *Journal of the American Medical Association, 269*(22), 2853–2859.

Stein, Z. (1990). HIV prevention: The need for methods women can use. *American Journal of Public Health, 80*(4), 460–462.

Stein, Z. (1993). HIV prevention: An update on the status of methods women can use. *American Journal of Public Health, 83*(10), 1379–1382.

Stevens, P. (1993). Lesbians and HIV: Clinical, research, and policy issues. *American Journal of Orthopsychiatry, 63*(2), 289–294.

Sunderland, A., Minkoff, H., Handte, J., et al. (1992). The impact of HIV serostatus on reproductive decisions of women. *Obstetrics & Gynecology, 79*(6), 1027–1031.

Toltzis, P. (1993). Rationales for treating the HIV-infected woman during pregnancy. *Clinical Perinatology, 29*(1), 47–60.

Torres, C., Gallison, M. (1993). Understanding the health care experiences of women with HIV/AIDS: A contextual perspective [unpublished research]. Rochester, NY: University of Rochester School of Nursing.

Touchette, N. (1993). Maternal-fetal HIV-1 transmission continue to confound. *The Journal of NIH Research, 5*, 44, 46–47.

Ukwu, H., Graham, B., Lambert, J., et al. (1992). Perinatal transmission of HIV-1 infection and maternal immunization strategies for prevention. *Obstetrics & Gynecology, 80*(3 [Pt 1]), 458–468.

Viscarello, R., Cullen, M., DeGennaro, N., et al. (1992). Fetal blood sampling in HIV-seropositive women before elective midtrimester termination of pregnancy. *American Journal of Obstetrics & Gynecology, 167*(4[Pt 1]), 1075–1079.

Wasser, S., Gwinn, M., Fleming, P. (1993). Urban-nonurban distribution of HIV infection in childbearing women in the United States. *Journal of Acquired Immune Deficiency Syndromes, 6*(9), 1035–1042.

Whipple, B. (1992). Issues concerning women and AIDS: Sexuality. *Nursing Outlook, 40*(5), 203–206.

Williams, A. (1991). Women at risk: An AIDS educational needs assessment. *Image: Journal of Nursing Scholarship, 23*(4), 208–213.

Wofsy, C. (1992). Therapeutic issues in women with HIV disease. In M. Sande & P. Volberding (Eds.), *The medical management of AIDS* (pp. 465–476). Philadelphia: WB Saunders.

Women's AIDS Network (1988). *Lesbians and AIDS: What's the connection?* San Francisco, CA: San Francisco AIDS Foundation.

Worth, D. (1989). Sexual decision-making and AIDS: Why condom promotion among vulnerable women is likely to fail. *Studies in Family Planning, 20*(6), 297–307.

Wright, T., Ferenczy, A. (1993). Viral testing for HPV: What does it tell us? *The Female Patient, 18*, 79–89.

9 Nursing Care of Chemically Dependent Clients

Jo Anne Staats

Major changes have occurred in the demographic composition of the HIV epidemic in the United States since the discovery of the virus in 1981. Although the infection was originally thought to affect primarily homosexual and bisexual men, it is now clear that injecting drug use is a major risk factor accounting for an increasing number of individuals with HIV infection. Injecting drug use is the principal mode of transmission of HIV infection to the heterosexuals. HIV infected injecting drug users (IDUs) have unprotected sex with women who subsequently become infected with HIV. These women, as well as women infected through injecting drug use, pass the virus to the fetus during pregnancy or the perinatal period.

EPIDEMIOLOGY

The National Institute on Drug Abuse (NIDA) has estimated that in the United States there are approximately 1.1 to 1.3 million IDUs (Coutinho, 1990). About half of these individuals may be actively using drugs at any given time (Friedland & Selwyn, 1990). IDUs account for the second highest number of persons with HIV infection (PWHIV) in the developed countries (Stimson, 1990). IDUs in New York City probably first became infected with HIV in the early 1970s, and since then the infection has moved rapidly through the IDU population (Des Jarlais et al., 1989).

As of October 1993, according to the Centers for Disease Control and Prevention (CDC), 24% of the total AIDS cases had been reported in individuals whose only risk factor was injecting drug use. Of these PWHIV, 75% were men and 25% were women. There were also 8193 women with AIDS (2% total AIDS

cases) whose only risk factor was having sex with an infected IDU. The incidence of HIV infection is higher among racial/ethnic minorities who are IDUs than among white persons.

In the United States, New York City has the highest cumulative total number of all AIDS cases, as well as the highest seroprevalence rate of HIV infection, among IDUs of any city (Table 9–1). The highest incidence of HIV seroprevalence is on the East Coast, with a lower incidence in the Midwest and Far West. However, the incidence of HIV infection is expected to increase in areas that currently have low rates. The history of HIV infection in New York City shows a zero seroprevalence rate in 1978, a 44% rate in 1980, and a 56% rate in 1984, with stabilization in 1987 to between 55% and 60% (Des Jarlais et al., 1989; American Public Health Association, 1990).

Des Jarlais and colleagues (1994) reported stability in HIV seroprevalence for a 9-year period (1984 through 1992) among IDUs in New York City. This observation may be related to the implementation of syringe exchange programs and/or increases in noninjecting heroin use, including smoking and intranasal use.

TRANSMISSION OF HIV INFECTION IN INJECTING DRUG USERS

HIV infection is transmitted from one IDU to another by the sharing of syringes and other drug paraphernalia. When IDUs insert a needle into a vein, but before they inject the drug into the bloodstream (mainlining), they draw blood back into the syringe to ensure that they are in a vein (booting) (Table 9–2). Instead of injecting into a vein, IDUs might

Table 9-1. Geographic Differences in HIV Infection Among Intravenous Drug Users

CITY OR AREA	RATE OF INFECTION IN IDUs (%)
New York City	61
Puerto Rico	59
Jersey City	50
Newark	50
Baltimore	29
Boston	28
Philadelphia	19
Other areas	≤10

Data from Evans, C.A., Beauchamp, D.E., Deyton, L., et al. (1989). Illicit drug use and HIV infection. In Report of the Special Initiative on AIDS of the American Public Health Association. Washington, DC: The Association.

also inject heroin under the skin (skin popping). Traces of blood always remain in the syringe and the needle. When uncleaned syringes and needles are shared, the blood is injected into the next user. HIV-infected blood is easily passed from one individual to another in this manner. The equipment (cooker) used to prepare the drugs may also be contaminated with infected blood and, when shared with another individual, may facilitate transmission. Transmission of HIV through semen from an infected IDU occurs when condoms are not used.

Among the population of IDUs, transmission of HIV is associated with a number of factors (Marmor et al., 1987; Schoenbaum et al., 1989). Both more frequent injections and more infections with used needles increase the likelihood of contracting HIV infection. IDUs who inject cocaine, which has a shorter half-life than heroin and requires more frequent injections, are at higher risk than heroin users. The sharing of needles with either acquaintances or strangers facilitates HIV transmission. For women, having frequent sex with heterosexual IDUs is an additional risk factor. Schoenbaum and colleagues (1989) also found that the presence of HIV antibody was independently associated with being black or Hispanic, having recently used drugs, frequenting shooting galleries, having a sex partner who uses drugs, and having a low income.

Crack, a purified form of cocaine, is smoked by inhaling the vapors given off when it is heated. It is readily available and inexpensive. Its use has been associated with trans-

Table 9-2. Drug-related Street Terminology

Mainlining	Injecting drugs directly into the vein
Skin popping	Injecting drugs intradermally
Snort	Short inhalation of heroin through the nose
Sniff	Short inhalation of cocaine through the nose
Booting	Process of drawing blood back into the syringe and mixing it with the drug before injecting
Spike	Needle
Works	Syringe, needle, and cooker
Cooker	Spoon or metal soda-can top that is used to prepare heroin for injection; the heroin is mixed with water, heated over a flame to dissolve it, cooled, and then drawn into the syringe through a piece of cotton
Shooting gallery	Place, frequently an abandoned building, where drugs are sold and bought along with the equipment needed for injecting; sex for drugs and money is also frequently available
Tracks	Needle marks on the skin
Speedball	Heroin and cocaine taken together
Freebase	Kit used to remove impurities from cocaine so that the fumes can be inhaled
Freeze	Cold feeling in the throat after sniffing cocaine
Line	Cocaine powder or flakes in a line on a smooth, hard surface so that it may be sniffed

Data from Narcotic and Drug Research, Inc. (1989). *AIDS: Medical management of the HIV infected/chemically dependent client.* New York: The Company.

Table 9–3. Substance Abuse Terminology

Addict	Person who is physically dependent on one or more psychoactive substances, whose long-term use has produced tolerance, who has lost control over his or her intake, and who would manifest withdrawal phenomena if discontinuation were to occur
Drug abuse	Any use of drugs that causes physical, psychologic, economic, legal, or social harm to the individual user or to others affected by the user's behavior
Physical dependence	Physiologic state of adaption to a drug or alcohol, usually characterized by the development of tolerance to drug effects and the emergence of a withdrawal syndrome during prolonged use
Polydrug abuse	Concomitant use of two or more psychoactive substances in quantities and with frequencies that cause the individual significant physiologic, psychologic, or sociologic distress or impairment
Relapse	Recurrence of alcohol or drug-dependent behavior in an individual who has previously achieved and maintained abstinence for a significant time beyond the period of detoxification
Tolerance	Physiologic adaptation to the effect of drugs, so as to diminish effects with constant dosages or to maintain the intensity and duration of effects through increased dosage
Withdrawal syndrome	Onset of a predictable constellation of signs and symptoms involving altered activity of the central nervous system after the abrupt discontinuation or rapid decrease in dosage of a drug

Data from Rinaldi, R.C., Steindler, E.M., Wilford, B.B., Goodwin, D. (1988). Clarification and standardization of substance abuse terminology. *Journal of the American Medical Association, 259,* 555–557.

mission of HIV (Inciardi et al., 1992; Schoenbaum et al., 1989). Inciardi and colleagues (1992) conducted an exploratory investigation of "sex for crack" exchanges that occurred in crack houses in Miami, Florida. They found that owners of the crack houses employed women to provide sex in exchange for crack. These women had frequent oral, vaginal, and/or anal sex with several men daily. Concurrent with these observations, structured interviews were conducted with 17 men and 35 women who were regular users of crack and had exchanged sex for crack or money during the preceding 30 days. It was found that almost one third of the men and 89% of the women had had 100 or more sex partners during the 30-day study period without using condoms.

Since 1981, New York City researchers have been studying behaviors that may be associated with HIV transmission at sexually transmitted disease clinics (Chiasson et al., 1990). One of their findings was that 4% of infected male subjects and 6% of infected female subjects had no identifiable risk factor. In this group, however, they did identify in-

dependent variables of crack use and crack-related sexual behavior.

SUBSTANCE ABUSE DEFINED

Substance abuse is a chronic, progressive disease that may be fatal if untreated. "The central dynamic of addiction is the loss of self-control evidenced by compulsive repetition of a dysfunctional behavior with negative consequences for the user, family members, friends, or associates" (American Nurses' Association, 1987, p. 4). Chemical dependency is characterized by an inability to control use of a substance, continued use of a substance despite the negative consequences, and development of tolerance to the substance and withdrawal effects (abstinence syndrome) when the substance is discontinued (Table 9–3). Phases of chemical dependency include the first stage, recreational use when there are no physical abnormalities; the second stage, purposeful but controlled use when physical abnormalities become apparent; and the final stage, binge use (Cartter et al., 1989). Rebound occurs when the effects of the drug begin to wear off. The phenomenon of rebound begins at baseline, when the drug enters the body. As the drug takes effect the high is reached, but when the amount of drug in the body diminishes, the user starts to "come down." Baseline is reached, and then the user "bottoms out" below baseline. The user takes in additional drug to prevent the extreme discomfort associated with rebound.

Patterns of drug use change with time. Before the 1970s, heroin use in the United States was largely contained within the ghettos. The early 1970s found some of those involved in the psychedelic drug culture turning to heroin (Casey, 1989). Then the Vietnam War introduced many middle-class men to the use of heroin and brought it into mainstream America.

Cocaine has been increasingly abused in the past two decades. This is partially the result of its decreased cost. In the past, it was viewed as a drug of the affluent, jazz musicians, and movie stars. A survey by the NIDA in 1974 revealed that approximately 5 million Americans had used cocaine at least once (Weiss & Mirin, 1987). By 1986, 22 million individuals had used cocaine.

Social problems, such as poverty, family dysfunction, and lack of educational opportunities, have long been thought to be the cause of chemical dependency. Current research indicates that some substance users have inherited a chemical imbalance that makes them vulnerable to depression, anxiety, or intense restlessness (Coleman, 1990). They use heroin, cocaine, and alcohol as a type of self-medication to alleviate these symptoms. An estimated one third to one half of chemically dependent individuals have this biologic abnormality. A biologic predisposition to substance use may explain why some individuals can dabble with drugs and never become addicted, whereas others become addicted almost immediately.

Researchers have identified a key gene linked to alcoholism in 77% of the subjects studied (Coleman, 1990). The gene is linked to the receptors for dopamine, a neurotransmitter involved in the sensation of pleasure. When alcohol use is stopped, depression occurs as a result of dopamine depletion. It is postulated also that cocaine floods the brain with dopamine and that long-term use of cocaine causes depletion of dopamine, leading to severe depression when cocaine use is stopped (Henneberger, 1990). Dopamine depletion may also be associated with heroin withdrawal.

POLYDRUG ABUSE

Of increasing concern is the phenomenon of polydrug use: using two or more substances for the purpose of potentiating the effects of several drugs or counteracting the negative effects of each substance. Cocaine, alcohol, opiates, and benzodiazepines are of greatest concern. A study of cocaine abusers found that 70% reported alcohol abuse and 43% reported sedative abuse (Kosten, 1991). Only 20% of those individuals who reported concurrent alcohol abuse had become alcoholic before using cocaine. For the rest who used alcohol, the alcohol was used to cope with the "crash" following cocaine use. Opioid abusers were excluded from the study. Another study of current opioid users demonstrated that 48% reported alcohol use, 29% cocaine use, and 23% sedative use (Kosten, 1991).

Multiple drug abuse presents problems within treatment programs. Cocaine use and alcohol use are common among methadone maintenance patients, often negating the effectiveness of treatment. Detoxification of clients who abuse multiple drugs requires careful management. It is recommended that only one drug at a time be withdrawn.

PHYSIOLOGIC EFFECTS OF HEROIN, COCAINE, AND ALCOHOL

Heroin, an opiate, is a central nervous system depressant. It can be snorted, smoked, or injected intradermally or intravenously. The effects of heroin are most intense after intravenous administration. Heroin is one of the most physically addicting of all drugs. Users inject themselves three to five times during a 24-hour period. Intravenous injection of heroin produces a euphoric feeling, a "rush," followed by relaxation that lasts several hours.

During this period, users are described as having a "nod."

Opiates, including heroin, produce suppression of the cough reflex and respiratory depression (Arif & Westermeyer, 1988). Other physical effects include miosis, constipation, and peripheral vasodilation. Rapid intravenous administration causes histamine release, resulting in itching, flushing, and sweating. Tolerance and physical dependence develop with chronic heroin use.

Cocaine is a central nervous system stimulant that produces heightened energy and self-esteem. It can be used intranasally (sniffed), smoked as freebase or crack, or injected intravenously (Engel, 1991). When inhaled, the effects of cocaine are felt in about 5 minutes and last 20 to 40 minutes. When crack is smoked, it is readily absorbed across the pulmonary vasculature and reaches the brain in 8 to 10 seconds (faster than with intravenous use); however, the "high" lasts only 2 to 5 minutes. Cocaine powder is water soluble and can be easily injected, resulting in a high that starts about 1 minute after injection and peaks in 5 minutes. "Speedball," a combination of cocaine and heroin injected intravenously, produces a calmer drug-induced euphoria. "Spaceball," is a combination of crack sprinkled with phencyclidine (PCP, or angel dust), has stimulant and hallucinogenic effects. Marijuana can also be combined with crack to produce a "turbo." Binges—episodes of frequent use of cocaine—maintain the euphoria and prevent the depressive crash that follows cessation of the drug. Psychologic and possibly physical addiction develops rapidly with continued use of cocaine.

Alcohol, a central nervous system depressant, is important in a discussion of injecting drug use because it is frequently used in combination with heroin and cocaine. Alcohol affects social behavior, cognition, motor performance, sexual activity, and respiration (Arif & Westermeyer, 1988). Use of alcohol leads to disinhibition of behavior. Continued drinking can lead to depression, somnolence, coma, and death. Tolerance and physiologic dependence develop with long-term alcohol use.

WITHDRAWAL

Few individuals can stop using heroin, cocaine, or alcohol without some type of treatment or support. The abrupt discontinuation of any of these substances results in withdrawal symptoms. The treatment approach may vary depending on the substance being used.

Discontinuation of heroin leads to symptoms of withdrawal 4 to 24 hours after the last dose. The symptoms intensify, peak in about 24 to 72 hours, and then decrease after 4 or 5 days. Symptoms of heroin withdrawal include anxiety, restlessness, irritability, lacrimation, generalized body aches, insomnia, perspiration, dilated pupils, gooseflesh, hot flushes, nausea and vomiting, diarrhea, fever, increased heart rate, and elevated blood pressure. Dehydration and weight loss may occur during this period. These symptoms are prevented by giving the drug of dependency or, in the case of heroin, administering another opiate in diminishing doses until withdrawal is accomplished.

Engel (1991) defines the cocaine abstinence syndrome that is associated with repeated use and cessation of cocaine. There are three phases: (1) crash, (2) withdrawal, and (3) extinction. "Crash" refers to the period immediately after a cocaine binge. Depression usually occurs 15 to 30 minutes after the final dose, and sleep overshadows the need for cocaine for the next 5 to 10 hours. Suicidal ideation and/or paranoia may be experienced. If a new binge is not started, this phase may last up to 4 days. During the withdrawal phase a sense of "being in control" and nearly normal affective functioning are gradually replaced by increasing cocaine craving and anhedonia. If cocaine is obtained, a binge will occur and the user will return to phase 1. A typical pattern of cocaine use would be 3- to 10-day cycles constituting 6 to 36 hours of cocaine use, 1 or 2 days of crash, 1 or 2 days of normalization, 1 or 2 days of resisting cocaine, and then a repeat of cocaine use. If abstinence is maintained through the first two stages for a period of 6 to 18 weeks, then the extinction phase has been reached. During this stage, less severe craving for cocaine occurs; however, it is still present and may be evoked by certain circumstances or objects. Cravings have been reported to last for months or years after the last use of cocaine.

Withdrawal from alcohol can be far more dangerous than heroin or cocaine withdrawal. The severity of the symptoms depends on the duration of alcohol use and the degree of intoxication. Typically, symptoms begin within 24 hours of alcohol cessation, peak within 2 or 3 days, and resolve within 1 to 2 weeks. Headaches, anxiety, involuntary twitching of muscles, tremor of hands, weakness, insomnia, and nausea are common early symptoms of withdrawal. Hypotension, fever, delirium (as evidenced by disorientation, delusions, and vivid visual hallucinations), and convulsions characterize more advanced withdrawal. Intravenous administration of diazepam or a similar tranquilizer is used during the early stages of alcohol withdrawal, followed by tapering doses or oral medications.

TREATMENT OF SUBSTANCE ABUSE

Various options exist for the treatment of chemical dependency. Some of the more common ones are detoxification programs, therapeutic communities, methadone maintenance programs, and self-help groups. If cocaine use has a biologic component, then drug therapy may be an effective treatment. Acupuncture, an alternative to current biomedical therapy, is gaining acceptance as a viable treatment option for chemical dependency.

Detoxification Programs

Detoxification programs may be affiliated with a hospital or may be independent. The length of stay varies from 3 days to more than 30 days, depending on the substance involved and the program. In New York City, for example, many inpatient cocaine detoxification programs last 3 days, whereas alcohol detoxification programs typically last 28 days. Programs requiring longer treatment offer counseling in addition to medical management of withdrawal.

Therapeutic Communities

Therapeutic communities (TCs) provide structured environments that are run by and for substance users. Synanon, the first TC, was founded in California in 1958 by Charles E. Dederich, a former alcoholic and active member of Alcoholics Anonymous (Sugarman, 1974). He developed the style of TCs: the confrontational groups, the verbal reprimand, and the principle of joint residence. Before entry into the community, individuals had to agree to conform to all rules and demonstrate their commitment to the community by doing something difficult but meaningful (such as yelling for help in front of other residents). In 1963, Daytop Village, modeled after Synanon, was started on the East Coast. Many TCs, based on these two early communities, have since been developed.

TCs require a lengthy time commitment (possibly up to 2 years). The theory of TCs maintains that the problem is not just one of addiction but rather a personality problem that leads to addiction. On admission to a TC, the individual is viewed as an infant who needs to learn adult ways, in place of addictive ways, to cope. Through a process of confrontational groups, sharing of chores, and increasing responsibilities and freedom, a personality restructuring is believed to occur.

With the advent of the AIDS epidemic, TCs have had to confront the problem of caring for members who are HIV infected or have AIDS. Many communities allow symptom-free HIV-infected persons to become members, but the TCs believe that they are not equipped to manage persons with HIV-related symptoms. Substance users who are HIV infected and have symptoms find it difficult to gain entrance to a TC. In response to this problem, Project Samaritan, Inc., opened a 66-bed health-related modified TC in New York City for HIV-infected substance users.

Methadone Maintenance

Methadone maintenance is used to treat heroin addiction. Methadone's effectiveness for this purpose was discovered in the early

1950s by Dr. Marie Nyswander, and her husband, Dr. Vincent Dole. Critics of methadone maintenance therapy contend that one addictive drug, methadone, is being substituted for another addictive drug, heroin. However, as one of the few treatments available for heroin addiction, methadone is widely used. The major advantage of methadone maintenance therapy is that it allows individuals to function normally in society.

Methadone is a synthetic drug that has properties similar to those of morphine. It can provide analgesia (when used for this purpose it is prescribed as Dolophine), suppress withdrawal symptoms for heroin, and remain effective with repeated administration (Jaffe & Martin, 1985). Because methadone is efficiently absorbed from the gastrointestinal tract, it can be administered by mouth. The effects of a maintenance dose of methadone last up to 30 hours, necessitating only once-a-day dosage.

Unlike other medications used to treat discase, the dispensation of methadone is controlled by the U.S. Food and Drug Administration and state regulations. Guidelines exist for daily dosage, frequency of clinic visits, dispensation of take-home methadone, and provision of counseling. Physicians cannot legally prescribe methadone for the treatment of chemical dependency (Newman, 1987; Novick et al., 1988). Publicly funded methadone maintenance treatment programs were started in the 1970s (Wesson, 1988).

The goal of methadone maintenance is to prevent withdrawal symptoms and to block the euphoric effects of other opiates. If an individual on methadone maintenance should take any opiate in any form, he or she would not experience a "high." On entering a methadone program, a person is assessed for the level of heroin use and started on a regimen of 10 to 40 mg of methadone per day. Dosage is based on clinical presentation and history of daily narcotic use. The dose is gradually increased, usually by increments of 10 mg, until a maintenance dose is reached, usually after 4 to 6 weeks. The usual maintenance dose is 60 to 80 mg per day, with a minimum effective dose of 40 mg; only rarely is more than 100 mg per day required (Dole, 1988).

During the induction phase the goal is to keep the person free of withdrawal symptoms. Symptoms of mild overdosage, which usually are eliminated with dose reduction, include sedation, sweating, and decreased libido (Arif & Westermeyer, 1988). Constipation is a frequent side effect that may not abate with dosage change or duration of therapy. The blood level of methadone for maintenance should be in the range of 150 to 600 mg/ml, although monitoring of the methadone dosage is usually based more on subjective reports than on blood levels (Dole, 1988). Miosis may be evident shortly after the methadone is taken and lasts several hours. Persons taking methadone feel a high about 20 to 30 minutes after administration but should not subsequently go into a nod, as occurs with heroin.

The use of cocaine by individuals on methadone maintenance has increased recently. The use of other substances (e.g., amphetamines, tranquilizers, and alcohol) is not uncommon. Urine testing is performed during treatment to detect the presence of these substances and to alert the staff to the need for intervention.

Certain medications can interfere with the metabolism of methadone and necessitate a methadone dose increase when treatment with one of these drugs is initiated. Rifampin, used in the treatment of tuberculosis, rifabutin, used as prophylaxis for and treatment of *Mycobacterium avium* complex infection, and phenytoin (Dilantin), an anticonvulsant, are frequently used. Any of these drugs may cause patients to complain that their methadone is "being eaten up." If an individual's methadone dose is not increased when one of these medications is initiated, symptoms of withdrawal will begin several days later. The methadone dose should be increased by 10 mg on the first day of rifampin, rifabutin, or phenytoin therapy and then by 10 mg every 1 to 2 days thereafter until oversedation is achieved. Patients may require a methadone dose up to 50% higher than their previous dose (Friedland & Selwyn, 1990). Other opiates, central nervous system depressants, tricyclic antidepressants, and anxiolytic agents also interfere with methadone metabolism to a lesser degree and require a dosage adjustment.

Table 9–4. Twelve-Step Program of Alcoholics Anonymous

1. We admitted we were powerless over alcohol—that our lives had become unmanageable
2. Came to believe that a Power greater than ourselves could restore us to sanity
3. Made a decision to turn our will and our lives over to the care of God as we understood Him
4. Made a searching and fearless moral inventory of ourselves
5. Admitted to God, to ourselves and to other human beings the exact nature of our wrongs
6. Were entirely ready to have God remove all these defects of character
7. Humbly asked Him to remove our shortcomings
8. Made a list of all persons we had harmed, and became willing to make amends to them all
9. Made direct amends to such people wherever possible, except when to do so would injure them or others
10. Continued to take personal inventory and when we were wrong promptly admitted it
11. Sought through prayer and meditation to improve our conscious contact with God, as we understood Him, praying only for knowledge of His will for us and the power to carry that out
12. Having had a spiritual awakening as the result of all these steps, we tried to carry this message to alcoholics, and to practice these principles in all our affairs

The Twelve Steps are reprinted with the permission of Alcoholics Anonymous World Services, Inc. Permission to reprint the Twelve Steps does not mean that A.A. has reviewed or approved the contents of this publication nor that A.A. agrees with the views expressed herein. A.A. is a program of recovery from alcoholism—use of the Twelve Steps in connection with programs and activities which are patterned after A.A., but which address other problems, does not imply otherwise.

Methadone maintenance does not control pain. Individuals receiving methadone, regardless of the dose, as treatment for heroin addiction are still able to experience pain. They require pain medication in higher and more frequent doses than a narcotic-naive individual would. In addition, adequate pain control is difficult to achieve when the methadone dose is more than 50 mg per day (Gayle Newshan, personal communication). In this circumstance, if long-term pain management is needed, the person may be weaned to 50 mg of methadone per day. When a person on methadone maintenance is admitted to the hospital, the hospital must confirm the patient's methadone dosage with the methadone program because the patient will require methadone while in the hospital. Clinicians should not assume that the patient is too sick for methadone; without the daily dose, the patient will experience withdrawal symptoms regardless of his or her medical condition.

Withdrawal from methadone maintenance is possible. This may be considered when an individual has been stabilized on methadone for a time and wants to be drug free. Depending on the maintenance dose of methadone, withdrawal should occur during a period of weeks to months and requires a gradual tapering of the dose (Arif & Wester meyer, 1988). Individuals who withdraw in this manner should be able to function normally and should experience no untoward effects.

Self-help Groups

Self-help groups are made up of individuals who have a common problem, chemical dependency, and whose goal is to live drug and alcohol free. The best-known of these groups is Alcoholics Anonymous (AA), from which Narcotics Anonymous (NA) and Cocaine Anonymous (CA) have evolved. Bill Wilson started AA in 1935 to help alcoholics achieve and maintain sobriety. Members of AA must admit they are alcoholics and recognize that they will always be alcoholics. They believe that recovery is a lifelong process. "'Living in Recovery' is a commitment to adopting a drug and alcohol free life-style that consists of a daily adherence to the values and concepts as set forth in the 12 step programs" (Narcotic & Drug Research, Inc., 1989, p. 104). Table 9–4 outlines the 12-step program of AA.

Chapters of AA, NA, and CA have been organized worldwide. In meetings, attenders share their experiences with drugs or alcohol and, through this process and with the help of a sponsor, obtain mutual support to remain drug or alcohol free. When an individual is in the early stages of recovery, daily meetings are strongly recommended. Because AA, NA, and CA are based on the premise of being drug and alcohol free, individuals on methadone maintenance or PWHIV receiving long-term pain medication may be excluded from these meetings. In some cities there are now meetings where such individuals are welcome. In addition, meetings are held for those who speak a language other than English and for gay and lesbian people in recovery. Al-Anon and Al-Ateen are groups for families of people who are actively using drugs or alcohol or who are in recovery.

Drug Therapy

Evidence suggests that long-term cocaine use alters neurophysiologic systems. Pharmacologic agents being studied include tricyclic antidepressants, anticonvulsants, neurotransmitter precursors, stimulants and dopamine agonists, serotonin reuptake blockers and agonists, neuroleptics, and opioid agonists/antagonists (Kleber, 1992).

Desipramine, a tricyclic antidepressant, has been the focus of much research. It has an effect on both the dopamine and catecholamine receptors and has few anticholinergic side effects. In studies of the drug a majority of patients showed extended periods of abstinence from cocaine, with a decrease in craving (Kleber, 1992). Improvement is observed approximately 2 to 3 weeks after desipramine is initiated. The starting dose is 50 mg/day with a rapid dose increase to 200 mg/day. Higher doses may be required. It is recommended that the drug not be started until several days after the most recent cocaine crash.

Amantadine, a presynaptic dopamine agonist, and bromocriptine, a postsynaptic dopamine agonist, may quickly ameliorate cocaine use and craving (Kleber, 1992). However, it appears that their effects may last only 3 weeks. They may be useful in combination with desipramine. Amantadine or bromocriptine therapy would be started concurrently with the use of desipramine; the former drug would begin action immediately and control symptoms until the latter drug became effective.

Methylphenidate has been tried but, with the exception of cocaine users who have a clear history of attention deficit disorder, appears to make cocaine abstinence worse (Kleber, 1992). Serotonin reuptake blockers, such as fluoxetine, appear to be well tolerated and may be effective in reducing cocaine use, craving, and depression (Batki et al., 1993). It is possible that different agents will be required for different groups of cocaine users.

Acupuncture

Acupuncture is a form of Chinese medicine that was developed more than 2500 years ago to relieve pain and stress. It involves insertion of thin needles into specific body points that control organ and body functioning. In the early 1970s Dr. Michael Smith identified that acupuncture could be used to treat heroin withdrawal and help individuals remain drug free. As a result, he started an acupuncture detoxification clinic at Lincoln Hospital in the South Bronx area of New York City. The program has been so successful that it has been replicated in many other countries.

Western scientists are not certain how acupuncture works. Possibly the needle insertion stimulates the body to produce endorphins, which are natural pain killers. Regardless of its mode of action, acupuncture is now being used to treat alcohol and cocaine addiction with the same reported success rates as with heroin. In the Lincoln Hospital program, patients are encouraged to receive daily acupuncture treatment for the initial 2 weeks of therapy and then maintenance treatments approximately three times a week indefinitely. Treatments involve inserting four or five needles in designated points on each ear and leaving them in place for 30 to 45 minutes. Many patients report a feeling of relaxation and a diminished desire to use their drug(s) after treatments. Counseling, along with NA, AA, or CA, is encouraged. Urine screening is done randomly.

The treatment of cocaine addiction by acupuncture is viewed as generally successful, and because few other treatment options exist, New York City has plans to establish acupuncture treatment clinics for cocaine addiction in a number of its municipal hospitals.

CHEMICAL DEPENDENCY AND HIV INFECTION

Even without the addition of HIV infection, chemical dependency has multiple negative effects on the body. Malnutrition, infectious diseases, trauma, and psychiatric disorders are common in substance users and may make disease processes caused by substance use difficult to differentiate from those caused by HIV infection. Table 9–5 lists more specific medical conditions that result from substance use.

Table 9–5. Medical Conditions Resulting From Substance Abuse

MEDICAL PROBLEM	COMMENTS
Heart and Lungs	
Cardiomegaly, cardiomyopathy	Direct toxic effect of alcohol from thiamine deficiency
Congestive heart failure	
Endocarditis	Results from IV drug use
Increased respiratory infections	Results from immunosuppression
Blood	
Anemia, leukemia, thrombocytopenia	Results from bone marrow suppression, vitamin deficiencies
Immune System	
Increased incidence of infection, AIDS	Results from injecting drug use; direct toxic effect on bone marrow and leukocytes, increased lifestyle stress and risk
Nervous System	
Withdrawal symptoms; seizures, tremors, hallucinations, delirium tremens, irritability, depression, paranoid ideation	Direct toxic effects and rapid decrease in drug blood levels
Cerebral atrophy and diminished functioning	Direct toxic effects and deficiencies—contributing factors
Psychiatric disorders	
Cerebellar disorders	
Neuropathies, palsies, gait disturbances	
Visual problems	
Digestive System	
Liver diseases (alcoholism, leading to hepatitis B, fatty liver, cirrhosis)	Direct toxic effects of alcohol; parenteral injection of hepatitis B virus
Pancreatitis	
Ulcers and inflammations of the gut, Mallory-Weiss syndrome, peptic ulcers, diarrhea, constipation	Direct irritation of intestinal mucosa by alcohol
Nutritional Deficiencies	
Pellagra	Niacin deficiency
Wernicke's encephalopathy	Thiamine deficiency
Dermatitis, cheilosis, stomatitis	Riboflavin deficiency
Anemia	Pyridoxine and folic acid deficiencies
Scurvy	Vitamin C deficiency
Endocrine System	
Hypoglycemia	Secondary to pancreatitis and deficiencies of gluconeogenesis
Hypercalcemia	From magnesium deficiency

From Narcotic and Drug Research, Inc. (1989). *AIDS: Medical management of the HIV infected/chemically dependent client.* New York: The Company.

Concern exists about the possibility that drug use will speed the progression of HIV infection in IDUs. However, studies have shown that progression of HIV infection is not more rapid among IDUs, regardless of whether they are currently using versus not using drugs, than among other groups (The Italian Seroconversion Study, 1992; Margolick et al., 1992; Selwyn et al., 1992). Other reports have associated continued injecting drug use with HIV progression (Des Jarlais, 1991). It is theorized that the cause of the progression is related to immunosuppression related to nonsterile injections and resulting stimulation of the immune complex. Continued drug injection may also lead to repeated reexposure to HIV. Currently there is no *in vivo* evidence that any psychoactive drug has a pharmacologic effect on the rate of progression of HIV infection (Des Jarlais, 1991).

HIV infection is associated with different opportunistic infections and malignancies in IDUs. The incidence of Kaposi's sarcoma, cytomegalovirus infection, and herpes simplex virus infection is lower among IDUs; *Pneumocystis carinii* pneumonia, cryptococcal disease, histoplasmosis, and extrapulmonary tuberculosis are more common (Friedland & Selwyn, 1990).

As of January 1993 the CDC expanded the case definition of AIDS to include bacterial pneumonia (two or more episodes in a 12-month period) and pulmonary tuberculosis regardless of CD4$^+$ T-cell count (CDC, 1992). Before this change, bacterial pneumonia, sepsis, and tuberculosis led to an increased non-AIDS mortality rate among HIV-infected IDUs (Selwyn & O'Connor, 1992). The new CDC change is expected to yield large increases in the number of IDUs meeting the new case definition of AIDS (Des Jarlais et al., 1992). The incidence of sexually transmitted diseases, infection with human papillomavirus, and cervical abnormalities demonstrated on Papanicolaou smears also is higher among HIV-infected female IDUs (Friedland & Selwyn, 1990).

Bacterial pneumonia tends to occur earlier in PWHIV and is viewed as a predictor of subsequent HIV-related illness (Selwyn & O'Connor, 1992). Regardless of HIV status, IDUs, if currently injecting, are at risk of acquiring a variety of bacterial infections, including pneumonia, endocarditis, and infections of the soft tissue, bones, joints, central and peripheral nervous systems, and peripheral vascular system, as well as having metastatic abscesses involving other sites. It is postulated that some of these infections are less likely to occur in individuals who employ skin-cleaning techniques before injecting (Vlahov et al., 1992).

IDUs are at high risk of having tuberculosis (TB). In New York City the incidence of pulmonary TB among IDUs is increasing. It was found that 57% of patients with both HIV infection and TB in New York City were IDUs (Friedland & Selwyn, 1990). A study of 169 homeless men in a congregate shelter in New York City found a high correlation among HIV seropositivity, injecting drug use, and active TB (Torres, 1990). Of these men, 22% had active pulmonary TB and 54% reported current active drug use. Of increasing concern in this population is the incidence of multi-drug-resistant TB (MDR-TB). MDR-TB results either from noncompliance with the TB medication treatment regimen, which leads to the development of resistant strains of *Mycobacterium tuberculosis,* or from exposure to an individual with MDR-TB (refer to Chapter 4).

Screening for TB is essential for any individual who is an IDU and therefore at risk of acquiring HIV infection. Drug treatment programs are required by federal regulations to perform tuberculin skin testing before admission. Further evaluation for clinical TB is recommended for an IDU with HIV infection who has a skin reaction of greater than or equal to 5 mm or for an IDU who is not infected but has a skin reaction of greater than or equal to 10 mm (CDC, 1990a). Chapter 4 reviews recommendations for prophylaxis and treatment.

When compliance might be an issue, health care personnel should arrange for direct observation therapy (DOT). In New York City the Department of Health has DOT workers who will go to the homes of individuals who might be noncompliant with TB medication. Methadone maintenance programs and congregate shelters have been successfully providing DOT on site (Selwyn et al., 1989; Torres et al., 1990). Currently, in New York City, methadone maintenance programs are mandated to provide DOT to all TB-infected clients.

Substance use and HIV infection can both cause central nervous system disease and dysfunction. It is essential to determine the cause of central nervous system symptoms because there may be a treatable condition. The differential diagnosis should include HIV-related dementia, opportunistic infections of the central nervous system, metabolic or toxic encephalopathy from some other cause, and the effects of substance use (Selwyn & O'Connor, 1992). A thorough history is essential. An assessment of level of consciousness might help differentiate between HIV-related dementia and drug use effects. Individuals with HIV-related dementia tend to maintain alertness until the later stages of disease, whereas drugs and alcohol alter the level of consciousness. A urine toxicology study should be done as part of the evaluation.

A dual diagnosis of psychiatric disorders and chemical dependency is not uncommon among the IDU population. Three patterns of dual diagnosis exist (Batki, 1990). In the first pattern the drug use causes the psychiatric problem. For example, cocaine psychosis is a result of cocaine use. In the second pattern a psychiatric condition predates substance use; possibly substance use is a form of self-treatment for the psychiatric condition. In the third pattern it is unclear which came first, the substance use or the psychiatric condition. The addition of HIV infection creates, in effect, a triple diagnosis. A dual or triple diagnosis involves a myriad of social, psychologic, and medical problems that complicate the provision of services. Differentiating the cause of the psychiatric symptoms will guide the treatment. HIV-related neuropsychiatric problems are discussed in Chapter 4.

Some constitutional symptoms are characteristic of both HIV infection and substance use. Unexplained fever, weight loss, fatigue, malaise, and diarrhea may be seen in both groups (Selwyn & O'Connor, 1992). Opiate addicts experience alternating constipation and diarrhea. Cocaine users frequently have anorexia and weight loss. Fevers may be a result of HIV infection or an indication of a bacterial infection in an IDU who has recently injected. Crack use leads to pulmonary problems that may easily be confused with *P. carinii* pneumonia. Lymphadenopathy is common in IDUs who are actively using drugs and is a frequent symptom in HIV-infected individuals. Posterior cervical lymphadenopathy is less common in IDUs, unless there are scalp lesions, and may be a useful indicator of HIV-related infection versus IDU-related infection.

RISK REDUCTION

Transmission of HIV infection may be prevented by the cessation of substance use and by abstinence from high-risk sexual activities. Failing these goals, IDUs need to know how to reduce the risk of transmitting HIV infection. Participating in needle exchange programs, cleansing syringes and needles with bleach, and using condoms are highly effective ways to prevent HIV transmission.

Studies have shown the IDUs are generally aware of the risk of needle sharing. In one methadone maintenance program and large detention facility in New York City, 97% of subjects interviewed recognized needle sharing as an AIDS risk factor (Selwyn, 1987).

Drug treatment offers IDUs the opportunity to stop injecting drug use—one high-risk behavior. Metzger and colleagues (1993) demonstrated that the HIV seroconversion rate is significantly lower for those individuals who remain in methadone maintenance than for those who do not. However, it was also found that methadone-maintained patients who continued to share needles were a more disturbed subgroup and probably required more intensive psychiatric services (Metzger et al., 1991).

Significant controversy surrounds syringe exchange programs and the instruction of users in how to clean their "works" with bleach. Many maintain that these programs encourage substance use, whereas others believe that these measures encourage risk reduction until the individual can enter a treat-

Table 9–6. Principles of Harm Reduction Model

1. Abstinence from drugs is not a realistic goal for many drug users.
2. Individuals can be taught how to reduce harmful consequences of drug use *if* they are approached in a nonjudgmental manner.
3. Examples of interventions to make drug use safer:
    a. Refer to needle exchange programs (if locally available).
    b. Teach how to clean injecting drug "works" with bleach.
    c. Instruct in risks of sharing drug works (not just HIV, but also hepatitis B, abscesses, and bacterial endocarditis).
    d. Instruct in proper injection technique (cleanse skin with alcohol, rotate sites if possible).
    e. Discuss alternate routes of administration (e.g., snorting heroin instead of injecting).

Data from Springer, E. (1991). Effective AIDS prevention with active drug users: The harm reduction model. *Journal of Chemical Dependency Treatment, 4*(2), 141–157.

ment program. In the United States, where 80% of active IDUs are not in treatment, too few treatment slots are available for the number of persons needing and wanting treatment, resulting in a wait for those who ask for it (CDC, 1990b).

The U.S. federal government's first comprehensive study of syringe exchange concluded that this intervention can help decrease the spread of HIV and recommended expansion of these programs (U.S. General Accounting Office, 1993). Syringe exchange program studies have been conducted in the Netherlands, Sweden, and Australia, and in the United States in Tacoma, Washington, New Haven, Connecticut, and New York City (Watters et al., 1994). Reports from these studies concluded that syringe exchange programs play a significant role in reducing the incidence of needle sharing and serve as a source of referrals into social services, medical services, and drug treatment (U.S. General Accounting Office, 1993; Watters et al., 1994). However, these programs have been less successful in changing sexual behaviors that incorporate the use of condoms (Dolan et al., 1990; Keffelew et al., 1990).

Where syringe exchange programs are unavailable, programs that instruct in the use of bleach for cleaning one's "works" and distribute individual bleach kits have been established. In many of these community-based organizations, recovered IDUs go into the community to teach and counsel active IDUs. This nontraditional type of outreach is believed effective in changing behavior with this group of individuals, who have little contact with a more traditional social service and medical care system (Stimson, 1990; CDC, 1990b).

The NIDA (National Institutes of Health), the Center for Substance Abuse Treatment (Substance Abuse and Mental Health Services Administration), and the CDC, on April 19, 1993, issued a bulletin updating recommendations to prevent transmission of HIV (CDC, 1993). The bulletin recommends bleach disinfection of needles and syringes for IDUs who continue to inject and states that sterile, never-used needles and syringes are safer than bleach-disinfected, previously used needles and syringes. The bulletin also recommends the use of full-strength household bleach to disinfect needles and syringes. Previously a solution of one part bleach to ten parts water was recommended. The recommendations were changed because of the difficulty of adequately cleaning the interior of needles and syringes.

There will always be IDUs who do not want to stop using drugs. The Harm Reduction Model is a new strategy developed to reduce the risk of HIV infection among this group (Springer, 1991). With this model, HIV/AIDS prevention takes precedence over stopping drug use. If drug users will not stop using drugs, then they should be encouraged to use drugs in a manner that will reduce the risk of HIV transmission (Table 9–6). Needle exchange and disinfection with bleach are part of the Harm Reduction Model. In addition, users should be taught safe injection techniques. Providers should also encourage users to try other routes of drug administration. Intranasal use is safer than injecting;

however, the drug effect will be slower than with injecting. Smoking produces a quicker effect than intranasal use, may be preferred by the user, and is safer than injecting. A criticism of this model is that, particularly with stimulants, heavy use of drugs clouds judgment, which leads to unsafe drug use; the individual becomes confused or intoxicated, or remembers but does not care about risk reduction (CIBA Foundation Symposium, 1992).

The correct use of condoms should be discussed with all IDUs and their partners. It should be stressed that entering drug treatment programs or cleaning their works does little to prevent the transmission of HIV infection unless safer sex is practiced also.

PAIN MANAGEMENT

Substance users have as great a need for adequate pain control as other patients. A study to define the pain syndromes and their management in PWHIV found little difference in the complaints of pain between IDUs and homosexual patients (Newshan & Wainapel, 1993). Abdominal and neuropathic pain occurred in approximately 50% of the patients, with equal frequency in IDUs and homosexual patients. Pain from esophagitis, headaches, Kaposi's sarcoma, postherpetic neuralgia, and backache was also reported.

It is important to remember that IDUs usually require higher and more frequent doses of opiates to manage pain. Every patient with chronic pain should be given medication on a regular basis rather than on an as-needed basis. This is particularly important with IDUs. An adequate amount and frequency of pain medication helps to relieve the anxiety experienced when patients with pain are made to wait for medication. Patients who use methadone require higher doses of pain medication. It is incorrect to try to control pain by increasing the methadone dose. Anxiety increases the pain experience, but anxiolytics, because of their potential for abuse, should be used with care in this population. Anxiety may be relieved with appropriate pain medication, relaxation exercises, therapeutic touch, acupuncture, or counseling.

Of concern to many practitioners is the issue of abuse of pain medication by IDUs. Some individuals with a substance use history seek medication for this purpose, and distinguishing between real pain and pain falsely reported by those seeking drugs can be difficult. Dal Pan and McArthur (1994) recommend that (1) single practitioners prescribe the medications, (2) "lost" prescriptions not be refilled, (3) narcotic prescriptions be carefully rationed, and (4) rescue doses of narcotic analgesics be limited on a monthly basis. It is important to evaluate all complaints of pain for a possible disease process that would respond to treatment. Requests for specific drugs (e.g., hydromorphone) that have a high street value should prompt concern that the drugs will be sold (Wesson et al., 1993). When possible, nonnarcotic pain relievers should be tried before narcotic pain relievers are prescribed. Drug users without pain frequently refuse the nonnarcotic medication, claiming that they have "tried it, and it doesn't work."

When substance users are started on a regimen of narcotic pain medication, the reason for its use and the treatment plan should be made clear. If the dosage is to be adjusted or tapered, this should be discussed with the patient beforehand. It is helpful to prescribe limited amounts of medication that only one provider can renew. Frequent visits to monitor progress and the patient's management of the medication are encouraged. If the patient expresses concern about potential abuse of the medication, the provider might consider having a family member or friend keep the medication and give it to the patient as needed. Family members and/or friends are also good sources of information regarding patient abuse of pain medication. A patient who is in recovery and requires pain medication should be encouraged to inform the treatment program or counselor, who may provide added support during this period.

RELAPSE PREVENTION AND MANAGEMENT

Relapses frequently occur with IDUs and should be anticipated. When relapse occurs, the goal is to get the client back to recovery as soon as possible. Relapse may mean one

Table 9–7. Events and Situations That Could Lead to Relapse

Parties	Rejecting help
Old friends	Not attending Alcoholic
Old relationships	Anonymous or Nar-
Fighting with family	cotic Anonymous
Isolation	meetings
Pressures becoming un-	Rationalizing problems
manageable	Lying consciously
Guilt	Feeling self-pity
Being oversensitive	Losing confidence
Living in the past	"I can do it by myself"
Anger becoming un-	attitude
manageable	Projecting
Daily routine	High expectations
"Don't care" attitude	Taking on too many
	projects
	Cravings

From Narcotic and Drug Research, Inc. (1989). *AIDS: Medical management of the HIV infected/chemically dependent client.* New York: The Company.

time only use (slip), repeated uses within a short period (binge), or a return to frequent or continual use.

Hall and colleagues (1991) identified three stages in the relapse process. The first stage is the "slip" after an episode of abstinence; the second is relapse itself, constituting continued use; and the final is a transition stage between the two. The authors referred to studies demonstrating that few individuals who slip do not return to pretreatment levels of drug use. Unfortunately, not enough is known to predict what interventions and support will help an individual to remain drug free after treatment.

Motivation to remain drug free appears to be crucial. Those individuals who are determined to avoid use of drugs seem to have fewer relapses than those who are less determined and are inclined to mix periods of abstinence with slips (Hall et al., 1991). Coping skills directed toward preventing relapse by identifying events and situations that could lead to relapse are of questionable benefit. The client may identify some of these events or situations (Table 9–7) as creating a high risk of having a relapse and may receive counseling on how to avoid, reduce, or manage the triggering events or situations. It may be more effective to teach skills directed toward developing a non-drug-using support network.

Drug users with concurrent depression and other psychiatric problems appear to have a high rate of relapse (Hall et al., 1991). These individuals should be identified while in treatment and should receive appropriate psychiatric counseling and medication.

HIV TESTING AND COUNSELING

Chapter 2 discusses issues and mechanisms for testing and counseling individuals at risk of acquiring HIV infection. Individuals with a history of injecting drug use, crack or alcohol use, or multiple, frequent sexual partners are considered at risk. These individuals may enter the health care system when they begin drug treatment, are hospitalized for an acute illness, or receive services from an outreach program. As with any person at risk, all the issues and implications of testing should be reviewed. Regardless of the person's HIV status, emphasis should be placed on discontinuing the risky behavior. Studies show that substance users enrolled in methadone maintenance treatment programs are interested in and seek HIV screening (Carlson & McClellan, 1987; Curtis et al., 1989). This information, and the knowledge that many IDUs are aware of risky behaviors, should encourage health care providers to discuss counseling openly.

PLANNING NURSING CARE

Assessment

The development of a nursing care plan for an HIV-infected IDU depends on an assessment of the individual's substance use. The health care worker must find out what drugs are used and in what amounts, the duration of use, the route, and what other risk behaviors are present. Without this information, adequate planning for care of the drug problem or the HIV infection is impossible (see Chapter 5 for nursing care planning).

A drug history should be taken in a thorough and nonjudgmental manner. The interviewer should explore his or her feelings about drug use before interacting with a client. The interviewer should not ask questions in a hurried manner that might imply that the interviewer is embarrassed or wants to conclude the session quickly. Genuine interest, concern, and a desire to help should be evident.

A drug history should elicit information on five aspects of substance use: substances used, routes of administration, patterns of use, treatment history, and medical and social complications of substance use (Selwyn & O'Connor, 1992). Information must be obtained regarding substances used. Be specific by actually asking about specific drugs, such as heroin, cocaine, "uppers," "downers," and alcohol. It also helps to be familiar with street terminology and to feel comfortable using it. Information on routes of administration, frequency of use, amounts used, and duration of use is important and must be obtained for each substance used, while keeping in mind that polydrug use is common. It is important to find out when each substance was last used.

It is hoped that obtaining a treatment history will ensure that referrals to drug treatment will not include programs that failed the individual in the past. It is important to find out from the patient why a specific treatment failed. When previous medical complications are assessed, the patient should be questioned about needle-related and drug-induced medical problems. Marital, family, and legal problems and unemployment are all important factors possibly related to drug use.

If it appears that the individual is not being truthful during the history taking, it may be useful to speak with family and/or friends. In many medical settings, social workers are an integral part of the health care team and may be able to help obtain this information.

Asking about the use of nonprescribed antibiotics and AIDS-related medications such as zidovudine, acyclovir, or ketoconazole is important. IDUs commonly purchase antibiotics on the street and use them for self-medication when not feeling well. Selwyn and associates (1989) reported that after an episode of high-risk behavior, IDUs may obtain AIDS treatment drugs on the street for "preventive" use.

The physical examination as discussed in Chapter 5 should support information obtained in the history. During the physical examination the nurse should be observant for recent injection marks (tracks). The most obvious locations are the arms and legs. Less obvious places are the neck, breasts, groin, feet, and dorsal vein of the penis. Urine toxicologic examination, which can detect opiates, cocaine, benzodiazepine, barbiturates, amphetamines, marijuana, and tricyclic antidepressants, should be an integral part of the health assessment. This should be done as soon as possible, because only the longest-acting substances are evident after several days.

Planning

Individuals with chemical dependency and HIV infection require a plan of care that addresses both problems. Many nurses have less difficulty in developing a plan for HIV infection than for chemical dependency. The goal of a nursing care plan for substance use should be to encourage the individual to enter treatment or, if they refuse treatment, to reduce high-risk behavior. If treatment is desired, a review of treatment options should be followed by a discussion of what might be the best choice for the client based on the drugs being used.

The nursing care plan for an individual who expresses an interest in drug treatment should include short-term goals that are reasonably attainable. Most substance users are easily frustrated and require fairly immediate gratification. The first, easily measurable part of the plan should be that the client either calls for an appointment or goes in person to the treatment program. This should be done as soon as possible, because it is common for substance users to express an interest in drug treatment one day and change their minds the next day. Once the substance user decides to seek treatment, this step may be the most difficult. Many view the first visit to a treatment program as an admission of having a problem—or, if this is not their first encounter with drug treatment, as a failure of previous drug treatment. If the plan of care is being developed in the clinic where the person receives care for the HIV disease, more frequent clinic visits might be scheduled to monitor success and offer encouragement. It is essential that strategies to cope with and prevent relapse be discussed. Individuals need to be reminded that no matter how sure they are that their problem is controlled, they are always at risk of having a relapse. Encouragement to "take one day at a time" is helpful.

For those individuals who are not interested in drug treatment, the plan of care must include harm reduction strategies. These may include referral to a needle exchange program, instruction in disinfecting needles and syringes, or a plan to switch routes of drug administration. If a community-based group that counsels active users is available, a referral should be considered.

Individuals with a substance use problem must want to stop using. A number of motivating factors can bring them to this point. Occasionally rejection by family makes substance users seek treatment. Sometimes services provided because of an AIDS diagnosis (e.g., housing, financial assistance) may make it easier to discontinue drug use. With adequate support, some drug users see the time from diagnosis to illness as a chance to "get it together." Having never thought they would live long enough to die of anything other than drugs, they see this time as extra time.

Health care providers are probably most frustrated by hospitalized substance users who continue to use drugs while in the hospital, "act out," and generally disrupt the unit. As stated before, there will always be drug users who do not want to stop using. Expecting them to stop "cold turkey" just because they are hospitalized is unrealistic. If they express an interest in drug treatment, a referral to a substance abuse counselor should be made immediately. If during the admission assessment it is discovered that the patient was using up to the time of admission, the issue of withdrawal must be addressed. Medication may be essential to control physical and/or psychologic symptoms of withdrawal. Failure to do so almost guarantees that the patient will obtain drugs from the outside. If a substance

abuse counselor has been consulted and appropriate medication has been prescribed but the patient continues to use unprescribed drugs and disrupt the unit, there are few solutions. Restricting visitors, particularly those suspected of bringing in drugs, and/or confining the patient to his or her room are last-resort options with varying degrees of success. It is important that all staff members who have contact with this patient are aware of the plan of care. "Splitting," playing off one staff member against another, is common and must be avoided.

If a patient began drug treatment while hospitalized, follow-up treatment must be arranged before discharge. If the patient is on methadone maintenance and was not enrolled in a methadone program before admission, arrangements for enrollment in a program must be made before discharge. If the patient was enrolled in a program, then the program leaders must be notified before discharge. In either situation the patient must be able to obtain methadone on the day after discharge; a prescription for methadone will not suffice.

Evaluation

Evaluating the plan of care determines its effectiveness and the need for changes. If the first step has been enrollment in a treatment program, confirmation may be made by having the patient return with a letter verifying attendance. All treatment programs require a signed letter requesting release of information before they will even acknowledge attendance by an individual at the program. Communication with the program is generally a good idea because it provides easy verification of attendance and compliance and more coordinated care. Many programs perform routine urine drug screening, which also helps to determine the success of treatment. When relapse is suspected, the individual should be confronted with the suspicion and the nursing care plan should be altered accordingly. When confronting a person, the nurse must be very specific about the reasons for thinking that the client is using: he or she appears high because of his or her behavior; physical examination reveals evidence of recent use; or someone has reported that the client has been using drugs. The plan for coping with the relapse should be delayed until the individual is no longer high.

When risk reduction for a person who does not want treatment has been discussed, follow-up visits should include questioning about specific measures taken by that individual.

NURSING RESEARCH RELATED TO HIV-POSITIVE CHEMICALLY DEPENDENT CLIENTS

Summary of Research

Nurse researchers have begun to explore pain phenomena in drug users with HIV disease. Newshan and Wainapel (1993) identified a higher incidence of pain caused by esophagitis and headaches among drug users, as well as the need for more frequent use of opiates for pain control than nonusers have. Hoyt and colleagues (1993) studied 71 hospitalized PWHIV to explore the differences in pain perception between chemically dependent and nondependent individuals. Their original hypothesis, that the two groups would demonstrate a significantly different perception of pain, was not supported.

Thorn and associates (1990) evaluated the compliance of IDUs and homosexuals in AIDS clinical protocols. Their results demonstrated that IDUs were as compliant as homosexuals when monthly clinic visits were scheduled but less compliant when twice-monthly visits were arranged.

Community-based long-term care delivery, in the presence of continued substance use, can pose numerous challenges to nurses. Schmidt (1992), in a review of 100 case consultations performed by clinical nurse specialists in a home care agency, identified illegal drug use as the reason for requesting a case consultation by a home care nurse in 12% of the requests.

Findings on research into harm reduction strategies from a nursing perspective have also been published. Vlahov and colleagues (1990; 1991a; 1991b; 1992) identified (1) an increased risk of HIV infection in needle-sharing behaviors in shooting galleries; (2)

the potential benefits of bleach and alcohol disinfection among IDUs in shooting galleries; and (3) the potential reduction in the frequency of serious bacterial infections associated with intravenous drug use by the use of alcohol swabs or other antiseptic agents before drugs are injected. Vlahov and associates (1991c) are also conducting a longitudinal study to identify risk factors for HIV infection among IDUs and the progression to AIDS.

Research Needed

Skinner and colleagues (1991) suggested specific areas of research and nursing in the area of HIV disease and psychoactive-substance users, including:

1. Determining a database of persons who use psychoactive substances
2. Exploration of HIV-associated behaviors linked to drug use
3. Epidemiologic studies to explain the sexual, contraceptive, and childbearing practices of users of any psychoactive substance
4. Investigation of the inherent effects of various psychoactive substances on the immune, neurologic, and endocrine systems

Additional areas to consider for nursing research include:

1. Identifying the learning needs of nurses caring for HIV-infected chemically dependent individuals
2. Comparing the knowledge, attitudes, and practices of nurses caring for IDUs and gay men with HIV disease
3. Exploring the differences in human responses between IDUs and other populations with HIV disease
4. Developing and testing strategies to enhance compliance among IDUs
5. Testing the efficacy of complimentary therapies for symptom control among IDUs
6. Exploring the attitudes of IDUs about nurses providing their care
7. Identifying service delivery strategies in

the presence of continued substance use

8. Evaluating the role of the professional nurse in addiction-related service settings, such as methadone maintenance programs and syringe exchange programs

9. Developing new strategies for harm reduction

CONCLUSION

Nurses must recognize that chemical dependency is a disease and requires nursing and medical intervention as does any other disease. The stigma of HIV infection only adds to the stigma of chemical dependency. With knowledge and understanding, nurses can greatly enhance the care given to substance users with HIV infection. IDUs should not be treated as pariahs. They deserve the same respect and dignity accorded other individuals.

REFERENCES

American Nurses' Association (1987). *The care of clients with addictions.* Kansas City, MO: The Association.

American Public Health Association (1990). *Illicit drug use and HIV infection* (2nd ed). Washington, DC: The Association.

Arif, A., Westermeyer, J. (1988). *Manual of drug and alcohol abuse.* New York, NY: Plenum Medical Book Company.

Batki, S.L. (1990). Drug abuse, psychiatric disorders and AIDS. *Western Journal of Medicine, 152*(5), 547–552.

Batki, S.L., Manfredi, L.B., Jacob, P., Jones, R.T. (1993). Fluoxetine for cocaine dependence in methadone maintenance; quantitative plasma and urine cocaine/benzoylecgonine concentrations. *Journal of Clinical Psychopharmacology, 13*(4), 243–250.

Carlson, C.A., McClellan, T.A. (1987). The voluntary acceptance of HIV-antibody screening by intravenous drug users. *Public Health Reports, 102*(4), 391–394.

Cartter, N.C., Petersen, L.R., Savage, R.B., et al. (1989). Providing HIV counseling and testing services in methadone programs. *AIDS, 4*(5), 463–465.

Casey, E. (1989). History of drug use and drug users in the United States. In *AIDS: Medical management of the HIV infected/chemically dependent client* (pp. 25–78). New York, NY: Narcotic and Drug Research Inc.

Centers for Disease Control (1990a). Screening for tuberculosis and tuberculosis infection in high-risk populations. *Morbidity and Mortality Weekly Report, 39,* 1–7.

Centers for Disease Control (1990b). Update: Reducing HIV transmission in intravenous drug users not in drug treatment—United States. *Morbidity and Mortality Weekly Report, 39,* 1–7.

Centers for Disease Control (1992). 1993 Revised classification system for HIV infection and expanded surveillance case definition for AIDS among adolescents and adults. *Morbidity and Mortality Weekly Report, 41*(RR-17), 1–19.

Centers for Disease Control and Prevention (1993). Use of bleach for disinfection of drug injection equipment. *Morbidity and Mortality Weekly Report, 41,* 418–419.

Chiasson, M.A., Stoneburner, R.L., Hildebrandt, D.S., et al. (1990). Heterosexual transmission of HIV associated with the use of smokable free-base cocaine (crack) [abstract No. Th.C.588]. *International Conference on AIDS, 6*(1), 272.

CIBA Foundation Symposium (1992). *AIDS and HIV Infection in Cocaine Users, 166,* 181–194.

Coleman, D. (1990, June 26). Scientists pinpoint brain irregularities in drug addicts. *The New York Times,* p. B5.

Coutinho, R.A. (1990). Epidemiology and prevention of AIDS among intravenous drug users. *Journal of Acquired Immune Deficiency Syndromes, 3*(4), 413–417.

Curtis, J.L., Crummey, C., Baker, S.N., et al. (1989). HIV screening and counseling for intravenous drug users. *Journal of the American Medical Association, 261*(2), 258–262.

Dal Pan, G., McArthur, J.C. (1994). Diagnosis and management of sensory neuropathies in HIV infection. *AIDS Clinical Care, 6*(2), 9–12, 16.

Des Jarlais, D.C. (1991). Potential cofactors in the outcomes of HIV infection in intravenous drug users. *NIDA Research* [monograph], *109,* 115–123.

Des Jarlais, D.C., Friedman, S.R., Novick, D.M., et al. (1989). HIV-1 infection among intravenous drug users in Manhattan, New York City, from 1977 through 1987. *Journal of the American Medical Association, 261*(7), 1008–1012.

Des Jarlais, D.C., Friedman, S.R., Sotheran, J.L., et al. (1994). Continuity and change within an HIV epidemic: Injecting drug users in New York City, 1984 through 1992. *Journal of the American Medical Association, 271*(2), 121–127.

Des Jarlais, D.C., Wenston, J., Friedman, S.R., et al. (1992). Implications of the revised surveillance definition: AIDS among New York City drug users. *American Journal of Public Health, 82*(11), 1531–1533.

Dolan, K., Stimson, G.V., Donoghoe, M.C. (1990). Differences in HIV rates and risk behavior of drug injectors attending syringe-exchange in England [abstract No. F.C.108]. *International Conference on AIDS, 6*(2), 116.

Dole, V.P. (1988). Implications of methadone maintenance for theories of narcotic addiction. *Journal of the American Medical Association, 260*(20), 3025–3029.

Engel, J. (1991). Cocaine: A historical and modern perspective. *Nebraska Medical Journal, 76*(8), 263–270.

Friedland, J., Selwyn, P. (1990). Intravenous drug use and HIV infection. *AIDS Clinical Care, 2*(4), 31–32.

Hall, S.M., Wasserman, D.A., Havassy, B.E. (1991). Relapse prevention. *NIDA Research* [monograph], *106,* 279–291.

Henneberger, M. (1990, August 24). Drug research surges after lull. *Newsday,* p. 8.

Hoyt, M.J., Nokes, K., Newshan, G., et al. (1993). The effect of chemical dependency on pain perception in persons with AIDS [abstract No. PO-B32-2275]. *International Conference on AIDS, 9*(1), 514.

Inciardi, J.A., Chitwood, D.D., McCoy, C.B. (1992). Special risks for the acquisition and transmission of HIV infection during sex and crack houses. *Journal of Acquired Immune Deficiency Syndromes, 5*(9), 951–952.

Jaffe, J.H., Martin, W.A. (1985). Opioid analgesics and antagonists. In A.G. Gillman, L.S. Goodman, T.W. Rall, F. Murad (Eds.), *Pharmacological basis of therapeutics* (7th ed) (pp. 532–581). New York: Macmillan.

Keffelew, A., Clark, G., Bacchelli, P., et al. (1990). Use of needle exchange programs by San Francisco drug users in methadone treatment [abstract no. F.C.107]. *International Conference on AIDS, 6*(2), 116.

Kleber, H.D. (1992). Treatment of cocaine abuse: Pharmacotherapy. *CIBA Foundation Symposium, 166,* 195–200.

Kosten, T.R. (1991). Client issues in drug abuse treatment: Addressing multiple drug use. *NIDA Research* [monograph], *106,* 136–151.

Margolick, J.B., Munoz, A., Vlahov, D., et al. (1992). Changes in T-lymphocyte subsets in intravenous drug users with HIV-1 infection. *Journal of the American Medical Association, 267*(12), 1631–1636.

Marmor, M., Des Jarlais, D.C., Cohen, H., et al. (1987). Risk factors for infection with human immunodeficiency virus among intravenous drug abusers in New York City. *AIDS, 1*(1), 39–44.

Metzger, D., Woody, G., De Philippis, D., et al. (1991). Risk factors for needle sharing among methadone-treated patients. *American Journal of Psychiatry, 148*(5), 636–640.

Metzger, D.S., Woody, G.E., McLellan, T., et al. (1993). Human immunodeficiency virus seroconversion among intravenous drug users in and out of treatment: An 18-month prospective follow-up. *Journal of Acquired Immune Deficiency Syndromes, 6*(9), 1049–1056.

Narcotic and Drug Research, Inc. (1989). *AIDS: Medical management of the HIV infected/chemically dependent client.* New York: The Author.

Newman, R.G. (1987). Methadone treatment. *New England Journal of Medicine, 317*(7), 447–450.

Newshan, G.T., Wainapel, S.F. (1993). Pain characteristics and their management in persons with AIDS. *Journal of the Association of Nurses in AIDS Care, 4*(2), 53–59.

Novick, D.M., Pascarelli, E.F., Joseph, H., et al. (1988). Methadone maintenance patients in general medical practice. *Journal of the American Medical Association, 259*(22), 3299–3302.

Schmidt, J. (1992). Case management problems in the home. *Journal of the Association of Nurses in AIDS Care, 3*(3), 37–44.

Schoenbaum, E.E., Hartel, D., Selwyn, P.A., et al. (1989). Risk factors for human immunodeficiency virus infection in intravenous drug users. *New England Journal of Medicine, 32*(13), 874–879.

Selwyn, P.A. (1987). Issues in the clinical management of intravenous drug users with HIV infection. *AIDS, 3*(suppl 1), S201–S208.

Selwyn, P.A., Alcabes, P., Hartel, D., et al. (1992). Clinical manifestations and predictors of disease progression in drug users with human immunodeficiency virus infection. *New England Journal of Medicine, 327*(24), 1697–1703.

Selwyn, P.A., Feingold, A.R., Iezza, A., et al. (1989). Primary care for patients with human immunodeficiency virus. *Annals of Internal Medicine, 111*(9), 761–763.

Selwyn, P.A., O'Connor, P.G. (1992). Diagnosis and treatment of substance users with HIV infection. *Primary Care, 19*(1), 119–156.

Skinner, A., Walls, L., Brown, L.S., Jr. (1991). AIDS-related behavioral research and nursing. *Journal of the National Medical Association, 83*(7), 585–589.

Springer, E. (1991). Effective AIDS prevention with active drug use: The harm reduction model. In M. Shernoff (Ed.), *Counseling chemically dependent people with HIV illness* (pp. 141–157). New York: Haworth Press.

Stimson, G.V. (1990, June). *The prevention of infection in injecting drug users: Recent advances and remaining obstacles.* Paper presented at the Sixth International Conference on AIDS, San Francisco, CA.

Sugarman, B. (1974). *Daytop Village: A therapeutic community.* New York: Holt, Reinhardt & Winston.

The Italian Seroconversion Study (1992). Disease progression and early predictors of AIDS in HIV-seroconverted drug users. *AIDS, 6*(4), 421–426.

Thorn, M., Staats, J., Torres, R. (1990). Evaluation of compliance of intravenous drug users and homosexuals in AIDS clinical trials [abstract No. S.D.782]. *International Conference on AIDS, 6*(3), 285.

Torres, R.A., Mani, S., Altholz, J., et al. (1990). HIV infection among homeless men in a New York City shelter. *Archives of Internal Medicine, 50,* 2030–2036.

United States General Accounting Office (1993). *Needle exchange programs: Research suggests promise as an AIDS prevention strategy* [GAO/HRD-93-60]. Washington, DC: The Author.

Vlahov, D., Munoz, A., Anthony, J.C., et al. (1990). Association of drug injection patterns with antibody to human immunodeficiency virus type 1 among intravenous drug users in Baltimore, Maryland. *American Journal of Epidemiology, 132*(5), 847–856.

Vlahov, D., Anthony, J.C., Celentano, D., et al. (1991a). Trends in HIV-1 risk reduction among initiates into intravenous drug use 1982–1987. *American Journal of Drug and Alcohol Abuse, 17*(1), 39–48.

Vlahov, D., Munoz, A., Celentano, D.D. et al., (1991b). HIV seroconversion and disinfection of injection equipment among intravenous drug users, Baltimore, Maryland. *Epidemiology, 2*(6), 444–446.

Vlahov, D., Anthony, J.C., Munoz, A., et al. (1991c). The Alive Study: A longitudinal study of HIV-1 infection in intravenous drug users—description of methods. *The Journal of Drug Issues, 21*(4), 759–776.

Vlahov, D., Sullivan, M., Astemborski, J., Nelson, K.E. (1992). Bacterial infections and skin cleaning prior to injection among intravenous drug users. *Public Health Reports, 107*(5), 595–598.

Watters, J.K., Estilo, M.J., Clark, G.L., Lorvich, J. (1994). Syringe and needle exchange as HIV/AIDS prevention for injection drug users. *Journal of the American Medical Association, 271*(2), 115–120.

Weiss, R.D., Mirin, S.M. (1987). *Cocaine.* New York: Ballantine Books.

Wesson, D.R. (1988). Revival of medical maintenance in the treatment of heroin dependence. *Journal of the American Medical Association, 259*(22), 3314–3315.

Wesson, D.R., Ling, W., Smith, D.E. (1993). Prescriptions of opioids for treatment of pain in patients with addictive disease. *Journal of Pain and Symptom Management, 8*(5), 289–296.

10

Infection Control

Nancy B. Parris

HIV infection is transmitted through sexual contact with infected persons and direct inoculation of contaminated blood products. It can also be transmitted perinatally from mother to neonate. AIDS is not casually or easily spread. Although only blood, semen, vaginal secretions, and possibly breast milk have been implicated in the transmission of AIDS by epidemiologic evidence, HIV has been isolated from many other body fluids, such as saliva, tears, cerebrospinal fluid (CSF), and urine. Therefore all body fluids are presumed to be potentially infective in the discussion of precautions that should be taken in the care of HIV-infected persons. This discussion of precautions taken in the workplace, however, refers only to blood and body fluid contact, because sexual contact is not relevant in this setting.

When providing patient care, all nurses and other health care workers must consider any patient to be potentially infected with HIV or other blood-borne pathogens. Therefore appropriate and sensible infection control precautions should be taken at all times. This chapter reviews precautions that should be followed with all patients infected with HIV regardless of whether they have clinical AIDS. The same precautions should be taken when in contact with *all* body fluids from *all* patients, to avoid percutaneous and mucous membrane exposure. Accidental needle-stick exposure poses the greatest hazard to health care workers; donning appropriate garb is not adequate protection. Too often a needle-stick injury has occurred when the nurse was in full isolation garb, feeling protected and comfortable, but gloves and a gown will not protect against a needle stick. Health care workers should use common sense in following the recommended guidelines but should never

become lackadaisical in their approach to infection control—a possibility whenever procedures are performed by rote.

When caring for any person requiring isolation precautions or when taking precautions with any patient's body fluids, the health care worker must always consider the patient. Observing good infection control practices and thereby minimizing the risk of exposure to infectious diseases is consistent with the objective of providing high-quality patient care.

PRECAUTIONS FOR NURSES

Precautions have been established that protect nurses and other health care workers from potential exposure to blood and other body fluids from patients with AIDS and HIV infection, thereby preventing the opportunity for tramsmission of HIV. Exposure refers specifically to percutaneous or mucous membrane contact with infected blood or other body fluids. Distinguishing exposure from routine contact is important, because ample data have continued to indicate that there is no risk of transmission of HIV from contact without exposure (Gerberding et al., 1987; Ippolito et al., 1993; Kuhls et al., 1987; Marcus et al., 1993). These studies have demonstrated that health care workers having prolonged contact with patients with AIDS did not show evidence of HIV infection.

Blood and body fluid precautions should be followed for all patients with diagnosed disease as well as for those with suspected HIV disease, whether or not it is symptomatic (CDC, 1991a, 1991b). The Centers for Disease Control and Prevention (CDC) suggested further that these protective barriers, referred to as "universal blood and body fluid precautions" or "universal precautions," be used con-

Table 10–1. Barrier Precautions

Gloves prevent contact with and exposure to:
   Body fluids
   Articles contaminated with body fluids
   Mucous membranes
   Nonintact skin
Protective clothing (i.e., **gowns or aprons**) protects:
   Clothes from soiling with body fluids
Masks and protective eyewear protect:
   Mucous membranes
   Nonintact skin from splashing or spraying
Hand washing prevents or reduces:
   Transient colonization with nonresident micro-
      bial flora
   Resident flora

Table 10–2. Gloves

Gloves must be worn:
   When there is a reasonable likelihood of hand
      contact with—
      Blood or other potentially infectious material
      Mucous membranes
      Nonintact skin
   When vascular access procedures are performed
   When contaminated items or surfaces are han-
      dled
Gloves must be changed:
   When they become—
      Contaminated
      Torn
      Punctured
   Between patients
   After each contact with each patient
Single-use, disposable gloves should never be:
   Washed
   Decontaminated
   Reused

sistently for all patients. In December 1991 the Occupational Safety and Health Administration (OSHA) published its final rule regarding occupational exposure to bloodborne pathogens, which mandates that health care workers implement universal precautions and that their employers provide appropriate resources for them to do so (Department of Labor, 1991). This rule will be reviewed in greater detail later in this chapter. "Body substance isolation" is an alternative system of precautions that accomplishes the same objective as universal precautions. These precautions are described in more detail later in this chapter. Use of precautions is especially important when the infection status of a patient is unknown.

The guidelines that follow in this chapter are similar to the CDC's blood and body fluid precautions, also called "disease-specific isolation precautions for patients with AIDS," and outline the measures to be followed. The recommended precautions are aimed at preventing the transmission of HIV (CDC, 1985, 1987a, 1987b, 1991a, 1991b; Garner & Hughes, 1987; Jackson & Lynch, 1989).

Because patients with AIDS are often infected with other organisms, appropriate precautions against transmission of those infections must also be taken. For many of the other infections, no additional precautions are required, because they are transmitted in the same way as HIV (e.g., hepatitis B) or because they are not transmitted from person to per-

son (e.g., toxoplasmosis). If the patient has pulmonary tuberculosis and has not yet received appropriate treatment, additional pre cautions will be needed to prevent the transmission of tuberculosis. Precautions to be taken with pulmonary tuberculosis will be addressed in this chapter; however, precautions to be taken with other infections are not addressed, and the appropriate precautions recommended by the CDC should be followed.

GUIDELINES FOR PRECAUTIONS

Gloves

When contact with a patient's body fluids is anticipated, appropriate protective barriers (i.e., gloves, cover gown, mask, and protective eyewear) should be used routinely to prevent percutaneous and mucous membrane exposure (Table 10–1). Disposable examination gloves should be worn when any blood or other body fluids are handled, but they are not necessary for direct care of patients where there is no contact with body fluids (Table 10–2). Gloves are also needed when one is touching mucous membranes and nonintact skin and for handling items or surfaces contaminated with body fluids. For example, examination gloves should be worn when the feces of an incontinent patient are handled and when the patient is cleaned after using the toilet, but they are not necessary when assessing vital signs of that patient or any other patient.

Gloves should be worn when the nurse is starting an intravenous infusion because of potential contact with blood. According to the CDC, gloves should be worn under the following circumstances: when phlebotomy is performed; when heel or finger sticks are performed on infants or children; when exposure to blood is anticipated; when the nurse has cuts, scratches, or other breaks in the skin; and during training in phlebotomy. The OSHA ruling, which in this case is more stringent than the CDC's recommendation, states that the only exception to glove use in the performance of vascular access procedures is for phlebotomy in volunteer blood donation centers. Gloves are not necessary when the intravenous bag, bottle, or tubing is changed, or when fluid is added to a burette; they are not needed for transport of a patient because any drainage or secretions should be adequately contained before transport. Gloves are not necessary for helping a patient ambulate or bathing a patient.

Gloves should be changed after each contact with each patient. Thorough hand washing after removal and disposal of the gloves is essential. Surgical or examination gloves should never be washed or disinfected for reuse. Either process may enhance penetration of fluids through undetected holes and may cause deterioration of the gloves.

Disposable examination gloves adequately protect the health care worker's skin from exposure to body substances and any microorganisms present as long as the gloves are not torn. Purchasing special gloves exclusively for use with HIV-infected patients is not necessary because they provide no additional protection and serve no practical purpose. The gloves should be properly fitted; rings that might tear through the glove should not be worn, and nails should not be so long as to poke through the gloves.

Differences in barrier effectiveness between latex and intact vinyl gloves have been studied in the past (Bienvenido et al., 1989; CDC, 1988b; Korniewicz et al., 1989; Zbitnew et al., 1989), and findings have suggested no statistically significant differences in leakage at low use levels (e.g., donning and removing gloves, using a washcloth, carrying a bedpan). In patient care activities requiring more manipulations, such as bandaging an amputation stump or connecting and disconnecting a Luer-Lok syringe to intravenous tubing, vinyl gloves demonstrated greater viral leakage than latex. Because latex gloves were found to fit better and therefore to allow for greater dexterity, they would be more desirable for the performance of those activities in which they are less prone to viral leakage. However, there has been an increase in reports to the U.S. Food and Drug Administration of allergic reactions to latex-containing medical devices, including gloves (Bubak et al., 1992; Culver, 1993; FDA, 1991). Reactions may range from a localized rash to anaphylaxis. Changing the brand of gloves may be an alternative for the nurse who is allergic to a particular brand of latex gloves, because it is possible that the allergy is related to chemicals used in manufacturing. If this approach is not effective, use of hypoallergenic gloves, glove liners, or powderless gloves, or overall avoidance of latex gloves, may be necessary. In summary, the type of glove should be appropriate for the task being performed, with attention paid to proper fit, so as not to stress the glove unnecessarily or tear it (Table 10–3).

Although it is recognized that gloves do not prevent needle-stick injuries, research indicates that they may provide some protection. One study indicated a significant reduction in the amount of blood on a needle as it passed through a latex or vinyl glove (Mast et al., 1993).

Hand Washing

Intact skin is an effective barrier against infection for health care workers. Hands should be washed immediately after being

Table 10–3. Guidelines for the Appropriate Use of Latex and Vinyl Gloves

Gloves are worn to provide a barrier that helps to:
    Protect the health care worker from acquiring infections
    Prevent the health care worker from transmitting infections to patients or others

Nonsterile Gloves
Should be worn when procedures are performed that involve the direct contact of the hands with the body
    fluids of a patient, during the care of a patient, or when soiled articles are handled
Should be procedure specific, that is, the gloves should be worn only *during* the procedure and then discarded
Vinyl Gloves
Applies to many routine procedures requiring gloves
Indications for use include carrying and emptying a bedpan or a suction canister
Latex Gloves
Applies only to procedures requiring a high degree of manual dexterity
Indications for use include cleaning up a blood spill and starting an intravenous line
Specialized Gloves for Chemotherapy
Should be worn only when procedures are performed that specifically require these gloves

Sterile Gloves (Latex)
Should be worn only when procedures are performed that require strict sterile technique
Should *not* be worn by persons who are outside the sterile field
Applies to all procedures performed in operating and delivery rooms and to specific procedures in other patient care areas
Indications for use, other than during surgery or delivery, include changing a wound dressing or inserting a
    Foley catheter

soiled with any body fluids, because hand washing is the single most important means of preventing infection (Table 10–4). This rule applies to all occasions of caring for patients with HIV infection, as well as for patients with any other problem or illness. Good hand washing, including cleaning underneath fingernails, between fingers, and beneath any allowable rings, is essential between patient contacts and immediately after removal of any type of gloves. During care of patients, jewelry should be kept to a minimum because it hinders good hand washing and use of gloves. Jewelry that has ridges or stones or that may interfere with proper hand washing should not be worn.

Proper hand washing includes use of warm running water, plenty of soap, friction over all surfaces of both hands, thorough rinsing, and paper towels to turn off faucets so as to avoid recontamination of hands. Special antimicrobial soaps are not necessary; most important is having a soap that is acceptable to staff members and that they will use.

Protective Clothing

Wearing protective gowns, aprons, or laboratory coats is recommended for contact that might cause the health care worker's clothing

Table 10–4. Hand Washing

Hands Should Be Washed:
Immediately after being soiled with any body fluids
Before contact with any patient
After gloves are removed
Between contacts with a single patient as needed

Proper Hand Washing Includes:
Use of warm running water
Plenty of soap
Friction over all surfaces of both hands
Thorough rinsing
Paper towels to turn off faucets if hands-free controls are not available

Hand Washing Should Include Cleaning:
Underneath fingernails
Between fingers
Beneath allowable rings

Table 10–5. Protective Clothing

Protective Clothing Includes:
Gowns
Aprons
Laboratory coats

Selection Depends on:
Task being performed
Degree of exposure anticipated

Protective Clothing Must Be Worn When Splashing of Blood or Body Fluids Is Likely, Such As:
Changing a wound dressing
Performing tracheal suctioning
Carrying a bedpan

Protective Clothing:
May be disposable or reusable
Must prevent blood or other body fluids from passing through to the nurse's skin or clothing
Must be removed and properly discarded once worn
Must be changed—
    Between patients
    When grossly soiled

to become soiled with body fluids (Table 10–5). AIDS is not transmitted by fomites, and therefore not through contaminated clothing, and wearing a protective garment is in part an issue of esthetics (Lovitt et al., 1992). In some instances a protective gown (i.e., a garment with sleeves) may provide a protective barrier for bare arms against splashing. As with the examples in the section on gloves, a cover gown is not routinely needed when the health care worker is taking vital signs or feeding a patient or helping with ambulation. On the other hand, use of a gown or apron might be desirable for emptying a bedpan, cleaning an incontinent patient of urine and feces, changing a dressing that involves a great deal of drainage, and performing any procedures that may generate splashes of body fluids. Cover gowns are not necessary when a patient is transported, because any drainage or secretions should be adequately contained before transport.

The choice of gown versus apron or laboratory coat should be determined by the task performed and the degree of exposure antic-

ipated. For example, gowns will provide more coverage than aprons, although aprons tend to be more "fluid proof." For minimal anticipated blood exposure to clothing, such as when phlebotomy is performed, a laboratory coat may be adequate. Although there is no industry standard for "fluid resistant" or "fluid proof" clothing, it is essential that the protective clothing prevent blood or other body fluids from passing through to reach the nurse's skin or clothing (Belkin, 1991). The clothing can be reusable or disposable; either is adequate as long as it protects clothes from contamination. Other factors to consider in the selection of appropriate clothing include its breathability, size, ease of dress, type of material, strength, flammability, and fasteners (Crow, 1991). Once worn, a gown or apron should be discarded in the proper receptacle and not reused.

Masks and Eye Protection or Face Shields

Masks and eye protection, or face shields, should reduce the incidence of contamination of the mucous membranes of the mouth, nose, and eyes (Table 10–6). Because AIDS is not transmitted by the airborne route, masks are not necessary as a routine precaution. However, in one documented case a health care worker was infected with HIV when blood from a patient with AIDS splashed into the worker's mouth. To prevent this type of exposure, the worker may wear a mask in certain instances as a barrier to cover the mouth and nose and protect any splashing body fluids. At the same time, protective eyewear or face shields should be worn as a barrier between the eyes and the patient's body fluids. Both should be worn to protect the health care worker's eyes, mouth, and nose during procedures that may generate droplets of blood or body fluids. Such procedures include suctioning a patient's fluids, assisting with bronchoscopy or endoscopy, and assisting with surgery in which high-powered drills may generate spraying of particles. The masks and eyewear should be worn only during the procedure for which they are indicated. The

Table 10–6. Mouth and Eye Protection

Mouth and Eye Protection Include:
Masks worn with goggles or glasses with side shields
Chin-length face shields
Combination mask with plastic eye shield

Mouth and Eye Protection Must Be Worn:
When splashing, spraying, or splattering of blood or body fluids is likely to result in exposure of the eyes, nose, or mouth
Only during the procedure for which they are indicated
When the procedures include—
  Suctioning of a patient
  Assisting with bronchoscopy or endoscopy
  Assisting with surgery involving high-powered drills

Prescription Eyeglasses May Be Worn:
As eye protection provided that they have side shields
With protective eyewear worn over them if they do not have side shields
With a mask to protect the nose and mouth

Discard After Use:
Disposable masks
Disposable face shields
Disposable combination masks with attached eye shields

Wash and Disinfect After Use:
Reusable goggles
Reusable face shields
Prescription eyeglasses if worn as eye protection

Table 10–7. Procedure Precautions

Needles and Sharps
Do not recap, bend or break.
Use a mechanical recapping device or one-handed technique when recapping is absolutely unavoidable.
Avoid accidental puncture injuries.

Cardiopulmonary Resuscitation
Use resuscitation bag or mask with one-way valve.

Transport
Standard procedures are adequate.

Dishes
Nondisposable dishes and utensils are adequate.

Laboratory Specimens
Standard procedures for all infective and potentially infective materials are adequate.

exception is during surgery, in which masks and protective eyewear are worn at all times, the mask serving to protect both the patient from the health care worker and the health care worker from the patient. The choice between protective eyewear and a face shield depends on the nurse's preference. Some favor goggles or glasses because the optics of the face shield may be slightly distorted by the curve of the plastic. Others prefer the face shield because it is one barrier item rather than two and allows better visualization of the health care worker's face. A combination mask and eye shield is also commercially available.

Protective eyewear not only should provide a shield in front of the eyes and be large enough to be worn over prescription eyeglasses but should also have protective sides and a top shield and be configured so that the bottom of the lenses angle toward the face for maximum protection. Prescription eyeglasses can be worn as eye protection only if they meet the criteria for protective eyewear and only if they are washed and decontaminated when soiled. Following these guidelines will prevent potential contamination of the health care worker's hands if he or she inadvertently touches the lenses. Some health care workers prefer goggles, which should be vented, although eyeglasses that satisfy the foregoing criteria are often more acceptable and less offensive to both patients and staff. Masks are worn once and discarded; reusable protective eyewear must be cleaned and disinfected after each use if eyewear is shared among staff. Subsequent users of the eyewear are thus protected not only from any organisms that may splash onto the front of the lenses but also from any infection the previous wearer may have.

Nurses are frequently involved in several hospital procedures and routines that require special precautions with patients to prevent exposure. Other situations cause concern to nurses regarding the potential for exposure (Table 10–7).

Needle and Sharps Disposal

To date, of the few cases of HIV infection in health care workers, most have occurred as a result of accidents with or improper handling of needles and "sharps." Gloves reduce the incidence of contamination of hands, but they cannot prevent penetrating injuries caused by needles or other sharp instruments. Therefore extreme caution should be taken to avoid any accidental injuries caused by needles, scalpels, or other sharp instruments or devices. Needles should never be recapped, bent, or broken and should not be handled in such a manner as to cause a puncture injury. In situations in which recapping or needle removal may be required, it must be accomplished with the use of a mechanical device protecting the hand, or by following a safe one-handed recapping technique. Once used, needles and sharps should be discarded immediately in a rigid puncture-proof container; they should never be left unattended on countertops or other surfaces. Disposal containers should be placed at convenient and accessible sites to encourage immediate disposal of needles and sharps after their use (Makofsky & Cone, 1993). Once filled, the sharps container should be closed securely and discarded with no further handling of the contents.

It is reported that at least 50% of needlestick injuries can be prevented by the elimination of exposed needles (Jagger & Pearson, 1991). Many devices are available to help reduce unnecessary exposure to needles. These include needle-free systems for intravenous lines and heparin locks, resheathing devices for syringes, and needle-free injectors. These devices have helped reduce the number of needle-stick injuries and have demonstrated increased acceptance among nurses who use them (Adams et al., 1993; Blackwell et al., 1992; Gartner, 1992; Linneman et al., 1991; Rutowski & Peterson, 1993; Skolnick et al., 1993; Whitby et al., 1991; Younger et al., 1992).

Any accidental needle stick, puncture injury, or exposure to broken skin from articles contaminated with blood or other fluids from any patient should be attended immediately. The site should be bled initially and then washed well with an antimicrobial soap. If the incident involves blood or body fluids splashed into the mucous membranes of the eyes, nose, or mouth, the area should be flushed immediately with water. The incident should be reported to the facility's occupational health department, with follow-up according to the CDC's recommended protocol (Table 10–8).

Cardiopulmonary Resuscitation

Although the risk of infection with HIV as a result of performing cardiopulmonary resuscitation is minimal and no cases of transmission of infection from mouth-to-mouth resuscitation have been documented, alternatives to direct mouth-to-mouth resuscitation should be available not only for use with patients who have HIV infection but for use with all patients. The available alternatives are a handheld resuscitator bag or a protective mask with a one-way valve. This equipment must be readily and constantly available on every unit or in every patient room, and in a consistent location (e.g., on the wall above the patient's bed) to prevent unnecessary lost time when the equipment is needed. Plastic mouth and nose covers with filtered openings may provide a degree of protection against transfer of oral fluids and aerosols. The use of these devices is more important in preventing exposure to other communicable diseases in addition to AIDS, because saliva has not been implicated in HIV transmission (Cummins, 1989; Emergency Cardiac Care Committee, 1989; Yeager, 1990).

Transporting the Patient

No special precautions are required in transporting a patient with AIDS or HIV infection. Any open draining wounds should be adequately covered before transport. If secretions and drainage are contained, the need for transport personnel to wear a gown or gloves will be obviated. Transport personnel need not wear a mask or protective eyewear, nor must the patient with HIV infection wear a mask.

Table 10–8. Postexposure Follow-up

Protocol for the follow-up of occupational exposures to biologic specimens of HIV seropositive individuals:
1. Clinical assessment and determination of HIV infection risk factors
2. Routine postexposure care
3. HIV antibody testing of employee and source patient for confirmation (with consent)
4. Counseling concerning the risk of HIV infection and prevention of its transmission, especially within first 6 to 12 weeks after exposure
5. Instructions to report all illness in the next 6 months

If the health care worker does not develop illness consistent with HIV infection:
1. HIV antibody testing at 6 weeks, 12 weeks, and 6 months after exposure
2. Prolonged HIV testing if the person has taken zidovudine prophylaxis
3. Stop follow-up and testing when consistent seronegative results are obtained

If the health care worker develops illness consistent with HIV infection:
1. Clinical assessment
2. HIV antibody testing (repeat monthly × 3)
3. Complete blood cell and differential counts
4. Consider other laboratory tests to rule out other causes of illness
5. Close follow-up

If the source individual is HIV seronegative:
1. Evaluate source for clinical manifestations of HIV/AIDS
2. Determine whether epidemiologic evidence suggests that source may have recently been exposed to HIV
3. Determine whether testing is desired by health care worker
4. Unless indicated, no further follow-up is necessary; if indicated, follow protocol noted above

If the source cannot be identified:
1. Evaluate the situation to determine appropriate follow-up on an individual basis

Data from the CDC (personal communication, Dec. 7, 1993) and Kuhls et al., 1987.

Dishes

Patients with HIV infection do not require any special dishes, glasses, or flatware for meals. Dishes, glasses, and utensils can be washed by following routine procedures used with all other dishes. Hot water and detergent should be used, and requirements set forth by local health departments for routine dishwashing should be followed.

Laboratory Specimens

All blood and body fluid laboratory specimens should be treated as infective, including laboratory specimens from patients with HIV infection. Specimen containers should be well constructed, with the lid always securely sealed to prevent leakage during transport. Care should be taken when the specimen is collected so that contamination of the outside of the container can be avoided. The container, once sealed, should be placed in a plastic bag for transport. The laboratory requisition should remain outside the bag so that it is not contaminated by the specimen. Once the specimen is bagged, the person transporting the specimen need not wear gloves because he or she should have no contact with the contents. Specimens from patients infected with HIV should not be identified as "AIDS specimens." Implementation of universal precautions eliminates the need for warning labels on specimens, because specimens containing blood and body fluids from all patients are handled as if infective.

Precautions for Other Infections

Because AIDS involves a deficiency in the immune system, many HIV-infected patients also have other infections. These infections are often opportunistic, in which event no additional precautions are required. However, certain infections require further precautions. Any additional isolation precautions required for the additional infections must be observed.

For example, if the patient has pulmonary tuberculosis, "tuberculosis isolation," or "AFB [acid-fast bacilli] isolation" procedures, as recommended by the CDC, are indicated (see below). A patient with diarrhea requires "enteric precautions," as described by the CDC, in addition to precautions against transmission of HIV.

Pregnant Women

Many female nurses and health care workers have questioned whether pregnant women should provide direct care for persons with HIV (PWHIV). The pregnant health care worker is at no greater risk of contracting HIV infection than the nonpregnant health care worker. However, if a pregnant woman is infected with HIV, the infant is at risk of acquiring infection through perinatal transmission. Meticulous adherence to the recommended precautionary techniques should be observed to prevent inadvertent exposure during routine patient care and subsequent risk of HIV infection. Furthermore, the pregnant health care worker is at no greater risk than a nonpregnant worker of acquiring other infections (e.g., cytomegalovirus) that the patient with AIDS may have.

TUBERCULOSIS PRECAUTIONS

Increases in the incidence of tuberculosis (TB) infection, the occurrence of outbreaks of TB, and cases of nosocomial spread of TB have been reported (Allen & Ownby, 1991; Beekmann et al., 1993; CDC, 1993a, 1993b, 1993c; Lutwick et al., 1993; McGowan, 1992; Pitchenik et al., 1992). Distribution of cases of TB within the United States is uneven, depending on various factors, including the presence of HIV infection (Castro & Dooley, 1993). PWHIV are of particular concern because they have a greater risk of TB infection. They have a greater likelihood of exposure to *Mycobacterium tuberculosis* than the general population and, once infected, will more probably progress to active disease because of their compromised immune system. Furthermore, an atypical picture of TB in HIV-infected persons often makes diagnosis difficult.

These patients frequently have nonreactive skin test results, atypical and nonspecific symptoms, chest radiographs suggestive of other diagnoses, and a high incidence of extrapulmonary and disseminated disease (Lutwick et al., 1993; Pitchenik et al., 1992). Further confounding the problem is the emergence of multidrug-resistant TB (MDR-TB), for which treatment becomes more challenging and risk of transmission possibly greater. Persons with HIV infection, patients with known exposure to MDR-TB, and patients with a history of noncompliance with TB therapy are among those at greater risk of being infected with MDR-TB strains.

Transmission

Clinical presentation of TB and specific drug treatment regimens are not addressed in this chapter; Chapter 4 deals with the clinical manifestations of TB. Those infection control interventions necessary to prevent transmission of disease are reviewed here (CDC, 1990b). Pulmonary TB, unlike HIV infection, is transmitted by the airborne route. Tiny droplet nuclei carrying the organism can be generated by sneezing, coughing, speaking, or singing by persons with active pulmonary or laryngeal TB. Persons with extrapulmonary TB and no active pulmonary disease, or those with infection (i.e., a positive skin test result) but no active disease are not infectious unless aerosols from extrapulmonary lesions are generated. TB infection, however, progresses to active disease at a particularly rapid pace, as noted in persons infected with HIV. The degree of infectiousness of a person with TB is correlated with the number of organisms expelled into the air, which in turn is related to the presence of pulmonary, laryngeal, or oral involvement; the presence of coughing or sneezing; a sputum smear with acid-fast bacilli; the patient's willingness or ability to cover his or her mouth when coughing or sneezing; the presence of cavitation on a chest radiograph; and the duration of adequate and appropriate chemotherapy (Department of Health and Human Services, 1993). MDR-TB is transmitted in the same manner and presents a similar clinical picture.

Table 10–9. Tuberculosis Precautions

Private room with negative airflow should have:
  Closed door
  Adequate air exchanges
  Nonrecirculating air vented to the outside
Masks that:
  Properly fit the face
  Filter out droplet nuclei
Nurses properly educated regarding:
  Patient assessment and early detection of disease
  Prompt initiation of precautions and isolation
  Importance of and compliance with routine employee skin testing

A higher mortality rate is noted with MDR-TB, which is probably related more to the patient's underlying immunosuppression and rapid progression of disease because of the failure of conventional drug treatments, than to an innately greater virulence of the resistant bacteria.

Environmental Controls

Early identification and treatment of TB infection and active disease are extremely important in controlling the transmission of the disease. Any patient seeking treatment who has respiratory symptoms (e.g., cough), and particularly those with night sweats, hemoptysis, fever, anorexia, and weight loss, should be considered potentially infected with *M. tuberculosis* and precautions should be taken immediately (Table 10–9). The importance of these precautions is underscored in facilities that have a high number of HIV-infected patients and in geographic areas where public health departments report increases of TB and where MDR-TB is prevalent. Patients with active or suspected disease should be placed in a properly ventilated private room with the door closed. Proper ventilation includes negative pressure with respect to the hall, adequate air exchanges (preferably at least six air exchanges per hour), and nonrecirculated air vented to the outside. Cohorting (patients with TB sharing a room with other TB patients) is not recommended because patients may be infected with different strains of the organism. In settings such as homes, where room pressures and air exchanges cannot be easily controlled, a room with a closed door, an open window, and a fan exhausting air out the window may create proper ventilation (CDC, 1990b).

Other engineering controls used in the hospital may include high-efficiency particulate air (HEPA) filters and ultraviolet lights. Health care facility personnel, including persons from the facilities, administration, and infection control departments, should determine appropriateness of isolation rooms for management of TB patients (CDC, 1990b).

Respiratory Protection

Health care workers providing care for patients with active TB should wear properly fitted face masks (respiratory protective devices) that can filter out droplet nuclei (DiPerri et al., 1993). Masks are to be worn when care is provided for the patient in his or her room and with a patient undergoing a treatment that may increase the risk of transmission of TB, until the patient has been adequately treated, shows clinical improvement, and is no longer considered infectious. Examples of treatments that increase the risk of spread include bronchoscopy, aerosol administration of medication, sputum induction, endotracheal intubation or suctioning, dental work, or other cough-inducing or aerosol-generating procedures. These treatments should be kept to an absolute minimum and performed in an adequate facility. When infectious, the patient should not be allowed to leave his or her room unless absolutely necessary and, while being transported, should wear a mask. The person transporting the patient may also need to wear a mask and should avoid elevators, waiting rooms, and other areas with other persons, including patients. The CDC, in its draft guideline for preventing the transmission of TB in health care settings, specifically recommends respiratory protective devices (respirator masks) that can filter particles 1 micrometer in size, with a filter efficiency $\geq 95\%$ (Department of Health and Human Services, 1993). The respirator should be checked for proper fit by the health care worker each time it is worn to ensure proper protection. Whether a powered air-purification respirator with an HEPA filter, as recommended by National Institute for Occupational Safety and Health in 1992, will be required by OSHA has yet to be determined. Data have not proved its effectiveness in the prevention of nosocomial transmission of TB (Makulowich, 1993). Nurses should remain in contact with infection control departments for updates regarding respiratory protective devices as specific recommendations and requirements continue to evolve.

Prevention

An effective TB program involves early detection, initiation of proper and timely precautions and isolation, and appropriate and adequate treatment of patients. Education of health care workers regarding good patient assessment and knowledge of precautions is essential in interrupting the spread of TB. Adherence to routine skin testing programs is not only important in protecting health care workers but should be mandatory (Tokars et al., 1992; Underwood et al., 1992).

UNIVERSAL PRECAUTIONS/BODY SUBSTANCE ISOLATION

The CDC has recommended infection control and isolation precautions for hospitalized patients for many years. Their last published guideline for isolation precautions in hospitals provided two alternative isolation systems: one that is category specific and includes the category "blood and body fluid precautions," and another that is disease specific, in which specific barrier precautions are indicated for each disease listed (CDC, 1988b). The purpose of disease-specific precautions is to minimize unnecessary precautions that occur with the category-specific system. In both of these systems, infectious diseases are listed and the precautions necessary to interrupt the transmission of each are indicated, either by category or by listing of all needed barriers. The concept includes posting a sign on the patient's door or by the bed, indicating precautions to be followed but not the patient's

diagnosis. One of the infectious diseases listed in this guideline is HIV disease, which falls into the blood-and-body-fluid category of precautions. The specific precautions needed to interrupt the transmission of HIV are outlined in this chapter.

Because a nurse or caregiver may not be aware that a patient is infected with HIV or has some other blood-borne infection such as hepatitis B, the CDC recommends that blood and body fluid precautions, or those barrier precautions necessary to interrupt the transmission of HIV and other blood-borne infections, be taken with all patients, or universally. These measures are now commonly known as "universal precautions" or "universal blood and body fluid precautions." Precautions are taken with blood, tissue, and body fluids associated with the transmission of blood-borne pathogens, which includes CSF, pleural fluid, peritoneal fluid, pericardial fluid, synovial fluid, and amniotic fluid. Feces, nasal secretions, sputum, sweat, tears, urine, and vomitus are included only if they contain visible blood, because the risk of transmission of HIV or hepatitis B virus from these materials is extremely low or nonexistent.

The CDC has always encouraged hospitals to tailor infection control recommendations to meet their own needs, and "body substance isolation" is such a system (Lynch et al., 1987). The concept of this system includes treating all blood and other body substances including feces, urine, and saliva, of all patients as potentially infective at all times, which is one way that this system differs from universal precautions. Signs are not placed on the individual rooms of patients with known infectious diseases to notify persons of the barrier precautions necessary in the care of that patient. Instead, a sign reminding all persons of barrier precautions to take with all patients is placed on *each* patient room, and health care workers do not know which patients have an infectious disease.

The purpose here is not to debate the merits of the two systems but to describe their basic differences. Both systems protect workers caring for patients both known and not known to have HIV or other infections. Both systems are currently in use at various institutions around the country. The basic concept behind both is the same, that of protecting the health care worker, protecting the patient, ensuring patient privacy, and protecting other patients from cross infection (Kephart et al., 1993). Which system is in place in any institution is secondary; more important is understanding the need to follow specific barrier precautions outlined herein with all patients, because that concept is truly universal.

OSHA'S BLOOD-BORNE PATHOGEN STANDARD

The U.S. Department of Labor OSHA, in an attempt to protect more than 5.6 million workers from occupational exposure to hepatitis B virus and HIV, issued its Blood-borne Pathogen Standard in 1991 (Pugliese, 1992). The standard covers full-time, part-time, temporary, and probationary employees in all health care facilities, including hospitals, clinics, dentists' and physicians' offices, blood banks, plasma centers, occupational health clinics, nursing (long-term care) homes, hospices, urgent care centers, clinical laboratories, mortuaries and funeral homes, and institutions for the developmentally disabled. The standard is performance oriented and thus allows employers the flexibility to develop worker protection programs that are unique to their particular setting and remain consistent to the intent of the standard (Turnbull & Balice, 1993) (Table 10–10).

The standard requires those employers to develop an exposure control plan identifying employees with occupational exposure; train all employees in occupational risks and methods to reduce risk; maintain records of employee training and medical evaluations; use warning labels and signs to identify hazards; implement methods to comply with provisions for worker protection, including universal precautions and safe handling of sharps, specimens, contaminated laundry, and regulated waste; provide voluntary hepatitis B vaccine at no cost to employees; provide medical evaluation after exposure incidents; provide personal protective clothing and equipment; and

Table 10–10. OSHA's Blood-borne Pathogen Standard

All health care employers are required to:
  Develop an exposure control plan
  Train all employees on occupational risks and risk reduction
  Maintain records of training and medical evaluations
  Use warning labels and signs
  Implement universal precautions
  Implement safe handling of sharps, specimens, and contaminated articles
  Provide hepatitis B vaccine
  Provide postexposure medical evaluations
  Provide personal protective clothing and equipment
  Institute additional precautions as necessary
All health care workers are required to:
  Comply with these practices and programs
  Use personal protective clothing and equipment as indicated
  Follow universal precautions

Data from Department of Labor (1991). Occupational exposure to bloodborne pathogens: Final rule. (29 CFR Part 1910. 1030.) *Federal Register, 56,* 64175-64182.

institute additional precautions for HIV and hepatitis B virus research and production facilities, if applicable. The requirements relevant to infection control and HIV infection are presented in this chapter, and it is important for nurses to be aware that their employer has an obligation to provide the resources and equipment as required within this ruling, and that the nurse has the responsibility to comply.

ENVIRONMENTAL CONSIDERATIONS

Although no environmentally mediated mode of HIV transmission has been documented, routine procedures and precautions should be followed with all patients (CDC, 1987a). Procedures for cleaning and disinfecting the patient's environment are generally those routinely used for all patients (Table 10–11). Although this section focuses on the hospital environment, the same principles apply to a long-term care facility and the home environment.

Table 10–11. Environmental Precautions

Cleaning the Room
Standard cleaning procedures are adequate.

Trash
Standard procedures for infective trash are adequate.

Linen
Standard procedures for soiled linen are adequate.

Sterilization and Disinfection
Standard procedures are adequate.

Cleaning the Room

Standard cleaning procedures are recommended both while a patient with HIV infection occupies the room and when the patient leaves the room because of discharge, transfer, or death. Neither HIV infection nor any other infections are transmitted as a result of soiled walls, ceilings, floors, countertops, and other environmental surfaces; therefore total decontamination or other extraordinary cleaning is not necessary. Any articles or surfaces visibly soiled with body fluids should be cleaned with a germicide solution as soon as possible after exposure. No special germicide is necessary for cleaning a surface contaminated with HIV. Disinfectant fogging is neither necessary nor recommended.

Waste

No epidemiologic evidence suggests that improper disposal of hospital waste has caused disease in the community. Therefore the identification of wastes for which special precautions are indicated is largely a matter of judgment about the relative risk of disease transmission, as well as a matter of compliance with local and state regulations. Trash contaminated with blood and body fluids from HIV-infected patients should be handled in accordance with the facility's policy for all infective or regulated waste. This policy must define infective waste or identify waste with the potential for causing infection during handling and disposal and for which some special precautions appear prudent. Although any item that has had contact with blood, exudates, or secretions is potentially infective, treating all such waste as infective is not usually considered practical or necessary. Blood, suctioned fluids, excretions, and secretions may be carefully poured down a drain connected to a sanitary sewer (i.e., a hopper, toilet, or utility sink). Sanitary sewers may also be used to dispose of other infectious wastes that can be ground and flushed into the sewer.

Handling waste defined as infective requires the use of a container that is closable, labeled with the biohazard symbol or colored red, and of sufficient strength to prevent leakage of contents. It is not necessary to use a double-bag procedure (i.e., two nurses removing the bag from the patient's room, one wearing protective garb and the other holding a cuffed outer bag into which the linen or trash bag is placed). Special handling of trash once it leaves the facility may be required by county or state regulations. This generally involves incineration or decontamination by autoclave before final disposal in a sanitary landfill. Disposal of trash from a patient with HIV disease is no different from routine handling of trash containing any infective material. Although certain trash may be identified as biohazardous, it is important that all trash be considered potentially infective and handled as such. This includes never placing sharps directly into the trash (other than a designated sharps disposal container), never reaching into a trash can to retrieve something inadvertently placed there, and using caution when handling all trash.

Soiled Linen

Soiled linen from a patient with HIV does not need to be handled any differently or separately from other soiled linen as long as it is properly and safely handled by all personnel coming in contact with it. It should be handled as little as possible and with minimal agitation to prevent gross microbial contamination of the air and of persons handling the linen. Soiled linen should be placed directly into the linen hamper at the location of use, not placed on the floor or on furniture in the patient's room. It should not be sorted or rinsed in the patient care areas. The only exception is in certain ambulatory health care units, such as psychiatric facilities, where patient clothing is laundered in designated areas on the unit, by the staff or the patient, as part of the daily activities. Any linen soiled with blood or other fluids should be placed in a leak-proof bag.

Laundry room staff members should handle all soiled linen in such a manner as to protect themselves from inadvertent exposure to any organisms contained within it, although risk of disease transmission is negligible. All laundry personnel handling soiled linen must wear protective garb, including gloves and water-resistant aprons. Linen washed with detergent in hot water (at least 71° C [160° F]) for 25 minutes, or in cool water ($\leq$70° C [158° F]) with a germicide suitable for low-temperature washing at proper use concentration, is decontaminated during the laundering; therefore the laundered linen can be used for any patient. There is no reason to dispose of or incinerate linen soiled with blood from a patient with HIV infection.

The greatest risk of infection to laundry room personnel is from contaminated needles or sharp instruments accidentally left with the linen and subsequently injuring someone. Therefore health care workers must ensure that instruments and articles are not inadvertently sent with the soiled linen.

Sterilization and Disinfection

Standard procedures for disinfection and sterilization of equipment, instruments, and other articles are recommended. No additional steps need be taken because properly followed disinfection or sterilization procedures destroy the HIV. Studies in the past have demonstrated that commonly used germicides rapidly inactivate HIV with routine use and at concentrations much lower than used in practice, and this continues to be true (CDC, 1987a; Gerberding & University of California, San Francisco, 1986). It is neither necessary nor recommended that separate equipment or instruments be used ex-

clusively for patients with AIDS or HIV infection.

Instruments or devices that enter sterile tissue or the vascular system of any patient or through which blood flows should be sterilized before reuse. Devices or items that come in contact with intact mucous membranes should be sterilized or should receive high-level disinfection whereby all vegetative organisms and viruses are killed, although bacterial spores are not (CDC, 1987a). Hospital policy and manufacturer's specifications regarding the use of any particular chemical sterilant should be followed. The chemical germicide or other method chosen for sterilizing or disinfecting a particular medical device depends on the manufacturer's specifications for compatibility of that device with the method or agent. At all times, instruments or devices should be thoroughly cleaned before being exposed to a chemical germicide or other method of sterilization or disinfection to ensure that all organic material (e.g., blood and mucus) is removed. Otherwise, sterilization or disinfection may not be achieved. Disposable instruments or devices should never be reused unless guidelines set forth by the manufacturer are followed. The importance of this point was underscored by an outbreak of AIDS in hospitalized infants in (what was then) the Soviet Union, in which disposable syringes, but not the needles, were reused. Similarly the CDC (1993d) has recommended that injection drug users use full-strength bleach to clean disposable needles and syringes because these items were not meant to be reused.

HIV is extremely fragile and is rapidly inactivated after drying. It has been demonstrated that high concentrations of HIV may survive in the environment for several days under laboratory conditions. Routine cleaning of the environment, proper cleaning of soiled surfaces, and proper cleaning and decontamination of instruments and devices prevent this survival time from being of any significance in the transmission of HIV. This finding does not create the need for any extraordinary cleaning or decontamination procedures but supports the need for adherence to proper procedures as described.

Blood or Body Fluid Spills

Gloves should be worn during cleanup and decontamination of a blood or body fluid spill. In most instances the proper procedure to follow is removal of visible material, most likely with a paper towel. The area should then be decontaminated, preferably with a solution of 5,000 parts per million of sodium hypochlorite (a 1:10 dilution of household bleach). For large spills of cultured or concentrated infectious agents in the laboratory, the contaminated area should be flooded with a liquid germicide before it is cleaned and then decontaminated with fresh germicide. If broken glassware is involved, a brush and dustpan or tongs, but never the hands, should be used to pick up the broken glass.

SPECIAL AREAS IN THE HOSPITAL

Patient care may vary significantly in different areas of the hospital, depending on the specific patient population (e.g., surgical units vs pediatrics, inpatient vs outpatient) or the procedure or purpose (e.g., operating room vs delivery room vs dialysis unit). Nonhospital settings can also be the sites of health care delivery. Precautions may differ depending on the area under consideration (Table 10–12).

Inpatient Areas

All the precautions described previously apply to inpatients. As inpatients, persons with any of the spectrum of HIV disease do not routinely require a private room to prevent the spread of their disease to other patients. Because of their immunocompromised status, however, they may need to be protected from other patients who have infections. If their condition is such that they cannot contain body fluids, persons with AIDS may be placed in an individual room. For example, the need for a private room may be due to a fulminating diarrhea that causes the patient to be incontinent of stool, or it may be due to central nervous system involvement that interferes with the patient's ability to handle personal secretions and excretions properly and hygienically. There are no special requirements as to positive or negative air balance for the room, because HIV is not airborne. Furthermore, there is no reason to restrict the patient to the room, unless the patient has pulmonary TB or some other infection requiring such restriction, or cannot contain or control his or her excretions and secretions. Unless restricted to the room for the aforementioned reasons, the patient may walk through the halls and use common lounges, treatment rooms, cafeterias, and lobby areas.

Separate toilet facilities are not required routinely for patients with AIDS, although they may be needed in certain instances, such as when the patient has diarrhea. No special procedure is needed for cleaning the toilet seat after its use by a patient with AIDS. Any toilet soiled with feces or urine should be cleaned by routine cleaning procedures before being used by another person, whether or not the person has AIDS.

Outpatient Departments

Essentially the same precautions apply in the outpatient departments as in the inpatient setting. Patients with HIV/AIDS may share a waiting area with other patients and may share bathroom facilities. Nurses should use appropriate barrier precautions; no additional precautions need be taken.

Table 10–12. Precautions for Special Areas in the Hospital

Special Areas
Inpatient units
Outpatient clinics
Emergency departments
Operating rooms
Labor and delivery rooms
Dialysis units

Precautions
Universal blood and body fluid precautions
Standard infection control procedures
Availability of manual resuscitation equipment
Special caution in handling sharps
Routine cleaning procedures
Plastic sleeve for dialysis

Operating Rooms

No additional preoperative precautions are necessary for patients with HIV/AIDS. The patient can be safely admitted to a multipatient preoperative room without risk of HIV infection to other patients. No special room is needed, nor is any special equipment required.

Because surgery involves exposure to large amounts of blood, the use of sharp instruments, and percutaneous and mucous membrane exposures, the operating room is an area of particular concern. During surgery, double gloving by the surgeon or other persons scrubbed for surgery is recommended (Gerberding et al., 1989). Puncture-resistant gloves are available, although their bulkiness may result in a loss of dexterity and for that reason are not widely used. All other protective barriers and precautions described previously also apply to the operating room. For example, a circulating nurse who is counting and handling bloody sponges should wear nonsterile gloves; protective eyewear should be worn by all persons scrubbed for surgery who are at risk of having blood or body fluids splashed into their eyes. Protective eyewear or face shields that protect the eyes from all sides are especially important in the operating room.

Extreme caution with all sharp instruments is important to prevent an accidental puncture injury that may result in exposure to the virus. To prevent accidental puncture injuries to the surgeon and scrub nurse during the operative procedure, surgeons can pick up and set down their own instruments from a Mayo stand set up for this purpose, rather than having them passed. Because a relatively high proportion of needlestick injuries among surgeons involve the index finger of the nondominant hand, protecting this digit may greatly reduce the risk of injury and subsequent infection (CDC, 1991a, 1991b; Lowenfels et al., 1989). A needle stick is most often caused by an attempt to grasp a needle or guide its tip, and therefore this practice should be avoided. A torn glove should be removed and replaced as soon as possible.

Postoperatively the patient may be admitted to the postanesthesia room for recovery.

Surgical instruments are washed and disinfected according to hospital policy for a "contaminated" or infected case; trash and linen are handled according to routine policy for infective trash and linen. Routine procedures for cleaning the room are carried out before the next patient arrives.

Labor and Delivery Rooms

Recommendations similar to those for operating room nurses should be followed in the labor and delivery rooms. A patient with HIV/AIDS may share a labor room with another patient. During and after delivery, health care workers should wear gloves and a gown when handling the placenta or infant until the blood and amniotic fluid have been removed from the infant's skin. Gloves and gown should also be worn during postdelivery care of the umbilical cord. Meconium aspiration should not be done by mouth suction.

Emergency Department and Emergency Transport

Emergency department and transport nurses encounter blood and body fluids under uncontrolled and emergent circumstances, which cause many opportunities for exposure. Universal precautions must be observed with *all* emergency department patients. Standard emergency department procedures and routines should be carried out with adequate and appropriate barrier precautions taken for patients with infections of any kind, including HIV infection (CDC, 1989; Holloway, 1986). A patient with HIV/AIDS infection in an emergency department or in an emergent situation is treated no differently from one in an inpatient setting. The same precautions are indicated in the same instances. As mentioned previously, manual resuscitation equipment (masks and bags) should be available to staff at all times so that mouth-to-mouth resuscitation of a patient with respiratory arrest is not needed.

Dialysis Units

PWHIV who have end-stage renal disease and are undergoing maintenance hemodialysis or peritoneal dialysis can be safely dialyzed when infection control precautions are used. When dialyzing all patients, health care workers should routinely follow universal blood-and-body-fluid precautions. A patient with HIV infection need not be isolated from other patients. During dialysis and especially when the patient is being attached to and removed from the dialyzer, there is considerable exposure to blood, and accidents that cause a great deal of blood splashing are not uncommon. Therefore additional protective measures should be taken for dialysis. A clear plastic bag with a hole at each end can be used to cover the arm and dialysis site (Corea, 1987). Then, if blood splashes, it is contained and should not contaminate anyone else. The dialyzer should be similarly covered with a plastic bag because it may rupture and cause blood to splash. Routine procedures for care and cleaning of the dialysis equipment should be followed, with no additional precautions for persons with HIV infection. The dialysis fluid pathways of the hemodialysis machine are generally disinfected with 500 to 750 ppm of sodium hypochlorite for 30 to 40 minutes or with a 1.5% to 2.0% solution of formaldehyde overnight. The dialyzer may be discarded after a single use. If the dialysis center has a dialyzer-reuse program in which a dialyzer is issued to a single patient and removed, cleaned, disinfected, and reused several times for that patient, HIV-infected patients can be included in the program. A dialyzer should never be used on more than one patient.

NONHOSPITAL (ACUTE CARE) SETTINGS

Psychiatric Facilities

PWHIV are treated in psychiatric facilities for either psychiatric disorders or problems resulting from central nervous system involvement with HIV. In this setting no special restrictions need be placed on patients with HIV infection (Table 10–13). They may share common rooms and dining facilities with other patients and staff. If the facility involves patients in their own food preparation, patients with HIV infection may participate and

Table 10–13. Precautions for Acute Care Settings

Settings
Psychiatric facilities
Long-term care facilities
Home care
Schools
Occupational settings

Precautions
Universal blood and body fluid precautions
Standard disinfection and cleaning procedures
Care with sharps
Attention to biting and injuries

share responsibilities and duties with other patients. Their laundry can be washed in machines provided for all patients. Patients with HIV infection should not be restricted from group events and activities or from using the facility's swimming pool. As in other health care settings, the patient may need evaluation for the presence of unacceptable behaviors or any changes that result in inappropriate actions such as biting or lack of control of secretions or excretions. A patient demonstrating these behaviors may need to be isolated or segregated from other patients until the behavior subsides or can be controlled. The patient may need further evaluation to determine whether additional precautions are indicated. This should be done on an individual basis, with no restrictions placed on any patient unless absolutely necessary.

Long-term Care Facilities and Nursing Homes

PWHIV can be safely cared for in long-term care facilities. No precautions in addition to those already mentioned are needed. Special attention should be paid to preventing decubiti or infection in patients with AIDS.

Home Care

Home care nurses may not know the HIV status of their clients. They should follow barrier precautions with all patients, as well as precautions similar to those mentioned pre-

Table 10–14. Disposal of Wastes for Home Care

Needle Disposal

Place needles, syringes, and sharps in a rigid, puncture-proof, nonbreakable container, such as a coffee can or a detergent or bleach bottle

Never recap needles or throw them directly into the trash

Keep the lid on the container

Label the container so as not to confuse with original contents

Keep out of reach of children

When full:

    Fill container to cover contents with a 1 : 10 dilution of household bleach

    Secure lid and seal with tape

    Place in a paper bag

    Place directly in garbage can on day of pickup

Disposal of Other Waste Materials

Place dressings, bandages, contaminated tissues, and other disposable items *excluding needles and sharps* in a plastic leak-proof bag

For disposal, tie up bag and place in garbage can

Dispose of feces, urine, sputum, and vomitus directly into the toilet and flush

Do not dispose of feces, urine, sputum, or vomitus into a sink or directly into the garbage

---

viously (Bryant, 1986; Lusby et al., 1986; Visiting Nurse Service, 1990). If running water is not available for hand washing, a waterless gel or commercially available solution should be used. The nurse should carry this product at all times. Some situations that may require the use of gloves include working with incontinent patients; changing disposable pads, diapers, dressings, or perineal pads; providing mouth care or urinary catheter care; and irrigating indwelling urinary catheters or cystostomy tubes. Examination gloves should never be reused. Rubber household gloves or general-purpose utility gloves used for housecleaning may be reused provided they are washed with soap and water before removal and decontaminated with a 1:10 dilution of household bleach if soiled with blood or body fluids. They should be discarded once they begin to deteriorate. Gowns, masks, and protective eyewear are seldom needed in home care. Some situations in which they may be useful are in removing or replacing dressings on large wounds with copious amounts of fluids; irrigating wounds, indwelling urinary catheters, or cystostomy tubes; suctioning the airway of a patient with copious secretions; or having direct sustained contact with a client who is coughing excessively and is unable to cover his or her own mouth.

As mentioned previously, avoiding needlestick injuries is of paramount importance. Needles or sharp instruments contaminated with blood should be disposed of safely. Laws concerning disposal of needles and sharps vary among states and should be consulted, but in all instances needles and sharps must be placed in a rigid, puncture-proof, unbreakable container. A coffee can with a lid or a detergent or bleach bottle works well as an improvised container. The lid should be kept on the container, which should be labeled and kept out of the reach of children. When the container is full, a 1:10 solution of household bleach solution should be poured into it until all contents are covered to decontaminate the contents. The lid should be secured with tape. The container should be placed in a paper bag and discarded on the day of trash collection by being placed directly into the garbage can, in a manner consistent with local public health regulations (Table 10–14).

A plastic leakproof bag can be used for disposal of dressings and other disposable items, excluding needles and sharps. Feces, urine, vomitus, sputum, and other body wastes can be flushed down the toilet. A 1:10

dilution of household bleach is the most practical agent for cleaning environmental surfaces in the home.

Nurses are responsible for educating informal caregivers of PWHIV about all of the precautions and procedures noted above. Because of the social, economic, and medical benefits of home care, the number of persons with AIDS who receive health care outside of hospitals is increasing. Persons infected with HIV and persons providing home care for those who are HIV-infected should be fully educated and trained regarding appropriate infection-control techniques. In addition, health-care providers should be aware of the potential for HIV transmission in the home and should provide training and education in infection control for HIV-infected persons and those who live with or provide care for them in the home. Such training should be an integral and ongoing part of the health-care plan for every person with HIV infection. Additional information on the nursing care of persons with AIDS in community settings can be found in Chapter 12. Chapter 5 presents a detailed account of the nursing management of AIDS in an adult client that is applicable to all settings.

School Settings

As few people as possible should be aware that a child has HIV infection; transmission is not casual and should not occur at the school. Therefore it is not necessary to inform teachers, administrators, parents, classmates, and other students of the child's diagnosis; they are not at risk of having HIV transmitted to them. When the child returns to school after a new diagnosis, a conference including the child's physician, the local public health officer, the school nurse, and the child's parents may be helpful. The only purpose of such a conference should be to deal with any special needs the child may have so that the nurse may more readily attend to the child if a problem occurs. The child may participate in regular school activities unless the child's physician deems restrictions necessary for medical reasons.

Children with poor hygiene who are unable to control their excretions and secretions may need to be restricted from certain classroom activities, but only children with severe illness or those exhibiting certain unacceptable behaviors, such as biting others, should be prohibited from attending school. HIV-infected children must be assessed periodically for changes in mental status that may have an impact on their behavior and hygiene.

If a child with HIV infection sustains an injury, the nurse should take the same precautions as do nurses in other outpatient settings when in contact with a child's blood and body fluids. These include wearing gloves when handling blood. Any objects contaminated with blood should be cleaned and disinfected immediately with a germicide.

In preschool areas, children should be prevented from sharing toys that they might place in their mouths. This is especially important for children infected with HIV, although the role of saliva in the transmission of AIDS is not clear. If toys that the children place in their mouths are used, they should be washed, disinfected, and rinsed well with water before being given to other children. If the toy is made of hard plastic or a similar substance, it can be washed with soapy water, soaked for 10 minutes in bleach or another disinfectant, and then rinsed well to remove all traces of the disinfectant. If made of soft cloth, the toy should be washed in hot soapy water with bleach added, preferably in an automatic washing machine. Common sense should prevail when dealing with similar objects. Child care workers should use disposable gloves to change diapers of young children. A plastic leakproof bag should be used for the disposal of diapers and gloves.

Occupational Settings

The barrier precautions previously mentioned should be followed by occupational health nurses handling a company's industrial emergencies and work-related problems for persons with AIDS or HIV infection. Such employees may continue to work without restriction unless their physicians indicate otherwise. Co-workers should not be informed of the person's diagnosis.

Table 10–15. Risk of HIV Infection

Risk of HIV infection to health care workers, to household contacts, or from employees with AIDS or HIV infection requires:

1. Actual percutaneous or mucous membrane exposure to blood or body fluids or
2. Sexual contact

RISK OF HIV INFECTION

Because of the high mortality rate associated with AIDS, health care workers caring for patients with HIV/AIDS and people living with persons with HIV/AIDS have concerns and fears about acquiring HIV infection. Many employees (especially health care workers) who might be infected with HIV have fears about the possibility of transmitting the virus to patients or co-workers (Table 10–15). Research on the risk of infection to health care workers and household contacts is ongoing.

Health Care Workers

Several studies have demonstrated that the risk of acquiring HIV infection from occupational exposure is extremely low (CDC, 1988a; Fahey et al., 1993; Flynn et al., 1987; Gerberding, 1989; Hadley, 1989; Ippolito et al., 1993; Kuhls & Cherry, 1987; Marcus et al., 1993; Marcus & Cooperative Needlestick Surveillance Group, 1988; McCray & Cooperative Needlestick Surveillance Group, 1986; Neisson-Vernant et al., 1986; Oksenhendler et al., 1986; Stricof & Morse, 1986; Weiss, 1992). By definition, "exposure" means actual percutaneous injury (e.g., a needle stick or a cut with a sharp object), contact of mucous membranes, or contact of skin with blood, tissues, or other body fluids to which universal precautions apply, including laboratory specimens that contain HIV, especially when the exposed skin is chapped, abraded, or afflicted with dermatitis or when the contact is prolonged or involves an extensive area, whereas "contact" refers to virtually any other interaction between the health care worker and the patient with HIV (CDC, 1990a). Contact may involve touching the patient, transporting the patient, performing a bed bath, giving postural drainage or physical therapy, and any other type of activity involved in providing routine care to a patient. No risk of acquiring HIV infection during routine contact with a patient with HIV/AIDS has been demonstrated, and a very low risk of infection (about 0.4%) is associated with percutaneous or mucous membrane exposure to the blood or body fluids of a patient with HIV infection. To date, more than 2,000 health care workers with percutaneous exposures to blood or mucous membranes of open wounds contaminated by blood or body fluids have been prospectively followed.

As of September 1993, a total of 39 health care workers in the United States, including 13 nurses, demonstrated documented HIV seroconversion after occupational exposure (34 had percutaneous exposure, 4 had mucous membrane exposure, and 1 had both percutaneous exposures; 36 had exposures to blood from an HIV-infected person, 1 to visibly bloody fluid, 1 to an unspecified fluid, and 1 to concentrated virus in a laboratory) (CDC, personal communication, 1993). An additional 81 health care workers, including 15 nurses, are reported to have possible occupational transmission of HIV. These individuals reported percutaneous or mucocutaneous occupational exposures to HIV-infected blood or body fluids, but seroconversion specifically resulting from an occupational exposure was not documented. Each of these individuals denied having risk factors other than the described work exposure. Of all of these individuals, those who did not have needle-stick exposures had not observed barrier precautions at the time of the exposure that resulted in infection; barrier precautions offer little protection to a health care worker after a needle-stick exposure. Despite these unfortunate cases, routine patient contact that does not involve actual exposure cannot result in infection with a virus transmitted from blood to blood.

The risk of HIV infection to health care workers after an exposure remains low. As stated previously, barrier precautions should prevent exposure, and infection cannot occur without exposure.

Prophylaxis

No effective vaccine against HIV has been developed, nor is there a proved prophylactic agent for postexposure treatment. Zidovudine (ZDV), also known as azidothymidine (AZT) and Retrovir, is a thymidine analog that *in vitro* has been shown to inhibit replication of some retroviruses, including HIV, by interfering with the action of viral ribonucleic acid–dependent deoxyribonucleic acid polymerase (reverse transcriptase) and possibly also by other mechanisms (CDC, 1990a; Yarchoan et al., 1988). Zidovudine has been used for treatment of adults with symptomatic HIV infection, including AIDS, and has been shown to increase the duration and quality of life of patients with advanced HIV infection and AIDS. It may delay disease progression in patients with less advanced HIV infection. Some institutions and physicians are now offering this drug for prophylaxis after occupational exposure to HIV.

A study to examine the efficacy of zidovudine prophylaxis for human beings after exposure to HIV included 84 health care workers with occupational percutaneous, mucous-membrane, or nonintact-skin exposure to HIV-infected blood (CDC, 1990a; Henderson & Gerberding, 1989). None was seropositive for HIV after at least 6 months of follow-up; 49 had been given zidovudine, the others a placebo. The absence of seroconversions in this small group is not unexpected, regardless of whether they took zidovudine, because the risk of infection is approximately 0.4%. There are a few reports of individuals who took zidovudine after occupational exposure and subsequently became infected with HIV, and although the circumstances surrounding the exposures and the time before prophylaxis was given vary considerably, it has been concluded that if zidovudine is protective, any protection afforded is not absolute (Gerberding, 1993; Lange et al., 1990; Looke & Grove, 1990; Tokars et al., 1992). Data involving studies of laboratory animals are limited and are inadequate to support or reject the hypothesis that zidovudine may be effective prophylaxis for human beings occupationally exposed to HIV. Studies are examining the toxicity of the agent when used for occupational postexposure prophylaxis (Gerberding, 1993; Tokars et al., 1992).

Various regimens are followed for zidovudine prophylaxis after occupational exposure. No data are available yet to determine the efficacy or compare the toxicity of dosages. The regimens may vary from a 100 to 200 mg dose given every 4 hours either five or six times daily (some protocols elect to skip the 4 AM dose) for 4 to 6 weeks. Some clinicians have used an initial dose of 400 mg; others have prescribed treatment from 4 days to 4 months. It is believed that the sooner the drug is started, the more chance it has to be effective; some institutions encourage health care workers to initiate treatment within 1 hour after exposure.

Zidovudine has some toxic and adverse effects, including granulocytopenia and anemia as the most frequently reported. Other symptoms include headache, nausea, insomnia, myalgia, diaphoresis, fever, malaise, anorexia, diarrhea, dyspepsia, vomiting, dyspnea, rash, and taste abnormalities. Less commonly reported side effects are polymyositis, peripheral neuropathy, and seizures.

Data from animal and laboratory studies are inadequate to establish the efficacy or safety of zidovudine for prophylaxis after occupational exposure to HIV. Reasons for using zidovudine as postexposure prophylaxis include the severity of the illness that may result from HIV infection, the documented antiviral effect in the treatment of persons with established HIV infection, the apparent reversibility of acute toxic effects when the drug is taken for short periods, and the suggestion from some animal studies that the drug may modify the course of some retroviral infections. Reasons not to use zidovudine for postexposure prophylaxis include a lack of data demonstrating efficacy for this purpose, limited data on toxic effects in uninfected persons, and carcinogenic effects in rats and mice.

Nurses and other health care workers need to be aware of the facts regarding use of zidovudine for postexposure prophylaxis so that they can make a timely decision if confronted with this situation. They must take into account the risks and the potential benefits. They should consider factors surrounding the exposure incident, including the type and route of exposure (percutaneous vs mucous membrane), the volume of fluid involved, and the concentration of virus in the source fluid (clinical vs research laboratory setting). Furthermore, the individual should be counseled regarding risks of exposure, the theoretical rationale for prophylaxis, limitations of current knowledge of the efficacy of zidovudine when used as postexposure prophylaxis, current knowledge of the toxicity of zidovudine and the limitations of this knowledge in predicting toxic effects in uninfected individuals who take the drug after occupational exposures, and the need for postexposure follow-up. If the health care worker decides to use zidovudine as postexposure prophylaxis, it should be initiated promptly after the exposure. Follow-up should include evaluation of drug toxic effects in the person and HIV seroconversion. Monitoring for seroconversion may have to be extended for a longer period than that of a person with HIV exposure who is not taking zidovudine.

Persons who take zidovudine should abstain from sexual intercourse or use an effective contraceptive because of the unknown but possible risk of teratogenesis associated with its use. Throughout the follow-up period, latex condoms should be used or abstinence from sexual intercourse should be practiced to prevent transmission of HIV to sexual partners.

HIV Screening of Patients

Much concern has been expressed about the need to identify patients with HIV/AIDS for the benefit of protecting health care workers. Although generally knowing everything possible about a patient's overall medical condition is desirable, nurses do not need to know a person's HIV antibody status to protect themselves; this is especially important because some patients who are infected with HIV may have a negative antibody test result. In many states, HIV antibody testing is illegal without the explicit consent of the patient, and in *all* instances posting a diagnosis on a patient's door breaches confidentiality and a

patient's right to privacy (see Chapters 13 and 14). Observing good hygiene, infection control practices, and barrier precautions protects health care workers whether or not they are aware of the patient's diagnosis.

Patients with HIV infection need the same good-quality nursing care that is provided for all patients. Fear of AIDS does not protect a nurse. Knowledge and understanding of the transmission of HIV help the nurse deal rationally with precautions and offer protection from exposure and subsequent potential infection. The procedures, benefits, and risks of HIV antibody testing of patients are discussed in detail in Chapter 2.

Household Members

Early studies demonstrated that, without sexual contact, household contacts of infected patients have little increased risk of HIV infection, and none at all when a few guidelines are followed (Bryant, 1986; Lusby et al., 1986, Visiting Nurse Service, 1990). Contact with blood and other body substances can occur in households, although transmission of HIV through this route is rare in household settings. Recently, however, two cases of transmission of HIV were reported by the CDC as the result of informal caregiver contact with blood, exudate, and other body secretions and excretions from an HIV-infected person in the household (CDC, May 20, 1994). In both instances, exposures occurred after the source-patients had developed AIDS; consequently, relatively high HIV titers may have been present in their blood. These two cases bring to eight the number of reports of household transmission of HIV not associated with sexual contact, injecting drug use, or breastfeeding. Of these eight cases, five were associated with blood contact (CDC, May 20, 1994). Informal caregivers who provide nursing care for HIV-infected patients in home settings should employ precautions to reduce exposures to blood and other body fluids and should be carefully trained by health care workers to provide safe care.

Good hygiene should be practiced to prevent transmission of all organisms within the home, especially to prevent infecting a person who has AIDS with an opportunistic organism. Razors, toothbrushes, and other personal articles that may come into contact with blood or body fluids should not be shared.

A person with HIV infection need not eat from any special dishes or with special utensils; routine washing in a dishwasher or soaking in hot soapy water removes and destroys the virus. As a matter of routine, household members should never eat from the same utensils or drink out of the same glass or cup.

The laundry of a patient with HIV disease does not have to be segregated, because HIV is destroyed by hot water and soap in a washing machine. If clothing is soiled with blood or body fluids, bleach should be added to the water. There have been no documented cases of transmission of HIV by fomites (inanimate articles) other than contaminated needles. Even if clothing is soiled with infected blood, transmission of the disease would not occur with such contact.

Employees With AIDS

Much concern has been expressed about workers, especially health care workers, with HIV/AIDS. A health care worker can transmit HIV to a patient only when the patient has severe trauma that would provide a portal of entry for the virus (e.g., during surgery), so that blood or serous fluid from the infected health care worker would have access to the open tissue of the patient. Such a circumstance is rare, as is the chance that a health care worker will infect a patient or another employee. Therefore each situation involving HIV infection in an employee should be handled individually. Precautions to prevent transmission of HIV from health care workers to patients are simple. *All* health care workers should wear gloves for direct contact with mucous membranes or nonintact skin of *all* patients. Health care workers who have exudative lesions or weeping dermatitis should refrain from direct patient care and from handling patient care equipment until the condition resolves itself. Termination of the worker's employment is not necessary, and work restrictions are rarely indicated. Protecting the employee's privacy and information about his or her diagnosis is important. Numerous companies and corporations have established policies permitting persons with HIV to continue working as long as they are physically able; the only limitations are situations that would increase the risk of infection to the HIV-infected employee. Recent court cases have resulted in rulings protecting a person with an infectious condition from employee discrimination under certain circumstances (see Chapter 14). This applies to persons with HIV infection because it is not casually transmitted or airborne.

As of December 1993, more than 11,000 reported cases of AIDS in the United States were in persons employed in health care (CDC, personal communication, 1993). This figure represents 4.7% of all reported cases, consistent with the percentage of the overall population employed in health care. There have been several studies of persons treated by HIV-infected health care workers, with tens of thousands of patients who had received care from HIV-infected health care workers, including dentists, physicians, obstetricians, and surgeons, followed up to determine whether any had become infected (Anonymous, 1993; CDC, 1993e; Dickinson et al., 1993; Rogers et al., 1993; von Reyn et al., 1993). The risk of transmission of a bloodborne pathogen from a health care worker to a patient is associated with the circulating titer of the pathogen in the blood, the procedures performed, the techniques and infection control precautions used, and the medical condition of the health care worker. There is only one documented case in which HIV was transmitted from an infected health care worker to patients. Six persons reportedly became infected with HIV after having received care from a dentist (CDC, 1991c). Despite this tragedy, data indicate that the risk of infection is extremely small, and whatever risk that exists can be reduced by appropriate use of infection control precautions.

The CDC does not recommend work restrictions for personal service workers (e.g., hairdressers, manicurists, or others providing services that involve casual contact with their clients) or food workers solely on account of HIV infection, because no cases of HIV transmission have been documented in these settings. Employees should not be restricted from using equipment and facilities in the workplace, including telephones, toilets, drinking fountains, eating facilities, and office equipment.

Few work situations warrant HIV antibody screening of employees, and such screening is generally inadvisable because it raises serious questions concerning employees' privacy rights (Lettau et al., 1992; Russo & LaCroix, 1992). The primary indications for screening include follow-up of an exposure incident and obtaining and storing blood of persons employed in laboratories who work with concentrated virus.

Fear of AIDS may cause employees, including health care workers, to refuse to work beside or perform services for persons infected with HIV. Such situations include health care workers who refuse to care for patients with AIDS, office employees who will not work with other employees who are infected, and employees who refuse to serve clients who have AIDS. In many of these situations, legal action has been taken against the employee. In some states the courts have maintained that the employer has an obligation to inform and educate the employee regarding the transmission of HIV if that employee is to work with clients or patients wth AIDS. If an employee does not work directly with persons with AIDS but, because of unfounded fear, refuses to perform a part of his or her job, education about HIV infection and its transmission should precede any corrective action on the part of the supervisor. An employee who refuses to work may be protected from dismissal or other disciplinary action only if the refusal is both reasonable and based on a good-faith belief in the existence of an imminent threat of serious injury or death. The most effective way to prevent refusal is by educating all employees about the transmission of HIV and methods of prevention in situations where it is possible (e.g., working with infected patients). Chapter 14 provides a detailed account of laws and rulings about employee rights and obligations, and Chapter 13 addresses the ethical obligations of nurses to provide care.

INFECTION CONTROL AND NURSING RESEARCH

A plethora of research topics on AIDS and nursing exists. The most important topics specifically related to infection control focus on behaviors and devices that increase or reduce the risk of exposure to the health care worker and that can be separated accordingly as those involving activities (e.g., compliance with universal precautions) and those regarding medical technology and protective medical devices. A considerable amount of research has been conducted in these areas; however, many questions remain unanswered.

Summary of Research

Although knowledge of and compliance with universal precautions help to decrease rates of contact with patients' blood, rates of compliance are lower than desirable and exposures, particularly percutaneous, continue to occur (Gauthier et al., 1991; Kristensen et al., 1992; Saghafi et al., 1992). Reasons for lack of compliance among health care workers, together with means to achieve greater compliance, should be evaluated. This evaluation may include studying resources, such as the availability of proper protective equipment of various sizes, ease of use, efficacy of protectiveness, cost, and application in actual clinical situations. The nurse's knowledge of universal precautions, risk of exposure and infection, and use of protective equipment plays an important role in compliance and should be studied further to determine educational needs of nurses. Furthermore, the nurse's attitude regarding the implementation, practical application, and necessity of universal precautions and the perceived risk associated with not following protocol is directly related to compliance and should be studied so that measures to achieve greater compliance, and thus lower exposure risks, can be employed.

Some of the issues related to protective garb, such as permeability of gowns and gloves and a lack of certain industry standards, were touched on earlier in this chapter. Further studies of the actual equipment and clothing are indicated to help establish guidelines.

Devices that eliminate sharps or effectively protect the health care worker from injuries from sharps need to be improved or developed, because percutaneous injury remains the greatest HIV risk to the health care worker. At least 800,000 accidental needlestick and sharp injuries occur annually, and 16,000 of those sharps (2%) are likely to be contaminated with HIV (Association for Practitioners in Infection Control [APIC], 1993). Although the risk of infection from such an exposure is less than 1%, the need to eliminate injuries from sharps, and thereby dramatically reduce the risk of infection, cannot be stressed enough. To a great extent, it is the responsibility of medical device manufacturers to improve available technology and replace high-risk devices (e.g., prefilled cartridges and intravenous needles) with safer products. Progress has been made with safer new devices currently available (e.g., rigid sharps containers, needleless intravenous systems, and resheathing syringes); however the speed of development of new devices must be accelerated. Clinical studies evaluating the safety, ease of use, benefit, and efficacy of improved products as they emerge, providing helpful feedback to manufacturers to further improve their products, are of paramount importance. It is essential that research geared toward the elimination of unnecessary and unsafe practices and devices continue. Additional research describing circumstances surrounding accidental sharps injuries and other exposures, such as when and how they occur, the devices involved, the specific circumstances of the incident, and other details pertaining to each incident, may help in identifying additional preventive measures.

Recommendations for Research

The APIC Governmental Affairs Committee has recommended the following in an effort to reduce unnecessary device-related risks, which provide fertile ground for nursing research, either alone or in collaboration with industry or as participants with other health care disciplines (APIC, 1993):

1. Use of alternative methods of performing medical procedures
2. Development of novel methods requiring fewer or no needles
3. Acceleration of the transfer of new technology into the workplace through funding of research, consortium studies, professional publication of clinical evaluations, and presentations at meetings
4. Formulation of coalitions and/or joint task forces to keep issues in the forefront to enhance collaboration among health care professionals, industry, and the government
5. Adoption of a nationwide database to evaluate injury-specific and device-specific data and their outcomes for prevention and education
6. Establishment of a central clearinghouse for development of criteria for each type of device and elimination of unnecessary and unsafe devices
7. Development of guidelines for standardized product evaluation to include quantitative and qualitative experience, packaging, user comments, cost, and impact on waste volume
8. Creation of a nationwide repository for product information, evaluation, and compatibility
9. Establishment of a nationwide surveillance system to assess intervention and outcome
10. Development of strategies to contain cost without impeding implementation of safer technology or without withdrawing and/or delaying introduced products

With these efforts it is hoped that medical devices in the future will substantially improve and that those posing a risk to the health care provider will be virtually eliminated. It is also anticipated that nursing practices will continue to evolve to ensure ease of compliance combined with optimal protection of the nurse.

SUMMARY

The importance of education regarding AIDS and HIV infection cannot be stressed enough. The nurse in practice must know and understand how HIV is transmitted and the simple and practical methods of prevention. Observing universal precautions with all patients is important, but even more important is understanding why the precautions have been established and how they halt transmission. Comprehension of these basic facts alleviates unfounded fears and enables people to deal more effectively and compassionately in any capacity with patients who have HIV infection. Nursing research in the area of infection control has focused on behaviors and devices that increase or reduce risk of exposure to health care workers. Further research in these same areas may answer some of the questions that nurses in practice have about their safety.

REFERENCES

Adams, K.S., Zehrer, C.L., Thomas, W. (1993). Comparison of a needleless system with conventional heparin locks. *American Journal of Infection Control, 21,* 263–269.

Allen, M.A., Ownby, K.K. (1991). Tuberculosis: The other epidemic. *Journal of the Association of Nurses in AIDS Care, 2,* 9–23.

Anonymous (1993). No HIV transmission from two surgeons and a dentist. *AIDS Clinical Care, 5,* 57.

Association for Practitioners in Infection Control (APIC) (1993). Position paper: Prevention of device-mediated blood-borne infections to health care workers. *American Journal of Infection Control, 21,* 76–78.

Beckmann, S.E., Osterholm, M.T., Henderson. D.K. (1993). Tuberculosis in the healthcare setting in the 1990's: From Bird Island to the Bronx. *Infection Control and Hospital Epidemiology, 14,*228–232.

Belkin, N.L. (1991). The protectiveness of protective clothing. *Infection Control and Hospital Epidemiology, 12,* 464–466.

Bienvenido, G., Yangco, M.D., Yangco, N.F. (1989). What is leaky can be risky: A study of the integrity of hospital gloves. *Infection Control and Hospital Epidemiology, 10,* 553–556.

Blackwell, B., Jagger, M., Hickey, S. (1992). Shielded safety syringes [letter and reply]. *Infection Control and Hospital Epidemiology, 13,* 571.

Bryant, J.K. (1986). Home care of the client with AIDS. *Journal of Community Health Nursing, 3,* 69–74.

Bubak, M.E., Reed, C.E., Fransway, A.F., et al. (1992). Allergic reactions to latex among health-care workers. *Mayo Clinic Proceedings, 67,* 1075–1079.

Castro, K.G., Dooley, S.W. (1993). *Mycobacterium tuberculosis* transmission in healthcare settings: Is it influenced by coinfection with human immunodeficiency virus? *Infection Control and Hospital Epidemiology, 14,* 65–66.

Centers for Disease Control (1985). Recommendations for preventing transmission of infection with human T-lymphotropic virus type III/lymphadenopathy-associated virus in the workplace. *Morbidity and Mortality Weekly Report, 34,* 681–695.

Centers for Disease Control (1987a). Recommendations for preventing HIV transmission in health-care settings. *Morbidity and Mortality Weekly Report Supplement, 36,* 1S–18S.

Centers for Disease Control (1987b). Human immunodeficiency virus infection in transfusion recipients and their family members. *Morbidity and Mortality Weekly Report, 36,* 137–140.

Centers for Disease Control (1988a). Update: Acquired immunodeficiency syndrome and human immunodeficiency virus infection among health care workers. *Morbidity and Mortality Weekly Report, 376,* 229–239.

Centers for Disease Control (1988b). Update: Universal precautions for prevention of transmission of human immunodeficiency virus, hepatitis B virus, and other bloodborne pathogens in health-care settings. *Morbidity and Mortality Weekly Report, 37,* 377–388.

Centers for Disease Control (1989). A curriculum guide for public-safety and emergency-response workers: Prevention of transmission of human immunodeficiency virus and hepatitis B virus. Atlanta, GA: CDC.

Centers for Disease Control (1990a). Public Health Service statement on management of occupational exposure to human immunodeficiency virus, including considerations regarding zidovudine postexposure use. *Morbidity and Mortality Weekly Report, 39,* 1–14.

Centers for Disease Control (1990b). Guidelines for preventing the transmission of tuberculosis in health-care settings, with special focus on HIV-related issues. *Morbidity and Mortality Weekly Report, 39,* RR-1, 7.

Centers for Disease Control (1991a). Estimates of the risk of endemic transmission of hepatitis B virus and human immunodeficiency virus to patients by the percutaneous route during invasive surgical and dental procedures. Atlanta, GA: CDC.

Centers for Disease Control (1991b). Revised recommendations for preventing transmission of human immunodeficiency virus and hepatitis B virus to patients during invasive procedures. Atlanta, GA: CDC.

Centers for Disease Control (1991c). Update: Transmission of HIV infection during an invasive dental procedure—Florida. *Morbidity and Mortality Weekly Report, 40*(2), 22–37.

Centers for Disease Control and Prevention (1993a). Recommendations for HIV testing services for inpatients and outpatients in acute-care hospital settings and technical guidance on HIV counseling. *Morbidity and Mortality Weekly Report, 42,* 1–17.

Centers for Disease Control and Prevention (1993b). Outbreak of multidrug-resistant tuberculosis at a hospital—New York City, 1991. *Morbidity and Mortality Weekly Report, 42,* 427–434.

Centers for Disease Control and Prevention (1993c). Tuberculosis morbidity—United States, 1992. *Morbidity and Mortality Weekly Report, 42,* 696–704.

Centers for Disease Control and Prevention (1993d). Use of bleach for disinfection of drug injection equipment. *Morbidity and Mortality Weekly Report, 42*(2), 418–419.

Centers for Disease Control and Prevention (1993e). Update: Investigations of persons treated by HIV-infected health-care workers—United States. *Morbidity and Mortality Weekly Report, 42,* 329–337.

Centers for Disease Control and Prevention (December 7, 1993). CDC Information Service [personal communication].

Centers for Disease Control and Prevention (May 20, 1994). Human immunodeficiency virus transmission in household settings—United States. *Morbidity and Mortality Weekly Report, 43*(19), 347–356.

Corea, A. (1987). Discussion of departmental policies, University of California Los Angeles Medical Center Dialysis Unit [unpublished].

Crow, S. (1991). Emperor's clothing for the contemporary healthcare worker. *Infection Control and Hospital Epidemiology, 12,* 308–310.

Culver, J. (1993). Sensitivity to latex in medical devices. *Journal of Hospital Occupational Health, 13*(1), 1–4.

Cummins, R.O. (1989). Infection control guidelines for CPR providers [editorial]. *Journal of the American Medical Association, 262,* 2732–2733.

Department of Health and Human Services (1993). Draft guidelines for preventing the transmission of tuberculosis in health-care facilities, second edition: Notice of comment period. *Federal Register, 58,* 52810–52854.

Department of Labor (1991). Occupational exposure to bloodborne pathogens: Final rule. (29 CFR Part 1910.1030.) *Federal Register, 56,* 64175–64182.

DiPerri, G., Cadeo, G.P., Castelli, F., et al. (1993). Transmission of HIV-associated tuberculosis to healthcare workers. *Infection Control and Hospital Epidemiology, 14,* 67–72.

Dickinson, G.M., Morhart, R.E., Klimas, N.G., et al. (1993). Absence of HIV transmission from an infected dentist to his patients: An epidemiologic and DNA sequence analysis. *Journal of the American Medical Association, 269,* 1802–1806.

Emergency Cardiac Care Committee of the American Heart Association (1989). Risk of infection during CPR training and rescue: Supplemental guidelines. *Journal of the American Medical Association, 262,* 2714–2715.

Fahey, B.J., Beekmann, S.E., Schmitt, M.M., et al. (1993). Managing occupational exposures to HIV-1 in the healthcare workplace. *Infection Control and Hospital Epidemiology, 14,* 405–412.

Flynn, N.M., Pollet, S.M., Van Horne, J.R., et al. (1987). Absence of HIV antibody among dental professionals exposed to infected patients. *Western Journal of Medicine, 146,* 439–442.

Food and Drug Administration (1991). Allergic reactions to latex-containing medical devices. *FDA Medical Alert,* MDA91-1 [and personal communication].

Garner, J.S., Hughes, J.M. (1987). Options for isolation precautions. *Annals of Internal Medicine, 107,* 248–250.

Gauthier, D.K., Turner, J.G., Langley, L.G., et al. (1991). Monitoring universal precautions: A new assessment tool. *Infection Control and Hospital Epidemiology, 12,* 597–601.

Gartner, K. (1992). Impact of a needleless intravenous system in a university hospital. *American Journal of Infection Control, 20,* 75–79.

Gerberding, J.L. (1989). Risks to health care workers from occupational exposure to hepatitis B virus, human immunodeficiency virus, and cytomegalovirus. *Infectious Disease Clinics of North America, 3,* 735–745.

Gerberding, J.L. (1993). Is antiretroviral treatment after percutaneous HIV exposure justified? *Annals of Internal Medicine, 118*(12), 979–980.

Gerberding, J.L., Bryant-LeBlanc, C.E., Nelson, K., et al. (1987). Risk of transmitting the human immunodeficiency virus, cytomegalovirus, and hepatitis B virus to health care workers exposed to patients with AIDS and AIDS-related conditions. *The Journal of Infectious Diseases, 156,* 1–8.

Gerberding, J.L., Littel, C., Brown, A., et al. (1989). Predictors of intraoperative blood exposures. Fifth International Conference on AIDS, Montreal, Quebec, Canada. Geneva: World Health Organization.

Gerberding, J.L., and University of California, San Francisco Task Force on AIDS (1986). Special report: Recommended infection-control policies for patients with human immunodeficiency virus infection—an update. *The New England Journal of Medicine, 315,* 1562–1564.

Hadley, W.K. (1989). Infection of the health-care worker by HIV and other blood-borne viruses: Risks, protection, and education. *American Journal of Hospital Pharmacy, 46,* S4–S7.

Henderson, D.K., Gerberding, J.L. (1989). Post-exposure zidovudine chemoprophylaxis for health-care workers experiencing occupational exposures to the human immunodeficiency virus: An interim analysis. *The Journal of Infectious Diseases, 160,* 321–327.

Holloway, N.M. (1986). AIDS awareness in the emergency department. *Critical Care Nurse, 6,* 90–93.

Ippolito, G., Puro, V., DeCarli, G. (1993). The risk of occupational human immunodeficiency virus infection in health care workers. *Archives of Internal Medicine, 153*(12), 1451–1458.

Jackson, M.M., Lynch, P. (1989). Infection prevention and control in the era of the AIDS/HIV epidemic. *Seminars in Oncology Nursing, 5,* 236–243.

Jagger, J., Pearson, R.D. (1991). Universal precautions: Still missing the point on needlesticks. *Infection Control and Hospital Epidemiology, 12,* 211–213.

Kephart, P.A., Roman, K.L., Myers, D.M. (1993). Universal precautions kit. *Infection Control and Hospital Epidemiology, 14,* 252.

Korniewicz, D.M., Laughon, B.E., Cyr, W.H., et al. (1989). Leakage of virus through used vinyl and latex examination gloves. *Journal of Clinical Microbiology, 28,* 787–788.

Kristensen, M.S., Wernberg, N.M., Anker-Moller, E. (1992). Healthcare workers' risk of contact with body fluids in a hospital: The effect of complying with the universal precautions policy. *Infection Control and Hospital Epidemiology, 13,* 719–724.

Kuhls, T.L., Cherry, J.D. (1987). Readers' forum: The management of health care workers' accidental parenteral exposures to biological specimens of HIV seropositive individuals. *Infection Control, 8,* 211–213.

Kuhls, T.L., Viker, S., Parris, N.B., et al. (1987). Occupational risk of HIV, HBV and HSV-2 infections in health care personnel caring for AIDS patients. *American Journal of Public Health, 77,* 1306–1309.

Lange, J.M.A., Boucher, C.A.B., Hollak, C.E.M., et al. (1990). Failure of zidovudine prophylaxis after accidental exposure to HIV-1. *The New England Journal of Medicine, 322,* 1375–1377.

Lettau, L.A., Blackhurst, D.W., Steed, C. (1992). Human immunodeficiency virus testing experience and hepatitis B vaccination and testing status of healthcare workers in South Carolina: Implications for compliance with U.S. public health service guidelines. *Infection Control and Hospital Epidemiology, 13,* 336–342.

Linnemann, C.C., Cannon, C., DeRonde, M., et al. (1991). Effect of educational programs, rigid sharps containers, and universal precautions on reported needlestick injuries in healthcare workers. *Infection Control and Hospital Epidemiology, 12,* 214–219.

Looke, D.F.M., Grove, D.I. (1990). Failed prophylactic zidovudine after needlestick injury. *Lancet, 335,* 1280.

Lovitt, S.A., Nichols, R.L., Smith, J.W., et al. (1992). Isolation gowns: A false sense of security? *American Journal of Infection Control, 20,* 185–191.

Lowenfels, A.B., Wormser, G.P., Jain, R. (1989). Frequency of puncture injuries in surgeons and estimated risk of HIV infection. *Archives of Surgery, 124,* 1284–1286.

Lusby, G., Martin, J.P., Schietinger, H. (1986). Infection control at home: A guideline for caregivers to follow. *The American Journal of Hospice Care, 3,* 24–27.

Lutwick, S.M., Abter, E.I.M., Chapnick, E.K., et al. (1993). Tuberculosis in patients infected with human immunodeficiency virus: A problem-solving approach. *American Journal of Infection Control, 20,* 156–158.

Lynch, P., Jackson, M.M., Cummings, J., et al. (1987). Rethinking the role of isolation practices in the prevention of nosocomial infections. *Annals of Internal Medicine, 107,* 243–246.

Makofsky, D., Cone, J.E. (1993). Installing needle disposal boxes closer to the bedside reduces needle-recapping rates in hospital units. *Infection Control and Hospital Epidemiology, 14,* 141–144.

Makulowich, G.S. (1993). Infection control update: Use of PAPRs to prevent TB transmission still debated by government agencies. *AIDS Patient Care, 7,* 286–287.

Marcus, R., Srivastava, P.V., Zalenski, R.J., et al. (1993). Risk of human immunodeficiency virus infection among emergency department workers. *The American Journal of Medicine, 94,* 363–370.

Marcus, R., and the Cooperative Needlestick Surveillance Group (1988). Surveillance of health care workers exposed to blood from patients infected with the human immunodeficiency virus. *The New England Journal of Medicine, 319,* 1118–1123.

Mast, S.T., Woolwine, J.D., Gerberding, J.L. (1993). Efficacy of gloves in reducing blood volumes transferred during simulated needlestick injury. *The Journal of Infectious Diseases, 168,* 1589–1592.

McCray, E., and the Cooperative Needlestick Surveillance Group (1986). Occupational risk of the acquired immunodeficiency syndrome among health care workers. *The New England Journal of Medicine, 314,* 1127–1132.

McGowan, J.E. (1992). Resurgent nosocomial tuberculosis: Consequences and actions for hospital epidemiologists. *Infection Control and Hospital Epidemiology, 13,* 575–578.

Neisson-Vernant, C., Afri, S., Mathez, D., et al. (1986). Needlestick HIV seroconversion in a nurse. *Lancet, 2,* 814.

Oksenhendler, E., Harzic, M., LeRoux, J.M., et al. (1986). HIV infection with seroconversion after a superficial needlestick injury to the finger. *The New England Journal of Medicine, 315,* 582.

Pitchenik, A.E., Fertel, D. (1992). Tuberculosis and non-tuberculosis mycobacterial disease. *Medical Clinics of North America, 76,* 121–171.

Pugliese, G. (1992). Occupational safety and health administration moves blood-borne pathogen compliance to the front burner. *American Journal of Infection Control, 20,* 167–169.

Rogers, A.S., Froggatt, J.W., Townsend, T., et al. (1993).

Investigation of potential HIV transmission to the patients of an HIV-infected surgeon. *Journal of the American Medical Association, 269,* 1795–1801.

Russo, G., LaCroix, S.J. (1992). A second look at the cost of mandatory human immunodeficiency virus and hepatitis B virus testing for healthcare workers performing invasive procedures. *Infection Control and Hospital Epidemiology, 13,* 107–110.

Rutowski, M., Peterson, S.L. (1993). A needleless intravenous system: An effective risk management strategy. *Infection Control and Hospital Epidemiology, 14,* 226–227.

Saghafi, L., Raselli, P., Francillon, C., et al. (1992). Exposure to blood during various procedures: Results of two surveys before and after the implementation of universal precautions. *American Journal of Infection Control, 20,* 53–57.

Skolnick, R., LaRocca, J., Barba, D., et al. (1993). Evaluation and implementation of a needleless intravenous system: Making needlesticks a needless problem. *American Journal of Infection Control, 21,* 39–41.

Stricof, R.L., Morse, D.L. (1986). HTLV-III/LAV seroconversion following a deep intramuscular needlestick injury. *The New England Journal of Medicine, 314,* 1115.

Tokars, J.I., Jarvis, W.R., Edlin, B.R., et al. (1992). Tuberculin skin testing of hospital employees during an outbreak of multidrug-resistant tuberculosis in human immunodeficiency virus (HIV)-infected patients. *Infection Control and Hospital Epidemiology, 13,* 509–510.

Turnbull, G.B., Balice, A.B. (1993). An innovative option to comply with 1992 OSHA Guidelines. *Infection Control and Hospital Epidemiology, 14,* 153–154.

Underwood, M.A., Berg, R., Bryant, J.K., et al. (1992). Commentary from the APIC guidelines committee on CDC guidelines for preventing the transmission of tuberculosis in health care settings, with special focus on HIV-related issues. *American Journal of Infection Control, 20,* 27–29.

Visiting Nurse Service Home Care and Administration (1990). Policy on universal precautions—infection control practice for all patient care [unpublished manuscript]. New York City.

von Reyn, C.F., Gilbert, T.T., Shaw, F.E., et al. (1993). Absence of HIV transmission from an infected orthopedic surgeon: A 13-year look-back study. *Journal of the American Medical Association, 269,* 1807–1811.

Weiss, S.H. (1992). HIV infection and the health-care worker. *Medical Clinics of North America, 76,* 269–280.

Whitby, M., Stead, P., Najman, J.M. (1991). Needlestick injury: Impact of a recapping device and an associated education program. *Infection Control and Hospital Epidemiology, 12,* 220–225.

Yarchoan, R., Thomas, R.V., Grafman, J., et al. (1988). Long-term administration of 3'-azido-2',3'-dideoxythymidine to patients with AIDS-related neurological disease. *Annals of Neurology, 23*(suppl), S82–S87.

Yeager, M. (1990). Concerns about contagious disease prompt infection controls for CPR. *Occupational Health and Safety, 59*(7), 51–52.

Younger, B., Hunt, E.H., Robinson, C., et al. (1992). Impact of a shielded safety syringe on needlestick injuries among healthcare workers. *Infection Control and Hospital Epidemiology, 13,* 349–353.

Zbitnew, A., Greer, K., Heise-Qualtiere, J., et al. (1989). Vinyl versus latex gloves as barriers to transmission of viruses in the health care setting. *Journal of Acquired Immune Deficiency Syndromes, 2,* 201–204.

11 Psychosocial and Psychiatric Aspects

Jacquelyn Haak Flaskerud

HIV disease generates a unique series of stresses for infected persons, sexual partners, family members, and health care professionals. It creates serious social and psychologic problems for everyone with whom the infected person has close contacts, including friends and employers. It causes stress in HIV-infected healthy people, in those with clinical disease, in the worried well, and in the general public.

HIV disease may also represent comorbidity in populations with preexisting mental illness. In these populations the prevalence of risk factors may be especially high. Hypersexuality and the practice of unsafe sex may be a particular risk, as may drug use and trading sex for drugs. HIV disease may also exacerbate preexisting mental illnesses such as major affective disorders and schizophrenia. Finally, HIV disease is associated with neuropsychologic dysfunctions. These may create extreme stresses and burdens for person(s) with HIV disease (PWHIV) and their loved ones. They also may produce a variety of psychiatric symptoms such as anxiety syndromes, mania, hallucinations, and paranoia. Whether because of stress, previous mental illness, or the viral infection itself, HIV disease produces psychosocial and psychiatric consequences that often require the intervention and support of nurses and other health-care givers.

UNIQUE FEATURES OF THE AIDS EPIDEMIC

The spectrum of disease caused by HIV infection includes a constellation of unique characteristics that make it a public health problem without contemporary counterpart. HIV disease is a relatively new communicable, sexually transmitted, eventually fatal disease.

It was first identified and occurs most frequently in socially stigmatized groups: homosexual men, injection drug users (IDUs), and ethnic people of color. The diagnosis of AIDS is a traumatic event because the disease is known to have a progressive course, no curative treatment, and an extremely poor prognosis. The complexity and multiplicity of problems confronting people with HIV infection and the psychologic fear it engenders affect every aspect of a person's life. Specific features of the AIDS epidemic contribute to the unique psychologic, social, and psychiatric aspects of the disease (Britton et al., 1993; Gillespie, 1992; Michels & Marzuk, 1993; Ostrow et al., 1991).

1. Persons with HIV disease are generally young. About 21% are in their twenties, 47% in their thirties, and 21% in their forties.
2. HIV disease is incurable, requires lifelong changes in behavior, and threatens a person's most intimate relationships.
3. The diagnosis of HIV infection may force the person's identification as a likely member of a stigmatized minority.
4. The social stigma and fear associated with the contagious aspect of the disease can cause others, even family members, to avoid social and physical contact with the infected person.
5. Because of moral disapproval and negative societal attitudes, there is a tendency to blame the infected person for the disease if he or she was exposed to the disease through sexual or drug use practices.
6. The entire continuum of HIV disease,

from exposure through infection to diagnosis, is characterized by extreme uncertainty, resulting in marked psychologic distress.

7. Persons with HIV disease are vulnerable to feelings of guilt, self-hatred, rejection, and ostracism, as well as to the commonly recognized feelings of fear, anxiety, depression, and anger that accompany other life-threatening illnesses.

8. There is a dynamic relationship between HIV disease and mental illness: HIV disease may exacerbate mental illness, and mental illness may perpetuate behaviors that facilitate transmission.

9. HIV disease is associated with the highest incidence of neurologic and neuropsychiatric morbidity of any serious common illness not primary to the nervous system.

10. AIDS is associated wth severe chronic physical disability that leaves persons debilitated and disfigured.

11. Health care professionals and the current patient treatment system for PWHIV are severely taxed and often overwhelmed by the complexity and multiplicity of problems associated with care of PWHIV. This situation is likely to worsen as the numbers of patients increase. In addition, fear and a lack of knowledge and sensitivity among health care workers are detrimental to patient care.

12. HIV disease has had a highly visible social and political impact. It has attracted a barrage of media attention that is not always accurate, is often stressful to PWHIV, aggravates public fears, and leads to attempts at repressive measures such as quarantines or mandatory HIV testing.

Because of these characteristics of both the disease and the epidemic, the care of PWHIV requires special attention to the psychologic, social, and psychiatric aspects of their disease. Also of concern to health care professionals are the stresses experienced by the worried well, by symptom-free seropositive persons, and by the sexual partners and families of PWHIV. The stresses that health care professionals themselves experience in giving care to PWHIV are a further consideration.

PSYCHOLOGIC RESPONSES TO HIV AMONG UNINFECTED PERSONS

HIV disease is occurring in a society that disapproves of homosexuality, drug use, and sexual promiscuity. This disapproval is accompanied by fear of contagion, prejudice, discrimination, stigmatization, and, in extreme cases, hatred and violence. It is within this social context that psychologic responses to HIV infection occur (Beevor & Catalan, 1993).

Psychologic responses to HIV occur in both persons who are and persons who are not infected. Many persons who are not infected are also not worried about being infected. The major psychologic responses of this group are denial and dissociation. Heterosexuals practice denial by underestimating their vulnerability to infection. Although they are very much aware of HIV disease, they do not consider it a threat to themselves. This underestimation of vulnerability is evidenced in the lack of behavioral change among heterosexual adolescents and young adults; in these groups the use of condoms and the number of sexual partners do not appear to have changed (Catania et al., 1992; Hein, 1993). Risk reduction practices appear to be limited among ethnic people of color, especially women (Eversley et al., 1993; Finelli et al., 1993; Kost & Forrest, 1992). Although a study of drugstore condom sales in the year after the surgeon general's report on AIDS showed a 20% increase in sales over the previous year, syphilis rates increased 25% in that year, with urban areas having the highest rates (Finelli et al., 1993; Moran et al., 1990).

Dissociation occurs among heterosexuals both by a physical separation of themselves from the so-called risk groups and by a psychologic dissociation with sexually transmitted diseases (STDs), drug use, and male-to-male sexual contact. Many people think of all of these conditions as so morally reprehensible that they would consider it an extreme insult to question a sexual partner about a history of sexually transmitted diseases, drug use, and sexual practices. Because of these two psychologic responses, dissociation and denial of HIV infection, heterosexuals might be characterized as unworried—but also as not vigilant and therefore vulnerable. These persons rarely seek HIV antibody testing or psychologic and social support related to their affective responses to AIDS (Beevor & Catalan, 1993).

Denial and dissociation may occur in homosexuals also. Several studies on both the East and West coasts have reported that homosexual men have significantly changed their sexual behavior in response to the threat of AIDS (Catania et al., 1992; Coates, 1990; van Griensven et al., 1993). However, other investigators have found that some gay men had misperceptions of risky behaviors and only a weak perception of their own vulnerability to HIV disease (Messiah et al., 1993). Furthermore, some men were engaging in risky behaviors but underestimated the risks associated with these behaviors because they knew their sexual partners. They believed the risk to be associated only with anonymous partners (Offir et al., 1993). Young gay men also were not practicing safer sexual behaviors, perceiving the disease to be that of an older generation of gay men (Hart et al., 1993; Silvestre et al., 1993). These groups might also be characterized as using psychologic responses of denial and dissociation with any perception of personal vulnerability.

Among gay and bisexual African American men, risk practices also continued; however, perception of risk was evident (Peterson et al., 1992). In addition to these psychologic responses, certain cognitive and affective responses among gay men and IDUs may be influencing their willingness to change their behavior (Offir et al., 1993). The value that gay men place on freedom of sexual expression may conflict with the sexual behavior change demanded by the AIDS epidemic. In the same way, among IDUs the value placed on sharing, closeness, and interaction may conflict with required changes in needle-sharing behaviors (Friedman et al., 1990). This may be especially true among women who,

because of gender role relationships, believe that they should share with a partner. Persons with these beliefs may choose not to change their risk behaviors (Wayment et al., 1993). Nevertheless, psychologic responses to the HIV epidemic may occur in these persons, who, although they are aware that their behaviors put them at risk, do not choose to change them. The psychologic responses of these persons may be anxiety based (Beevor & Catalan, 1993). Their responses may include generalized anxiety and panic attacks, obsessive-compulsive behavior, hypochondriasis, and anxiety-based physical symptoms related to perceptions of risk.

In another group of persons, the psychologic response to the HIV epidemic is characterized by extreme anxiety, even though they have no known risk behaviors (Fullilove, 1989; King, 1990). For some, anxiety is relieved by reassurance and a negative HIV antibody test result. However, other persons in this group are not persuaded by laboratory evidence and are convinced that they have symptoms of HIV disease. These persons are in need of psychotherapy that relates their perception of symptoms to anxiety.

Finally, a variety of other responses may occur in persons who have HIV antibody seronegativity. Such persons may have a false sense of security that could foster continued high-risk behavior (Otten et al., 1993). Some persons feel that they are immune to the virus. Other seronegative persons, involved in high-risk behaviors, have ongoing anxiety related to their uncertainty regarding their HIV antibody status. Still others vacillate between periods of hope and despair regarding their HIV status. Persons who are not infected but are engaged in high-risk behaviors may require ongoing intervention and repeated HIV testing (Valdiserri et al., 1993). This intervention should include counseling, education, and behavior change strategies.

PSYCHOSOCIAL STRESS ON PERSONS WITH THE SPECTRUM OF HIV DISEASE

Persons who are infected with HIV have a variety of psychologic and social stresses that may differ in degree of severity depending on

Table 11–1. Psychosocial Assessment

1. Psychosocial history	5. Life-cycle phase
2. Current distress and crisis	6. Illness phase
3. Past and current coping	7. Individual identity
4. Social support needed and available	8. Experience with loss and grief

stage of illness and whether or not symptoms have begun. As noted earlier, the stresses associated with HIV disease are compounded by the youth of the population affected; the high mortality rate and accompanying anxiety and depression; the social stigma, fear, ostracism, and discrimination associated with diagnosis of the disease; the debilitation, disfigurement, and symptoms of the disease; and its contagious nature.

Psychosocial Assessment

Gathering information about persons across the spectrum of HIV infection in various categories of psychosocial adjustment can assist the health care professional in anticipating reactions, needs, and vulnerability to psychologic dysfunction and in designing an appropriate psychosocial intervention plan (Beckett & Shenson, 1993; Beevor & Catalan, 1993; Britton et al., 1993; Cote et al., 1992; Green, 1993; Kelly & Murphy, 1992; Ostrow et al., 1991; Perry et al., 1993; Regan-Kubinski & Sharts-Engel, 1992; Sadovsky, 1991). Psychosocial assessment should be done frequently with persons with HIV infection and especially at the various crisis points in the disease spectrum.

Psychosocial History. The person's history of interpersonal relationships, education, and career can provide insight into vulnerability to psychologic dysfunction. Use of nonprescribed drugs and alcohol, prior psychiatric care, and preexisting mental illness are other indicators of possible psychologic dysfunction. Psychologically healthy individuals usually have stable jobs and stable interpersonal relationships. Psychologically vulnerable HIV-infected persons may have preillness behaviors that include drug use and

multiple sexual contacts. The presence of a personality disorder, as in IDUs, or of a previous psychiatric disorder is more apt to result in severe psychologic symptoms and a maladaptive response to the stresses of illness (see Table 11–1).

Current Distress and Crisis. What specific threats and losses is the person experiencing currently? What aspect of the illness is the most distressing and bothersome to the individual at the present time? The person's level of anxiety, fear, and behavioral disorganization will change from one time to the next and will be related to the duration, intensity, and precipitant of the current crisis.

Coping. The person who is facing HIV disease will call into action previous patterns of understanding problems and methods of resolving them. Knowing which approaches have been successful for this person in the past and which approaches are currently being tried will give an indication of how he or she will attempt to cope with the illness and how successful that attempt might be. It will also give direction for providing support to the person's coping responses.

Social Support. What sources of support are available to the person? Family? Spouse? Lover? Friends? Social groups? What is the person's social identity? To which cultural or subcultural groups does he or she belong? What are the possibilities for support within that social identity? Gender, age, ethnicity, and route of exposure all affect the amount and kind of social support available and needed by PWHIV. Fewer organized resources are available for women, African Americans and Latinos, and IDUs. Furthermore, the needs of these groups differ from one another and from those of gay white men. The following questions should be asked: What types of support and assistance do PWHIV need? Practical assistance? Social interaction? Emotional support? How can that assistance be provided?

Life-Cycle Phase. People have different goals, resources, skills, and social roles depending on their age. The majority of

PWHIV are in their twenties, thirties, and forties. Young adults are not developmentally prepared to confront their mortality. Those in their twenties have fewer resources and skills than those in their forties. The former are involved in the psychosocial tasks of establishing independence, autonomy, and adult identity. At times of illness this age group typically becomes intensely reinvolved with the family of origin, emotionally and financially. Older persons (those in their thirties and forties) have more resources (money, housing, insurance) and have established independent adult roles. At times of illness they are more likely to depend on a spouse or lover and friends for support.

Illness Phase. People's needs for psychosocial support differ according to their phase of illness. Stresses on the person are different in the HIV testing, AIDS diagnosis, treatment, and after-treatment phases. They also differ depending on the person's clinical syndrome: an opportunistic infection, a neoplasm, or a central nervous system (CNS) disease. PWHIV fear CNS disease more than other clinical syndromes; the associated memory loss and mood changes result in depression, anger, and strain on their social network (Getzel & Mahony, 1990; Gillespie, 1992). Emotional reactions and methods of coping differ in response to the illness phase and the clinical syndrome.

Individual Identity. An individual's personal identity also affects his or her reaction to a life-threatening illness. The person's sources of self-esteem, valued achievements, and future goals make up that person's identity. These and the individual's orientation to living and search for meaning all play a role in how the person perceives and combats the illness.

Loss and Grief. The losses that the individual has had, is currently having, and anticipates having as a result of the illness determine the kind of psychosocial support needed. Persons may be currently grieving a loss and going through the grief process.

They may have had previous experiences with loss and grief and feel some recognition and equanimity toward the process, or they may have had no previous experience and are anxious and fearful about anticipated losses and the grieving process.

An assessment of the person with HIV disease in these various areas will provide the health care professional with the information needed to design a psychosocial intervention plan. This plan can be individualized to meet the specific needs of persons as they move through the various phases of the disease spectrum and the phases of their emotional and social responses to the illness. The common psychosocial crises that occur in PWHIV have been identified, and intervention strategies have been designed to support them during these crises.

Psychologic Stresses

The major psychologic stress on PWHIV is the knowledge that they have a fatal disease with the potential for a rapid decline to death. Most frequently, psychologic reactions are of fear, anxiety, and depression, which are compounded by the uncertainty of the course of the disease. Social stresses on PWHIV include exposure, stigma, rejection, abandonment, and isolation. Common psychologic reactions are guilt, fear, anger, and suspicion (Bennett, 1990; Britton et al., 1993; Getzel & Mahony, 1990; Hedge, 1990; Hintze et al., 1993; Kelly & Murphy, 1992; Regan-Kubinski & Sharts-Engel, 1992). Psychologic reactions have been reported to reach levels of clinical psychopathology in 20% of subjects in different studies of gay men and IDUs (Britton et al., 1993; Castro et al., 1989; Catalan & Riccio, 1990; Folkman et al., 1993; Michels & Marzuk, 1993).

Crisis Points. Certain crisis points in the course of the disease precipitate intense anxiety, fear, and depression (Andrews et al., 1993; Grothe et al., 1993; King, 1990; Ragsdale & Morrow, 1990; Snyder et al., 1992; Sohier, 1993; Twiname, 1993; Valente et al., 1993) (Table 11–2). The initial intense crisis

Table 11–2. Crisis Points and Emotional Response

CRISIS POINTS	EMOTIONS AND BEHAVIORS	INTERVENTIONS
HIV seropositivity	Anxiety; panic; depression; hopelessness; suicidal ideation and attempts; somatic complaints	Suicide assessment
AIDS diagnosis	Intense anxiety; fear; anger; guilt; impulsive behavior; suicidal ideation and attempts	Crisis intervention Pharmacotherapy
Treatment	Depression; weakness; alienation; dysphoria; fear of disfigurement; disability; pain	Individual therapy Education Resource provision
Treatment termination	Anxiety; fear	Stress reduction techniques
New symptoms	Hypochondriasis; demanding and dependent behavior; anxiety	Support groups Support assistance
Recurrence and relapse	Depression; dependence; apathy; isolation; suicidal ideation; dysphoria; fear of abandonment	Clergy; attorney
Terminal illness	Deterioration; decline; ambivalence; dependence; disinterest; resolution	

is at the time of confirmation of HIV seropositivity. Risks, benefits, and the components of comprehensive pretest and posttest HIV counseling are addressed in depth in Chapter 2. Psychologic responses are described here. For symptom-free persons with seropositivity, significant adverse reactions in the form of depression, anxiety, and preoccupation with AIDS are reported commonly (Kelly & Murphy, 1992; Perry et al., 1993). Suicide risk is reported to be high also in persons recently found to be infected with HIV (Beckett & Shenson, 1993; Cote et al., 1992; Kelly & Murphy, 1992). The devastating effects of seropositive test results include feelings of panic, depression, and hopelessness.

Interpersonal and social responses may also be devastating. Many individuals lose their sexual partners because of disclosure of seropositive results. In addition, discrimination in employment and housing, loss of insurance benefits, and social ostracism may occur. Persons receiving HIV-positive test results may require prolonged counseling; they also need a variety of social, medical, and psychiatric support services. Perry and colleagues (1993) found that counseling during the HIV testing process provided an opportunity to identify those most at risk for psychopatho-

logic abnormalities: those with a history of current depression, anxiety, cognitive symptoms, and drug use.

During the long asymptomatic phase of HIV infection, many persons do not have severe distress (Ragsdale & Morrow, 1990). Those with sustained psychopathologic problems have been identified as those who at the time of HIV testing demonstrated depression, anxiety, and cognitive symptoms within clinical ranges and as those who use drugs (Perry et al., 1993). In general during the asymptomatic phase, most persons live with a degree of hope and an absence of anxiety (Kelly & Murphy, 1992). These findings are a change from earlier times in the epidemic and are thought to be related to a greater understanding of the difference between HIV infection and AIDS and to the knowledge that HIV disease involves a long asymptomatic stage.

When HIV-infected people begin having symptoms of disease, they experience all the psychologic and social stresses associated with AIDS (Ragsdale & Morrow, 1990; Twiname, 1993; Valente et al., 1993). Probably each development (for instance, the appearance of symptoms) that signals to the person further deterioration toward AIDS and eventually death has the potential of stimulating a psychologic crisis (Linn et al., 1993). The same existential issues that accompany a diagnosis of other life-threatening illnesses occur with AIDS. The normal response to an AIDS diagnosis is characterized by disbelief, numbness, a feeling of being already dead, and denial, followed by anger, turmoil, disruptive anxiety, and depressive symptoms. High levels of anxiety can exist for 2 to 3 months after diagnosis and can take the form of panic attacks, agitation, tachycardia, impulsive behaviors such as sexual acting out, and suicidal ideation.

The treatment phase is often accompanied by weakness, depression, alienation, and dysphoria. Patients fear disfigurement, debilitation, and pain. Treatment may include isolation procedures that make patients feel alienated and socially abandoned. The termination of treatment often brings on increased anxiety and fears of renewed disease progression. Hypervigilance with body functions and the appearance of new symptoms can result in hypochondriasis, demanding behavior toward medical personnel, and excessive dependence on health-care givers.

Recurrence or relapse of disease is often accompanied by feelings of hopelessness, helplessness, sadness, low self-esteem, discouragement, loss of control, dependence, isolation, and suicidal ideation. Patients fear being abandoned by health-care givers who might decide that continued treatment is futile. This stage may be accompanied by cognitive impairment because of CNS disease. The terminal phase of illness is marked by deterioration and decline and can be accompanied by ambivalence, dependence, disinterest, or resolution.

Suicide Assessment. The potential for suicide has been recognized at several crisis points in HIV infection and disease (Beckett & Shenson, 1993; Flaskerud, 1992; Gillespie, 1992). Increased risk of suicide is associated with HIV antibody testing and learning of a seropositive status, with a diagnosis of AIDS, and with later stages of illness characterized by pain and dementia (Cote et al., 1992; McKegney & O'Dowd, 1992; Pergami et al., 1992; Perry et al., 1993; Twiname, 1993; Wolcott et al., 1989). The suicide rate of men aged 20 to 59 years with AIDS in New York City in 1985 was 36 times that of men of the same age without this diagnosis and 66 times that of the general population (Marzuk et al., 1988). In 1992, Cote and associates reported the suicide rate in the United States among male PWHIV to be 7.4 times higher than men in the general population.

PWHIV who have the most current suicidal ideation are those with asymptomatic and those with early symptomatic disease (McKegney & O'Dowd, 1992; O'Dowd et al., 1993; Twiname, 1993). In addition PWHIV who are more likely to kill themselves are those with previous depressive episodes, adjustment disorders, personality disorders, alcohol abuse, high levels of environmental stress, inadequate counseling before and after the HIV antibody test, and poor support networks (O'Dowd, 1993; Pergami et al., 1992; Wolcott et al., 1989). Several groups whose behavior puts them at risk of acquiring HIV infection are also those who are more at risk of committing suicide. IDUs frequently have preexisting personality or affective disorders (Wolcott et al., 1989). Gay men and lesbians have been reported to attempt suicide two to three times as often as their heterosexual counterparts, and racial stigma has been linked with suicide (Grossman, 1991; Hall & Stevens, 1988).

Assessment of suicide risk should accompany any of the crisis points in the HIV disease spectrum (Beckett & Shenson, 1993). Assessment should include the following:

1. A history of affective disorder and drug use
2. Amount of pain and disability being experienced
3. An investigation of a plan and method for suicide
4. An evaluation of the extent, availability, and supportiveness of the person's social network
5. Whether significant others have committed suicide
6. Whether the person is suffering grief and loss
7. Socioeconomic status (housing, employment, insurance)

8. Spirituality
9. An investigation of an assisted suicide plan

PWHIV contemplating suicide may have made suicide pacts with friends and loved ones, and they may be grieving the loss of friends who died of AIDS. They may be experiencing the loss of independent functioning accompanied by a loss of self-esteem. They may also be facing an existential crisis in which life has ceased to have meaning. Any or all of these factors may be motivation for suicide (Beckett & Shenson, 1993).

Crisis Intervention. During the crisis points, PWHIV need a full range of psychosocial interventions, including immediate crisis intervention or individual therapy, or both, to deal with feelings of extreme anxiety, fear, and anger and with impulsive behavior and suicidal thoughts and behaviors. PWHIV disease should be encouraged to express their anxiety, fear, sadness, and anger and to grieve, with the understanding that grief can be a healing process (Lazzari et al., 1993; Sohier, 1993). Pharmacotherapy should be used for intense anxiety, depression, hopelessness, and insomnia. Whenever possible, health-care givers should support and enhance the person's coping behaviors and not work in opposition to them unless they are dangerous or destructive. Clients also need ongoing psychosocial support in the form of support groups to dispel self-blame and guilt, provide reassurance, share information and experiences, and reduce feelings of isolation and loneliness (Kendall, 1992). Experience with PWHIV in support groups and research on levels of distress in persons in different stages of HIV spectrum disease suggest that separate support groups should be developed: one for persons with early symptoms, one for persons with Kaposi's sarcoma, and one for other PWHIV. Such suggestions are based on the differing levels of anxiety and areas of concern among these groups (Ragsdale & Morrow, 1990).

Infected people need education regarding the disease and its treatment, liaison with community resources to help them resolve practical problems, and instruction in stress and anxiety reduction techniques such as relaxation. They also need supportive intervention from a social network that includes family, friends, health care professionals, volunteers, an attorney, and clergy who can offer encouragement, comfort, concern, compassion, affection, and legal and spiritual assistance.

All these interventions play a role in the treatment of PWHIV during crisis stages. Which will take priority at any given time depends on individual response and can be determined by psychosocial assessments of the person at crisis points. Given the heterogeneity of the population of HIV-infected individuals, no single therapeutic strategy is likely to be universally efficacious (Perry, 1990). If possible, the HIV-infected person should be assigned a primary caregiver, primary care nurse, or case manager to coordinate service needs and provide a central and familiar person the client can see to ensure continuity of care throughout the course of the illness, hospitalizations, community care, and referrals.

Psychologic Conflicts. People with HIV disease are subjected to an unusual number of psychologic, or internal, conflicts (Table 11–3). Some of these conflicts revolve around transmission of the disease: who the person got it from or to whom he or she might have transmitted it. Emotional responses to these internal conflicts can be directed toward self and others and can involve anxiety, depression, fear, anger, suspicion, and guilt (Folkman et al., 1993; Hintze et al., 1993; Sadovsky, 1991).

Similar concerns and conflicts are evident in the person's efforts to protect himself or herself from the risk of infection. Fear of associating with others, anger at and suspicion of others who might transmit infection, and guilt and loneliness from abandoning friends for self-protection are all involved in this conflict. People may also experience guilt over their previous lifestyles, especially if they have had a number of anonymous sexual partners or have used injection drugs or other recreational substances (Kendall, 1992). Getzel and Mahony (1990) reported bargaining to go

Table 11–3. Internal Conflicts and Emotional Responses

PSYCHOLOGIC CONFLICTS	EMOTIONS AND BEHAVIORS	INTERVENTIONS
Transmission	Anxiety; depression; fear; anger	Education
		Resource provision
Protection from infection	Suspicion; guilt	Support groups
Previous lifestyle	Internalized homophobia or societal prejudices; bargaining to go straight; preexisting affective symptoms	Stress reduction techniques
Personal relationships	Loneliness; frustration; rejection; abandonment	

straight or denying a homosexual identity as part of a search for a magical cure among PWHIV in group therapy in New York City. For IDUs, the presence of preexisting personality or affective disorders compounds the psychologic problems of HIV disease (Wolcott et al., 1989). Strong feelings of guilt and self-blame among PWHIV can cause them to internalize society's prejudicial attitudes toward the group(s) to which they belong and lead them, in turn, to stigmatize others. Among homosexuals this is called internalized homophobia, but it may happen in any group toward which society expresses disapproval, such as drug users, prostitutes, and persons with multiple sexual partners.

Finally, many conflicts occur over continuing personal relationships, especially those which have a sexual focus. Fears of social abandonment, isolation, and loneliness accompany giving up intimate sexual relationships. This is especially true if sexual relationships were used to provide interpersonal contacts (Kendall, 1992).

Certain sexual practices (e.g., anal intercourse) among gay men and ritual needle sharing among IDUs may have functioned to integrate the person into the homosexual or drug-using community (Wayment et al., 1993). Giving up these practices and making major lifestyle changes may result in an emotional crisis. Restraints on sexual or drug use behavior may demand new social skills for negotiation, limit setting, or partner rejection, as well as new psychologic skills for tolerating frustration, managing anxiety, and creating or enhancing self-reassurance and self-control.

Some of the psychologic conflicts can be

resolved through individual or group education that focuses on transmission and protection from infection by means of an intervention that involves cognitive-behavioral skills training (Kelly & Murphy, 1992). Others can be resolved through support groups and finding reassurance, shared experiences, and intimacy among persons with the same concerns (Kendall, 1992), which include the need to share unacceptable feelings, obtain positive reinforcement, and explore options to enhance the quality of daily life. Support groups can also help prevent loneliness and isolation and can identify ways for members to reach out to family and friends (Kelly & Murphy, 1992). Community resources can help people build social networks and develop sustained relationships that are not predicated on sex or drug use and sharing. The use of anxiety reduction and stress reduction techniques, such as relaxation or other behavioral techniques, can assist individuals in dealing with their fears and anxieties (Kelly & Murphy, 1992).

Social Stresses

Persons with HIV disease are subject to an unusual number of social conflicts and stresses (Folkman et al., 1993; Green, 1993; van Servellen et al., 1993) (Table 11–4). The first of these may involve public identification as a member of a highly stigmatized group (Grossman, 1991). Social stigmatization is attached to both of the largest transmission groups for HIV infection: men who have sex with men and IDUs. Persons who have considered their sexuality or drug use to be private matters are now subject to exposure

Table 11–4. Social Stress and Emotional Response

SOCIAL CONFLICTS	EMOTIONS AND BEHAVIORS	INTERVENTIONS
Disclosure and exposure	Fear of abandonment, isolation, and rejection	Support groups
		Stress reduction techniques
Stigma	Guilt; anger; suspicion	Resource provision
Employment and insurance	Insecurity because of loss of job and health benefits	Financial counseling
Social support limitation; distance from family	Loneliness; alienation	

and possible rejection by family and friends. Because the diagnosis is HIV infection, they may be abandoned by friends who accept their sexual preference or drug use but are afraid of the disease (Grossman, 1991). At a time when people most need social support, comfort, compassion, and closeness, they might be left alone and isolated. Confiding the diagnosis to family and friends is often not a matter of personal choice. The appearance of symptoms or a diagnosis of AIDS is often difficult to hide because of obvious physical signs, such as frequent illness and infections, disfigurement, weight loss, and debilitation.

Persons with asymptomatic disease are faced with a dilemma as to whether to confide in friends, family, and health care workers, because stigmatization and social rejection are likely to result from receipt of this information (Hays et al., 1993). In one study among persons with an AIDS diagnosis, one third had not discussed their health problems or sexual orientation with their families or employers, but among persons in the early symptomatic stage, two thirds had not done so (Ragsdale & Morrow, 1990). Among those who had disclosed information, one fourth had negative reactions: condemnation or outright rejection. Among African American men with HIV, negative reactions were even more common (Ostrow et al., 1991). These reactions occurred most frequently among confidants but were also found among employers and health care workers. Limandri (1989) reported that what persons seek from disclosure is compassion, understanding, and information. Participating in a support group can provide the opportunity to practice telling others

in an environment that is least likely to be rejecting.

PWHIV have been confronted with a variety of problems involving employment and insurance. Some individuals have been fired from their jobs because employers and co-workers feared they would contract AIDS. In some cases this discrimination has extended to the families of PWHIV. Others have had to leave jobs because of physical disability. In many instances health insurance is lost when the job is lost. PWHIV are often young and have limited experience with medical insurance policies. Many are, in fact, new in the work force and employed by small companies with no insurance coverage. In addition, some insurance companies have tried to avoid covering PWHIV because of the high costs of care. Many PWHIV are without financial security, material resources, and insurance. Community resources that they might need include Social Security Disability Insurance, Supplemental Security Income, and Medicaid. These should be applied for immediately, and arrangements should also be made for legal assistance and personal assistance in the home, such as visiting nurse services and "buddies" to assist with chores and shopping.

Finally, many PWHIV have limited social support networks (Green, 1993; Ostrow et al., 1991). Often the family is not involved with the person, or family members live in distant places. The reason could be alienation from the family because of lifestyle or relocation in a large urban area, such as New York, San Francisco, or Los Angeles, that is far from where the family lives. Some families abandon a relative with HIV when they learn of the diagnosis. This action could be the result of a desire to avoid social stigma, an incorrect belief that homosexuality or drug use itself causes HIV and that the disease is a just retribution, or fear of contagion. Such a situation leaves the infected person at a crucial time without a family to assist with basic physical needs and to provide emotional support, and it forces greater dependence on spouses, lovers, and friends. Community resources can help to meet basic physical needs of PWHIV at home through practical services such as shopping and housekeeping. Some clergy and churches assist visiting parents and siblings in finding places to stay when they come from out of town. The gay community and gay service agencies in large cities have organized a variety of supportive services for persons with limited or distant social support networks. These services include case management, which provides social service, nursing service, insurance counseling, client advocacy, and emotional and physical support through a "buddy" system (Green, 1993; Sonsel, 1989).

Political and social organizations that offer specialized services are less commonly available to drug users who have AIDS, women and children with AIDS, and persons with hemophilia and other blood transfusion recipients with AIDS (Bussing & Burket, 1993; Green, 1993; Stowe et al., 1993). The social network and support resources of drug users usually consist of other drug users and family; they have no organized community for support (Friedman et al., 1990; Stowe et al., 1993). Close liaison with drug rehabilitation programs and self-help groups of former addicts may provide some supportive service for IDUs with AIDS (Metzger et al., 1993). Women with AIDS are often IDUs or the sexual partners of IDUs. Specialized AIDS services for women are extremely limited, but supportive services are sometimes provided through other women's organizations that focus on domestic violence, rape, and homelessness and through reproductive and family planning clinics (Eversley et al., 1993; Shayne & Kaplan, 1991). Children with AIDS most frequently have parents with AIDS and a very limited support network. Andrews and colleagues (1993) reported a strong attachment between mothers with HIV and their children but also a bond of secrecy between them, which might preclude active involvement in social services and support groups. A few hospitals have begun support groups for children who have siblings or parents with AIDS. Nonspecific children's services might be useful also. Persons with hemophilia have supportive medical and social resources to deal with their hemophilia, and these resources might be mobilized to assist with problems associated with AIDS, but there are few specialized AIDS services (Bussing & Burket, 1993). HIV-seropositive men with hemophilia have been reported to have increased depression, anxiety, and anger-hostility symptoms requiring both clinical intervention and social support (Dew et al., 1990). Blood transfusion recipients have extremely limited AIDS support services and have been reported to have high rates of depression (Cleary et al., 1993). In addition, both persons with hemophilia and other blood transfusion/blood product recipients may feel betrayed by the medical system because of the means of their infection with HIV.

As can be noted from the foregoing discussion, the psychosocial stresses on persons with AIDS are overwhelming and result in psychologic reactions that may vary in severity. These stresses call for a range of psychologic, social, economic, and legal interventions, and at any given time in the course of a person's disease they may call for all the interventions and services discussed in this section.

PSYCHIATRIC DISORDERS AND HIV

Psychiatric morbidity in HIV occurs through a variety of mechanisms (El-Mallakh, 1992; Jacobsberg & Perry, 1992). The most common types of psychiatric disorders found in the clinical care of PWHIV are displayed in Table 11–5. These disorders are based on criteria from the *Diagnostic and Statistical Manual of Mental Disorders, Third Edition, Revised,* published by the American Psychiatric Association. The discussion of psychologic and social stresses presented above notes that persons may have severe psychologic reactions to a diagnosis of HIV and to the societal consequences of the disease. These psychologic

Table 11–5. Psychiatric Disorders in HIV

DISORDERS	INTERVENTIONS
Adjustment disorders	Crisis intervention
Major affective disorders	Psychosocial therapy
Anxiety disorders	Pharmacotherapy
Organic mental disorders	Education
Delirium	Social and economic
Organic mood disorders	support
Organic delusional disorders	
Personality disorders	
Substance abuse disorders	

Table 11–6. HIV and Organic Mental Disorders

Dementia
HIV-1–associated dementia complex
Dementia associated with opportunistic infections
   and neoplasms

Infections
Fungal
   Cryptococcal disease
   Candida abscess
Protozoal
   Toxoplasmosis
Bacterial
   Mycobacterium avium-intracellulare
Viral
   Cytomegalovirus
   Herpesvirus
   Papovavirus (papillomavirus)

Cancers
Primary cerebral lymphoma
Disseminated Kaposi's sarcoma

reactions may reach pathologic levels (Britton et al., 1993). Reactive depression or anxiety disorders and adjustment disorders may occur in response to crisis points in the illness or stresses engendered by it (Rosenberger et al., 1993; Snyder et al., 1992). These reactive disorders may be transitory and may respond to crisis intervention, short-term psychosocial therapy, pharmacotherapy, and education (Michels & Marzuk, 1993).

However, HIV disease can occur also in persons with preexisting mental illness and may represent a situation of comorbidity (Batki, 1990; Catalan & Riccio, 1990; Chuang et al., 1992; El-Mallakh, 1992; King, 1990; Sacks et al., 1992). Persons with substance abuse disorders, schizophrenic disorders, major depression, and bipolar disorders who also have HIV disease exemplify instances of comorbidity. Several investigators have found that PWHIV who have preexisting mental disorders are also those who have the most severe and pathologic reactions to their HIV disease (Dew et al., 1990; Fell et al., 1993; Perry et al., 1993; Rosenberger et al., 1993). In addition, currently existing mental illness may facilitate the behaviors involved in transmission of HIV: injection drug use, hypersexuality, and the practice of unsafe sex may be high in mentally ill persons (Empfield et al., 1993; Kelly et al., 1993; Sacks et al., 1992; Susser et al., 1993). Unprotected sexual activity with multiple partners who are chosen casually is frequent. Impulsive and hypersexual behaviors, especially among persons with bipolar and depressive disorders and those who use recreational drugs, may be high. Finally, the existence of mental disorders in PWHIV complicates the diagnosis of reactive disorders and neuropsychologic disorders associated with HIV (Batki, 1990). It also complicates treatment. Psychosocial and educational interventions are appropriate for this group of PWHIV but are considerably more difficult to implement. Pharmacologic treatments may also be indicated.

Another cause of HIV-related psychopathology is the neuropsychologic complications and direct effects of the disease on the CNS (Catalan & Thornton, 1993; Dilley, 1992; El-Mallakh, 1992; Flaskerud, 1992; Snyder et al., 1992). HIV-associated diseases of the CNS are displayed in Table 11–6 and may be due to metabolic derangements; space-occupying lesions, including tumors or abscesses; cerebral infections; side effects of medication; and the direct cytopathic effects of the virus on the CNS. The clinical manifestations of these disorders are discussed in depth in Chapter 4.

Neuropsychologic symptoms in PWHIV infection are associated with subcortical dysfunction and include apathy, withdrawal, loss of memory and concentration, impaired cog-

Table 11–7. Symptoms of HIV Associated Dementia

EARLY SYMPTOMS	LATE SYMPTOMS
Cognitive	
Memory loss	Global dementia
Impaired concentration	Confusion
Mental slowing	Distractibility
Confusion of time or person	Delayed verbal response
Behavioral	
Apathy, withdrawal, "depression"	Vacant stare
	Restlessness
Agitation, confusion, hallucinations	Disinhibition
	Organic psychosis
Motor	
Unsteady gait	Slowing; truncal ataxia
Bilateral leg weakness	Weakness, especially legs
Loss of coordination	
Tremor	Spasticity, hyperreflexia tremor

nition, mental and motor slowing, and depression or mania (Baumann, 1993; Singer, 1992; Swanson et al., 1993a, 1993b). The early and late symptoms associated with HIV-1–associated dementia complex are displayed in Table 11–7. Neuropsychologic disorders may precipitate acute stress reactions resulting in psychiatric morbidity and suicidal ideation (Gillespie, 1992).

The differential diagnosis of neuropsychologic disorders, preexisting mental disorders, and reactive disorders is complicated in PWHIV disease (Baumann, 1993; El-Mallakh, 1992; King, 1990; Singer, 1992). Many affective, behavioral, cognitive, and somatic symptoms such as depressed mood, apathy or agitation, loss of concentration, and insomnia may be present in any of the three categories of disease. Symptoms of neuropsychologic disorders and psychiatric disorders such as schizophrenia also may overlap (Dilley, 1992; Flaskerud, 1992; Singer, 1992). In both types of disorders, paranoia, hallucinations, and catatonia may be present.

Impaired cognition and memory, sensory and perceptual deficits, and motor impairment are the major areas of nursing problems associated with CNS-related HIV disease

(Baumann, 1993; Flaskerud, 1992; Swanson et al., 1993b). These areas are covered in depth in Chapter 5, along with their related nursing diagnosis, management and health teaching, referrals, and nursing care evaluation. These areas of nursing problems also most clearly differentiate CNS-related HIV disease from other psychiatric syndromes. The most typical differentiating symptoms are failures in cognition, specifically: defects in memory, retention, and recall; difficulty in dealing with abstract concepts; and problems in grasping, retaining, and following instructions or completing several-step tasks (Singer, 1992). Although some psychologic and psychiatric syndromes may include distraction and selective memory loss, clients will have clear orientation and no difficulty with abstraction or following instructions (Bornstein et al., 1993). Furthermore, sensory and perceptual deficits that may occur in other psychiatric syndromes may include sensory hallucinations but will not include impaired vision. Likewise, motor impairment in other psychiatric syndromes may include the extrapyramidal side effects of antipsychotic drugs but will not include paresis and palsy.

Several studies have been conducted that add direction and clarity to the neuropsychologic assessment of cognitive abnormalities. The use of mental status examinations that the nurse can employ as a quick screening device for cognitive dysfunction has been supported (Crum et al., 1993; Cummings, 1993; Hilton et al., 1990). It should be noted that these studies concluded that mental status examinations such as the Mini-Mental State Exam and the Neurobehavioral Rating Scale are useful for screening or identifying persons with cognitive difficulties but not for making a diagnosis (Baumann, 1993; Crum et al., 1993; Hilton et al., 1990). The Neurobehavioral Rating Scale has been recommended by nurses because it measures both behavior and cognition (Hilton et al., 1990). Nurses should consider seriously the addition of a short mental status examination to their assessment of PWHIV. One note of caution should be made: Satz and colleagues (1993) reported that low educational level might confound the presence of cognitive abnormalities. These inves-

Table 11–8. Psychopharmocology and HIV

MEDICATION GROUP	USE	SIDE EFFECTS	PRECAUTIONS
Antidepressants	Depression Pain of neuritis	Sedation Anticholinergic effect	Monitor level of sedation Dries mucous membranes and may contribute to GI candidiasis
Stimulants	Depression Cognitive deficits—improves concentration, memory, attention Increases appetite	Anxiety Sleeplessness Drug-induced psychosis	Take into account drug history
Antipsychotics	Psychotic symptoms Agitation Severe anxiety	Extrapyramidal reactions	Exacerbates motor symptoms
Benzodiazepines	Anxiety Agitation	CNS toxic effects Sedation	Monitor for multiple benzodiazepines in use May exacerbate cognitive deficits

tigators suggest that little education might lower the threshold for neuropsychologic abnormalities and signify the need for earlier treatment.

The psychiatric treatment of persons with reactive psychologic disorders to HIV, comorbid psychiatric disorders and HIV disease, and neuropsychiatric syndromes has common characteristics (Swanson et al., 1990). Education of the patient and family about the relationship of HIV disease and psychiatric symptoms should include an explanation of common reactive syndromes; cognitive and perceptual disturbances; and cyclic and schizophreniform symptoms. Psychosocial treatment and support should include mobilizing family, friend, self-help group, and financial support networks; regulating stressors and modifying behavior; monitoring personal emotional health and crises; and providing realistic hope and referrals for spiritual care.

Psychopharmacologic treatment is useful also, in conjunction with the treatment of medical conditions. Concerns about drug interactions should be taken into account; however, psychopharmacologic agents can provide substantial symptom relief for PWHIV and should not be totally avoided (Angrist et al., 1992; Fernandez, 1990; Jacobsberg &

Perry, 1992; Shader & Greenblatt, 1993). They have been used safely with PWHIV for years with relatively few problems even when medical pharmacotherapy includes the use of antiretroviral agents or active treatment for opportunistic infections (Dilley, 1992). Because of the early effects of HIV on the CNS and the possibility of neurologic dysfunction, psychotropic medications should be used in the lowest dose possible. Some PWHIV appear to be sensitive to the anticholinergic side effects of antidepressants and neuroleptics (Michels & Marzuk, 1993). Furthermore, changes in medication regimens should be made slowly. Table 11–8 displays general categories of psychopharmacologic medications and their use, side effects, and precautions. Finally, close attention should be given to the psychiatric and neurologic side effects of antiretroviral, antibiotic, and chemotherapeutic agents used in the treatment of the spectrum of HIV disease. These are detailed in Appendix III. Many of the side effects mimic psychiatric and neuropsychiatric disorders. Some of these drugs cause anxiety, irritability, racing thoughts, insomnia, and frank mania. The side effects of these drugs should be compared with psychotropic drugs to ensure that one drug does not potentiate the side effects of the other.

Table 11–9. Psychosocial Stresses on Lover or Spouse

STRESSES	INTERVENTIONS
Guilt over transmission	Lover-spouse support groups or couples groups
Fear of contagion	
Anxiety, fear, depression over life-threatening illness	Individual therapy
Disrupted relationship equilibrium	Community resources
Decisions regarding treatment	Attorney, clergy, liaison psychiatry
Conflicts with family and hospital staff	Bereavement groups
Anticipatory and postmortem grief	

A comprehensive treatment plan for PWHIV includes psychopharmacologic treatment, psychosocial interventions, and education to deal effectively with mental disorders, neuropsychologic disorders, and reactions to psychologic and social stresses. Added to the picture of psychosocial stresses and the need for appropriate psychologic and social services to PWHIV are the psychosocial stresses on lovers, spouses, friends, and children of PWHIV and their needs for services and support.

PSYCHOSOCIAL STRESSES ON THE LOVER, SPOUSE, OR SEXUAL PARTNER

A diagnosis of HIV disease has widespread consequences that affect the entire social support network of PWHIV. Affected most immediately and extensively is the lover, spouse, or sexual partner. This person experiences both psychologic and social effects of having a partner with HIV infection (Britton et al., 1993; Brown & Powell-Cope, 1991, 1993; Cowles & Rodgers, 1991; Martin & Dean, 1993; McCann & Wadsworth, 1992; McGaffic & Longman, 1993; Powell-Cope & Brown, 1992) (Table 11–9). One psychologic stress experienced by the lover or spouse of an infected person might be guilt about possibly having transmitted the disease. Another is fear of being infected through sexual contact with the infected person (Martin & Dean, 1993; McCann & Wadsworth, 1992). These issues can be discussed in support groups for the spouse, lover, or sexual partner or in support groups for couples in which one partner has HIV disease. Through sharing experiences, support groups help members avoid self-blame and guilt. They also provide information on contagion and transmission, as well as a safe setting in which members can discuss frankly the needed changes in sexual practices.

The psychologic stresses related to a diagnosis of a life-threatening illness and the premature death of a young adult can cause the same existential crisis, anxiety, and depression in the lover or spouse as it does in the infected person (Brown & Powell-Cope, 1993; McCann & Wadsworth, 1992). Among gay men especially, the loss of loved ones can occur frequently, sometimes without any time to recuperate from previous losses and sometimes unrelentingly for a long period (Martin & Dean, 1993; McGaffic & Longman, 1993). Some social networks have been decimated by AIDS, which has led to chronic bereavement in survivors. Often bereavement is accompanied by significant physical and psychologic symptoms. Despair over a loved one's death from AIDS can reach suicidal proportions (Martin & Dean, 1993). Lovers and spouses should seek individual counseling to assist them in dealing with their crisis, as well as with the ongoing sadness, fear, and anxiety that can accompany impending death in a young partner. Support groups can also provide emotional support to spouses and lovers.

Various interpersonal stresses affect the spouse or lover of PWHIV. Major stresses occur because the equilibrium of the relationship is disrupted (Brown & Powell-Cope, 1991). A relationship based on interdependence, mutual support, autonomy, and egalitarianism may be severely threatened when one partner becomes emotionally and physically dependent, unable to contribute financially, limited in the ability to provide support, and impaired in cognitive functions. Spouses and lovers can find themselves involved in activities that drain them physically, emotionally, and financially (McCann & Wadsworth, 1992). Caring for the partner with HIV can require losing time from work, constantly supervising the PWHIV, assisting with all aspects of daily living, and providing emotional support, comfort, compassion, and affection (McCann & Wadsworth, 1992). The diagnosis of HIV disease also requires a change in sexual activities, both to prevent transmission of infection and in response to decreased sexual desires because of illness. All these changes in the relationship can be intensely stressful and demoralizing to the spouse or lover. Again, support groups for lovers and spouses or for couples can help resolve some of these issues through sharing of experiences. They also provide information on community resources to assist lovers and spouses in the care of the partner.

Stresses associated with frequent and prolonged hospitalization of the partner can range from the logistics of visiting, to making sure that the partner's financial and insurance resources remain adequate, to making decisions about the partner's medical treatment (McGaffic & Longman, 1993; Sadovsky, 1991). The lover or spouse is often called on to make decisions when the partner's mental status is compromised or when the partner is extremely ill (Haas et al., 1993). Decisions about life support and the disposition of property often fall to the spouse or lover. Early in the illness the partner with AIDS and the lover or spouse should discuss the partner's wishes regarding treatment, life support, funeral, burial, and disposition of property (Haas et al., 1993). Lovers must obtain a durable power of attorney to carry out these decisions.

Decisions made by the PWHIV and his or her partner can create conflicts with hospital staff and with the extended family and can cause additional stress on the lover or spouse (Britton et al., 1993). Decisions regarding treatment and life support may conflict with the course of action that the hospital staff believes is necessary or indicated. These conflicts can often be resolved with the assistance of the psychiatric consultation-liaison team, hospital chaplain, and hospital attorney. These same persons can assist in mediating conflicts between the spouse or lover and the patient's family. Sometimes the partner of the PWHIV is blamed for the disease (Britton et al., 1993). Conflicts are more common when families are emotionally distant from the patient and do not realize the extent and depth of the relationship between the patient and the lover in a gay relationship. Disputes can arise over treatment issues, burial, and disposition of property. In addition to helping resolve conflicts, hospital liaison psychiatrists, clergy, and attorneys can assist lovers or spouses of patients in preparing for these situations and taking the necessary steps to implement decisions.

Finally, lovers and spouses of PWHIV must face anticipatory grief over the loss of a partner and postmortem grief when the partner dies (Brown & Powell-Cope, 1993; Martin & Dean, 1993; McGaffic & Longman, 1993). Sometimes a bereaved gay partner is denied a rightful place at funerals and memorial services. There may be disputes over wills and life insurance. HIV support groups in large cities focus specifically on bereavement and the grief process. These groups encourage persons to grieve—to express sadness, fear, loneliness, anger, and guilt—with the understanding that grief is a healing process that is important to the recovery of the bereaved.

PSYCHOSOCIAL STRESSES ON FAMILY, CHILDREN, AND FRIENDS

The families, children, and friends of PWHIV often need supportive care (Table 11–10). For gay men, friends may represent

Table 11–10. Psychosocial Stresses on Families

STRESSES	INTERVENTIONS
Preexisting conflicts	Supportive interventions
Revelation of lifestyle	of consultation-liaison
Guilt over lifestyle	team, clergy, attorney
Fear of social stigma	Support groups
Conflict with PWHIV's	Community resources
lover	
Physical, emotional,	
and financial drain	
Loss and grief	

a reconstituted family (Britton et al., 1993). All the emotional and social reactions that occur with the PWHIV, lovers, and spouses also occur with families and friends: shock, denial, anxiety, anger, fear, guilt, and depression (Bor, 1990, 1992; Lippman et al., 1993; Ostrow et al., 1991; Schmidt, 1992; Solomon, 1990; Takigiku et al., 1993; Turner et al., 1993). Thus families are often viewed as emotionally "coinfected" because they have similar psychologic symptoms. Families experience conflict under the best of circumstances; a chronic, eventually terminal illness strains family relationships and requires nurturing of a sick member at a time when families might least expect or be equipped to do so.

Preexisting conflicts between the family and the PWHIV regarding lifestyle or sexual preference may have resulted in the family's emotional and geographic distance from the patient (Lippman et al., 1993; Sohier, 1993; Takigiku et al., 1993). In other cases the distance is only geographic and results from the person's having relocated to a major metropolitan area. Either situation makes the family's relationship with the PWHIV difficult and imposes stress on the family. Families who are emotionally distant by choice may feel ambivalent about the PWHIV or may reject him or her, leading to psychologic turmoil that includes anger, bitterness, anxiety, embarrassment, and despair (Bor, 1992; Lippman et al., 1993). Anger at the PWHIV may be generated by the thought that the person's behavior (i.e., sexual activity or injection drug use) is killing him or her; however, families are often unwilling to express anger toward a family member with a terminal illness. Families who are geographically distant experience severe situational stresses in attempting to visit with no place to stay and in being unable to provide emotional and physical assistance because of distance. Families should know that most large cities that are AIDS epicenters have local services available to family members even if they are from out of town.

Some families have other stresses. The diagnosis of HIV disease may be their first knowledge that their relative is homosexual, is a drug user, or has had multiple sexual partners (Hargrave et al., 1991; Kaminsky et al.,

1990; Lippman et al., 1993; Morales, 1990; Ostrow et al., 1991; Sohier, 1993). This news is greeted with shock, anger, bewilderment, rejection, and sometimes guilt. In this case families experience double grieving: for their relative's behavior or identity and for his or her terminal illness. Parents may feel guilty if they believe that they are responsible for their child's lifestyle. This is especially true of mothers who traditionally have been blamed by society for their children's actions. Knowledge of a relative's homosexuality, drug use, or promiscuity may cause conflict and divided loyalties within a family. Sometimes certain family members, usually siblings, have known of the person's lifestyle but have kept it secret from parents (Bor, 1992). As a result they have felt isolated from their own support system. Sometimes a mother has kept such information secret from a father. Family members kept in the dark might feel hurt because they were not informed earlier. In other families no one has preexisting knowledge, but when the person's lifestyle is revealed, some in the family decide to accept it and others to reject it. Fears and suspicions are aroused and loyalties are threatened.

When the PWHIV is also an IDU, other kinds of family conflicts occur (Bor, 1990). Some families serve as enablers of the person's drug use by providing support, housing, and money. Such families may feel guilty that they are responsible for the person's disease. In other cases the diagnosis of HIV disease reveals to the family that a person is still using drugs. Under these circumstances families feel hurt, anger, and betrayal.

Mothers who are infected with HIV experience the stresses of caring for children, guilt over eventually abandoning their children, and emotional and physical fatigue from the care of children who are also infected (Andrews et al., 1993). When the PWHIV is a young child, other stresses and conflicts occur within the family. In families in which parents are also infected, siblings may feel fear and insecurity about who will care for them (Bor, 1990). They may also feel resentment and anger toward the PWHIV because of the lack of attention given to them by the family during the PWHIV's illness.

In all these situations, families need compassionate, supportive, constructive assistance from clergy, health-care givers, and the psychiatric consultation-liaison team to deal with their feelings, work together, help the PWHIV cope, and assist in the PWHIV's care. They can also use assistance with such practical needs as housing and transportation and can benefit from sharing feelings and experiences in a support group for families. Support groups for children and younger siblings of PWHIV can assist them in coping with their special issues. Recurring themes are fear of transmission, dealing with bereavement and grief, relating positively to children, and coping with discrimination and stigmatization (Andrews et al., 1993; Bor, 1990, 1992).

As mentioned in the previous section, families sometimes perceive the lover of the PWHIV as having too much control in treatment decisions (Britton et al., 1993). Families have to adjust to the lover's role as equivalent to that of a spouse. This is especially difficult if they have not met or known each other previously. Because the lover's role and responsibilities are socially ambiguous, they often must be clarified before families and lovers can work together for the well-being of the PWHIV.

Another social stress that families face is whether to disclose the diagnosis of HIV disease to friends and then which friends to tell (Powell-Cope & Brown, 1992). Having a child or sibling with HIV disease subjects the family to the powerful threat of social stigma and rejection by friends, neighbors, co-workers, and schoolmates (Andrews et al., 1993; Bor, 1992; Hargrave et al., 1991; Ostrow et al., 1991). Children and adolescents are often kept in the dark about a parent's or sibling's HIV disease in an effort to protect them from social stigma and rejection. They may be confused and distressed about being excluded from a family problem. On the other hand, rejection and taunting by schoolmates and neighbors are real possibilities if the family member's disease becomes known. In addition, adolescents may suffer embarrassment because they are in the process of confronting their own sexuality.

The consequence of social rejection and stigma is that families lack the social support they would normally receive when a family member has a life-threatening illness (Andrews et al., 1993; Ostrow et al., 1991; Takigiku et al., 1993). In addition, during their bereavement some of the emotional support that usually accompanies mourning may not be available to them. When the diagnosis is not disclosed to others, pain often becomes intensified and sorrow is prolonged. In some ethnic groups stigmatization is particularly intense (Carrier, 1989; Kaminsky et al., 1990; Morales, 1990; Ostrow et al., 1991). Whether to tell friends can present a major conflict. Because of this situation, support groups become an important part of a family's social network (Lippman et al., 1993). In addition, clergy can take the lead in establishing an atmosphere of compassion and concern among their parishioners so that the traditional social support of religion is available.

The prolonged pain and debility of the PWHIV is another stress to families (Schmidt, 1992). In some instances the PWHIV pressures the family to help him or her commit suicide. Prolonged debility brings with it a great need for physical, emotional, and financial assistance. It can deplete family resources and drain family members emotionally and physically (Andrews et al., 1993; Bor, 1990, 1992). Often families must make difficult decisions about life support or whether to continue to provide food and fluids (Haas et al., 1993). The provision of emotional support, physical assistance, financial assistance, and community resources is essential to supportive care of the family.

Families and friends also face fears of contagion and transmission and will benefit from education regarding the disease. Friends who have been involved in behaviors or circumstances similar to those of the PWHIV may feel vulnerable because they identify with the ill person. In addition, they might want to be supportive but not know how. For many the diagnosis of AIDS in a friend leads to difficult reappraisals and evaluations of their own lifestyles and behaviors (Martin & Dean, 1993). As noted earlier, some gay social networks have been decimated by AIDS. In these instances bereavement is chronic, and some individuals wonder whether anyone will be left in the network to care for them.

Issues of bereavement affect both family and friends. Since PWHIV are usually young, lovers, spouses, family, children, and friends are dealing with loss and grief in the context of an untimely, undeserved, and unjust illness and death (Bor, 1992; Hargrave et al., 1991). John Kennedy said at the death of his infant son that "it is an unnatural thing for parents to bury a child." These issues, as well as sadness, anger, anxiety, guilt, and loss, must be dealt with as part of the grief process. For many survivors of PWHIV the grief and healing process is long (Martin & Dean, 1993; McGaffic & Longman; 1993; Sohier, 1993). Sadness, hurt, anger, and guilt can go on for a significant period after the death. Families must deal with the ambivalence of grief and anger, as well as the confusion and pain caused by social rejection. In some survivors suicide is a concern; in others, guilt over transmission or over survival is an issue. Ongoing involvement in family support groups for as long as 2 years has been found especially beneficial (McGaffic & Longman, 1993). The services of mental health counselors and clergy can greatly facilitate the grief process.

SPIRITUAL NEEDS

Throughout the discussion of psychosocial stresses on PWHIV and on their partners, families, children, and friends, references have been made to the need for the services of clergy. The spiritual needs of PWHIV, their loved ones, and caregivers involve existential concerns about self-identity; the meaning of life, adversity, and individual destiny; the need for love and acceptance; and sometimes the need for reconciliation and forgiveness. Spiritual needs of PWHIV present a special challenge to nursing care, particularly in the face of organized religion's condemnation and rejection of homosexuals, drug users, and sexually promiscuous persons (Andrews et al., 1993; Bellemare, 1988; Bennett, 1990; Broadley, 1993; Carson, 1993; Carson & Green, 1992; Cherry & Smith, 1993; Coward & Lewis, 1992; Graydon, 1988; Hart, 1993; Kendall, 1992; Saynor, 1988; Sohier, 1993; Tibesar, 1986).

Spirituality, or the spiritual dimension of an individual's life, involves questions about the meaning of life, hope, self-identity, and self-worth. It can also embody forgiveness and reconciliation. In contrast to religious practice and organized religion (although these are meant to serve the spiritual needs of their members), spirituality does not involve a particular creed, liturgy, or theism. The spiritual needs of PWHIV and their significant others include a profound need for meaning and hope. Most people create a self-identity and a sense of self-worth from their professional and personal relationships and the consequent productivity and satisfaction engendered. These relationships give their lives meaning, a sense of purpose, direction, and value. HIV disease threatens an individual's meaning and hope with physical debility, anxiety, loss of personal relationships, social alienation, rejection, and loss of job and productivity. PWHIV often must reestablish the sense that their life has value, direction, and purpose. The significant others of PWHIV also experience anxiety, personal and social isolation, alienation, and an unacceptable and abrupt death of a loved one from a controversial disease.

Traditionally people turn to the clergy, religion, and pastoral care to help them meet their spiritual needs. Many PWHIV, however, view organized religion and its value system as oppressive and irrelevant. Their experiences with organized religion often have been negative, and they are alienated from the religious community. Many have lived without spiritual comfort and support. When they feel spiritual needs, they may not recognize them as such or they may repress or deny them.

The ultimate spiritual concerns of PWHIV include questions of self-identity (Who am I now?), questions about the meaning of life (Is there any value or purpose to this suffering? Is there a reason to go on living?), questions about adversity (Is life essentially cruel and unfair?), questions about destiny (Why did this happen to me?), and questions about being or existence (Has my life made a difference? Have I made a contribution to the world? Will I be remembered?). PWHIV also ask other questions that relate directly to AIDS, its stigma, and social ostracism. Ques-

Table 11–11. Spiritual Needs and Care of Persons With AIDS

SPIRITUAL NEEDS	SPIRITUAL CARE
Meaning, value, hope, purpose, direction	Know spiritual concerns and issues
	Strengthen person's sense of worth, identity, and dignity
Love, acceptance	Provide compassionate, accepting care
Reconciliation with family, church	Listen
Rituals and practices of organized religion	Provide assistance in locating clergy, a religious community

tions about AIDS as a punishment for homosexuality, for using drugs, or for enjoying life can leave PWHIV guilt ridden.

To deal with all these questions, both PWHIV and their loved ones have a need for spiritual care (see Table 11–11). Often that care comes from clergy and is known as pastoral care. However, health care workers can also provide spiritual care. Knowing the spiritual concerns of the PWHIV is the first step. Approaching the PWHIV with compassion, nurturance, and support is the second. Spiritual care for PWHIV must respect their conscience and integrity, accept and affirm their lives and their relationships, and break through the perception that spirituality is the preserve of the religious. Spiritual care involves strengthening the person's sense of meaning, purpose, worth, dignity, and identity. A sense of meaning and hope is life affirming and nourishing, whereas the collapse of a person's meaning system is a primary motivation for suicide.

In addition to meaning and hope, PWHIV need love and acceptance. Filling this need is sometimes difficult for significant others and health care workers because sick or dying people are often irascible, demanding, hostile, and unreasonable. The assistance of clergy and the religious community with these needs can be invaluable. Not only can they provide PWHIV with the love and acceptance needed, but they can also support health-care givers and significant others in meeting these spiritual needs on a consistent basis.

A third step in providing spiritual care is being available to listen. Health care workers can be open to discussions about faith, belief, meaning in life, and mortality. They can help PWHIV review their lives, identify what has given them meaning and hope in the past,

and plan experiences that will provide purpose and identity in the present and future. Sometimes PWHIV request help in reconnecting with traditional faith and organized religion. Some ask for the ritual and practices of a particular religion. These practices provide comfort and give the person a sense of continuity with his or her past. They can decrease feelings of anxiety, isolation, and alienation by offering an experience of community. The health care worker can find clergy who are willing to work with PWHIV and their families in approaching the spiritual dimension of the illness. Clergy can assist PWHIV in reconciling with their families and their church. They can encourage PWHIV, their families, and their congregations to forgive one another. Members of a congregation or religious community can be an important support system, providing spiritual, emotional, physical, and financial assistance (Hart, 1993). Furthermore, acceptance by a religious congregation can help PWHIV and their families and loved ones counter the feelings of guilt and sin that have been associated with the disease.

Spiritual well-being has been associated with hardiness and with long-term survival (Carson, 1993; Carson & Green, 1992; Rabkin & Remien, 1993). Therefore providing spiritual care may mean more than just spiritual and psychosocial comfort; it may involve physical strength and physiologic competence as well. An understanding and supportive response to the spiritual needs of the PWHIV can benefit the person's overall health, well-being, and longevity. Responding to clients' spiritual needs will help them to live a life of meaning and purpose. It will also help them to die with dignity and a sense of completion. Health care workers can provide spiritual care

Table 11–12. Psychosocial Stresses on Nurses and Other Health Care Workers

STRESSES	INTERVENTIONS
Contagion and transmission	Education
Discomfort with homosexuality and drug use	Adequate staff and resources
Intensive complicated care	Psychosocial support groups
Facing own mortality	Crisis intervention and individual support
Repetitive grief	Clear institutional policies and treatment goals
Conflicts over goals of treatment	Personal stress reduction

or can facilitate the provision of spiritual care to their clients. In addition, health care workers must be aware of their own spiritual and psychosocial needs in caring for PWHIV.

PSYCHOSOCIAL STRESSES ON NURSES AND OTHER HEALTH CARE GIVERS

Caring for persons with HIV disease puts enormous stress on health care workers (Table 11–12). This is especially true of nurses who spend a great deal of time with patients and have close contact with them through performing supportive care and procedures. Nurses of PWHIV and other health care workers are subject to a wide range of emotional, social, and work-related stresses, some of which are also experienced by patients, lovers, spouses, families, children, and friends of the PWHIV and some of which are unique to health care givers. In general, their reactions can be characterized as pertaining to disease and death, sexuality and intimacy, and the burdens and rewards of caretaking (Bennett et al., 1991; Butters et al., 1993; Gallop et al., 1992; Getzel & Mahony, 1990; Klonoff & Ewers, 1990; Miller, 1991; Silverman, 1993; Stein et al., 1991; Trudeau, 1991; van Servellen & Leake, 1993). Chapter 16 provides personal accounts of some of these reactions by nurses.

Initially nurses and other health care workers have anxiety and concerns about contagion and transmission (Gallop et al., 1992; Silverman, 1993). They are in contact with the patient's body fluids, administer medications and intravenous fluids, change beds, bathe patients, and provide toilet care. Their concerns include fears of personal exposure (e.g., needle sticks) and exposure of other staff members. In addition, they have concerns about appropriate infection control procedures. This extends to fears of introducing infection to the PWHIV, of cross-infection of other patients, and of adequately teaching infection control procedures to families, friends, lovers, and spouses of patients. Anxiety may decrease with the introduction of adequate and accurate information concerning AIDS and infection control procedures (Gallop et al., 1992). Willingness to work with PWHIV and take appropriate precautions, as well as behavior toward PWHIV, improve when nurses are exposed to support groups or group interventions that include affective components (Gallop et al., 1992; Stein et al., 1991). The fear of transmission has had social consequences for health care workers, some of whose spouses or lovers have urged them to quit their jobs to avoid infection of themselves and their families. Others have experienced social stigma and avoidance by friends because they work with PWHIV (Silverman, 1993).

Stresses on nurses also result from the uncertainty and discomfort they feel in relating to drug users, prostitutes, sexually promiscuous persons, homosexuals, and the lovers of gay PWHIV. Personal values, cultural background, and religious ideals are challenged by the different backgrounds of these patients. Again, through education and with the assistance of the consultation-liaison psychiatric team or mental health consultants, nurses may become more comfortable discussing sexuality openly. This ability includes knowing enough about bisexuality and homosexuality to understand the issues and problems related to HIV transmission and being able to discuss sexual precautions and answer questions of lovers and family. Several studies have measured health care workers' attitudes toward homosexuals and AIDS. Both physicians and registered nurses have demonstrated homophobic and AIDS-phobic attitudes and behaviors (Gallop et al., 1992; Silverman, 1993).

The intense physical care and emotional needs of hospitalized PWHIV can cause health care workers to become overtaxed, stressed, fatigued, and fearful of being overwhelmed by the burden of the intensive, complicated care (Lego, 1994; Stein et al., 1991; van Servellen & Leake, 1993). Enormous demands are made on their energies by the frequent necessity to meet immediate needs and by serious time pressures and overwork. In addition, they feel stressed because inattention to other responsibilities and other patients is necessitated by the seemingly all-encompassing needs of the AIDS population (Miller, 1991). These stresses increase each day because of the mushrooming incidence of the disease and tax institutional resources to the limit. In some institutions the quality and comprehensiveness of training programs have been questioned because students are taking care of only PWHIV and have no experience with patients who have other problems.

Nurses have become overwhelmed by caring for PWHIV day after day. Infection control procedures often leave them feeling isolated, and they are emotionally and physically drained by the intensive physical and psychologic needs of the patients. AIDS brings to the nurse's attention the constant responsibility for intense, complex monitoring of the sights, sounds, smells, and suffering of life-and-death struggles (Lego, 1994; Stein et al., 1991). Nursing care problems of the patient with AIDS can include concurrent needs for attention to respiratory distress, pain, nausea and vomiting, diarrhea, bleeding, fatigue, motor weakness, breakdown of skin, breakdown of oral mucous membranes, nutritional deficits, fluid volume deficit, alteration in mental status, and acute psychologic distress. Nurses have found it especially difficult to deal with patients' anger and seemingly unreasonable demands in complex nursing care situations. Other health care workers also are often fatigued and overtaxed by the immediate demands of acute situations as well. For instance, interns are called on to manage acute crises in the illness; they perform such procedures

as arterial blood gas measurements, taking blood samples for culture, lumbar punctures, and bone marrow biopsies. They also feel isolated from the rest of the staff and resentful that residents and attending physicians avoid discussing life-sustaining treatment with patients and families and leave do-not-resuscitate orders up to them (Silverman, 1993).

Dealing with patients with AIDS has a special impact on health care workers because they and the patients are usually about the same age (Stein et al., 1991). Identification and a sense of personal vulnerability to disease and death are elicited when patients are young, hitherto healthy persons who face rapid physical deterioration and death (Martindale & Barnett, 1992; Robbins et al., 1992). Health care workers are forced to recognize the fact of their own death and dying and are faced with the need to reexamine the meaning and quality of their lives (Silverman, 1993). Some handle these feelings with denial and distancing tactics; others identify with their patients. Physicians have expressed the level of distress they feel when diagnosing *Pneumocystis* pneumonia as "pronouncing a death sentence." The age of the patients has evoked the feeling that "it's like telling your brother that he's going to die." An especially difficult situation is discussing life-sustaining treatments with a patient whom the health care worker has just met and who may need immediate intubation. These situations take their toll on health care workers in cumulative stress, depression, and psychic fatigue.

Nurses often become intensely involved with PWHIV because of the time and closeness of the nursing care demanded (Trudeau, 1991). To some degree they become the patient's family, and some nurses have been asked to hold the durable power of attorney for the patient and make decisions regarding treatment, disposition of property, and burial. This relationship is highly stressful when the patient dies, and nurses and physicians react much more strongly than they would with patients who have relied more on family and friends for support. Repetitive grief and demoralization occur because of the high mortality rate for AIDS (Stein et al., 1991).

The traditional goals of nursing and medical care impose additional stresses on health-care givers. In general, these goals are to cure, to prolong life, and to improve the quality of remaining life when its duration is beyond control. PWHIV fall into the second and often the third category. Prolonging life and improving quality of life become the prime focus of service. However, even these goals cannot be carried out without personal conflict, ambiguity, and disagreements among staff. Many of the treatments for HIV disease produce debilitating and distressing side ef-fects, so that prolonging life and improving quality of life can be at odds. Often treatment fails. Health care workers become involved in questions about whether the treatment regimen is justified; they become pessimistic and wonder, "What's the use?" Their pro-fessional identity as persons who improve patients' lives is called into question, which results in a feeling of professional impotence. Sometimes health care workers feel anger at colleagues for what they consider lack of involvement with or support for the patient. On the other hand, some staff members may emphathize with the desire of a PWHIV for suicide; they may even be supportive of med-ically assisted suicide on request. These con-flicts can result in anxiety, depression, and anger among staff.

The care of the PWHIV presents a chal-lenge to the nurse's competence, to profes-sional and personal values, and to ethical con-victions. So that the psychosocial needs of health personnel caring for AIDS patients can be met, a multifaceted program of institu-tional support is required (Butters et al., 1993; Frost et al., 1991; Gallop et al., 1992; Lego, 1994; Silverman, 1993; Stein et al., 1991; Wil-liamson, 1991).

1. All staff members should receive regu-larly scheduled educational and informational updates on HIV and its treatment. These ed-ucational programs must be repeated at in-tervals to reinforce and update information. Especially important is instruction on (a) transmission and contagion, (b) bisexuality and homosexuality, (c) drug use, drugs in use, and needle sharing, (d) assessment of mental status and recognition of delirium, (e) moni-toring of cognitive dysfunction and adjust-

ment of expectations for the patient's inde-pendent adherence to procedures and treat-ment, and (f) hospital and community re-sources to assist patients and families.

2. Clear, consistent policies and proce-dures should be developed regarding infec-tion control, the ethical and professional re-sponsibility to care for PWHIV, and HIV test-ing. Such policies, adhered to by all staff, will decrease anxiety about transmission and en-sure correct and appropriate behavior toward patients. Professionals most likely to experi-ence occupational exposure (e.g., nurses and surgeons) should be involved in developing these policies.

3. Clear, consistent, and explicitly stated agreement among all hospital staff on the goals of treatment for PWHIV will ensure a common approach and feelings of support for other staff members. This agreement on goals might address the issues of prolonging life through the use of available treatment; en-hancing the quality of life for both patient and family through excellence in symptom control and attention to psychologic, social, spiritual, legal, and financial needs; and providing sup-portive care until death.

4. Regular and as-needed small-group meetings to provide emotional support for staff specifically related to the care of PWHIV and their families will promote a sense of shared experience and social and professional group support to health care workers. Nurses and physicians should be encouraged to dis-cuss issues of grief and loss in this safe envi-ronment.

5. Easy access to mental health consultants who can provide emotional support for pa-tients and staff members can be helpful in crisis situations. Referrals can be made for staff desiring more long-term psychologic support.

6. Adequate institutional resources and support to provide the level of nursing and medical care needed will prevent staff from becoming overwhelmed, fatigued, and over-taxed by the care of PWHIV.

7. On a personal level, nurses and other health care workers can implement several measures that can reduce their stress at work and away from work. At work they can:

- Work regular (consistent) hours or shifts
- Take lunch and coffee breaks
- Take brief respite breaks (look out the window, wash hands and face, massage face, do isometric exercises)
- Acknowledge and reward work well done by one another

Away from work they can:

- Exercise, eat, and drink in moderation
- Create meaningful relationships and commit time to maintain them
- Develop an absorbing hobby or diversional activity
- Not bring work home
- Take regular vacations

Several psychosocial issues that usually arise separately are combined in the treatment of patients with AIDS, creating unusually difficult problems. These include fears of contagion, disease, and death in young persons; negative social attitudes and personal prejudices; overworked, fatigued, and overwhelmed health care workers; and overtaxed institutional resources (Silverman, 1993; Stein et al., 1991). Such difficult problems require institutions to provide a set of supportive guidelines for nurses and other health care professionals in the care of persons with HIV disease.

PSYCHOSOCIAL TASKS OF HEALTH CARE WORKERS TREATING PERSONS WITH AIDS

In caring for persons with AIDS, nurses and other health care workers engage in a variety of psychologic, social, and educational tasks to ensure that patient needs are met. Nursing models that emphasize care of the whole person provide guidelines for the nurse in meeting the physiologic, psychosocial, and educational needs of the patient:

- Accept, value, and provide longitudinal psychosocial and physical nursing care and medical care to the patient.
- Support the patient's capacity for hope, self-determination, independence, and control.
- Provide accurate medical information

concerning treatment alternatives, benefits and risks, and the rationale for suggested interventions.
- Provide accurate information regarding health-enhancing behavioral options (e.g., diet, rest, excercise, prevention of infection) in a sensitive, nonjudgmental manner.
- Understand common psychosocial issues surrounding AIDS, and provide assistance or referral for problems.
- Familiarize oneself with community psychologic, social, educational, political, and financial resources and appropriate referrals for patients, lovers, families, children, friends.
- Recognize and ensure treatment of neuropsychiatric syndromes common to AIDS.
- Control symptoms, reassure patients that this will be done, and provide supportive care or comfort measures.
- Carry out patients' decisions concerning life-sustaining treatment and reassure them that they will not be abandoned.
- Recognize the stress that co-workers experience in caring for patients with AIDS and work to minimize it.
- Assist survivors with bereavement support and grief counseling.

NURSING RESEARCH IN PSYCHOLOGIC AND PSYCHIATRIC ASPECTS OF HIV DISEASE

Summary of Research

Nurses have made important contributions to research in the area of psychosocial aspects of HIV disease. To date, this research has been largely descriptive. Nursing research has described the stresses and supports of the person with HIV disease, their partners, families, and children, and the stresses on nurses themselves (Andrews et al., 1993; Brown & Powell-Cope, 1991, 1993; Linn et al., 1993; Powell-Cope & Brown, 1992; Ragsdale & Morrow, 1990; Sohier, 1993; van Servellen et al., 1993; van Servellen & Leake, 1993, 1994). In addition, some of these studies have related stress to a particular phase of illness associated with symptom severity and quality of life or self-care activities (Linn et al., 1993; Ragsdale et al., 1992; Ragsdale & Morrow, 1990; Valente et al., 1993). Spiritual characteristics of long-term survivors also have been described (Carson, 1993; Carson & Green, 1992). In the case of caregiver stress, investigators have studied the various components of burden related to illness progression and the most stressful aspects of clinical management (Brown & Powell-Cope, 1991, 1993; Schmidt, 1992). The stress of bereavement on survivors has been detailed as well (McGaffic & Longman, 1993; Sohier, 1993).

The psychiatric aspects of HIV disease have been less well studied by nurses, although measures of psychopathology are sometimes used in studies of psychosocial stress (Valente et al., 1993; van Servellen et al., 1993). The neuropsychologic aspects of HIV disease also have not been studied extensively. The research that has been done describes and relates HIV disease stage to neuropsychiatric symptoms (Swanson et al., 1993a, 1993b). Other studies in this area have focused on establishing the validity of instruments that might be easily incorporated into nursing practice to measure both cognitive and behavioral dysfunction (Baumann, 1993; Hilton et al., 1990). Studies such as these provide an important baseline for future research on cognitive dysfunction and guidelines for nursing assessment and intervention.

Nurses have made the largest contribution to the study of psychosocial stress by investigating their own stress in relation to the care of PWHIV, their own attitudes, fears, and lack of knowledge, and the effect of providing this care on their practice (Alexander & Fitzpatrick, 1991; Bond et al., 1990; Breault & Polifroni, 1992; Campbell et al., 1991; Currey et al., 1990; Dow & Knox, 1991; Downes, 1991; Huerta & Oddi, 1992; Kemppainen et al., 1992; Martindale & Barnett, 1992; Scherer et al., 1989; Strasser & Damrosch, 1992; Swanson et al., 1990; Tesch et al., 1990; Young et al., 1990). In general, these studies have been atheoretical surveys. A number of intervention approaches have been described and sometimes tested: education, group discussion, psychosocial support groups, and

guidelines for staff support (Baer & Longo, 1989; Flaskerud et al., 1989; Pasacreta & Jacobsen, 1989; van Servellen et al., 1988; Young, 1988). There is an absence, however, of experimental evidence that these psychoeducational supportive interventions modify attitudes and fears. Because no studies have indicated which of the many situational factors in HIV care is the most stressful to care providers, it is not clear what kinds of information, support, and psychotherapeutic interventions are needed most.

Psychosocial and psychiatric interventions have not been studied extensively. Although most research assumes a role for social support in buffering stress, few studies have documented the use of a specific support protocol as an intervention. Notable exceptions were three studies of support groups, one for PWHIV and two for nurse caregivers (Kendall, 1992; Lego, 1994; Stein et al., 1991).

Interventions for remediating cognitive impairment and the stresses on informal caregivers have not been investigated in PWHIV, although they have been recommended on the basis of cross-sectional, descriptive studies (Swanson et al., 1993a, 1993b). Health care workers who are caring for PWHIV can look to these studies and to nursing research on elderly persons with cognitive dysfunction for models of care. Several nurses have documented the effectiveness of an assisted modeling and validation program to enhance self-care skills, memory, and concentration in elderly persons (Beck et al., 1991; McEvoy & Patterson, 1986; Roper et al., 1991; Tappen, 1988).

The studies reviewed here provide a beginning base for a science of psychosocial and neuropsychiatric nursing practice. However, many important dimensions of this area of practice still need extensive study.

Research Needed

The major need is for research that designs and tests interventions for the mental health needs of PWHIV. At each stage of illness—for instance, HIV testing, the appearance of symptoms, or cognitive disturbance—studies are needed that will guide the type of therapy needed. Cognitive, behavioral, and supportive therapies may all be useful; however, intervention outcome studies are needed to determine which therapeutic components are most effective for whom and at what stage of illness.

For persons in whom psychopathology develops in response to HIV or who are experiencing the comorbidity of HIV and psychiatric illness, investigations of concurrent psychologic and medical treatment seem warranted. Recently Burack and colleagues (1993), on the basis of a sample of 330 gay or bisexual men, proposed the influence of clinical depression on decreases in the CD4$^+$ T-cell count. Conversely, Lyketsos and colleagues (1993), in a larger sample (n = 1718) followed for 8 years, did not find a relationship between depression and the rate of CD4$^+$ cell decline, AIDS-related symptoms, and time to death. Additional research to examine the effect of depressive symptoms on HIV progression with time seems important. Studies of the response to therapy for depression and HIV disease progression are needed also. Finally, continued risk behaviors in populations with psychopathology demand research into behavioral interventions to decrease transmission in this population.

Remediating cognitive impairment in persons with HIV should also be a focus of research. Again, studies of concurrent medical and psychoeducational supportive therapies seem warranted. Direction for these interventions may be taken from the research literature on early descriptive work with HIV and on interventional research conducted on cognitive abnormality in elderly persons. There is a substantial body of literature on interventions to improve coping with other chronic illnesses that can undoubtedly serve as a useful template for guiding research on the stresses of HIV for those with the disease and their caregivers.

Meeting the psychosocial, psychiatric, and neuropsychologic needs of PWHIV may call for a variety of interventions based on differences in population groups: gay men, women, children, persons with hempohilia, ethnic people of color, homeless persons, those with preexisting mental illness, IDUs, and so forth.

Each of these groups might be responsive to different aspects of treatment. Intervention outcome studies are needed to determine which therapeutic approach works best for each group.

In approaching the psychosocial stresses of PWHIV, many investigators use general stress process models to guide their studies. In this model, social support is cited as a mediator of the stress process and is generally measured in terms of social support network availability and perceived satisfaction with that support. Support may be conceptualized as emotional, problem solving, and instrumental. The majority of studies do not find a buffering effect for social support when it is conceptualized and measured in this way (Green, 1993). Support groups as an intervention are rarely studied, and yet they are always recommended as a therapeutic approach to reducing stress for PWHIV, partners, families, and nurses. Extensive research needs to be done in this area. Currently, it is assumed that social support is linked to psychologic well-being (because it is included as a component of the stress process model!), and it is prescribed on the basis of that assumption. The following are some of the studies needed to clarify our conceptualizations and prescriptions in this area:

- Support needs of different social, cultural, gender, and sexual-preference groups
- Support needs across the spectrum of HIV disease
- Essential components of successful support groups for specific populations
- Importance of various network components (e.g., friends, family) for gay men, women, African Americans, Latinos, children, and other groups
- Support needs of informal caregivers
- Hypothesis testing studies of the outcomes of differentiated and specific support interventions

Studies that take into account the full diversity of the HIV-infected population and the many different requirements and opportunities of the subgroups within it would facilitate appropriate supportive interventions being made for all. In the meantime, studies that employ global social support measures or that prescribe the same will continue to befuddle this whole field of research.

Finally, there have been enough descriptive cross-sectional surveys of nurses' HIV-related stresses as reflected in their attitudes, fears, and behaviors. To study the stress of AIDS caregiving on health care workers, researchers must take a new direction and attempt a new set of studies that take a theoretical and comparative perspective:

- Longitudinal studies using sequential measurement of caregiver symptoms to assess cumulative effects and changes with time
- Controlled observations of the physical, psychologic, and social aspects of HIV-related work and stress
- Investigations using standardized measures as well as psychodiagnostic interviews (1) to assess physical symptoms, anxiety, depression, and behavioral and cognitive symptoms and (2) to determine whether health care workers are experiencing a stress-related disorder
- Comparative longitudinal studies that specify and quantify the stresses that providers experience in relation to the cumulative effects of care and to the type of care required for HIV disease and persons with other life-threatening disease
- Evaluations of intervention programs for caregivers with matched comparison groups of providers not receiving the particular intervention
- Hypothesis testing studies that investigate the preexistence of undiagnosed occupational, physical, and psychiatric morbidity in health care workers involved in intensive caregiving to PWHIV.

SUMMARY

The diagnosis of AIDS presents psychologic and social dilemmas, conflicts, and stresses for everyone intimately involved with the PWHIV, for less intimately involved acquaintances, and ultimately for society. An awareness of these stresses on the people involved, of the psychosocial supports needed and available, and of new developments in the treatment of HIV disease and care of patients will assist the nurse in giving optimal nursing care. In addition, nurses should care for themselves and request from their institutions and one another the support they need to battle HIV disease. Nursing research in the psychologic and psychiatric aspects of HIV disease has focused principally on identifying the stresses on PWHIV, on their partners, families, and friends, and on health care workers. Research is needed on interventions into psychologic and social stresses, treatment of psychiatric disorders and neuropsychologic dysfunction, and interventions for PWHIV and their caregivers.

REFERENCES

Alexander, R., Fitzpatrick, J. (1991). Variables influencing nurses' attitudes toward AIDS and AIDS patients. *AIDS Patient Care, 5*(6), 315–320.

Andrews, S., Williams, A.B., Neil, K. (1993). The mother-child relationship in the HIV-1 positive family. *IMAGE: Journal of Nursing Scholarship, 25*(3), 193–198.

Angrist, B., D'Hollosy, M., Sanfilipo, M., et al. (1992). Central nervous system stimulants as symptomatic treatments for AIDS-related neuropsychiatric impairment. *Journal of Clinical Psychopharmacology, 12*(4), 268–272.

Baer, C.A., Longo, M.B. (1989). Talking about it: Allaying staff concerns about AIDS patients. *Journal of Psychosocial Nursing and Mental Health Services, 27*, 30–32.

Batki, S.L. (1990). Drug abuse, psychiatric disorders, and AIDS: Dual and triple diagnosis. *Western Journal of Medicine, 152*, 547–552.

Baumann, S.L. (1993). Problems in the mental health assessments of persons with HIV. *Journal of the Association of Nurses in AIDS Care, 4*(4), 36–44.

Beck, C., Heacock, P., Mercer, S., et al. (1991). Measurement of dressing performance in persons with dementia. *American Journal of Alzheimer's Care and Related Disorders and Research, 29*(7), 30–35.

Beckett, A., Shenson, D. (1993). Suicide risk in patients with human immunodeficiency virus infection and acquired immunodeficiency syndrome. *Harvard Review of Psychiatry, 1*, 27–35.

Beevor, A.S., Catalan, J. (1993). Women's experience of HIV testing: The views of HIV positive and HIV negative women. *AIDS Care, 5*(2), 177–186.

Bellemare, D. (1988). AIDS: The challenge to pastoral care. *Journal of Palliative Care, 4*(4), 58–60.

Bennett, C., Miche, P., Kippax, S. (1991). Quantitative analysis of burnout and its associated factors in AIDS nursing. *AIDS Care, 3*, 181–192.

Bennett, M.J. (1990). Stigmatization: Experiences of persons with acquired immune deficiency syndrome. *Issues in Mental Health Nursing, 11*, 141–154.

Bond, S., Rhodes, T., Philips, P., et al. (1990). HIV infection and AIDS in England: The experience, knowledge and intentions of community nursing staff. *Journal of Advanced Nursing, 15*, 249–255.

Bor, R. (1990). The family and HIV/AIDS. *AIDS Care, 2*(4), 409–412.

Bor, R. (1992). The impact of HIV/AIDS on the family. *AIDS Care, 4*(4), 453–456.

Bornstein, R.A., Pace, M.A., Rosenberger, P., et al. (1993). Depression and neuropsychological performance in asymptomatic HIV infection. *American Journal of Psychiatry, 150*(6), 922–927.

Breault, A.J., Polifroni, E.C. (1992). Caring for people with AIDS: Nurses' attitudes and feelings, *Journal of Advanced Nursing, 17*, 21–27.

Britton, P.J., Zarski, J.J., Hobfoll, S.E. (1993). Psychological distress and the role of significant others in a population of gay/bisexual men in the era of HIV. *AIDS Care, 5*(1), 43–54.

Broadley, R.C. (1993). Spiritual support at the end of life. *HIV Frontline, 13*, 6–7.

Brown, M.A., Powell-Cope, G. (1991). AIDS family caregiving: Transitions through uncertainty. *Nursing Research, 40*(6), 338–345.

Brown, M.A., Powell-Cope, G. (1993). Themes of loss and dying in caring for a family member with AIDS. *Research in Nursing and Health, 16*, 179–191.

Burack, J.H., Barrett, D.C., Stall, E.D., et al. (1993). Depressive symptoms and CD4 lymphocyte decline among HIV-infected men. *Journal of the American Medical Association, 270*, 2568–2573.

Bussing, R., Burket, R.C. (1993). Anxiety and intrafamilial stress in children with hemophilia after the HIV crisis. *Journal of American Academy of Children and Adolescent Psychiatry, 32*(3), 562–567.

Butters, E., Higginson, R., George, R., et al. (1993). Palliative care for people with HIV/AIDS: Views of patients, carers and providers. *AIDS Care, 5*(1), 105–116.

Campbell, S., Maki, M., Willenbring, K., et al. (1991). AIDS-related knowledge, attitudes, and behaviors among 629 registered nurses at a Minnesota hospital: A descriptive study. *Journal of the Association of Nurses in AIDS Care, 2*(1), 15–23.

Carrier, J.M. (1989). Sexual behavior and spread of AIDS in Mexico. *Medical Anthropology, 10*, 129–142.

Carson, V.B. (1993). Prayer, meditation, exercise, and special diets: Behaviors of the hardy person with HIV/AIDS. *Journal of the Association of Nurses in AIDS Care, 4*(3), 18–28.

Carson, V.B., Green, H. (1992). Spiritual well-being: A predictor of hardiness in patients with acquired immunodeficiency syndrome. *Journal of the Professional Nurse, 8*(4), 209–220.

Castro, F., Coates, T., Ekstrand, M. (1989, June). Prevalence and predictors of depression in gay and bisexual men during the AIDS epidemic: The San Francisco men's health study. Presented at the 5th International AIDS Conference, Montreal, Canada.

Catalan, J., Riccio, M. (1990). Psychiatric disorders associated with HIV disease. *AIDS Care, 2*(4), 377–380.

Catalan, J., Thornton, S. (1993). Whatever happened to HIV dementia? *International Journal of STD/AIDS, 4*(1), 1–4.

Catania, J.A., Coates, T.J., Kegeles, S., et al. (1992). Condom use in multiethnic neighborhoods of San Francisco: The population-based AMEN (AIDS in Multi-Ethnic Neighborhoods) Study. *American Journal of Public Health, 82*, 284–287.

Cherry, K., Smith, D.H. (1993). Sometimes I cry: The experience of loneliness for men with AIDS. *Health Communication, 5*(3), 181–208.

Chuang, H., Jason, G.W., Pajurkova, E.M. (1992). Psychiatric morbidity in patients with HIV infection. *Canadian Journal of Psychiatry, 37*(2), 109–114.

Cleary, P., Van Devanter, N., Rogers, T.F., et al. (1993). Depressive symptoms in blood donors notified of HIV infection. *American Journal of Public Health, 83*(4), 534–539.

Coates, T.J. (1990). Strategies for modifying sexual behavior for primary and secondary prevention of HIV disease. *Journal of Consulting and Clinical Psychology, 58*(1), 57–69.

Cote, T, Biggar, R., Dannenberg, A.L. (1992). Risk of suicide among persons with AIDS. *Journal of the American Medical Association, 268*(15), 2066–2068.

Coward, D.D., Lewis, F.M. (May 13-17, 1992). The lived experience of self-transcendence in gay men with class IV HIV infection. Paper presented at the 17th Annual Oncology Nursing Society Congress, San Diego, CA.

Cowles, K.V., Rodgers, B.L. (1991). When a loved one has AIDS: Care for the significant other. *Journal of Psychosocial Nursing, 29*(4), 7–12.

Crum, R.M., Anthony, J.M., Bassett, S.S., et al. (1993). Population-based norms for the mini-mental state examination by age and educational level. *Journal of the American Medical Association, 269*(18), 2386–2391.

Cummings, J. (1993). Mini-mental state examination: Norms, normals, and numbers. *Journal of the American Medical Association, 269*(18), 2420–2391.

Currey, C.J., Johnson, M., Ogden, B. (1990). Willingness of health-professions students to treat patients with AIDS. *Academic Medicine, 65*, 472–474.

Dew, M.A., Ragni, M., Nimorwiez, P. (1990). Infection with human immunodeficiency virus and vulnerability to psychiatric distress. *Archives of General Psychiatry, 47*, 737–744.

Dilley, J.W. (1992). Management of neuropsychiatric disorders in HIV-spectrum patients. In M.A. Sande & P.A. Volberding (Eds.), *The medical management of AIDS* (3rd edition) (pp. 218–233). Philadelphia: W.B. Saunders.

Dow, M.G., Knox, M.D. (1991). Mental health and substance abuse staff: HIV/AIDS knowledge and attitudes. *AIDS Care, 3*(1), 75–87.

Downes, J. (1991). Acquired immunodeficiency syndrome: The nurse's legal duty to serve. *Journal of Professional Nursing, 7*(6), 333–340.

El-Mallakh, R.S. (1992). AIDS dementia-related psychosis: Is there a window of vulnerability? *AIDS Care, 4*(4), 381–387.

Empfield, M., McKinnon, K., Cournos, F., et al. (1993). HIV seroprevalence among homeless patients admitted to a psychiatric inpatient unit. *American Journal of Psychiatry, 150*, 47–52.

Eversley, R.B., Newsetter, A., Avins, A., et al. (1993). Sexual risk and perception of risk for HIV infection among multiethnic family-planning clients. *American Journal of Prevention Medicine, 9*(2), 92–95.

Fell, M., Newman, S., Herns, M., et al. (1993). Mood and psychiatric disturbance in HIV and AIDS: Changes over time. *British Journal of Psychiatry, 162*, 604–610.

Fernandez, F. (1990). Psychopharmacological interventions in HIV infections. *New Directions for Mental Health Services, 48*, 43–53.

Finelli, L., Budd, J., Spitalny, L.C., et al. (1993). Early syphilis: Relationship to sex, drugs, and changes in high-risk behaviors from 1987–1990. *Sexually Transmitted Diseases*, *20*(2), 89–95.

Flaskerud, J.H. (1992). Psychosocial and neuropsychiatric care. *Critical Care Nursing Clinics of North America*, *4*(3), 441–420.

Flaskerud, J.H., Lewis, M.A., Shin, D. (1989). Changing nurses' AIDS-related knowledge and attitudes through continuing education. *Journal of Continuing Education in Nursing*, *20*, 148–154.

Folkman, S., Chesney, M., Pollack, T., et al. (1993). Stress, control, coping, and depressive mood in human immunodeficiency virus–positive and –negative gay men in San Francisco. *Journal of Nervous and Mental Disorder*, *18*(17), 409–416.

Friedman, S.R., Des Jarlais, D.C., Sterk, C.E. (1990). AIDS and the social relations of intravenous drug users. *The Milbank Quarterly*, *68*(suppl 1).

Frost, J.C., Makadon, H.J., Judd, D., et al. (1991). Care for caregivers: A support group for staff caring for AIDS patients in a hospital-based primary care practice. *Journal of General Internal Medicine*, *6*, 162–167.

Fullilove, M. (1989). Anxiety and stigmatizing aspects of HIV infections. *Journal of Clinical Psychiatry*, *50*(suppl 1), 5–8.

Gallop, R.M., Taerk, G., Lancee, W.J., et al. (1992). A randomized trial of group interventions for hospital staff caring for persons with AIDS. *AIDS Care*, *4*(2), 177–185.

Getzel, G.S., Mahony, K.F. (1990). Confronting human finitude: Group work with people with AIDS. *Journal of Gay and Lesbian Psychotherapy*, *1*(3), 105–120.

Gillespie, F.J. (1992). Neuropsychopathology of HIV/AIDS. *British Journal of Nursing*, *1*(5), 222–225.

Graydon, D.N. (1988). AIDS: Observations of a hospital chaplain. *Journal of Palliative Care*, *4*(4), 66–69.

Green, G. (1993). Editorial review: Social support and HIV. *AIDS Care*, *5*(1), 87–104.

Grossman, A.H. (1991). Gay men and HIV/AIDS: Understanding the double stigma. *Journal of the Association of Nurses in AIDS Care*, *2*(4), 28–32.

Grothe, T.M., Illeman, M.L. Molaghan, J.B. (1993). Mapping the roller coaster ride. *HIV Frontline*, *11*, 3–5.

Haas, J.S., Weissman, J.S., Weissman, J.S., et al. (1993). Discussion of preferences for life-sustaining care by persons with AIDS. *Achives of Internal Medicine*, *153*, 1241–1248.

Hall, J.M., Stevens, P.E. (1988). AIDS: A guide to suicide assessment. *Archives of Psychiatric Nursing*, *1*(2), 115–120.

Hargrave, R., Fullilove, M., Fullilove, R.E. (1991). Defining mental health needs for Black patients with AIDS in Alameda County. *Journal of the National Medical Association*, *83*(9), 801–804.

Hart, C.W. (1993). "Our minister died of AIDS": Pastoral care of a congregation in crisis. *Journal of Pastoral Care*, *47*(2), 109–115.

Hart, G.J., Dawson, R.M., Fitzpatrick, M., et al. (1993). The treatment-free incubation period of AIDS in a cohort of homosexual men. *AIDS*, *7*(2), 231–239.

Hays, R.B., McKusick, L., Pollack, L., et al. (1993). Disclosing HIV seropositivity to significant others. *AIDS*, *7*(3), 425–431.

Hedge, B. (1990). The psychological impact of HIV/AIDS. *AIDS Care*, *2*(4), 381–383.

Hein, K. (1993). "Getting real" about HIV in adolescents. *American Journal of Public Health*, *83*(4), 492–494.

Hilton, G., Sisson, R., Freeman, E. (1990). The neurobehavioral rating scale: An interrater reliability study in the HIV seropositive population. *Journal of Neuroscience Nursing*, *22*(1), 36–42.

Hintze, J., Templer, D.I., Cappelletty, G.G., et al. (1993). Death depression and death anxiety in HIV-infected males. *Death Studies*, *17*(4), 333–341.

Huerta, S.R., Oddi, L.F. (1992). Refusal to care for patients with human immunodeficiency virus/acquired immunodeficiency syndrome: Issues and responses. *Journal of Professional Nursing*, *8*(4), 221–230.

Jacobsberg, L.B., Perry, S. (1992). Psychiatric disturbances. *The Medical Clinics of North America*, *76*(1), 99–106.

Kaminsky, S., Kurtines, W., Hervis, O.O., et al. (1990). Life enhancement counseling with HIV infected Hispanic gay males. *Hispanic Journal of Behavioral Science*, *12*(2), 177–195.

Kelly, J.A., Murphy, D.A. (1992). Psychological interventions with AIDS and HIV: Prevention and treatment. *Journal of Consulting and Clinical Psychology*, *60*(4), 576–585.

Kelly, J.A., Murphy, D.A., Bahr, G.R., et al. (1993). Factors associated with severity of depression and high-risk sexual behavior among persons diagnosed with human immunodeficiency virus (HIV). *Health Psychology*, *12*(3), 215–219.

Kemppainen, J., St. Lawrence, J.S., Irizarry, A., et al. (1992). Nurses' willingness to perform AIDS patient care. *Journal of Continuing Education in Nursing*, *23*(3), 110–117.

Kendall, J. (1992). Promoting wellness in HIV-support groups. *Journal of the Association of Nurses in AIDS Care*, *3*(1), 28–38.

King, M.B. (1990). Psychological aspects of HIV infection and AIDS: What have we learned? *British Journal of Psychiatry*, *156*, 151–156.

Klonoff, EA., Ewers, D. (1990). Care of AIDS patients as a source of stress to nursing staff. *AIDS Education and Prevention*, *1*, 338–348.

Kost, K., Forrest, J.D. (1992). American women's sexual behavior and exposure to risk of sexually transmitted diseases. *Family Planning Perspective*, *24*, 244–245.

Lazzari, C., de Ronchi, D., Volterra, V., et al. (1993). Death and dying during AIDS: Psychotherapeutic interventions. *AIDS Patient Care*, *7*(3), 166–168.

Lego, S. (1994). AIDS-related anxiety and coping methods in a support group for caregivers. *Archives of Psychiatric Nursing*, *8*(3), 200–207.

Limandri, B.J. (1989). Disclosure of stigmatizing conditions: The discloser's perspective. *Archives of Psychiatric Nursing*, *3*(3), 69–78.

Linn, J.G., Monning, R.L., Vsin, B.S., et al. (1993). Stage of illness, level of HIV symptoms, sense of coherence and psychological functioning in clients of community-based AIDS counseling centers. *Journal of the Association of Nurses in AIDS Care*, *4*(2), 24–32.

Lippman, S.B., James, W.A., Frierson, R.L. (1993). AIDS and the family: Implications for counselling. *AIDS Care*, *5*(1), 71–78.

Lyketsos, C.G., Hoover, D.R., Guccione, M., et al. (1993). Depressive symptoms as predictors of medical outcomes in HIV infection. *Journal of the American Medical Association*, *270*, 2563–2567.

Martin, J.L., Dean, L. (1993). Effects of AIDS-related bereavement and HIV-related illness on psychological distress among gay men: A 7-year longitudinal study, 1985–1991. *Journal of Consulting and Clinical Psychology, 61*(1), 94–103.

Martindale, L., Barnett, C. (1992). Nursing faculty's knowledge and attitudes toward persons with AIDS. *Journal of the Association of Nurses in AIDS Care, 3*(2), 9–13.

Marzuk, P.M., Tierney, H., Tardiff, K., et al. (1988). Increased risk of suicide in persons with AIDS. *Journal of the American Medical Association, 259*(9), 1333–1337.

McCann, K., Wadsworth, E. (1992). The role of informal carers in supporting gay men who have HIV-related illness: What do they do and what are their needs? *AIDS Care, 4*(1), 25–34.

McEvoy, C.L., Patterson, R.L. (1986). Behavioral treatment of deficit skills in dementia patients. *The Gerontologist, 26*, 475–478.

McGaffic, C.M., Longman, A.J. (1993). Connecting and disconnecting: Bereavement experiences of six gay men. *Journal of Association of the Nurses in AIDS Care, 4*(1), 49–57.

McKegney, F.P., O'Dowd, M.A. (1992). Suicidality and HIV status. *Clinical and Research Reports, 149*(3), 396–398.

Messiah, A., Bucquet, D., Mettetal, J.F., et al. (1993). Factors correlated with homosexually acquired human immunodeficiency virus infection in the era of "safer sex." *Sexually Transmitted Diseases, 20*(1), 51–58.

Metzger, D.S., Woody, G.W., McLellan, T., et al. (1993). Human immunodeficiency virus seroconversion among intravenous drug users in and out of treatment: An 18-month prospective follow-up. *Journal of Acquired Immune Deficiency Syndromes, 6*, 1049–1056.

Michels, R., Marzuk, P.M., (1993). Progress in psychiatry. *New England Journal of Medicine, 329*(9), 551–560; 628–638.

Miller, D. (1991). Occupational morbidity and burnout: Lessons and warnings for HIV/AIDS carers. *International Review of Psychiatry, 3*, 439–449.

Morales, E.S. (1990). HIV infection and Hispanic gay and bisexual men. *Hispanic Journal of Behavioral Sciences, 12*(2), 212–222.

Moran, J.S., Janes, H.R., Peterman, T.A., et al. (1990). Increase in condom sales following AIDS education and publicity, United States. *American Journal of Public Health, 80*(5), 607–608.

O'Dowd, M.A. (1993). Suicidal behaviors and AIDS. *HIV/AIDS Mental Hygiene, 3*(1), 1–4.

O'Dowd, M.A., Biderman, D.J., McKegney, F.P. (1993). Incidence of suicidality in AIDS and HIV-positive patients attending a psychiatry outpatient program. *Psychosomatics, 34*(1), 33–40.

Offir, J.T., Fisher, J.D., Williams, S.S., et al. (1993). Reasons for inconsistent AIDS-preventive behaviors among gay men. *Journal of Sex Research, 30*(1), 62–69.

Ostrow, D.G., Whitaker, R., Frasier, K., et al. (1991). Racial differences in social support and mental health in men with HIV infection: A pilot study. *AIDS Care, 3*(1), 55–62.

Otten, M.W., Zaidi, A.A., Wroten, J.E., et al. (1993). Changes in sexually transmitted disease rates after HIV testing and posttest counseling, Miami, 1988 to 1989. *American Journal of Public Health, 83*(4), 529–533.

Pasacreta, J.V., Jacobsen, P.B. (1989). Addressing the need for staff support among nurses caring for the AIDS population. *Oncology Nurses Forum, 16*, 659–663.

Pergami, G.C., Catalan, A., Riccio, J., et al. (1992). Risk of deliberate self-harm and factors associated with suicidal behaviour among asymptomatic individuals with human immunodeficiency virus infection. *Acta Psychatrica Scandinavica, 86*, 70–75

Perry, S., Jacobsberg, L., Card, C.A.L., et al. (1993). Severity of psychiatric symptoms after HIV testing. *American Journal of Psychiatry, 150*(5), 775–779.

Perry, S.W. (1990). AIDS in psychiatry. *Psychiatry*. Philadelphia: J.B. Lippincott.

Peterson, J.L., Coates, T.J., Catania, J.A., et al. (1992). High-risk sexual behavior and condom use among gay and bisexual African-American men. *American Journal of Public Health, 82*(11), 1490–1494.

Powell-Cope, G., Brown, M.A. (1992). Going public as an AIDS family caregiver. *Social Science and Medicine, 34*(5), 571–580.

Rabkin, J.E., Remien, R. (1993). Resilience in adversity among long-term survivors of AIDS. *Hospital and Community Psychiatry, 44*(2), 162–167.

Ragsdale, D., Kotarba, J.A., Morrow, J.R. (1992). Work-related activities to improve quality of life in HIV disease. *Journal of the Association of Nurses in AIDS Care, 3*(1), 39–44.

Ragsdale, D., Morrow, J.R. (1990). Quality of life as a function of HIV classification. *Nursing Research, 39*(6), 355–359.

Regan-Kubinski, M.J., Sharts-Engel, N. (1992). The HIV-infected woman: Illness cognition assessment. *Journal of Psychosocial Nursing, 30*(2), 11–15.

Robbins, I., Cooper, A., Bender, M.P. (1992). The relationship between knowledge, attitudes and degree of contact with AIDS and HIV. *Journal of Advanced Nursing, 17*, 198–203.

Roper, J., Shapira, J., Chang, B. (1991). Agitation in the demented patient: A framework for management. *Journal of Gerontological Nursing, 17*(3), 17–21.

Rosenberger, P.H., Bornstein, R.A., Nasrallah, H.A., et al. (1993). Psychopathology in human immunodeficiency virus infection: Lifetime and current assessment. *Comprehensive Psychiatry, 34*(5), 521–525.

Sacks, M., Dermatis, H., Looser-Ott, S., et al. (1992). Seroprevalence of HIV and risk factors for AIDS in psychiatric inpatients. *Hospital and Community Psychiatry, 43*(7), 736–737.

Sadovsky, R. (1991). Psychosocial issues in symptomatic HIV infection. *American Family Physician, 44*(6), 2065–2072.

Satz, P., Morgenstern, H., Miller, E.N., et al. (1993). Low education as a possible risk factor for cognitive abnormalities in HIV-1: Findings from the multicenter AIDS cohort study (MACS). *Journal of Acquired Immune Deficiency Syndromes, 6*(5), 503–511.

Saynor, J.K. (1988). Existential and spiritual concerns of people with AIDS. *Journal of Palliative Care, 4*(4), 61–65.

Scherer, Y.K., Haughy, B.P., Wu, Y.B. (1989). AIDS: What are nurses' concerns? *Journal of the Association of Nurses in AIDS Care, 3*(4), 33–41.

Schmidt, J. (1992). Case management problems and home care. *Journal of the Association of Nurses in AIDS Care, 3*(3), 37–44.

Shader, R.I., Greenblatt, D.J. (1993). Use of benzodiazepines in anxiety disorders. *The New England Journal of Medicine, 328*(19), 1398–1405.

Shayne, V.T., Kaplan, B.J. (1991). Double victims: Poor women and AIDS. *Women and Health, 17,* 21–37.

Silverman, D.C. (1993). Psychosocial impact of HIV-related caregiving on health providers: A review and recommendations for the role of psychiatry. *American Journal of Psychiatry, 150*(5), 705–712.

Silvestre, A.J., Kingsley, L.A., Wehman, P., et al. (1993). Changes in HIV rates and sexual behavior among homosexual men, 1984–1988/92. *American Journal of Public Health, 83*(4), 578–580.

Singer, E.J. (1992). Cognitive dysfunction in an HIV-infected patient. *Hospital Practice, May 15,* 91–100.

Snyder, S., Reyner, A., Schmeidler, J., et al. (1992). Prevalence of mental disorders in newly admitted medical inpatients with AIDS. *Psychosomatics, 33*(2), 166–170.

Sohier, R. (1993). Filial reconstruction: A theory of development through adversity. *Qualitative Health Research, 3*(4), 465–492.

Solomon, K. (1990). Facing AIDS with my mother. *The Body Positive, 3*(1), 22–25.

Sonsel, G.E. (1989). Case management in a community-based AIDS agency. *Quality Review Bulletin, 15*(1), 31–36.

Stein, E., Wade, K., Smith, D. (1991). Clinical support groups that work. *Journal of the Association of Nurses in AIDS Care, 2*(2), 29–36.

Stowe, A., Ross, M.W., Wodak, A., et al. (1993). Significant relationships and social supports of injecting drug users and their implications for HIV/AIDS services. *AIDS Care, 5*(1), 23–33.

Strasser, J., Damrosch, S. (1992). Graduate nursing students' attitudes toward gay and hemophiliac men with AIDS. *Evaluation and the Health Professions, 15*(4), 115–127.

Susser, E., Valencia, E., Conover, S. (1993). Prevalence of HIV infection among psychiatric patients in a New York City men's shelter. *American Journal of Public Health, 83*(4), 568–570.

Swanson, B., Cronin-Stubbs, D., Colletti, M. (1990). Dementia and depression in persons with AIDS: Causes and care. *Journal of Psychosocial Nursing, 28*(10), 33–39.

Swanson, B., Cronin-Stubbs, D., Zeller, J.M., et al. (1993a). Characterizing the neuropsychological functioning of persons with human immunodeficiency virus infection. Part 1. Acquired immunodeficiency syndrome dementia complex: A review. *Archives of Psychiatric Nursing, 7*(2), 74–81.

Swanson, B., Cronin-Stubbs, D., Zeller, J.M., et al. (1993b). Characterizing the neuropsychological functioning of persons with human immunodeficiency virus (HIV) infection. Part II. Neuropsychological functioning of persons at different stages of HIV infection. *Archives of Psychiatric Nursing, 7*(2), 82–90.

Swanson, J.M., Chenitz, C., Zalar, M. (1990). A critical review of human immunodeficiency virus infection and acquired immunodeficiency syndrome–related research: The knowledge, attitudes, and practices of nurses. *Journal of the Professional Nurse, 6,* 341–355.

Takigiku, S.K., Brubaker, T.H., Hennon, C.B. (1993). A contextual model of stress among parent caregivers of gay sons with AIDS. *AIDS Education and Prevention, 5*(1), 25–42.

Tappen, R.M. (1988). Revitalization: A developing approach to nursing care of the cognitively impaired. *Florida Nurse, 32*(2), 7.

Tesch, B.J., Simpson, D.E., Kirby, B.D. (1990). Medical and nursing students' attitudes about AIDS issues. *Academic Medicine, 65*(7), 467–469.

Tibesar, L.J. (1986). Pastoral care: Helping patients on an inward journey. *Health Progress, 67,* 41–47.

Trudeau, M. (1991). Dark nights and bright mornings: Caring for a person with AIDS. *Journal of Psychosocial Nursing and Mental Health Services, 29*(1), 32–33.

Turner, H.J.A., Hays, R.B., Coates, T.J. (1993). Determinants of social support among gay men: The context of AIDS. *Journal of Health and Social Behavior, 34*(1), 137–153.

Twiname, B.G. (1993). The relationship between HIV classification and depression and suicidal intent. *Journal of the Association of Nurses in AIDS Care, 4*(4), 28–35.

Valdiserri, R.O., Moore, M., Gerber, A.R., et al. (1993). A study of clients returning for counseling after HIV testing: Implications for improving rates of return. *Public Health Reports, 108*(1), 12–18.

Valente, S.M., Saunders, J.M., Uman, G. (1993). Self-care, psychological distress, and HIV disease. *Journal of the Association of Nurses in AIDS Care, 4*(4), 15–27.

van Griensven, G.J.P., Samuel, M.C., Winkelstein, W., Jr. (1993). The success and failure of condom use by homosexual men in San Francisco. *Journal of Acquired Immune Deficiency Syndromes, 6*(4), 430–431.

van Servellen, G.M., Leake, B. (1993). Burn-out in hospital nurses: A comparison of acquired immunodeficiency syndrome, oncology, general medical, and intensive care unit nurse samples. *Journal of Professional Nurses, 9*(3), 169–217.

van Servellen, G.M., Leake, B. (1994). Emotional exhaustion and distress among nurses: How important are AIDS-care specific factors? *Journal of the Association of Nurses in AIDS Care, 5*(2), 11–19.

van Servellen, G.M., Lewis, C.E., Leake, B. (1988). Nurses' responses to the AIDS crisis: Implications for continuing education in nursing. *Journal of Continuing Education in Nursing, 19,* 4–8.

van Servellen, G., Padilla, G., Brecht, M.L., et al. (1993). The relationship of stressful life events, health status and stress-resistance resources in persons with AIDS. *Journal of the Association of Nurses in AIDS Care, 4*(1), 11–22.

Wayment, H.A., Newcomb, M.D., Hannemann, V.L. (1993). Vitamin A status in HIV infection. *Nutrition Research, 13,* 157–166.

Williamson, P.R. (1991). Support groups: An important aspect of physician education. *Journal of General Internal Medicine, 6,* 179–180.

Wolcott, D.L., Fawzy, F.I., Namir, S. (1989). Clinical management of psychiatric disorders in HIV spectrum disease. *Psychiatric Medicine, 7*(2), 107–127.

Young, E.W. (1988). Nurses' attitudes toward homosexuality: Analysis of change in AIDS workshops. *Journal of Continuing Education in Nursing, 19,* 9–12.

Young, M., Henderson, M.M., Marx, D. (1990). Attitudes of nursing students toward patients with AIDS. *Psychological Report, 67,* 491–497.

Community-Based and Long-Term Care

12

Peter J. Ungvarski and Joan Schmidt

When planning for the health care needs and social services of persons with HIV disease (PWHIV), nurses must look at the full range of services that may be required throughout the course of illness. In June 1988 the members of the Presidential Commission on the HIV Epidemic pointed out in their final report that continued focus on AIDS, rather than the entire spectrum of the HIV epidemic, has left the United States unable to deal effectively with the epidemic. Most important, the report looked at health care delivery "through the lens of the HIV epidemic and found gaping holes, huge problems" (Gebbie, 1989, p. 869). In essence, the HIV epidemic has vividly exposed the many weaknesses inherent in health care in the United States.

Gebbie (1989) noted that the HIV epidemic has revealed major deficits, such as (1) failure to offer each child born a comprehensive health and health education program, which would provide a basis for a healthy adult life; (2) failure to construct a coherent system of delivering illness care services and a method of paying for such services; and (3) failure to understand the dangers of creating a permanent underclass, a drug-linked culture that does not participate in the ordinary obligations, and benefits, of our social service system. In fact, the HIV epidemic has shown that there is no such thing as a "health care system" in the United States (Ungvarski, 1989). The definition of the word "system" implies an interdependence and interrelationship between elements, which forms a collective entity. In the United States we have the antithesis to this definition: a fragmented array of health care services provided by federal, state, local, nonprofit, voluntary, and proprietary agencies. The United States and the Re-

public of South Africa are the only developed industrialized countries that do not ensure that all citizens have access to basic health care (Lundberg, 1991).

In many respects, the phrase "health care system" is a misnomer. What is actually provided in the United States is a system of acute care, not health care. Essentially, an individual who becomes seriously ill is provided a bed in a hospital. The emphasis is on hospitals, with limited focus on long-term care and virtually no investment in primary care or prevention. The latter is available to those who can afford it and who seek it out.

The consequence for Americans without health insurance is an increase in morbidity and mortality rates. Burstin and associates (1992), in a study of 51 hospitals in New York State, found that uninsured patients were at greater risk of suffering medical injury as a result of substandard medical care. Franks and colleagues (1993) studied 4,694 Americans prospectively and concluded that lacking health insurance is associated with an increased risk of death. Both these studies underscore the inequities that currently exist in health care service delivery and the urgent need for reform in the United States.

AIDS AS A CHRONIC DISEASE

In 1989 the concept was introduced that AIDS should be viewed as a chronic disease (Fee & Fox, 1992). This approach was based on the premise that antiretroviral agents plus preventive and suppressive therapies for opportunistic infections would significantly prolong life, even if the underlying HIV infection cannot be cured. However, Fee and Krieger (1993) argued that the chronic disease model alone is inadequate to describe the complexities of HIV disease because, unlike other chronic diseases such as diabetes and heart disease, HIV is infectious. They proposed that health professionals describe HIV as a chronic infectious disease, thus reflecting the need to be concerned about the prevention of new infections, as well as the health care needs of those who are already infected.

If HIV is to be treated as a chronic infectious disease in the 1990s, the focus must shift from the acute care, inpatient setting to ambulatory care (Imperato, 1990). However, in a nationwide survey of 401 nurse executives to determine the availability of health care services for people with AIDS, Sowell et al. (1990) found that acute care services were still the most widely available. Only half of the urban hospitals and one third of the rural hospitals offered comprehensive, chronic ambulatory care services, and such services were neither available nor planned by 60% of the hospitals. Home care services were more prevalent: 91% of the nurse executives indicated that their communities offered home health care and hospice care and 59.9% provided case management services. Only 47.9% of those surveyed stated that their communities had long-term care services for people with AIDS, and 52.1% said that long-term care was neither available nor planned. The authors of this study concluded that nurse executives must exercise leadership in their communities to advocate more community-based services.

COMMUNITY NURSING CENTERS

The 1980s saw the growth of community nursing centers as a source of primary health care, including services for people with HIV/AIDS. A study conducted by the National League for Nursing (NLN) used the following characteristics to define a nursing center: "1) a nurse must occupy the chief management position in the center; 2) accountability and responsibility for client care and professional practice remain with the nurse; and 3) nurses are the primary providers seen by clients visiting the center" (NLN, 1992, p. 1). The NLN estimates there are approximately 250 nursing centers in the country; of the 98 centers

that responded to the NLN survey, 2% specialize in the care of PWHIV/AIDS.

Nursing centers offer health care services to populations that historically have been underserved. In the NLN survey of the nursing centers' clients, 52% were white, 31% black, 13% Latino, and 2% Asian, indicating that 46% of the clients served were from minority populations. The centers are also providing health care to uninsured persons. When the NLN reported how services were compensated, 27% paid out of pocket and 13% were uncompensated. Medicare covered 11%, Medicaid 13%, private insurance 19%, and others 17%.

One example of a nursing center that specializes in HIV/AIDS is the Denver Nursing Project in Human Caring. This project opened in 1988 to provide comprehensive services to PWHIV and their significant others. Nurses use Jean Watson's philosophy and science of human caring as the basis for practice (Lyne & Waller, 1990). Watson believes that nursing educators and clinical staff need to work together "to transform the system from a sick care system to a human care-healing model" (Darbyshire, 1992, p. 44). For clients to have a consistently available nurse to guide them through the health care maze and the unpredictable course of HIV/AIDS, the Denver caring center utilizes nursing care partnerships (Schroeder & Maeve, 1992). The effectiveness of the nursing care partnerships was evaluated by three methods: a nursing focus group, a client survey, and a random chart review. The nursing care partnerships have resulted in increased satisfaction for both clients and nurses. However, the clients' primary criticism was the nurses' lack of knowledge of the social service system and how to make appropriate referrals.

Realizing and acknowledging these issues, the nurse can appreciate that planning care for an HIV-infected person from the time of diagnosis through the course of illness, can be not only difficult but also frustrating. What is needed in the early stages of HIV infection is clinical monitoring through primary care and psychosocial services, and in the later stages, acute care, home care, long-term residential care, and hospice care are required. Many individuals have limited access to primary care and support services; they may be refused access to long-term residential care because they are infected with HIV. Lack of entitlement and the inability to pay, unfortunately, are barriers to care that are shared by most HIV-infected persons.

Additionally, HIV-infected individuals require health care that is delivered by knowledgeable, competent health care providers. Stone and associates (1992) examined more than 800 AIDS hospitalizations in 40 hospitals in Massachusetts and found the relative risk of death was more than twice as high at hospitals with lower AIDS familiarity than at hospitals more experienced in AIDS care. The need to disseminate HIV/AIDS care information continues even as we progress through the second decade of this disease. This chapter not only discusses the various aspects of planning care in a nonacute setting but also attempts to describe the realities related to access and delivery of services.

CASE MANAGEMENT

Because the United States has no system of health care, and because the average consumer has great difficulty in understanding and negotiating the complexities of entitlements such as private insurance policies, Medicaid, and Medicare, case management has become a necessity. Case management is not new. At the turn of the century, public health programs provided community service coordination that was the forerunner of case management (American Nurses' Association [ANA], 1988). Coordination of services has always been the focus of public health nursing (ANA, 1988).

After World War II, the term "case management" was used to describe the community services necessary for care of discharged psychiatric patients (Grau, 1984). The term first appeared in social welfare literature in the early 1970s, followed closely by mentions in the nursing literature (ANA, 1988). In more recent years, the U.S. government policy on health care has moved toward programs that offer a comprehensive, coordinated continuum of care at the community level. In 1981

Table 12–1. Team Members Involved in Case Management of a Person With HIV Infection

1. Client and significant other(s)
2. Primary physician
3. Consulting physicians (e.g., ophthalmologist managing cytomegalovirus retinitis)
4. Hospital-based staff, including resident physicians, nurses, nutritionists, pharmacists, and discharge planners
5. Home care staff, including visiting nurse, homemakers, home attendants, home health aides, continuous care nurses in the home, and special teams providing in-home infusion therapy
6. Case workers and managers from AIDS organizations, Medicaid programs, child welfare agencies, drug treatment programs, and health clinics
7. Mental health professionals
8. Clergy

the Omnibus Budget Reconciliation Act and Medicare prospective reimbursement program encouraged case management to provide community-based alternatives to institutional placement.

The ANA (1988) defined case management as a system of elements including (1) health assessment, (2) planning, (3) procurement of services, and (4) monitoring to ensure that the multiple service needs of the client are met. Ideally, case management should not only optimize the client's self-care capability through the efficient use of resources but also stimulate the creation of new services. The goals of case management are to provide high-quality care, minimize fragmentation of care across many settings, enhance the quality of the client's life, and contain cost (ANA, 1988; Morrison, 1990). The best situation is to have a single designated case manager. However, because of the complex needs of clients with HIV disease and the numerous players involved with care, what actually takes place is multiagency case management (Table 12–1). To achieve the client's goals, the various health care professionals managing the case should be aware of each other's capabilities and limitations and should develop a milieu of cooperation.

Synonymous terms for case management include case coordination, service management, care management, and managed care. Case management can provide facilitating functions, gatekeeping functions, or a combination of both. Facilitating functions include assisting the client and significant other in obtaining the needed services in a maze of complex rules and regulations. The gatekeeping role of case management ensures that the client and significant others receive appropriate and cost-effective health care.

Less clearly defined is who should actually provide case management, and there are no delineated job requirements for the position. Case management models vary and include a single designated case manager, an interdisciplinary team, or a mutliagency team. In reality, the ubiquitous, monolithic case manager does not exist.

The ANA (1988) defined the component parts of case management in the framework of the nursing process. In this model, interaction with the client, family, and significant others, and with various providers, is followed by assessment, planning, implementation, and evaluation. Professional nurses are uniquely qualified to be case managers because of their theoretical background in the biologic and social sciences and the humanities; their knowledge of health maintenance, disease processes, and medications; and their experience in collaboration as part of the health care team (ANA, 1988).

Regardless of the professional discipline of persons hired to perform case management, they should be provided with the necessary education, reference tools, and resource persons to understand the complex biobehavioral and psychobehavioral responses that individuals experience during the course of HIV disease. They should be good listeners and not individuals who make quick value judgments without a total picture of the situation. As part of their role preparation, they should be taught the etiquette and value of telephone case management; they should be told that the telephone is an invaluable asset and should not be viewed as an interruption. Above all, case managers should keep in mind that they are not the client's only advocates. Advocacy based on a collaborative process, with mutual respect, will do more to obtain

the needed services than will an adversarial approach.

Assessment

The collection of baseline data provides the framework on which the case manager structures the plan of care. Assessment is an interaction with the client, significant others, family members, and service providers. It is a time to introduce the role of the case manager and to establish a relationship between the case manager and the other parties. It is wise to remember that first impressions are lasting.

Comprehensive evaluation includes, but is not limited to, collection of data that describe (1) demographic and personal characteristics, (2) support persons, (3) functional status of the client, (4) clinical needs of the client, (5) family information, (6) legal issues, (7) social data, (8) financial data, and (9) summary of service providers, both individuals and agencies, that are involved in the case (see Appendix V for a detailed assessment outline). The primary purposes of the assessment are to identify the client's care needs and problems, to evaluate what needs are being met, and to determine what should be improved.

Ideally the initial interview should take place with the client and significant others in the client's home. The presence of a significant other is especially important when there is a potential for discrete or undiagnosed cognitive impairment of the client. For the initial interview, the home setting provides the case manager with an opportunity to assess the home environment and community resources. Although at the initial assessment the client may be relatively healthy and independent, this information will provide a basis for future evaluation of the feasibility of in-home service, should the need arise. If the initial assessment is performed at the hospital or in an office, the case manager should arrange an in-home visit at a later date for assessment purposes.

Planning

The cardinal rule for the development of a service plan is that the client and significant others actively participate in developing the plan, which must include mutual goals. Involvement of the client in setting goals is probably the rule that health care professionals most frequently ignore. Unilateral setting of goals by the case manager will eventually lead to labeling the client as noncompliant. In this case the true statement would be, "This client was noncompliant with the case manager's wishes"! For example, if the case manager decides that home attendant services are indicated, even though the client views them as intrusive and can still manage on his or her own, much time and effort will have been wasted when the home attendant arrives and the client refuses service. It is important to keep in mind that the plan of care belongs to the client, not the case manager.

The plan of care should also include measurable objectives, the steps to be taken to meet these objectives, and a time frame. Documentation throughout the process is important, and constraints on achieving goals or meeting time frames should be recorded. The case manager should realize that problems with the care plan are inevitable and should not view them as personal failure. Internalization of problems can lead to frustration and anger and can impede the process.

The final requirement of the planning process is selection of the services needed. In the case of the HIV-infected person, this may be limited because access to institutional long-term care has been limited throughout the HIV/AIDS epidemic. In many areas nursing homes and psychiatric facilities that will accept an HIV-infected person are scarce. Gaining access to addiction treatment services may be even more difficult. Day care is virtually non-existent. Home care and hospice care, although available in most areas, may not be adequate or safe for the client's needs. The case manager, from time to time, may reach a dead end when other service providers reject the referral.

Implementation

In the implementation phase of the case plan, access to services is accomplished by completion of applications and contact with providers. Advocacy for entitlements will require providing all necessary information, and educating the client and significant others to prevent future denial of services or financing.

The case manager should anticipate problems and conflicts during the process of implementation: for example, checks don't arrive on time, transportation is delayed, home care workers fail to arrive, and clients miss appointments. A backup plan is needed for such situations: petty cash for food until checks can be traced, alternative transportation or appointment rescheduling, and someone to stay with the client until a replacement home care worker is available. The more service providers involved with a case, the greater is the likelihood that problems will arise.

The case manager should watch for and avoid duplications in service. As the number of AIDS service organizations increases, so does the number of duplicative services provided. For example, if a client moves into supportive housing for PWHIV that provides health care monitoring and psychosocial support services, as well as food and shelter, there is little need to provide for medical appointments, counseling, friendly visitors, or volunteer "buddies" as previously required.

Evaluation

Evaluation should be ongoing and planned, and it should not be left to chance or until a crisis. Planned visits to the client at specified intervals, or at least telephone audits to verify services and to identify problems, can be invaluable tools in preventing a major crisis. Educating the client and significant others about the importance of self-care is essential in providing services and containing costs.

Unnecessary services should not be continued for the sake of convenience. Likewise, the case manager should not provide services as "gifts" in an attempt to win the client's confidence. Overservicing a client and significant others is antithetical to achieving and maintaining independence.

Family members or significant others providing care may experience role fatigue. Plans of care that specify intervals of re-

Table 12–2. Constraints on Case Management

1. Case management usually is limited to the provision of services to persons with diagnosed AIDS, thus excluding persons who are HIV seropositive and in the earlier stages of disease.
2. Usually health care facilities and organizations are not reimbursed for case management.
3. Communication channels between case managers and other service providers are not always well established.
4. Power struggles can emerge between case managers from different agencies.
5. There is a lack of specialized training and resource materials that prepare case managers to interpret and understand the complex clinical problems of their clients, such as clinical needs related to opportunistic infections, research protocols, drugs, and alternative therapies.
6. Many case managers do not adequately involve the client in the plan of care.
7. Many case managers are unprepared to deal with an HIV-seropositive person who chooses to continue to engage in unsafe sexual activity or use drugs or who wishes to become pregnant and have a baby.
8. Undiagnosed HIV-related cognitive impairment can complicate the decision-making process.
9. Confidentiality laws may leave case managers reluctant to provide adequate information to other service providers involved in the case.
10. Hospitals are not experienced with outpatient case management and are not familiar with solutions to problems that face persons with HIV infection or AIDS when they are at home in the community.
11. Emphasis on cost saving may result in conflict over supplies and medications prescribed by case managers and denied by third-party payers.

spite to prevent psychologic or physical fatigue are usually successful. Periods of respite care vary from a few hours a week to a long weekend once every few months. Redefining goals and modifying the care plan will be based on the ongoing assessment of the needs of the client and significant others. See Table 12–2 for constraints on case management.

HOME CARE

In 1981 the only option for care of PWHIV was acute care hospitalization. Nursing responded to the need, however, and by 1984 the first program of home care services for PWHIV was organized and implemented at the Visiting Nurse Association and Hospice of San Francisco. This was followed 1 year later by the development of a formalized program of home care services at the Visiting Nurse Service of New York (VNSNY). Today, VNSNY operates the largest home care program of its kind in the world for PWHIV, with an average daily census of more than 1,700 clients.

Home care providers have responded to the growing health care needs of PWHIV by designing special programs and adapting current ones to meet their needs. Home care is especially appropriate and effective for PWHIV. It enables them to remain in familiar surroundings, thus providing maximum emotional support for them and their significant others. It provides maximum independence and control over decision making in the least restrictive setting. Home care can improve the quality of life significantly and can give PWHIV the greatest use of their remaining time (Ungvarski, 1988). It promotes the participation of significant others in the plan of care. Finally, it provides an opportunity for case finding and health teaching in the community (Ungvarski, 1987). Health teaching is especially important in preventing transmission of not only HIV but also tuberculosis, which has become a major HIV-related illness.

One misconception of home care is that it consistently costs substantially less than institutional care. The cost of service in the home (excluding supplies such as medications, dressings, and intravenous infusion equipment) can range from about $140 to $1,000 per day (New York City Department of Health, 1989). In addition, estimates comparing home care costs with institutional care rarely include total costs of care and may fail to include the average daily cost of rent, food, and utilities.

Master and colleagues (1993) recently reported the costs of hospital alternative care for Medicaid recipients with AIDS enrolled in a health maintenance organization in Boston, Massachusetts. They reported the average costs as $90 per patient per month for case management; $328 per patient per month for home intravenous therapy; and $405 per patient per month for home nursing and support services. However, it is important to note that in a health maintenance organization with capitated monthly expenditures, the costs of services are usually distributed among all patients enrolled, whether or not they actually utilize the services that are available. Additionally, in a capitated program of case management, costs cited may not reflect the actual needs of the client but be limited to what is allowed by the dollar amount allocated to each client per month.

Another misconception is that home care is intended to take over or take away the care and responsibility for the PWHIV from the significant others. Nothing could be further from the truth. Home care is specifically designed to support the client and significant others in self-care activities and is not a system of care to take over custody of the client. In this respect, home care may be inappropriate for individuals who require continuous care in an institutional setting and may not be feasible with an insurance plan that has capitated monthly costs.

Many health care professionals throughout the United States place undue pressure on home care agencies to accept all PWHIV who are referred, because there are virtually no other options for long-term care outside the hospital. Therefore it is important for all health care professionals to understand the purposes of home care, as well as its limits and constraints, which are predominately governed by reimbursement issues.

As previously stated, home care is a supportive system of care for the client and significant others. Therefore, in addition to educating the client in self-care, the significant other, often referred to as the informal caregiver, must be educated as the most important

provider of care. Formal caregivers include professional and paraprofessional health care workers who participate in the plan of care (Table 12–3). The informal and formal caregivers should work together to develop a plan of care that is mutually agreeable, is designed to meet the needs of the client and significant others, and is realistic about the care that can be safely provided by the home care agency.

Case Management Issues and Home Care

Schmidt (1992) reviewed 100 consultations that took place at the VNSNY and found that the case management problems for PWHIV fell into four general categories: client/significant others, housing and community, support services, and nurses' needs (Table 12–4). Nurses identified psychiatric and other mental health issues as their number one case management problem in the home.

Cognitive impairment resulting from the neurotropic effects of HIV disease or an opportunistic central nervous system infection is a grossly underdiagnosed problem in the HIV-ill population. Once the client is home, the visiting nurse or paraprofessional home care worker is often the first person to detect cognitive and motor impairment. In the case of clients who live alone, forgetting to take medications or miscalculating doses can lead to disastrous problems such as overmedication or the worsening or recurrence of an opportunistic infection because of inability to comply with a suppressive therapy regimen. In addition, home care is not the best milieu for the cognitive stimulation therapy necessary to keep the client at an optimal level of functioning. Home care in conjunction with a program of day care is most desirable.

Because there are few long-term care options for HIV-ill persons with psychiatric disorders, acute care facilities may withhold psychiatric diagnoses when making home care referrals. Once the client is at home, paraprofessional home care workers, as well as families and significant others, are often reluctant or unable to cope with combative, assaultive, or self-destructive behaviors. In some

Table 12–3. Formal Caregivers Providing Home Care Services

CATEGORY OF STAFF	FUNCTIONS
Professional staff	
Physician	Provides for medical care (usually through periodic office or clinic visits and telephone contact with the visiting nurse)
Visiting nurse (usually the case manager)	Provides orders for nursing care and coordinates all professional and paraprofessional services needed; promotes and teaches self-care to client and significant others
Medical social worker	Provides for necessary concrete social services as well as counseling
Therapists	Provide maintenance or restorative therapies and teach self-care to client and significant other
Specialists	Provide specific services (e.g., respiratory therapists for aerosolized pentamidine or clinical nurse specialist for problems in case management)
Paraprofessional staff	
Housekeeper	Provides chore services such as shopping, cleaning, laundry, meal preparation (no personal care)
Personal care assistants (also referred to as home attendants or personal care attendants)	Provide, in addition to chore services, assistance with bathing, dressing, toileting, ambulating, and traveling to and from appointments
Home health aides	In addition to the above, assist with many nursing tasks such as taking temperatures, providing special exercises, taking care of and providing safety with oxygen therapy
Homemakers	Usually provide chore services and child care services; may provide child care in the presence of an ill parent or may also act as a surrogate parent, staying 24 hours when the parent is hospitalized

These definitions and functions often vary from state to state.

Table 12–4. Case Management Issues and Home Care: Summary of 100 Consultations

CATEGORY OF PROBLEMS	FREQUENCY	CATEGORY OF PROBLEMS	FREQUENCY
Client/significant others		Support services—cont'd	
Psychiatric/mental health	13	Clients not home for service	6
Parenting	12	Inadequate service authorization on	6
Illegal drug use	12	admission	
Client safety (impaired cognition)	7	Nurses' needs	
Financial (including Medicaid access)	7	Medical/nursing management of specific AIDS-indicator disease	11
Housing/community	6	Medication questions	8
Support services		Medication noncompliance	6
Level of in-home service	10	Clinical care related to tuberculosis	6
Accessing community resources	9	Do not resuscitate orders	
Referral process to Medicaid home care	7	Emotional support (an ongoing process)	3
Lack of care partner (emergency backup)	7		

Though 100 consultations were reviewed, the numbers cited exceed 100 because several consultations involved multiple problems.
From Schmidt, J. (1992). Case management problems and home care. *Journal of the Association of Nurses in AIDS Care, 3*(3), 37–44.

instances this behavior can pose a real threat to the safety and welfare of the home care staff.

Home care agencies have begun to recognize that PWHIV need specialized mental health services (Pessin et al., 1993). The VNSNY and the Visiting Nurse Association of Boston use psychiatric clinical nurse specialists to provide counseling and support to clients and significant others in the home. Psychiatric nurses also work with the home care staff to develop a safe plan of care. However, it is important to realize that there are clients who cannot be maintained safely in the community because they pose a danger to themselves or others, need 24-hour supervision, and have no significant others who can provide backup for the home care staff. Long-term care facilities would be the most appropriate setting for such clients, but if local long-term care facilities are unwilling or unable to accept such individuals, then the only safe plan of care would be to return the client to the hospital.

Family cases referred for home care services provide a unique challenge. Among the possible situations are (1) infection of husband and wife, (2) infection of both parents and children, (3) the presence of uninfected children in the same household with infected parents and siblings, (4) infection of multiple generations of individuals in the same household, and (5) infection of a gay couple, with both partners being severely ill. In the case of households with children present, home care nurses need to assess whether parent(s)' functional limitations prevent them from caring for their children. Extended family members may be able to assist with child care; if not, referrals for homemaker services will be necessary (when available).

Legal assistance is often required for planning wills and guardianship. Referrals will be necessary to assist survivors (e.g., grandparents, aunts, uncles) in caring for HIV-ill children whose parents have died or are in prison. In the absence of planned guardianship or relatives willing to provide child care, referrals to foster care agencies will be necessary. By the end of 1995, it is projected that an estimated 24,600 children and 21,000 adolescents in the United States will be left orphaned by HIV/AIDS (Michaels & Levine, 1992).

Management of Illegal Drug Use

Evidence suggests a failure to diagnose alcohol and drug dependencies when clients are referred for home care services (Hurley and Ungvarski, 1994). With the initiation of services, the problem becomes evident and directly affects the client's ability to comply with prescribed medical and nursing regimens, as well as the willingness of paraprofessional workers to go into the home to provide services. Even when the HIV-infected individual is alcohol or drug free, the significant other(s) may be overtly using substances, which, again, leads to reluctance of paraprofessionals to enter the home or may result in abusive behavior toward home care workers. When the problem of drug or alcohol use is diagnosed by professional home care staff, treatment options for referral are limited. Alcohol and drug treatment programs that meet the needs of homebound clients are almost nonexistent. In the absence of a treatment plan for the chemical dependency, home care may not be feasible.

Home care agencies are able to provide services to active substance abusers if clients are willing to cooperate with a plan of care (Schmidt, 1992). Such a plan should include the stipulation that clients and significant others do not engage in substance use or drug trafficking while home care workers are present. Clients also need to be told that home care workers cannot be involved in the procurement of drugs or alcohol.

Staff members need to be educated about how to set limits on manipulative behaviors such as repeated requests for money. If clients have no money for food, they can be referred to food pantries or AIDS organizations that provide food. Another issue that staff may find disturbing is the clients' use of profanity. If clients use profanity to express themselves, it is unrealistic to expect them to alter their vocabularies, especially in their own homes. Staff should acknowledge legitimate expressions of anger and frustration. However, nurses should set limits on verbal abuse that is directed toward them or another person. Any threats of violence directed toward home care workers need to be reported to a supervisor immediately.

Case conferences are an effective way for home care agencies to set up a contract with the client and significant others. During the case conference, the agency explains what services it can provide and what is expected of the client and significant others. It is important for home care staff to outline what behaviors are acceptable and unacceptable, and what behaviors (such as threats of violence) may lead to termination of home care services.

Home care staff will have to rely on the assistance of other community agencies when they encounter child neglect or abuse, incest, or truancy. A parent who repeatedly succumbs to the need to spend all available money on drugs and is unable to provide food for the children may require intervention from agencies that provide protective services for children. Such services are usually more readily available than are treatment resources for the parent's drug addiction. Situations of abuse are not restricted to those involving substance use. Client abuse by family members or lovers also occurs and may necessitate referral to community-based agencies that provide protective services for adults.

Housing and Community Problems

Home care cannot be provided in inadequate or unsuitable housing. Examples of HIV-ill persons with unsuitable housing include (1) persons with diarrhea who are housed in single-room occupancy hotels (often referred to as welfare hotels), have no bathroom or sink in the room, and are required to use distant, shared bathroom facilities; (2) those with significant weight loss who live in places without facilities for cooking and food storage and are too weak to go out for meals; (3) those who require intravenous therapy but have neither a telephone to use in case of a medical emergency nor a refrigerator where solutions and drugs can be stored; and (4) clients who can no longer walk and live in buildings with broken or no elevator service.

The provision of home care services may require that the client be relocated to more suitable housing or that home care be delayed until necessary services are provided.

Home care cannot be provided in unsafe housing. Examples of unsafe housing include (1) buildings in which previous home care staff have been accosted or mugged; (2) buildings where entrances and hallways are used as "shooting galleries" for injection drug users or where crack and cocaine are sold; (3) buildings designated by local police departments as high-crime areas; and (4) homes in which overt drug using and trafficking takes place in the presence of home care staff. Although most home care agencies in large urban areas provide an escort service for visiting nurses, this service is expensive, is not directly reimbursable, and therefore is extremely limited. Escort service is not usually provided for paraprofessionals, so they may refuse to provide service to clients in unsafe environments. This should not be misconstrued as refusal to care for a PWHIV, a commonly encountered misinterpretation. In some cases, home care workers can arrange to be met by the family or significant others and escorted to and from the home. If staff is unable to provide care because the environment is judged unsafe, clients will need a referral to community housing organizations to help find safe, affordable housing.

Support Services

In the absence of previous experience, it is not uncommon, while the client is in the hospital, for the significant others to agree to participate in the home-based plan of care. However, once faced with the harsh realities of intense levels of physical care and emotional support needed in the home, the significant others or family members may withdraw active participation. Some family members or significant others will insist that a client be returned home with home care services but may themselves be unable to participate in care because they live far away. The participation of family and significant others is the foundation of safe home care. Reimbursement for services varies with the payer source—for example, private insurance, Medicaid, or Medicare—and from state to state in the case of Medicaid. Capitations on the amount of service often require that significant others participate. If they do not, modification of the original plan and referral to an institution for long-term care may be necessary.

Many AIDS organizations provide buddy services. Buddies are usually volunteers who visit clients once or twice a week. The buddy can run errands, maybe cook a meal and eat with the client, or, if the client is strong enough to go out, take the client for a walk or ride or out to the movies. The use of buddies is a good way to increase socialization for clients who have little support; they can also provide respite for significant others.

Problems of Medical Follow-up

When home care service is provided to persons covered by Medicaid, their hospital-based medical care is often provided by house staff (residents in training). At the time of home care referral, the resident providing the initial medical orders is usually not assuming the role of primary care physician. Once the client is at home, the visiting nurse may find no physician willing to modify or provide orders for the medical portion of the plan of care. Visiting nurses spend an inordinate amount of time attempting to arrange ongoing medical care for Medicaid recipients receiving home care. In the absence of medical supervision, the visiting nurse may have to return a client to the acute care facility to obtain medical orders or prescriptions, which otherwise could be obtained by a telephone call to a primary care physician. Many states regulating home care require physician's orders at specified intervals, but there is no legislation requiring physicians to provide a continuum of medical care to persons receiving home care. Ironically the burden of ensuring adequate medical care for the person receiving home care is on the professional nurse. Visiting nurses try to network with clinical nurses to communicate with physicians and obtain orders, because, unlike the physicians,

the clinic nurses are a consistent presence with greater knowledge of the clients.

Managing client care at home and planning for care are directly related to the individual client's problems, which result from the numerous AIDS-indicator diseases that may develop in a PWHIV. Chapters 4 and 5 detail specific individual responses to HIV disease and the related nursing care.

ALTERNATIVE/COMPLEMENTARY THERAPIES

Alternative therapies, also known as complementary or unconventional therapies, are defined as medical interventions that are not generally taught by U.S. medical schools or offered by U.S. hospitals (Eisenberg et al., 1993). Traditional Western medicine focuses on the treatment of disease; proponents of alternative therapies stress the need to treat the person with a holistic approach that recognizes the interaction of the mind, body, and spirit (Strawn, 1989). This interaction is now being studied through the field of psychoneuroimmunology, a theoretical framework that analyzes the relation between cognition, mood, and emotions and the neurologic and immune systems (Groer, 1991). It is believed that changes in one area can influence other systems in either a positive or a negative way.

The alternative/complementary therapies (ACTs) may be divided into four general categories: (1) spiritual and psychologic, (2) nutritional, (3) drug and biologic, and (4) physical forces and devices. See Table 12–5 for a listing of the most common ACTs. An in-depth discussion of each of these therapies is beyond the scope of the chapter. However, it is important for nurses to realize (1) why clients use ACTs, (2) how frequently ACTs are used, especially by people with HIV disease, and (3) the nursing implications when clients use ACTs.

Murray and Rubell (1992, p. 62) stated that people seek out ACTs because they find conventional medicine to be overly technologic, impersonal, and costly, and they are attracted by the opportunity to "take charge of their health." Greenblatt et al. (1991) and Irish (1989) cited disillusionment and distrust

Table 12–5. General Categories of Alternative/Complementary Therapies

CATEGORY	THERAPIES
Spiritual and psychologic	Creative visualization, guided imagery, faith healing, hypnosis, laughter therapy, meditation, reframing and positive affirmations
Nutritional	Bach flower remedies, herbal therapies, vitamin and mineral supplements, dietary regimens such as vegetarian and macrobiotic
Drug and biologic	Homeopathy, oxygen therapies including ozone therapy, urine therapy, non-FDA-approved medications
Physical forces and devices	Acupuncture, acupressure, chiropractic, crystals, massage therapy, Reiki, reflexology, relaxation techniques, therapeutic touch, yoga

of conventional medicine as motivating factors. Abrams (1990) traced the roots of the alternative therapy movement for HIV infection to frustration with the slow pace of research and despair over the limited effectiveness of antiretroviral agents. Clients may use alternative therapies to ameliorate either the symptoms of HIV infection or the side effects of medications (Anderson et al., 1993). Although ACTs may offer clients a sense of hope and control, Strawn (1989) was careful to emphasize the need to distinguish healing from cure, so that clients do not blame themselves for an outcome that fails to meet their expectations. Critics of ACTs argue that placing responsibility for healing with the client, rather than with a specific treatment or physician, may result in guilt and depression for the client (Monaco, 1989).

Practitioners of conventional Western medicine have recently begun to recognize the widespread use of ACTs in the United States. In a nationwide study of 1,539 randomly selected adults, Eisenberg and colleagues (1993) found that 34% of those surveyed had used ACTs in the previous year, and that fewer than 3 in 10 had informed their medical doc-

tors about their use of ACTs. Use of ACTs was most common in persons 25 to 49 years of age who had some college education. Rates of ACT use ranged from 23% to 53% in all socioeconomic groups.

Several studies have documented the use of ACTs by people with HIV/AIDS. In a study of 50 patients with AIDS in Chicago, 36% used ACTs, including acupuncture, imagery, massage therapy, megavitamins, acupressure, and unapproved medications (Hand, 1989). A San Francisco clinic population survey of 197 found that 29% used ACTs and that 31% of these individuals were also enrolled in clinical trials (Greenblatt et al., 1991). Anderson and colleagues (1993) surveyed 184 HIV-infected patients in Philadelphia, and found that 40% used ACTs. Of those using ACTs, 38% did not tell their regular health care providers, and 42% of those patients who were participating in clinical trials used ACTs during the trials. Kassler and associates (1991) found that 22% of 114 clients used herbs and that several were taking herbs at dosages that could cause adverse effects.

A high percentage of clients who use ACTs do not inform their regular health care providers. Greenblatt et al. (1991) stated that clients may not disclose this information because of fear of embarrassment or disapproval. It is important for nurses to incorporate questions about ACTs into their health care assessments. Irish (1989) suggested asking the following question in a nonjudgmental manner: "What other practices or beliefs are important to your health maintenance program?" (p. 306). This information should be documented in the client's record and shared with other health care providers. If the nurse is unfamiliar with the particular ACT, he or she may ask the client for an explanation or request the client's permission to contact the ACT practitioner to discuss the therapy. Other nurses may use ACTs in their own practice, including therapeutic touch and acupuncture (Newshan, 1989; Sanders, 1989). It is important to keep an open mind and try to understand why the ACT is important to the client. If practitioners of conventional therapies open dialogue with ACT providers, it will improve communication, reduce the likelihood of conflicts, and help to meet the needs of the clients (Anderson et al., 1993).

As with any therapy, nurses need to be aware of the possible side effects of ACTs and to assess whether the ACT may be causing adverse effects. Adverse effects are most likely to occur when ACTs are ingested. Clients following a macrobiotic diet may have nutritional deficiencies in vitamins C, B_2, B_{12}, D, iron, folic acid, and calcium (Irish, 1989). Kassler et al. (1991) researched the possible adverse effects of various herbal remedies. These included central nervous system excitation or depression; anticoagulation; gastrointestinal disturbances such as nausea, vomiting, or diarrhea; photosensitivity; dermatitis; diuresis; and electrolyte disturbances. Because there is no quality control for herbal products, preparations may vary in the dosage of active ingredients or the presence of additives. If a client is taking both prescribed medications and ACTs, it may be difficult to determine the source of newly reported symptoms: is it a prescribed medication, an ACT, or a new opportunistic infection? If a nurse suspects that an ACT may be causing adverse effects, he or she should discuss the situation with the client, the ACT provider, and the traditional health care practitioner.

Nurses may find themselves in a dilemma when clients reveal their use of ACTs but refuse to inform their physicians or other health care providers. This problem may arise when clients enrolled in clinical trials are also using ACTs. The use of ACTs while in clinical trials may confound the study results. ACTs may affect the efficacy of the trial drug. Side effects may be attributed to the study drug when in fact they are being caused by the ACT (Greenblatt et al., 1991). Clients may insist on their right to use both ACTs and trial drugs, especially if they feel improvement in their clinical status. In this situation the nurse should consult with his or her supervisor to discuss the most effective way to handle this problem without destroying rapport with the client.

Since alternative therapies are not usually reimbursed by insurance, most clients pay the entire cost (Eisenberg et al., 1993). If a client is on a fixed income, the ACT may result in considerable expense. Nurses may act as sounding boards for clients who are trying to decide the most beneficial ways to allocate limited resources.

DRUG UNDERGROUND AND BUYERS' CLUBS

Nurses in the community may also discover that clients are taking medications not approved by the U.S. Food and Drug Administration (FDA). Because they were discouraged by the slow pace of FDA research in the 1980s, consumer groups set up ways to access medications not yet approved in the United States (Abrams, 1990). These groups publish newsletters and offer information through hotline numbers. Home care nurses may find medications in the home with handwritten labels, or they may find drug information that is written in a language other than English (Schmidt, 1992). As with any medication, the nurse needs to notify the health care provider and monitor the client for side effects, but because these medications are not approved in this country, it may be difficult to find information. The National AIDS Information Clearinghouse maintains a database with information on medications available both in the United States and abroad (telephone number 1-800-458-5231). It can supply information on nonapproved medications, known side effects, and available clinical trials.

It is important for nurses to distinguish the drug underground and buyers' clubs from expanded drug access. Expanded drug access may be approved by the FDA when a drug has proved beneficial in clinical trials but has not yet received final FDA approval. The FDA will give drug companies authorization to release the medication to physicians who call an "800" number and complete the necessary paperwork. Expanded access provides a way for clients to access trial drugs through a physician when the client may not meet the eligibility criteria for a clinical trial.

PARTICIPATING IN RESEARCH

Clients infected with HIV may debate about whether to participate in a clinical drug or treatment trial at any point during the course of illness. The nurse can assist the client in reaching a realistic decision about whether to participate. Clinical research trials may be established to study the efficacy of a drug or HIV-related treatments that are psychologic, social, or epidemiologic in nature. The nurse's role in these types of research could be as principal investigator, collaborator, or data collector. The nurse clinician should be prepared to offer clients information about clinical trials and help them enroll if they so decide. Although all research has similarities, the risk/benefit ratio is greater in drug trials and therefore the need for safeguards is greater.

A clinical trial is a study that tests new drugs and other treatments to determine safety and effectiveness (U.S. Department of Health and Human Services, 1989). The drug approval process occurs through the cooperation of the FDA, the National Institutes of Health (NIH), and the pharmaceutical manufacturer. The FDA reviews the data supplied by NIH and the pharmaceutical manufacturer and requests additional information until it is certain that the drug is safe and effective. NIH consists of 13 institutes, one of which is the National Institute of Allergy and Infectious Diseases (NIAID).

In 1987, NIAID established the AIDS Clinical Trial Group to conduct collaborative clinical trials for AIDS therapies. By 1990, there were 47 group centers, usually located in major medical centers in geographic areas where the incidence of HIV infection is high. In 1989 NIAID created 18 Community Programs for Clinical Research on AIDS to test AIDS-related drugs and vaccines. The expressed purpose of the programs is to "reach out to population groups that have been underrepresented in AIDS research" (NIAID, 1990, p. 11).

In some communities there is also a growing movement to test drugs in other community settings such as the Community Research Initiative (AIDS Treatment Resources, 1990). The initiative offers HIV-positive clients the opportunity to take drugs that have uncertain effectiveness and that probably have not yet been tested within the formal FDA approval mechanism. Drugs with some demonstrated effectiveness can also be made

available to a private physician for clients who cannot participate in a clinical trial or who have failed approved therapies; this process may be considered a parallel track. However, some physicians may not utilize this option because of the paperwork involved.

Despite the extensive network of clinical trials, activist community groups such as the AIDS Coalition to Unleash Power (ACT-UP) charge that many clients with HIV infection are routinely excluded from drug trials because of lifestyle, gender, or pregnancy status. These charges seem founded when the demographics of the subjects participating in clinical trials are examined. The overwhelming majority of the subjects are white, gay men living in urban settings (Perryman, 1990); the numbers of persons with HIV infection in those geographic areas do not proportionately reflect this same distribution.

Before a drug reaches the marketplace for general distribution, it must pass through numerous steps. The overall goal of this process is to ensure that the drug is safe and effective. Hundreds and sometimes thousands of chemicals must be made and tested to find one that can achieve the desirable results without unacceptably serious side effects (Cohn, 1988). The development of a new drug involves three stages of research: (1) preclinical research that focuses on development, information synthesis, and animal testing, (2) human testing divided into phases I, II, and III, and (3) postmarketing research.

The most important stages in new drug development are the three phases of clinical research in humans. Phase I trials are concerned with learning more about the safety of the drug. These trials are usually conducted with healthy volunteers who are paid for their services. The subjects submit to a variety of tests to determine what the drug does in the human body: how it is absorbed, metabolized, and excreted; its effect on different body parts; and the side effects that occur as the dose is increased. A main reason that drugs fail to proceed to phase II is evidence of toxicity at doses too small to produce any beneficial effects (Flieger, 1988).

The purpose of phase II trials is to determine whether the drug is effective in treating the disease or condition for which it is intended. These studies recruit a few hundred patients and attempt to determine short-term side effects and risks in people whose health is impaired. Most of the phase II trials are randomized, controlled trials that are often double blind. When this methodology is used, potential subjects are randomly divided into two groups, with one group (experimental group) receiving the experimental drug and the other group (control group) receiving a placebo. When the research is double blind, neither the patients nor the health care providers know which patient is receiving the placebo and which is receiving the experimental drug. By the end of phase II trials, the researchers know whether the drug has a therapeutic effectiveness and its short-term adverse and other side effects (Flieger, 1988). The FDA can quickly terminate phase II trials when there is evidence that the experimental group is receiving major benefit over the control group. This is the situation that occurred when zidovudine was tested.

Phase III studies are designed to provide information about optimal dosage rates and schedules. Because thousands of patients are enrolled, more information about the drug's safety and effectiveness is learned. Although phase III studies are controlled, they more closely approximate the conditions of ordinary medical practice. Not all drugs go through all the phases (AIDS Treatment Resources, 1990). The evidence of safety and effectiveness of zidovudine (formerly known as azidothymidine [AZT]) was so great that phase III studies were not required before the FDA approved the drug for general use. During the same 4- to 6-month period of phase II testing, only one AIDS patient died while being treated with zidovudine, whereas 19 died while being given a placebo. Consequently, zidovudine was prematurely approved (without completion of phase IIII trials) for compassionate reasons and made widely available.

Patients and health care providers have identified five major benefits of clinical trials: (1) having a chance to help others, (2) obtaining access to top-quality health care, (3) gaining power for oneself by taking positive ac-

tion, (4) being helped by a new drug, and (5) receiving financial assistance (most drugs are provided without charge by the pharmaceutical company, and associated laboratory and other diagnostic tests are usually covered by the agency funding the research study). There are three major risks associated with participating in clinical trials: (1) the treatment may not have benefits, (2) it may actually be harmful, and (3) the drug may have harmful side effects (Department of Health and Human Services, 1989). In addition, in many studies the participants are not allowed to take other drugs while they are subjects. A comprehensive checklist of questions that the client needs to have answered before making a decision about participating in research is included in Appendix VI.

After drugs are approved for general use, postmarketing surveillance continues. The FDA and the pharmaceutical firm must monitor adverse reactions to drugs. To help track the performance of their products, many drug firms rely on their sales personnel (Ackerman, 1988). The nurse should communicate with these salespersons by sharing ideas and seeking information about the drugs. The FDA has an "adverse drug reaction" form that should be completed whenever a health care provider notices an unusual or adverse reaction to a drug or treatment. However, physicians or other health care providers are not legally required to report these adverse drug reactions to the FDA. It is estimated that fewer than 10% of adverse drug reactions are reported by physicians and an even smaller percentage by other health care providers. To increase the number of adverse reaction reports, the FDA is educating physicians, pharmacists, and nurses about how reactions should be reported. Reporting has been made easier by the creation of hotlines and more rewarding by the provision of significant information about the drug (Ackerman, 1988).

Many pharmaceutical firms encourage open communication by providing scientific information about their product. Anecdotal reports may result in the discovery of new uses for established drugs. For example, naltrexone, a drug approved for treating heroin addicts, may be effective in the treatment of Kaposi's sarcoma and has been used by physicians to treat this tumor without knowledge of the FDA or without formal testing. This use is legal because once the FDA has released a drug into the marketplace, no law requires that physicians dispense it only for approved uses (Ackerman, 1988). However, this information about results in the treatment of Kaposi's sarcoma would be useful to other physicians who are not aware of this application of naltrexone.

INSTITUTIONAL LONG-TERM CARE

Throughout the HIV epidemic, home care has played by far the most significant role, not only because care at home is so often preferred by consumers, but also because the service has so much potential for flexibility (Wyatt, 1990). However, as with any chronic disease, variables associated with the life of the affected individual may necessitate care in a setting other than the home. These variables range from the lack of a suitable home in which to provide care to the lack of a significant other to provide the needed care. Options to home care include skilled nursing facilities (SNFs), often referred to as nursing homes, day care, and residential care with supportive services. Although the demand for these alternatives has been self-evident and is increasing, the supply has remained pitifully low and, in some areas, nonexistent.

Care in a Skilled Nursing Facility

According to Benjamin and Swan (1989), when case managers explore the option of nursing home care for persons with HIV disease, they find not a solution but a service gap, because many SNFs are reluctant to provide care to this client population. Reasons frequently cited for refusal of nursing homes to accept persons with HIV disease include (1) increased costs of infection control measures and staffing, (2) poor Medicaid reimbursement levels, (3) an unprepared workforce, (4) a philosophic orientation toward geriatric care, (5) homophobia among administrators or staff members, (6) already high occupancy rates, and (7) possible loss of referrals of non-

HIV-infected residents (Taravella, 1990). Linsk and colleagues (1993) surveyed nursing home administrators in Illinois and found that major concerns were the ability to recruit staff to care for PWHIV, and staff fear and apprehension.

As a further illustration of the short supply, by March 1990 in New York City, with 9,602 people with AIDS, approximately 130 dedicated AIDS skilled nursing beds were available at three facilities (Taravella, 1990). By the end of 1992 there were 530 skilled nursing home beds for people with AIDS in all of New York State (New York State Department of Health, 1993). The plans for the future are not promising. Through 1993 there will be an anticipated 1,513 skilled nursing beds for persons with HIV illness in the entire United States (Taravella, 1990).

One of the first SNFs in the United Sates to admit a PWHIV was the Human Resources Health Center located in Dade County, Florida. According to Diana Liebisch the director of nursing at that time, admission of people with AIDS to the facility was considered part of its mission, and the staff struggled through fear and confusion, changing care regimens as new information became available and adjusting policies to meet the challenge (Harvard AIDS Institute, 1989). By 1989 the facility had served 169 people with AIDS and has expanded its capabilities.

Kane and Smith (1989) were the first to study the integration of people with AIDS into nursing homes. The study was conducted in 16 nursing homes in Minnesota, equally divided between eight SNFs willing to take or already having admitted people with AIDS, and eight SNFs that did not have plans to admit people with AIDS. Kane and Smith (1989) interviewed 100 nursing home residents, 100 family members of residents, and 100 nursing home staff members. They also interviewed the administrator, director of nurses, and director of social work at each of the 16 facilities, as well as four people with AIDS who were residents in the SNFs studied.

In facilities receptive to admitting PWHIV, the staff was more knowledgeable and held more positive attitudes than the staff in comparison homes. The SNFs that had admitted PWHIV did not encounter negative reactions of residents or family members, and staff did not resign as anticipated. An interesting finding was the fear among the residents and their families and among the staff about the reactions of the others. The residents and their families were fearful that the staff would quit, and the staff members were fearful that families would move the residents to other SNFs; neither fear materialized. The universal concerns over HIV contagion and infection control practices were noted also but were certainly not limited to the nursing home setting.

In interviews with people with AIDS in nursing homes, Kane and Smith (1989) reported that the most significant concerns were (1) lack of training or familiarity of some staff members with high-tech equipment, (2) quality of meals, (3) quality of activities, (4) lack of telephones, (5) routines that prohibited sleeping late, and (6) concern about the reactions of non-AIDS residents. The concerns of the PWHIV regarding a lack of skill with particular equipment are understandable, but the same problem can occur in other health care settings as well. Complaints about meals, schedules, and activities are common among elderly nursing home residents as well as people with AIDS (Kane & Caplan, 1990).

The clinical needs of clients with HIV infection remain the same regardless of the setting. For example, clients with toxoplasmosis will require suppressive therapy to prevent recurrence, assistance with personal care, and physical and occupational therapy, whether they are in a hospital or nursing home, or at home. Dementia is the primary clinical condition that requires the supportive and protective environment of an SNF (Benjamin & Swan, 1989; Kator & Cunningham McBride, 1990). The dementia seen in many of the clients with AIDS can result in bizarre behavior, violent acting out, decline in self-care skills, and delusional thinking (Dunn, 1990). Both staff and residents should be informed about these behaviors as a consequence of disease and taught how to respond appropriately.

As with other health care settings, nursing home staff need preparation to meet the clinical needs of HIV-infected persons with specific opportunistic diseases. They must be trained in such techniques as infusion therapy to suppress opportunistic infections and prophylaxis to prevent infections. Flexibility must be introduced into a system of care traditionally dominated by exclusionary rules.

On the basis of 8 years' experience admitting people with AIDS to the Palm Beach County Home and General Care Facility, in Palm Beach County, Florida, Dunn (1990) recommended that planning for SNF care includes (1) developing procedures specific to the needs of people with AIDS, (2) increasing social services, (3) providing support group therapy, (4) offering addiction recovery therapy or meetings at the facility, (5) developing policies and plans for handling substance abuse in the facility, and (6) providing necessary education and support groups for staff.

The concerns and needs of the members of the nursing staff in nursing homes are the same as those expressed by their colleagues in other settings. History has demonstrated that with education and experience these fears can be decreased.

Day Care

An underdeveloped option for long-term care of PWHIV is a day care and treatment program. In August 1988 the Village Nursing Home in New York City opened the first day care program designed specifically for PWHIV. The goals of the program are rehabilitation, socialization, and recreation (McNally & Mason-Beck, 1989). The program also provides meals and respite for the family and significant others.

Day care for clients with AIDS dementia complex can be an important part of the plan of care because of the socialization experience. Including cognitive stimulation and exercise therapy can also improve mental and motor dysfunction associated with the neurotropic effects of HIV. Supervision of medications in this type of program can help ensure compliance. Infusion therapy can be provided at a reduced cost, because the nurse can care for several clients at one time.

For clients who have no significant others, live in substandard housing, and have difficulty providing for themselves, the day care program can function as a coordinator of care and case manager for a variety of services (Wyatt, 1990). Combining day care with home care in the evenings and on weekends for clients with high-level care needs is another option for a plan of care.

In addressing the need for flexibility in the continuum of long-term care, the Village Nursing Home, in addition to its day care program, has implemented a home care program and plans to open an SNF dedicated to caring for PWHIV. This will provide a true "system" of long-term care, allowing clients to move from one service level to another as needed.

Residential Care

In July 1983 the gay community and health care professionals in San Francisco opened the world's first AIDS residence (Harvard AIDS Institute, 1989). Today this program, known as the Shanti Project, operates several residences in San Francisco. The program's chief goal is to provide high-quality, long-term, low-cost housing for displaced persons living with AIDS or severe HIV disease who are able to live independently and cooperatively with needed support services in a group setting. The staff work closely with other AIDS agencies to provide the medical and social services needed by the residents. Residents requiring home care receive services from the Hospice of San Francisco and Visiting Nurse Association.

In New York City in 1983, members of the gay community recognized the need for housing that was supportive of the needs of PWHIV and formed the AIDS Resource Center, which initially offered donations to individuals for rent and food. Today the AIDS Resource Center operates two types of supportive housing programs for PWHIV: a congregate living facility and scatter-site apartments.

The congregate living facility, known as Bailey House, has 44 private rooms for clients. Case management, support groups, and on-site health supervision by a professional nurse and a visiting physician are provided. The scatter-site housing program offers a series of apartments throughout the boroughs of New York City. Services are similar to those at Bailey House except that no on-site health supervision is offered. Clients in both settings who require home care receive services from the Visiting Nurse Service of New York.

One of the most prevalent case management problems in residential programs is substance use, including alcohol, crack and cocaine, marijuana, and heroin. The problem becomes obvious when the resulting behaviors are property destruction, physical and verbal abuse of residents and staff, and unsafe sex. The problem of substance use is not limited to self-identified drug users. In fact, many of the problems of substance use may not be addressed until after the client takes residence in the facility. Case management should include nondiscriminatory rules regarding behaviors that are not allowed and clear communication of the consequences of breaking the rules. Above all, the staff must be willing to enforce the prearranged limits and must do so consistently. A practice of vacillating and making exceptions give mixed messages to the clients and encourages them to test the rules.

A recurrent issue encountered by clients in congregate living facilities is the constant reminders that they have HIV infection. Clients must deal with grieving, both actual and anticipatory, which in most situations is handled through support groups. Volunteers and a program of recreation, as well as availability of religious and spiritual counseling, are important adjuncts to quality living by the residents. Other case management issues to be considered include (1) residents' bringing guests back to their rooms to have sex, (2) homophobia and fear of injection drug users among residents, (3) managing and supervising clients with progressive dementia, and (4) preferential treatment received and given by both staff and residents.

HOSPICE CARE

Since the opening of St. Christopher's Hospice in England in 1967, hospice care has received considerable attention worldwide. By

1980 the Health Care Finance Administration had approved 26 hospice demonstration programs to study the efficacy and economics of hospice care in the United States. Since then, hospice care has become integrated into the schema of health care in the United States.

Hospice care in the United States has emerged as a model of home care for terminally ill individuals. A prevalent misconception is that a hospice is a place to institutionalize a dying person. Although all certified hospice programs are required to have inpatient beds available, their use is usually limited to short periods for respite care and symptom control. This basic lack of understanding led to demands, early in the AIDS epidemic in the United States, to place PWHIV in hospices.

The major appeal of hospice care is the concept of interdisciplinary and holistic case management as the ideal health care model. Hospice care emphasizes the quality of life for terminally ill individuals through symptom control (palliative care) and expert psychologic and spiritual care. Most clinicians would agree that this ideal approach to care should be applied to all health care settings. If one goes one step farther, all health care professionals should emphasize quality-of-life issues through symptom control and expert psychologic and spiritual care. Although most health care professionals have formally studied death and dying, few have formally studied, with hospice experts, the basics of symptom control, especially pain control. Therefore they are limited in applying this concept to client care, irrespective of the clinical setting.

Until 1983 the cause of AIDS remained unknown, and until March 1987 no treatment of HIV infection was available. Consequently, in the early years of the epidemic, AIDS was viewed as a rapidly progressing terminal illness. Through clinical research, the development of antiviral agents, and improved methods of treating and preventing opportunistic infections, the clinical picture has changed dramatically. Today the needs of the HIV-ill person can be more appropriately described as a continuum of care for chronic illness. This is not meant to imply that hospice care is not needed; it should be available to

those individuals who wish it. However, barriers to hospice care for PWHIV remain. First, federally established reimbursement rates do not reflect the actual costs associated with case management and the clinical needs of HIV-infected individuals. Second, national, state, and local hospice organizations have had to redefine palliative care as it relates to AIDS. Among the issues are (1) continuation of intravenous therapy for palliative reasons, for example, ganciclovir to prevent blindness as a result of cytomegalovirus retinitis, (2) periodic transfusions to correct anemia, and (3) continuation of expensive suppressive medicines specific to HIV-related illnesses. Third, hospice staff members usually do not have the technical preparation to provide the high-tech services often needed by this client population.

Hospice care, regardless of the stage of HIV illness, is unacceptable to many PWHIV because they are young and because they believe that a cure is imminent (Martin, 1991; Ungvarski, 1988). They often choose to pursue aggressive medical treatment and to participate in research protocols (Ungvarski, 1989). Commenting on knowledge, self-determination, and decision making, Derek Hodel (1990), executive director of the People with AIDS Group, summarized: "The truth is, a lot of people with AIDS don't want to be 'self-empowered.' They want to stay alive" (p. 30). Consequently, although the care providers and significant others may clearly see the benefits of and need for hospice care, they should not be surprised if PWHIV reject this model of care.

Hospice care focuses on the quality rather than the quantity of life. Therefore the foundation of hospice care is symptom control, that is, taking control of a particular symptom and preventing its recurrence, rather than allowing the symptom to control the individual's life and detract from it (MacFadden, 1988). Pomerantz and Harrison (1990) identified common symptoms seen in end-stage HIV illness as (1) pain, (2) diarrhea, (3) nausea and vomiting, (4) dehydration, (5) urinary incontinence, (6) fever, (7) respiratory problems including chest pain, cough, and hypoxemia, (8) decubitus ulcers, (9) delirium and dementia,

(10) weight loss, and (11) depression, anxiety, and fear. Chapter 5 includes nursing management information that incorporates the symptom control, and Chapter 11 covers the psychosocial aspects of care, including grief and bereavement. The following discussion is limited to medical interventions that may be employed to control symptoms of end-stage HIV illness.

Schofferman (1988) identified pain resulting from peripheral neuropathy as the most commonly encountered pain requiring palliative treatment. Price and Brew (1990) described the pain, thought to be related to HIV infection of nerve or dorsal root ganglia, as painful paresthesias and burning, especially in the feet. It may prevent walking by some individuals, and it is not generally relieved with zidovudine. Treatment is with tricyclic antidepressants, such as desipramine or imipramine and analgesics. Newer antiretroviral nucleoside drugs, such as dideoxyinosine (ddI) and dideoxycytidine (ddC), also cause axonal neuropathies, and individuals with underlying neuropathy may be particularly vulnerable to this adverse affect of ddI and ddC (Price & Brew, 1990).

Pain assessment is extremely important to determine the specific plan of care for PWHIV. For example, if pain is related to a tumor such as Kaposi's sarcoma that is pressing on a bone, nerve, or hollow viscus, management may include chemotherapy to reduce tumor size. Likewise, if pain is due to extensive lesions, such as esophageal lesions associated with infection with herpes simplex virus, the plan of care should include antiviral therapy for the infection in addition to analgesia. According to Schofferman (1988), treatment of pain in PWHIV follows the same general guidelines as in patients with cancer. Constipation, a common side effect of narcotic analgesics, is seen less often in AIDS because of the high incidence of diarrhea (Pomerantz & Harrison, 1990; Schofferman, 1988).

Nausea and vomiting may be the consequence of opportunistic diseases or their treatment. Initial control of these symptoms may be achieved by parenteral administration of medication or use of suppositories. Metoclopramide, prochlorperazine, or trimethoben-

zamide may be used to control nausea and vomiting (Pomerantz & Harrison, 1990). A more recently approved antiemetic that may be prescribed is dronabinol. It is classified as a cannabinoid—a synthetic form of active substances found in marijuana.

The assessment of diarrhea should include such causes as side effects of drugs, malabsorption, lactose intolerance, and development of a gastrointestinal opportunistic infection. If none of the preceding is identified as the cause of diarrhea, such agents as loperamide and diphenoxylate with atropine may be administered. Dehydration accompanying diarrhea requires oral fluid replacement to the extent tolerated.

In addition to fluid intake, Pomerantz and Harrison (1990) recommended controlling fever with two tablets of aspirin alternated with two tablets of acetaminophen every 2 hours. In the presence of low platelet counts or idiopathic thrombocytopenic purpura, commonly seen in HIV infection, aspirin administration is contraindicated. In the presence of severe anemia and neutropenia in persons taking zidovudine, acetaminophen may be contraindicated.

Respiratory problems may be alleviated by oxygen administration for air hunger, analgesia for chest pain, and antitussive agents for cough. Although placement of a Foley catheter may result in urosepsis, its benefit for a patient with urinary incontinence may outweigh the risk. Although prevention of decubitus ulcers is every nurse's priority, they may occur. The primary focus is prevention of ulcer extension and secondary infection, because in most cases little healing will take place.

Delirium and dementia may be the result of advanced HIV infection, sepsis, and fever, or in some cases the result of adverse drug effects. Pomerantz and Harrison (1990) suggested that effective treatment can be achieved with the combination of haloperidol and diazepam.

Symptom control is an art as well as a science, and health care professionals who lack the education and experience are strongly encouraged to seek consultation for their clients from hospice staff. This is especially true with pain control. According to Rogers (1989), many studies have demonstrated that patients often suffer needlessly because of undermedication, which occurs because health care professionals have insufficient knowledge of the pharmacology of analgesics and because they fear they may be fostering narcotic abuse. Bohnet (1986) pointed out that until the symptoms are controlled or managed, no other concern of the client can be realistically addressed by nursing assessment or intervention.

HIV NURSING RESEARCH IN COMMUNITY-BASED AND LONG-TERM CARE

Summary of Research

Research concerning the advanced practice roles of clinical nurse specialists, nurse practitioners, and nurse midwives has not only provided emerging models of care but also validated the effectiveness of nurses in the case management of HIV-infected individuals. Clinical nurse specialists have demonstrated flexibility in role functions by serving as direct care providers, consultants, and case managers in both in-patient and community-based settings (Layzell & McCarthy, 1993; McCann, 1991; Sherman & Johnson, 1991). Aiken and colleagues (1993) compared HIV-related primary care service delivered by physicians with that delivered by nurse practitioners and found not only comparable levels of care but fewer problems reported by patients who were receiving care from nurse practitioners. De Ferrari and associates (1993) examined a midwifery model of care for pregnant HIV-infected women and found high levels of continuity of care.

Wright and colleagues (1993) evaluated case management activities performed by nurse case managers in the California Pilot Care and Waiver Projects for HIV/AIDS patients. The authors found that these programs provide vehicles for the coordination and linkage of community services for PWHIV and function as a service delivery model using nurse case management for PWHIV with symptoms. This survey validated the interdis-

ciplinary case management model in a community-based HIV population. Sowell and associates (1992) examined the effects of case management on controlling hospital costs of the care of people with AIDS. The authors identified not only lower hospital-based charges for case-managed clients but increased survival time between HIV diagnosis and death.

A major emphasis on HIV care in the community and in the home has occurred throughout the first decade of the AIDS epidemic in the United States. Salsberry and colleagues (1993), in an ongoing investigation, are studying the problems that this change in health care delivery has engendered for agencies providing this care, as well as the agencies' responses to these problems. Their preliminary findings suggest that home care agencies may not be well positioned to meet the cyclic needs of HIV patients, that care is becoming increasingly fragmented, with multiple agencies seeking to patch together a program of comprehensive services, and that the policies of home care agency may limit the number of HIV-infected patients eligible for home care.

Brown and Powell-Cope (1991) studied the social context of AIDS family caregivers in the home. Their findings revealed uncertainty as a dominant theme, with a core category of transitions through uncertainty as well as subcategories of concern, including managing and being managed by HIV disease, living with loss and dying, renegotiating relationships, "going public," and containing the spread of HIV disease.

Nursing research has also focused on assessment tools to identify the specific health care needs of PWHIV/AIDS. Berk and colleagues (1992) adapted the Peters (1988) Community Health Intensity Rating Scale so that it could be applied to patients in a hospital or dedicated HIV clinic or to patients receiving home care or long-term care. The authors collected content-related validity evidence and produced a set of specifications for environmental, psychosocial, physiologic, and health behaviors assessment.

Nokes and associates (1994) developed the HIV Assessment Tool (HAT), a visual analog scale, to rate HIV-related symptom severity and general well-being of PWHIV. The instrument can be used to relate HIV symptoms to disease progression and to evaluate the effectiveness of nursing interventions.

Hurley and Ungvarski (1994) conducted a retrospective study of the home health care needs of adults with AIDS. In addition to identifying physiologic and psychologic needs (see Chapter 5), problems identified included inadequate nutrition, issues related to compliance with prescribed medications, inadequate in-home support systems, inadequate facilities and utilities in the home, financial concerns, and lifestyles that included drug and/or alcohol abuse. The authors concluded that the home health care needs of people with AIDS are multifaceted in nature and extend well beyond the clinical manifestations of HIV disease.

Nurse researchers have also studied the problem of accessing community-based HIV/AIDS services in rural areas of the United States. Gay men often move from rural to urban areas in other states to lead an openly gay lifestyle; if they become HIV infected, they may return home to be cared for by their families. Smith and associates (1990) studied the problem of migrating home for HIV/AIDS care and concluded that because these individuals are diagnosed and reported in large urban areas in other states, the actual numbers of PWHIV are underestimated in many states. Ultimately the result is underfunding of services for HIV-infected individuals residing in rural areas. Davis and Stapleton (1991) and Davis and associates (1992a, 1992b) studied the phenomenon of HIV-infected persons in rural areas and identified the fact that many of the individuals who move back home are not terminally ill and return home for a variety of reasons. The authors concluded that nurses in rural areas need to be prepared to care for persons living with HIV/AIDS and must begin to educate and prepare local agencies and community groups.

Swan and associates (1992) studied the average number of nursing care hours required by PWHIV in an SNF. They demonstrated that the needs of PWHIV reflect greater nursing care time, which results in higher costs for this population in nursing homes.

Nursing theory–based managed care has also been examined to explore the applicability of models developed by Orem, Parse, and Watson (Holzemer, 1992; Nokes & Carver, 1991; Schroeder & Maeve, 1992). Schroeder (1993) was able to demonstrate the cost-effectiveness of a theory-based nurse-managed center for PWHIV/AIDS utilizing Watson's model of human caring.

Research Needed

Nursing research in the area of community-based and long-term care for PWHIV/AIDS is needed to identify the psychologic, physiologic, environmental, and health-related behaviors of clients. Areas for further study include:

1. Identification of human responses, both physiologic and psychologic, that clients manifest in various community-based settings
2. Congruency studies of health care needs identified by clients through self-reporting, in comparison with those identified by nurses providing their care
3. Development and validation of assessment tools to identify client needs in various care settings
4. Identification of the availability and utilization of community-based resources
5. Identification of the impact of caregiving on family systems
6. Identification of factors that influence access to health care, such as insurance, finances, housing, community safety, and care in rural areas
7. Identification of issues that impede an individual's ability to comply with prescribed therapies, such as drug and alcohol use and limited education
8. Comparison of the cost of nursing care in various community-based settings
9. Evaluation of patient outcomes to compare nurse-managed versus non-nurse-managed care
10. Evaluation of the efficacy and costs of

alternative/complementary therapies prescribed by nurses

11. Evaluation of patient outcomes related to care provided by advanced practice nurses compared with nurse generalists or physicians

SUMMARY

Planning for the long-term care needs of the client with HIV disease ranges from primary care with scheduled follow-up in the early phase of diagnosis to provision of home care, long-term residential care, or hospice care in the later stages. Health care professionals responsible for case management can improve access to these services if they are familiar with the capabilities and limitations of the various service providers.

In August 1990 the National Commission on AIDS submitted its first annual report to the President and Congress. Among their findings were that (1) the belief that Medicaid will pay for health care needs of PWHIV is a "Medicaid fantasy"; (2) for medically disenfranchised persons and those unable to pay, no system of care exists; and (3) health care in the United States has been unresponsive to the needs of HIV-infected people. The report emphasizes that at the end of the first decade of the HIV-AIDS epidemic in the United States, there is still no national policy or plan, and no national voice.

Unquestionably the health care professionals intimately involved in HIV AIDS education, care, and research have begun to address the clinical needs of this client population and have clearly articulated what needs to be done to address the problems of care. The federal government must take a more active role. "The development of a comprehensive system with linkages to research protocols, existing community-based services, hospitals, drug treatment programs, local health departments, and long-term care facilities, based on a foundation of adequate support, is long overdue and should be a top priority for the federal government" (National Commission on AIDS, 1990, p. 167).

REFERENCES

Abrams, D.I. (1990). Alternative therapies in HIV infection. *AIDS, 4*(12), 1179–1187.

Ackerman, S. (1988). Watching for problems that testing may have missed. In *New drug development in the United States* (DHHS publication No. [FDA] 88-3168) (pp. 51–53). Rockville, MD: U.S. Department of Health and Human Services.

AIDS Treatment Resources (1990). *Deciding to enter an AIDS/HIV drug trial.* New York: AIDS Treatment Resources, Inc.

Aiken, L.H., Lake, E.T., Semann, S., et al. (1993). Nurse practitioner managed care for persons with HIV infection. *Image: Journal of Nursing Scholarship, 25*(3), 172–177.

American Nurses' Association (1988). *Nurisng case management.* Kansas City, MO: The Association.

Anderson, W., O'Conner, B.B., MacGregor, R.R,, Schwartz, J.S. (1993). Patient use and assessement of conventional and alternative therapies for HIV infection and AIDS. *AIDS, 7*(4), 561–566.

Benjamin, A.E., Swan, J.H. (1989). Nursing home care for persons with HIV illness. *Generations, 13*(4), 63–64.

Berk, R.A., Poe, S.S., Baigis-Smith, J.A. (1992). Healthcare needs scale for patients with HIV/AIDS: Content validation. *Journal of the Association of Nurses in AIDS Care, 3*(3), 10–18.

Bohnet, N.I. (1986). Symptom control. In M. O'Rawe Amenta & N.L. Bohnet (Eds.), *Nursing care of the terminally ill* (pp. 67–80). Boston: Little, Brown.

Brown, M.A., Powell-Cope, G.M. (1991). AIDS family caregiving: Transitions through uncertainty. *Nursing Research, 40*(6), 338–345.

Burstin, H.R., Lipsitz S.R., Brennan, T.A. (1992). Socioeconomic status and risk for substandard medical care. *Journal of the American Medical Association, 268*(17), 2383–2387.

Cohn, J. (1988). The beginnings: Laboratory and animal studies. *New drug development in the United States* (DHHS publication No. [FDA] 88-3168) (pp. 8–11). Rockville, MD: U.S. Department of Health and Human Services.

Darbyshire, P. (1992). The core of nursing. *Nursing Times, 88*(36), 11–15.

Davis, K., Cameron, B., Stapleton, J. (1992a). Impact of HIV patient migration to rural areas. *AIDS Patient Care, 5*(5), 225–228.

Davis, K.A., Ferguson, K.J., Stapleton, J.T. (1992b). Moving home to live: Migration of HIV-infected persons to rural states. *Journal of the Association of Nurses in AIDS Care, 3*(4), 42–47.

Davis, K., Stapleton, J. (1991). Migration to rural areas by HIV patients: Impact on HIV-related healthcare use. *Infection Control and Hospital Epidemiology, 12*(9), 540–543.

De Ferrari, E., Paine, L.L., Gregor, C.L., et al. (1993). Midwifery care for women with human immunodeficiency virus disease in pregnancy: A demonstration project at the Johns Hopkins Hospital. *Journal of Nurse Midwifery, 38*(2), 97–102.

Department of Health and Human Services (1989). *AIDS clinical trials: Talking it over.* Bethesda, MD: National Institutes of Health.

Dunn, S. (1990). Providing care in a county nursing home AIDS unit. In V.E. Fransen (Ed.), *Proceedings: AIDS prevention and services workshop* (pp. 116–119). Princeton, NJ: Robert Wood Johnson Foundation.

Eisenberg, D.M., Kessler, R.C., Foster, C., Norlock, F.E., Calkin, D.R., Debanco, T.L. (1993). Unconventional medicine in the United States. *New England Journal of Medicine, 328*(4), 246–252.

Fee, E., Fox, D.M. (1992). Introduction: The contemporary historiography of AIDS. In E. Fee, D.M. Fox, (Eds.), *AIDS: The making of a chronic disease* (pp. 1–19). Berkeley: University of California Press.

Fee, E., Krieger, N. (1993). Thinking and rethinking AIDS: Implications for health policy. *International Journal of Health Services, 23*(2), 323–346.

Flieger, K. (1988). Testing in "real people." *New drug development in the United States* (DHHS publication No. [FDA] 88-3168) (pp. 13–14, 17). Rockville, MD: U.S. Department of Health and Human Services.

Franks, P., Clancy, C.M., Gold, M.R. (1993). Health insurance and mortality: Evidence from a national cohort. *Journal of the American Medical Association, 270*(6), 737–741.

Gebbie, K.M. (1989). The President's Commission on AIDS: What did it do? *American Journal of Public Health, 79*(7), 868–870.

Grau, L. (1984). Case management and the nurse. *Geriatric Nursing, 5*(8), 372–375.

Greenblatt, R.M., Hollander, H., McMaster, J.R., Henke, C.J. (1991). Polypharmacy among patients attending an AIDS clinic: Utilization of prescribed, unorthodox, and investigational treatments. *Journal of Acquired Immune Deficiency Syndromes, 4*(2), 136–143.

Groer, M. (1991). Psychoneuroimmunology. *American Journal of Nursing, 91*(8), 33.

Hand, R. (1989). Alternative therapies used by patients with AIDS. *New England Journal of Medicine, 320*(10), 672–673.

Hart, L.K., Freel, M.I., Milde, F.K. (1990). Fatigue. *Nursing Clinics of North America, 25*(4), 967–976.

Harvard AIDS Institute (1989). *Alternatives to hospital care for people with HIV infection* (Invitational Conference, November 8–10, 1989). Cambridge, MA: Harvard Schoool of Public Health.

Hodel, D. (1990, October 31). All fired up or just all fired. *Outweek, 70,* 30–31.

Holzemer, W.L. (1992). Linking primary health care and self-care through case management. *International Nursing Review, 39*(3), 83–89.

Hurley, P.M., Ungvarski, P.J. (1994). Home healthcare needs of adults with HIV disease/AIDS in New York City. *Journal of the Association of Nurses in AIDS Care, 5*(2), 33–40.

Imperato, P.J. (1990). Acquired immunodeficiency syndrome: The agenda for the 1990s. *New York State Journal of Medicine, 90*(3), 115–116.

Irish, A. (1989). Maintaining health in persons with HIV infection. *Seminars in Oncology Nursing, 5*(4), 302–307.

Kane, R.A., Caplan, A.L. (1990). Everyday ethics: Resolving dilemmas in nursing home life. New York: Springer Publishing Company.

Kane, R.A., Smith D. (1989). *Multiple perspectives on AIDS and the nursing home: A pilot study and recommendations for research* (report No. PB 90-101320). Rockville, MD: Agency for Health Care Policy and Research.

Kassler, W.J., Blanc, P., Greenblatt, R. (1991). The use of medicinal herbs by human immunodeficiency virus–infected patients. *Archives of Internal Medicine, 151*(11), 2281–2288.

Kator, M.J., Cunningham McBride, L. (1990). Developing a long-term care facility program for AIDS patients. *Pride Institute Journal of Long-Term Home Health Care, 9*(1), 15–19.

Layzell, S., McCarthy, M. (1993). Specialist or generic community nursing care for HIV/AIDS patients? *Journal of Advanced Nursing, 18*(4), 531–537.

Lindemer, S. (1990). Writing as therapy. *Coping, Living With Cancer, 4*(1), 31.

Linsk, N.L., Cick, P.J., Gianfrani, L. (1993). The AIDS epidemic: Challenges for nursing homes. *Journal of Gerontological Nursing, 19*(1), 11–22.

Lundberg, G.D. (1991). National health care reform: An aura of inevitability is upon us. *Journal of the American Medical Association, 265*(19), 2566–2567.

Lyne, B.A., Waller, P.R. (1990). The Denver Nursing Project in Human Caring: A model for AIDS nursing care and professional education. *Family and Community Health, 13*(2), 78–84.

MacFadden, D.K. (1988). Symptom control in AIDS. *Journal of Palliative Care, 4*(4), 42–45.

Martin, J.P. (1991). Issues in the current treatment of hospice patients with HIV disease. *The Hospice Journal, 7*(12), 31–40.

Master, R.J., Gallagher, D., Rivard, M., et al. (1993). An HMO for Medicaid-covered patients with AIDS (PWAs) [abstract No. PO-B38-2392]. *International Conference on AIDS, 9*(1), 534.

McCabe, E. (1992). Ozone therapies for AIDS. *AIDS Patient Care, 6*(6), 254–255.

McCann, K. (1991). The work of a specialist AIDS home support team: The views and experiences of patients using the service. *Journal of Advanced Nursing Practice, 16*(7), 832–836.

McNally, L., Mason-Beck, L. (1989). Day treatment for persons with AIDS. *Generations, 13*(4), 69–70.

Michaels, D., Levine, C (1992). Estimates of the number of motherless youth orphaned by AIDS in the United States. *Journal of American Medical Association, 268*(24), 3456–3461.

Monaco, G. (1989). Counseling patients about dubious and rip-off remedies for AIDS and ARC. *PAAC-NOTES, 1*(3), 80–84.

Morrison, C. (1990). Case management and the determination of appropriate care settings. In Agency for Health Care Policy and Resources Conference Proceedings. *Community-based care of persons with AIDS: Developing a research agenda* (DHHS publication No. PHS 90-3456) (pp. 75–82). Washington, DC: U.S. Government Printing Office.

Murray, R.H., Rubel, A.J. (1992). Physicians and healers—unwitting partners in health care. *New England Journal of Medicine, 326*(1), 61–64.

National Commission on AIDS (1990, August). *Annual report to the President and the Congress.* Washington, DC: U.S. Government Printing Office.

National Institute of Allergy and Infectious Diseases (1990). *NIAID AIDS research.* Bethesda, MD: The Institute.

National League for Nursing (1992, May 13). Community nursing centers: A promising new trend in American health care. New York: The League.

New York City Department of Health (1989) *HSA/New York City AIDS Task Force Report.* New York: The Department.

New York State Department of Health (1993, June). *AIDS: 100 questions and answers.* New York: The Department.

Newshan, G. (1989). Therapeutic touch for symptom control in persons with AIDS. *Holistic Nursing Practice, 3*(4), 45–51.

Nokes, K.M., Carver, K. (1991). The meaning of living with AIDS: A study using Parse's theory of man-living-health. *Nursing Science Quarterly, 4*(4), 175–179.

Nokes, K.M. Wheeler, Kendrew, J. (1994). Development of an HIV assessment tool. *Image: Journal of Nursing Scholarship, 26*(2), 133–138.

Perryman, S. (1990). AIDS: Perspective of a black woman as an epidemic among the myriads. *Body Positive, 3*(7), 37–38.

Pessin, N., Lindy, D., Stricoff, D.J., et al. (1993). Integrating mental health and home care services for AIDS patients. *Caring, 12*(5), 30–34.

Peters, D.A. (1988). Development of a community health intensity rating scale. *Nursing Research, 37*(4), 202–207.

Pomerantz, S., Harrison, E. (1990). End-stage symptom management. *AIDS Patient Care, 4*(1), 18–20.

Price, R.W., Brew, B. (1990). Management of the neurologic complications of HIV-1 infection and AIDS. In M.A. Sande & P. A. Volberding (Eds.), *The medical management of AIDS* (2nd ed.) (pp. 161–181). Philadelphia: W.B. Saunders.

Rogers, A.G. (1989). Analgesics: The physician's partner in effective pain management. *Virginia Medical, 116*(4), 164–170.

Salsberry, P.J., Nickel, J., O'Connell, M.O., et al. (1993). Home health care services for AIDS patients: One community's response. *Journal of Community Health Nursing, 10*(1), 39–51.

Sanders, P. (1989). Acupuncture and herbal treatment of HIV infection. *Holistic Nursing Practice, 3*(4), 38–44.

Schmidt, J. (1992). Case management problems and home care. *Journal of the Association of Nurses in AIDS Care, 3*(3), 37–44.

Schoefferman, J. (1988). Pain: Diagnosis and management in the palliative care of AIDS. *Journal of Palliative Care, 1*(4), 45–46.

Schroeder, C. (1993). *Cost-effectiveness of a theory-based nurse-managed center for persons living with HIV/AIDS* (publication No. 15-2548). New York: National League for Nursing.

Schroeder, C., Maeve, M.K. (1992). Nursing care partnerships at the Denver Nursing Project in Human Caring: An application and extension of caring theory in practice. *Advances in Nursing Science, 15*(2), 25–38.

Sherman, J.J., Johnson, P.K. (1991). Nursing case management. *Quality Assurance and Utilization Review, 6*(4), 142–145.

Smith, J., Landau, J., Bahr, R. (1990). AIDS in rural and small town America: Making the heartland respond. *AIDS Patient Care, 4*(3), 17–21.

Sowell, R.L., Fuszard, B., Gritzmacher, D. (1990). Services for persons with AIDS [Nurse executives report]. *Journal of Nursing Administration, 20*(7/8), 44–48.

Sowell, R.L., Gueldner, S.H., Killeen, M.R., et al. (1992). Impact of case management on hospital charges of PWAs in Georgia. *Journal of the Association of Nurses in AIDS Care, 3*(2), 24–31.

Stone, V.E., Seage, G.R., Hertz, T., Epstein, A.M. (1992). The relation between hospital experience and mortality for patients with AIDS. *Journal of the American Medical Association, 268*(19), 2655–2661.

Strawn, J. (1989). Complementary therapies: Maximizing the mind-body connection. In J. Meisenholder & C. La Charite (Eds.), *Comfort in caring: Nursing the person with HIV infection* (pp. 181–198). Glenview, IL: Scott, Foresman.

Swan, J.H., Benjamin, A.E., Brown, A. (1992). Skilled nursing facility care for persons with AIDS: Comparison with other patients. *American Journal of Public Health, 82*(3), 453–455.

Taravella, S. (1990). Who will provide long-term care for AIDS patients? *Modern Health Care, 20*(12), 38–39.

The Presidential Commission (1988, June). *Report of the Presidential Commission on the Human Immunodeficiency Virus Epidemic.* Washington, DC: U.S. Government Printing Office.

Ungvarski, P.J. (1987). AIDS and long-term care. *Caring, 6*(10), 44–47.

Ungvarski, P.J. (1988). Testimony on home care. In *The Presidential Commission on the Human Immunodeficiency Virus Epidemic: Hearing on care of HIV-infected persons— January 13–15, 1988.* Washington DC: U.S. Government Printing Office.

Ungvarski, P.J. (1989). Developing long-term plan of care for the HIV epidemic. *Caring, 8*(11), 4–8.

Wright, J., Bakken Henry, S., Holzemer, W.L., et al. (1993). Evaluation of community based nurse case management activities for symptomatic HIV/AIDS clients. *Journal of the Association of Nurses in AIDS Care, 4*(20, 37–47).

Wyatt, A. (1990). AIDS and the long-term care continuum. *Pride Institute Journal of Long-Term Home Health Care, 9*(1), 6–14.

13 Ethical Issues Related to the Care of Persons With HIV

Judith M. Saunders

The human face of AIDS should be ever before us. Respecting personal dignity and autonomy, respecting the need for confidentiality, reducing discrimination, and minimizing intrusiveness should all be touchstones in the development of HIV/AIDS policies and programs.

> *AIDS: An Expanding Tragedy, Final Report of the National Commission on AIDS* (1993, p. 12)

Ethical controversies within the context of HIV/AIDS have been influenced by the nature of the stigmatized population in the United States most affected by this disease: gay men, injection drug users, people of color, and people of poverty. Controversy has permeated discussions of HIV/AIDS since the first case of HIV/AIDS was diagnosed in 1981, and very often the controversy has been rooted in claims about whose perspective is morally correct. The controversies have been evident in bitter, often polarized, positions as individuals and groups affected by HIV/AIDS have taken stands on the right way to respond to this world pandemic, with one group advocating mandatory testing and isolation of HIV-seropositive individuals while other groups have advocated education and voluntary testing.

The disease occurred after scientific and technologic advances in medicine already had fueled debate about moral or ethical choices regarding the circumstances of life, death, reproduction, initiation and withdrawal of treatment, genetic manipulation of personal traits, and scientific integrity (Harron et al., 1983). No aspect of health care has been left untouched by the controversies about values and rights of human life, issues about life and

death, allocation of public funds for research and treatment, mandatory testing for HIV antibodies, informed consent, profit versus treatment, duty of health care workers (HCWs) to provide care, access of women, children, and minorities to involvement in research, honesty in research endeavors, and rights of patients to specify their own treatment course. Most of the topics were not unique to ethical controversy within the context of HIV/AIDS, but the nature of the illness and its affected population provided an urgency and intensity of debate not commonly encountered in debates before 1981. Walters (1988) cautioned that beneficence, justice, and autonomy must all be considered important in examining the public policy that governs society's response to AIDS.

This debate has not been waged in "center ring" by experts who entertained an interested and passive audience in the wings. Not waiting for an invitation, patients and their families voiced their concerns, AIDS activists sat at the conference tables and refused to leave, and HCWs asked hard questions out of fear and concern. New partnerships were formed between clinicians and their patients (Institute of Medical Ethics, 1992). Streets became theaters where actors/activists engaged the media to take messages of right and wrong to the public; they defied churches as the source of moral right and demanded new answers to old questions. HIV/AIDS has made many contributions to health care and to the way that moral issues are defined and debated.

While the knowledge base of ethics continues to draw heavily from normative ethics and associated principles, such as autonomy or utility, other views have gained attention. This chapter describes the knowledge base of

Table 13–1. Common Terms and Their Definitions

TERM	DEFINITION
Normative ethics	Application of moral reasoning to determine what ought to be done in a specific situation
Principle	Fundamental source of justification of judgments reached in situations
Dilemma	Moral reasoning indicating a choice between equally unappealing solutions
Rule	Specific guideline to actions for ethical principles and values (professional codes contain rules)
Rights	Justified claims that individuals/groups hold: their just due
Value	What an individual feels is important that provides a basis for ethical decisions

ethics: principles, rights, situation ethics, feminist ethics, and the ethics of caring. Ethical decision making is presented after a discussion of these ethical approaches. Together, approaches to ethics and ethical decision making should guide clinicians in their deliberations of ethical problems and encourage reflective responses.

The chapter considers ethical issues within the following topic areas: HIV/AIDS and the workplace; access to care; decisions about whether to accept or refuse treatments; and suicide, rational suicide, and assisted suicide. Case illustrations are provided to clarify specific ethical problems or to demonstrate the complexity of some dilemmas. A final section considers nursing research and ethics with specific suggestions for research that is needed.

MAJOR ETHICAL APPROACHES

Moral reasoning, or ethics, is that body of philosophical knowledge that deals with moral human conduct. All people struggle to weigh right and wrong in a given situation. Our deliberations reflect personal values that provide a sense of the right way to behave in ordinary human interaction, and as nurses we learned these values from our families, our teachers, our religions, and our own experiences, observations, and judgments about what is right and what is wrong. These values form the basis of our personal and traditional codes of conduct.

The terms "ethics" and "moral reasoning" will be used interchangeably in this chapter to refer to a body of knowledge that has evolved from moral philosophy and that applies analytic and critical approaches to moral problems and judgments (Beauchamp & Childress, 1989; Davis & Aroskar, 1991). Ethics invites a person to use reasoning rather than emotions in the process of forming judgments about what is right or wrong in the situation being considered. Table 13–1 defines terms that are pivotal to ethical discussions.

Principles of Ethics

Normative ethics is applied ethics—that is, the application of moral reasoning to determine which course of action is most acceptable. The two major theories that provide the basis of most moral reasoning are deontology and utilitarianism. Utilitarianism (also called teleology) gauges the worth of the actions by assessing the short-term and long-term consequences of actions. Deontology is concerned with duty and considers how actions are accomplished, not only their consequences. Whereas utilitarianians assert that the principle of utility justifies the other principles of ethics, deontologists consider an array of principles, even if they cannot always specify the utility. For example, when considering whether or not to tell a patient that she has terminal-phase lung cancer, the physician deontologist would believe that truth telling is most important, whereas the physician utilitarian would base the decision on the consequences of telling the truth versus concealing the prognosis.

To understand what is at stake in problem situations, such as keeping confidential a patient's plan of suicide, the nurse examines the principles most involved in the situation. This understanding will help point the way to actions that are morally correct in the situation; however, individuals may perceive different

Table 13–2. Definitions of Often Cited Principles and Rules of Ethics

PRINCIPLE OR RULE	DEFINITION
Autonomy	Self-governance. The autonomous person determines his or her own course of action in accordance with a plan chosen by self, with the capacity to understand consequences of the action.
Beneficence	Duty to help others further their important and legitimate interests.
Justice	Fair distribution of benefits and burdens in society. Justice requires a fair distribution of scarce resources, or a balance of claims and needs.
Nonmaleficence	Duty to prevent harm, remove harm, and provide benefit.
Utility	Balances benefits and harms and looks to the short-term and long-term consequences of the actions.
Paternalism	Duty to act for another person, when qualified, when the action is for the other person's good and she or he is unable to act for self. Used when autonomy is compromised.
Confidentiality	A rule that imposes duties not to disclose certain information. Person who discloses confidential information has the burden of proof to justify the conditions of disclosure.
Fidelity	Loyalty between humans, often in the context of voluntary relationships.
Sanctity of human life	Human life has an inherent value. A moderate interpretation is the usual practice, and this allows refusal of lifesaving treatments.
Truth telling, or veracity	Duty to tell the truth and not lie.

principles as having priority in the situation, so controversy may exist among individuals. Table 13–2 presents a brief definition of principles and rules of ethics and provides an accessible, quick reference to these terms.

Autonomy. Perhaps the U.S. heritage of rugged individualism has contributed to our society's high value on self-regulation, or right to autonomous behavior. The autonomous person makes decisions and determines actions to follow after selecting a plan. A person is a free agent—free to choose actions that either benefit or harm the self without constraint from others. However, not everyone qualifies to act as an autonomous agent. Those who cannot clearly understand the situation and the potential consequences of the chosen action are often termed "ineligible" to act as autonomous agents. This ineligibility may be temporary, such as when one's thinking is clouded by trauma or medications. In some cases, the ineligibility may be more durable, such as during childhood, or for individuals whose severe confusion prevents simple problem solving.

Because people are social beings, their in-dividual actions occur within a social context, so effects of their actions on others and on their community must also be considered. Regard for others automatically implies that certain circumstances might warrant constraints on personal autonomy. For example, when the action can harm others, then arguments are advanced that constraints are justified.

Autonomy is an important principle in many health care situations. For example, autonomy is important when a nurse determines whether a person (1) needs a guardian or conservator, (2) can provide informed consent for a procedure, (3) has the ability to refuse treatments, and (4) should have involuntary suicide prevention interventions.

Beneficence. The moral principle of beneficence calls forth the duty to provide benefit to others—that is, to help others when we are in a position to do so. Determining when doing good becomes a duty (moral obligation), rather than a commendable but not obligatory act (moral option), is difficult. Most ethicists recognize that limitations do exist on the duty of people to take positive action to promote good, but they debate how to decide the nature and degree of these limitations. Beauchamp & Childress (1989) argued that, in general, Person A has a duty of beneficence toward Person B when each of the following circumstances is present:

1. Person B is at significant risk of loss or damage.
2. Person A needs to act to prevent this loss.
3. Person A's action is likely to prevent loss or damage.
4. Person A incurs no significant risk in taking the action.
5. Person B will likely gain more than the potential harm that would come to Person A through the action taken.

Beneficence is especially important in health care when one is (1) assessing the nurse's duty to provide care, (2) informing others that they have been exposed to harmful substances or conditions, or (3) informing someone that a person plans to harm him or her.

Justice. The principle of justice is concerned with a fair distribution of society's burdens and benefits. Justice centers around deciding what should be distributed and what reasoning will guide those actions. Giving people their just due means, first, that a legitimate claim exists for the benefit being awarded; the benefit is not awarded to someone who does not deserve it, and those who deserve it receive their reward. This simple guideline still leaves room to argue about how that deserving claim should be established. Is a person deserving because of (1) equal stature with others who have a claim? (2) An established need for the benefit? (3) The amount of work extended? (4) Significant contributions made to society? (5) Or particular merit? (Beauchamp & Childress, 1989). For example, let us suppose that gene therapy is available for early HIV intervention. This therapy can effectively stop disease progression, but it is delivered through bone marrow transplant. How will people be qualified to receive this therapy? Who will have no access to this treatment? Who will make the decision?

Distributive justice is important when the resource (e.g., material, procedure) is particularly scarce or when the competition is great, such as gene therapy. Another example involves Bob, a 30-year-old man who lives in the Northwest. Bob said that his physician had informed him that he would die if he did not have either a heart transplant or an artificial heart installed. He was informed also that he would not be given a high priority for either of these procedures because he did not have a family, was gay, and did not have insurance.

The principle of distributive justice informs public policy on the distribution of budget allocations between research and treatment efforts. A less macro level of distributive justice in health care is determining which staff will be assigned to specific patients, such as the more experienced and competent staff to sicker or to more prominent patients.

Nonmaleficence. The principle of "nonmaleficence" calls for preventing harm and undoing harm. This principle is not absolute, and ethicists recognize that temporary suffering might be inflicted to cause a subsequent remedy or to prevent worse harm. Inflicting harm, however, always requires a moral justification. Even a risk of harm is to be avoided if possible, and actions that carry with them potential harm are considered carefully. Some ethicists restrict their interpretation of nonmaleficence to inflicting no harm, while using the principle of beneficence broadly to include preventing harm and removing harm (Beauchamp & Childress, 1989). The principle of nonmaleficence is important in considering diverse issues such as euthanasia, implementing clinical trials of a new drug, or refusing to care for patients with HIV disease.

Utility. The principle of utility examines the anticipated consequences of an action to judge its merit. This principle seeks actions that accomplish the greatest good for the largest number, or the least harm for the greatest number. Utility, then, weighs benefits against harm in a situation and tries to determine actions that will maximize benefits while minimizing harms. An action that is perceived as being too harmful in its long- or short-term consequences will be rejected.

As a principle, utility is one among many, not the supreme principle of the utilitarians—that is, it does not have greater priority than any other principle. Nor does the principle of utility always weigh the interest of society against the interests of an individual, but other principles (autonomy, beneficence, and nonmaleficence) are called on more often in considering the interests of the individual.

The principle of utility is pivotal in examining the costs and benefits of any particular action. Costs are often considerations of financial consequences, whereas the term "risk" is used when potential human harm is considered. The cost-benefit approach is important in examining research proposals as well as considerations of public health measures, such as mandatory testing for HIV antibody.

Paternalism. Paternalism involves acting on behalf of another person to prevent or restrict harm in circumstances where the person is unable to act for self. If Person A has Person B's permission to act in that situation, then Person A's behavior is not considered paternalistic. In paternalistic behavior, Person A intends to look out for the good and general welfare of Person B, and cannot be self-serving. Paternalism always needs to be justified because it always violates an existing moral rule. Typically, the justification for paternalistic action arises because Person B is perceived as being unable to act for self—because something has compromised Person B's autonomy.

Truth Telling. The duty to tell the truth seems to be both a simple and a clear responsibility appropriately associated with a morally right action. Is this duty unconditional, or are there instances where telling the truth might be harmful to others? Telling the truth is sometimes confused with the way that the truth is told. For example, it has been argued that telling someone that he or she has a terminal illness such as end-stage cancer or AIDS will take hope away from the person, so telling only a "partial truth" has been advocated. Shneidman (1980), on the

other hand, pointed out that the argument that hope should not be removed may be offered to protect the teller more than the patient, and he advocates that physicians, nurses, and other HCWs be taught how to be attentive to "what to tell whom, under what circumstances, and to what end." Shneidman explained that the truth should not be used as a weapon of attack but should be delivered with sensitivity to what the person can manage and use at the time, and perhaps the telling should be continued on another day when the person is ready to hear and use more information.

Shneidman, unlike Collins (1981), did not advocate withholding truth from patients "for their own good." Both withholding truth and telling such a partial truth that meaning is distorted are considered tantamount to lying, and both are common practices between nurses and their patients. Consider the patient who has said on many occasions, "When I progress to AIDS, I will kill myself, rather than witness my own costly deterioration." Will the truth of his diagnosis of AIDS do more harm than good—specifically, will the truth trigger a premature death through suicide or cause the patient to end his life saddened and without hope?

Whereas many people agree that truth telling is not an absolute duty (i.e., a duty without any constraints), fewer people agree on the criteria for determining when truth telling might be or would be harmful. First, a clear agreement on the nature of truth is not always reached, especially in the context of illness and its treatment. Second, predicting individual response to specific information is not a science, and many would argue that, as an art form, it is fairly primitive.

A different arena for considering issues and problems associated with truth telling has been labeled as whistle-blowing. "Whistle-blowing" refers to making public another's unethical and/or illegal practices and often pits an individual against a corporation or government agency. Telling the truth in these situations also has overtones of disloyalty to those being accused of unethical or illegal practices. The whistle-blower often has much to risk, such as job loss, in coming forward with the truth.

In health care, truth telling is involved with decisions about delivering bad news to patients or their families. Another issue in truth telling in health care involves informing the patient or research study participant about risks associated with specific procedures or medication.

Confidentiality. The rule of confidentiality imposes a duty on specific persons not to disclose certain information. There is an issue of privilege between the person and the information—for example, nurses are privileged to have certain information about patients to deliver effective care, and they are responsible for safeguarding that information to ensure that it does not go to nonprivileged persons. Confidentiality is a duty to the person and is not assigned to the information itself, outside of the person or persons who hold the information. For example, the nurse has confidential information about the results of John's HIV test. The slip of paper with that information blows out the nurse's car window and is retrieved by another person, Belinda. Belinda, who knows John socially, does not necessarily have a duty of confidentiality to John. Nurses who discuss their patients in public places, such as the cafeteria, elevator, or bus, risk violating their duty to hold in confidence privileged information.

Nurses, physicians, and other HCWs have a responsibility to keep the patient's information private, but there are times when keeping information confidential might pose risks to others and the staff's duty to keep information confidential therefore conflicts with the duty to protect others. For example, in the 14 months since James's diagnosis of AIDS, he has been in and out of hospitals and is again an inpatient. His condition is steadily deteriorating. James has been divorced for 4 years and has two children (aged 7 and 6 years), whom he sees often. He and his ex-wife are friendly. Only his ex-wife knows that he is gay. His parents live in the city and visit often; all the family members believe that James has leukemia. James has refused to tell his ex-wife that he has AIDS. Staff members are uncertain about what they should do—whether to maintain James's privacy or to respect James's ex-wife's and former gay lover's right to know of their exposure to HIV infection.

Fidelity. Fidelity is the duty to hold an agreement or promise. This rule is important in considering agreements not only between nurses and their patients but also between nurses and their employers. For example, an employer violates fidelity in a situation where the employer, on learning that an employee has been found to have HIV antibodies, terminates that employee solely because of the test results.

Sanctity of Life

Sanctity of life, also referred to as respect for life, is the view that life has an intrinsic value and that each individual is valuable and unique (The Hastings Center, 1987). A strong commitment to sanctity of life gives priority to this duty over other duties. If sanctity of life is valued absolutely over all other values, then individuals cannot refuse lifesaving treatments and suicide is never an acceptable option. In a society where sanctity of life is an absolute duty, the most abhorrent crime would be the crime of taking a life, and capital punishment would therefore be unthinkable. Sanctity of life is generally not held to such a rigid standard. The strongest sanctity-of-life view is a religious conviction that life is sacred, so individuals may not dispose of it as they choose. Even this view allows individuals in life-threatening circumstances to refuse treatment that would extend their lives, but not to commit suicide.

Today, we honor an individual's right to use or to forego life-sustaining treatment. Less agreement exists on the circumstances, if any, under which an individual has a right to seek death deliberately by independent action or with the active assistance of another person. Sanctity of life is a major consideration in shaping these judgments.

Situation Ethics

Proponents of situation ethics reject ethical rules that are applied to all situations. Instead, situation ethics looks to the situation for moral action guides and denies that any guide to decision making can be universally applied. Rules and guides for past actions provide examples of how similar situations have been handled in the past but do not impose an obligation on the person to act in a similar way in the current situation. For example, one nurse addressed the issue of when suicide is acceptable by asserting: "It depends on each case. There are no rules for when suicide is acceptable. You must judge each situation on its own merits" (Valente et al., 1993).

In considering the merits of situation ethics, one has to ask whether any moral rules are absolute and universal. Beauchamp and Childress (1989) offered several examples of rules that might be absolute and therefore preclude the usefulness of situation ethics: (1) act as a caring physician, and (2) avoid murder, when murder is defined as *unjustified* killing. Situation ethics has not gained strong support as an approach to ethical knowledge.

Rights and Responsibilities

Discussions of ethics often include assertions of individual and group rights, such as the assertions that all humans have a right to the respect of others, that a person has a right to voice his own opinion, or that a person's right to privacy is greater than another person's right to know. These discussions often reflect strong emotions but may not reflect positions that have been thoughtfully considered. Sometimes, when discussions surrounding moral rights cannot be resolved easily, people turn to legal experts for guidance, and yet the two types of rights are not the same. Curtin and Flaherty (1982, p. 4) defined a human right as "a person's just due." Other ethicists have asserted that there are no universally accepted human rights (Beauchamp & Childress, 1989). Nonetheless, this language—the language of "rights"—persists and has proved useful in examining some ethical issues. Beauchamp and Childress (1989) wrote of a moral right as a claim that is justified by ethical principles and rules; they pointed out that rights can be either negative or positive—that is, one can have the right to do or have something, or the right to *refuse* something. Not all claims are considered a

moral right, and whether or not a claim is truly a moral claim may be difficult to establish. The determination of a claim as a moral one, rather than as a want, may influence the assignment of the responsibility to respond to that claim.

When someone has a claim, or a right, to a form of conduct, a parallel responsibility or obligation is usually inferred. For example, if everyone has a moral right to health care, then who has the responsibility, or duty, to provide access to that care? Moreover, if patients have a right to privacy, then nurses share with other health care workers a responsibility to protect patient confidentiality. Brown (1987) pointed out that the American Nurses' Association (ANA) Code for Nurses charges nurses with this obligation for their patients. Other claims cannot be linked so easily with obligations, nor can responsibility be attached so easily to specific groups or individuals.

Because all individuals and groups have some rights, these rights will compete or conflict with each other on some occasions. Nurses have a right to pursue their own religious beliefs; however, even though these beliefs may condemn the lifestyles of some of their patients, these patients also have a right to respect. In other instances, nurses may find their values in conflict with circumstances in the work setting. For example, nurses have the right to adequate resources to deliver care in a manner that is safe for themselves and their patients and may disagree with their employers about what resources are adequate for accomplishing this. Trauma nurses may believe that their work requires puncture-resistant gloves for adequate protection, but the hospital administration may believe that the added margin of safety is too small to warrant such a large increase in the cost of gloves. Typically, most nurses learn more about their responsibilities than they learn about their rights as nurses.

Curtin (1990) described nursing as a moral art that encompasses professional obligations derived from the covenant that it has with the public to provide care and to improve quality of life among those seeking nursing services. Meeting this covenant requires nursing to be proactive and involves both individual and collective obligations.

Ethics of Caring and Feminist Ethics

As interest in moral reasoning has been strengthened during recent decades, concerns have also surfaced about the adequacy of ethical principles in guiding our understanding of and responses to current problems. Gilligan's study (1982) of female moral development and reasoning helped to focus the criticism that current principle-based approaches to moral reasoning devalued relationship issues while overemphasizing logic. Noddings (1984) developed an ethics-of-caring ideal that emphasized relationship (how we meet each other morally) and human affect and that rejected the universality of principle-based ethics. In the ethics-of-caring model, one does not assess a situation by considering autonomy, beneficence, and justice; instead, one considers commitment, reciprocity, grasping the other's reality, and self-maintenance. Others have added to our understanding of the concept of caring, our knowledge of caring as an ethical model, and the relationship between caring and practice (Benner & Wrubel, 1989; Bishop & Scudder, 1987; Condon, 1992; Neil & Watts, 1991; Stevenson & Tripp-Reimer, 1989; Watson, 1988).

Questions have emerged about caring as an ethical ideal to assist us in interacting effectively with ethical problems. Hoagland (1991) argued that the Noddings formulation (1984) of caring does not allow an adequate analysis of oppression and does not support a vision of change.

Women's experiences with oppression, indifference, and hostility parallel the experiences of those affected by HIV infection. Because of these experiences, feminist ethicists criticize traditional ethical approaches as being ineffective in addressing such oppression (Card, 1991). Jaggar (1991) asserted that feminist ethics ensure that the moral experiences of men and women are regarded respectfully. Jaggar (1991) also set the agenda of feminist ethics as examining issues such as domination, control, domestic and international inequities, gender privilege, public and private realms, and the actual as well as the hypothetical.

Both the ethics of caring and feminist ethics move from the universal to the contextual, and both place a priority on understanding and preventing domination. These emerging ethical approaches may provide insights and useful new formulations of moral action.

RESOLVING ETHICAL DILEMMAS

Nurses confront ethical problems each day in their personal and professional lives, and they recognize that understanding definitions of principles will not, by themselves, be sufficient for ethical problem solving. An ethical problem or dilemma occurs when the nurse is aware of a conflict among competing rights, such as the following: (1) the patient is seeking assistance in deciding the "right" course of action; (2) the staff members disagree about the right actions; (3) the patient and family want one course of action, whereas the staff members advocate another; and (4) conflict exists among legally sanctioned family and either life partners or friends who are close enough to be considered family about the best course of action for a patient who cannot make decisions for himself or herself. Many resources exist to help people resolve these conflict situations: available literature, specialists (such as ethicists), or ethics committees at a hospital or organizational level. Legal solutions to ethics problems are not always satisfactory resolutions because legal actions are rooted in traditions different than those of ethical concerns—that is, what is legally sanctioned is not always right.

Resources to Help in Formulating Actions

Ethics Committees. Some hospitals, long-term care agencies, and ambulatory care resources have formed either nursing or interdisciplinary ethics committees to assist staff, patients, and families in deciding actions for ethical problems and dilemmas (Albrizio et al., 1992; American Hospital Association, 1985; Schultz & Moore, 1993; Stoll & Mason, 1993). If your agency or organization does not have a resource (such as an ethicist or an ethics committee), you may want to explore establishing one. Exploring various options helps the nurse choose the type of resource that best matches his or her own agency. One of the most comprehensive ethics programs is at Mt.

Sinai Hospital in New York City and includes the following features: full-time nurse ethicist; a nursing ethics committee; monthly nursing ethics seminars; regularly scheduled meetings between the AIDS center nurse clinicians and the nurse ethicist; and inclusion of ethics in nursing grand rounds on AIDS (Stoll & Mason, 1993). Most resources are less extensive but include an educational program on ethics for nursing staff and routine meetings to discuss ethical concerns that arise in caring for patients with HIV disease.

Other Resources. The American Nurses' Association (ANA) established the Center for Ethics and Human Rights, and this office actively addresses topics that concern nurses as they respond to clinical issues of ethics and human rights.* Several state nursing associations, such as the California Nurses' Association, have established ethics committees and may offer members direct consultation for ethical problems. The ANA and some state nursing associations have published position papers on common ethical problems that nurses encounter. Organizations also have published position papers or codes for nurses to guide nurses in their care of people affected by HIV disease.

Models of Ethical Decision Making

Cameron (1993) described the model of decision making for ethical problems that people living with AIDS use. This three-step model includes the following three questions: What should I believe? Who should I be? What should I do?

Most nurses use models based on principles to formulate action plans and to resolve clinical dilemmas. These models include the following steps: (1) describe the situation, including who was involved (and their roles), when the major events occurred, and the setting(s); (2) identify the ethical principles (e.g., values, rules) involved; (3) discuss proposed solutions and what each of the solutions is

*Colleen Scanlon is the director of this center. She can be reached at 202-554-4444, ext. 294, American Nurses' Association, 600 Maryland Ave., S.W., Suite 100 West, Washington, DC 20024-2571.

trying to accomplish; (4) identify alternative actions available; and (5) decide the possible outcomes of these actions, including identification of the way that moral principles would be affected (Aroskar, 1980; Curtin, 1978).

Gadow (1990) recommended that a decision-making model be based on advocacy nursing, in which advocacy is directed toward assisting patients in their own actions, not in doing for them. This decision-making model is more accurately described as advocacy for patient autonomy. The decision-making process includes the following five steps: (1) assessing the patient's ability for self-determination, (2) determining the nature of the nurse-patient relationship, (3) disclosing the nurse's views on the situation, (4) determining the patient's values, and (5) determining other, individual values that may have an impact on the patient in considering the situation. This decision-making model emerges from autonomy and focuses on the individual in context, similar to the ethics-of-caring model.

Most groups develop operating rules to facilitate their discussions. First they reduce pressures on individuals to arrive at a consensus. They also encourage disagreements to surface and be heard. At the same time, they encourage individuals to examine consequences of their own proposed actions while also hearing other's concerns. As the group examines the problem, they often discover unresolved clinical problems, rather than ethical problems or dilemmas.

CHOOSING TO ACCEPT OR REFUSE TREATMENTS

Although making choices about medical treatment has grown more complex each year, the right of the individual to choose an unpopular or harmful procedure has grown more acceptable. Freedom of choice remains so highly valued in American society that autonomy seems to be the cornerstone principle that other principles are measured against. Conflict is most apparent when consequences of harmful choices are examined (autonomy vs utility), when one person's autonomy negatively affects another, or when one person's autonomy interferes with another's rights and responsibilities. Determining whether a person can act autonomously is challenging when the individual has intermittently diminished capacity, demonstrated by forgetfulness, short attention span, confusion, or disorientation. Agich (1990) cautioned that respecting autonomy in long-term care for chronically ill and elderly patients means offering some meaningful options from a limited array of actions. The role of autonomous choice when the available choices are not meaningful to the person has received scant attention in ethics. Finally, the nurse's role in advising patients about their choices must be considered. These issues will be discussed under the following headings: (1) accepting and refusing recommended treatments, (2) gaining access to unrecommended treatments, and (3) determining the staff's role in patient choice.

Accepting and Refusing Recommended Treatments

Usually, individuals are free to accept or to refuse the medical treatments recommended by their physicians and other health care staff. The person's right to determine whether treatments match personal values does not necessarily cease when the person is no longer able to choose. For example, advance directives and durable power of attorney are two methods of soliciting choice from the able person in anticipation that she or he might not always remain able. These directives allow the individual to make personal preferences known.

Ideally the patient, without constraint, chooses options in partnership with the physician and the nurse, who share their expert knowledge with the patient. Conflicts arise because many situations fall outside this ideal situation and force caregivers to struggle with conditions that limit autonomy.

Gaining Access to Unrecommended Treatments

Example. Franklin knew that he was in a late stage of AIDS. His CD4$^+$ T-cell counts,

taken last year, had fallen to 10. An anxious guardian of his own health care, Franklin believed that a new antiviral treatment might be worth trying, although his condition had not been improved by other single or combined antiviral agents. When Franklin asked his physician to prescribe this new treatment, which was in clinical trials, his physician responded: "With 10 T-cells, why bother trying? That is sort of like taking out insurance after the house has been bombed." This response was not a tactful refusal. Franklin persisted, asserting his right to try the medication. He pointed out that the drug's merits were described in *BETA (Bulletin of Experimental Trials Activity)*. Franklin did try the drug, but the struggle further damaged his relationship with the physician, so Franklin requested a different physician in his health maintenance organization.

Issues Related to Example. HCWs are not required to prescribe or participate in treatments that they believe will either harm patients or simply be ineffective. The physician or nurse has many issues to consider in responding to a patient's request for a specific treatment. One issue is the patient's challenge of the stance that the HCW is the expert and should know what is best for him or her. Another issue is considering the consequences of participating in an activity perceived as ineffective or harmful. The nurse and the physician might be able to participate in a treatment that they have judged harmful by monitoring the patient for adverse effects to provide some degree of safety. Preserving a long-standing and effective relationship with the patient might be another consequence that would influence a decision to participate in an activity perceived as harmful or ineffective.

The balance of power and control within a patient-HCW relationship is a dynamic force that varies according to the issue being considered and the resources of the persons involved. The HCW will exert more control when safety and ethical wrongdoing are perceived but can afford to soften influence when less is at stake in the situation.

Determining the Staff's Role in Patient Choice

In Gadow's model (1990) of ethics and decision making, the nurse is an active participant, and the nurse's view of the situation is offered to patients who need to choose a course of action. This is a major departure from the typical practice of trying to present information objectively to reduce pressure on patients. Gadow (1990) stated that her recommendation is based on autonomy as pivotal in nursing action. In some situations the nurses' and other HCWs' duty to protect patients may necessitate actions that seem to limit patient autonomy.

Example. Rosa and her husband, Bill, had used drugs throughout their 3 years of marriage, when Bill was identified as having HIV disease. He died within a few weeks after the diagnosis was made, and Rosa found herself both widowed and pregnant. She already had two other young children. She agreed to be tested, and results were positive. She entered a drug rehabilitation program and has been clean and sober for 2½ years. She is proud of being a good mother to her three healthy children despite the challenges of her failing health, severe fatigue, and repeated episodes of infection. On her last visit the home health nurse was distressed with Rosa's deteriorated condition and questioned whether Rosa was able to provide a safe environment for her children. The nurse wondered whether to initiate proceedings to have the children placed in foster care. The home health nurse had not discussed her concerns and recommendations with Rosa because she wanted to consult with her team first.

Issues Related to This Example. The nurse acted out of beneficence. Aware that Rosa neglected her own needs to provide what her children needed, the nurse was concerned with protecting both Rosa and the children. A major issue in the team discussion was Rosa's capacity to make an informed decision, because she had increasing problems with attention span and forgetfulness. The team also considered the importance to Rosa of being a good parent and the excellent relationship that she had with her children.

The team ended with the following plan of care: (1) the physician would initiate a neurobehavioral assessment of Rosa; (2) the home health aide's services would be increased to 5 days a week; (3) the social worker would work with Rosa to see whether she had family and/ or friends who could help her with shopping and during evenings and weekends; (4) the nurse would encourage Rosa to start planning for the placement of her children once she became too sick to care for them; and (5) the nurse would help Rosa keep an energy log to allocate her limited energy to activities that mattered to her. What had seemed initially to be a recommendation for paternalistic action from staff revealed a complex situation requiring actions that attended to both clinical and ethical domains. The final plan tried to include meaningful options for Rosa and her children.

HIV AND THE WORKPLACE

For many nurses the workplace not only provides a source of income necessary for personal and family needs but also reinforces self-perception and a sense of worth. At work, nurses do not have a free choice of colleagues nor of their activities. Expectations of the workplace include an environment of mutual respect, adequate resources to complete nursing tasks, and a safe environment.

Health care settings have all the expectations and obligations of other types of work settings, and in addition they are expected to be safe for all and to be healing environments for patients. The public expects those who work in health care settings to provide an environment where fears can be stilled, not intensified, and where illness can be cured, not contracted.

The ethical issues surrounding HIV and the workplace encompass questions of how to establish and maintain a safe environment for patients and HCWs, and how to safeguard rights when nurses' and other HCWs' rights conflict with patients' rights. Addressing these issues encompasses the scope of ethical knowledge and pits clinical knowledge against public fears and concerns. The following discussion of HIV and the workplace is organized around protecting HCWs, protecting patients, and work setting ethical issues.

Protecting Health Care Workers

Example. In 1985 Barbara Fassbinder, RN (1993), was on duty in the emergency room of a small Wisconsin hospital when a patient was brought in by two people who did not seem to know the patient very well. The patient was in acute distress and soon went into respiratory arrest. During the unsuccessful attempt to resuscitate the patient, Ms. Fassbinder disconnected an arterial line and held a pressure bandage in place for 10 minutes. She noticed blood on her finger and wiped it away, but it was about 45 minutes before she was free to wash her hands. Neither she nor other staff wore gloves during this procedure because they were not performing sterile procedures. A few months later, Ms. Fassbinder was confirmed as the first HCW to have a work-related HIV infection that was not secondary to a percutaneous exposure.

Scope of Risk of HIV Infection to HCWs in Hospitals. The Centers for Disease Control and Prevention (CDC) extensively studies the risk of transmission of HIV after an HCW's percutaneous exposure. A report from the U.S. Office of Technology Assessment (1992) provided the following summary: Of 1,989 HCWs who reported 2,119 exposures, six HCWs have undergone seroconversion as a result of occupational percutaneous exposure. This clearly indicates a very low rate of risk per exposure, specifically, 0.30%. The risk rate for nonpercutaneous exposures such as Ms. Fassbinder's is much smaller. Although the risks are small, the stakes are high because the disease is life-threatening, and it is these stakes that have fueled nurses' fears. Despite such widespread fears of HIV infection, studies have shown that nurses and other HCWs do not use universal precautions consistently, a measure that would prevent most, though not all, exposures (Naccache et al., 1993; Willy et al, 1990). In an effort to reduce their risk at work, many nurses and physicians continue to call for mandatory testing of patients in situations where they fear increased risk of exposure— for example, during surgery (Colombotos et al., 1991).

Ethical Issues. The health care agency has a responsibility to provide a reasonably safe work environment for its employees, which includes access to adequate equipment and supplies for nurses to use in barrier precautions. This responsibility now has the weight of law: the Occupational Safety and Health Administration (OSHA) requires health care settings to implement universal precautions and to provide infection control plans along with personal protective equipment, worker training, and postexposure follow-up (U.S. Office of Technology Assessment, 1992).

During the first decade of the AIDS epidemic, the types of exposure that posed risk of HIV infection in the workplace were well documented. Universal precautions and safe management of sharps provided adequate protection to nurses and other HCWs. It is the nurse's responsibility to be aware of this body of knowledge and to apply reasonable precautions to work situations. For example, hepatitis B virus is much easier to contract after exposure than is HIV; a vaccine is available to nurses, but many nurses fail to be vaccinated.

Nurses must use reasonable precautions to protect themselves as they provide care to patients. To determine precautions needed, the nurse must assess the circumstances of the nurse-patient care situation. For example, whereas HIV can be contracted only if the virus enters the bloodstream of the nurse or HCW, tuberculosis is spread through airborne droplets in sneezes and coughs. Because individuals with AIDS have a high incidence of tuberculosis infection, nurses need to use adequate barriers to protect themselves and other patients from tuberculosis as well as other infectious illnesses. The nurse's general moral responsibility to provide knowledge-based care is framed in the ANA Code for Nurses (1985), which gives nurses the duty to maintain competence in nursing. It also assigns to individual nurses the responsibility for his or her own judgments and actions.

Testing of Patients in Acute-Care Settings. A practice with popular support is not necessarily a morally supportable practice. A national survey of physicians and registered nurses reported strong support among physicians and nurses for mandatory testing of surgical patients (Colombotos et al., 1991). The Oncology Nursing Society's position paper on HIV-related issues (Halloran et al., 1988, p. 214) states: "Before there can be restriction of an individual's autonomy, it must be demonstrated that such restrictions will result in an overriding benefit to the cause of a larger societal good." The CDC (1993) recently updated the recommendations for HIV testing of patients in acute care settings because of recent surveys and reports that estimated that 77% of HIV-infected patients with primary diagnoses other than HIV/AIDS were hospitalized in 11% of the nation's hospitals. The CDC did not support mandatory testing but recommended that voluntary, confidential testing be offered to patients, with caution that testing is not a substitute for universal precautions and other infection control programs. The CDC's recommendations emphasized conditions of voluntary testing that had been identified by Walters (1988): (1) counseling to help people understand the test results, (2) establishment of an environment of nondiscrimination, and (3) protection of the confidentiality of test results.

Earlier studies reported variations and abuse in HIV testing in hospitals because patients were tested without their permission, patients lacked risk factors, and physicians misinterpreted the test results (Henry et al., 1988a, 1988b). These abuses disregarded the patient's autonomy, while also increasing the patient's potential harm, because confidentiality was not protected adequately. If voluntary testing programs are initiated in acute care settings, then policies and procedures must ensure voluntariness (not coercion), confidentiality, the patient's right to refuse recommended testing without penalty, available counseling, and continued staff compliance with the full infection control program, including universal precautions. These policies

and procedures will help to ensure that patients have the tools they need to support their right to autonomy; those who voluntarily agree to be tested and are found to have HIV seropositivity may benefit from early treatment measures, which are now available. Chapter 2 provides a complete discussion of HIV testing and counseling procedures.

While the HCW's risk of infection from patients is minimal, it is a greater risk than that of patients in becoming infected from their HCWs. Nurses have a right to safety, so they must have access to the protective devices (masks, gloves, gowns, soap) needed for their own safety. Nurses must exercise adequate professional judgment about the protection required for the specific situation.

Testing of Pregnant Women and/or Newborn Infants. The rapid increase of HIV/AIDS among women has brought new challenges in providing access to care for women and their children, and in pitting women's rights against those of their babies. Some child-care providers advocate routine involuntary screening of all newborn infants, or pregnant women, whereas other clinicians wonder whether the clinical benefits can justify the significant loss of freedom that women incur (*AIDSline*, 1992).

An ongoing anonymous survey conducted by the CDC has found that 1 of 667 women who delivers a baby has HIV antibodies, and the percentage of pregnant women who agree to voluntary testing varies greatly from one program to another (*AIDSline*, 1992). One question that needs to be answered in deciding the public worth of a proposed routine screening program is, How would HIV-infected mothers and infants benefit from such a program? Another question to explore is, What are the potential harmful effects of the testing program, especially for women who learn that they have HIV?

Dumois (1993) argued eloquently about the dangers to women and their babies if mandatory routine testing is initiated for infants. These dangers include denial of privacy to women, increased harm to women, potential harm to infants because of denial of treatments, and the lack of established benefits for infants as a result of proposed early intervention.

Protecting Patients in Health Care Settings

Example. Bob is an obstetrician/gynecologist who shares a practice with six other physicians. His practice is varied and includes occasional gynecologic surgery. His colleagues and his patients have been aware of his homosexuality. When Bob learned that he was infected with HIV, he told his colleagues but not his patients. Soon after he learned of his seropositivity, *Pneumocystis carinii* pneumonia developed. He responded well to treatment and soon felt well enough to resume practice. In the interim, his colleagues met and decided that it was not wise for him to resume practice unless he limited his activities and obtained informed consent from his patients. Bob disagreed, saying that he had a right to privacy, that he posed no danger to his patients, and that his partners were being unreasonable and greedy.

Should any constraints be placed on Bob's activities? Which activities should he continue and which should he curtail or stop? Should he obtain informed consent from his patients, and if this is justified in Bob's case, is it justified for all HCWs? Who should decide these issues, inasmuch as Bob and his partners all have something to gain or lose with almost any decision made?

Scope of Risk of HIV Infection to Patients. Before 1985, when routine screening of all blood donations was instituted, the patients' main risk of HIV infection in health care settings was from blood transfusions. More recently, the public became frightened of contracting HIV infection from HIV-seropositive HCWs when six patients of a Florida dentist with HIV were infected by him. How they were infected remains unconfirmed, although a most likely source was inadequately cleaned instruments. Studies to determine the risk to patients in receiving care from HIV-infected HCWs have confirmed that the risks are very low: the CDC has estimated that 13 to 128 patients may have been infected during a span of 10 years, although

only six have been confirmed (CDC, 1993; El-Mallakh et al., 1992; Lo & Steinbrook, 1992; U.S. Office of Technology Assessment, 1992). Figure 13–1 shows the source of infection reported by the CDC in 92 HIV-seropositive patients among 19,036 patients treated by 57 HIV-seropositive HCWs.

Despite the low risk of patient infection from HIV-infected HCWs, public and political action has been noteworthy through media coverage, bills introduced in Congress, and recommendations about HCW-patient contacts from government agencies. Many nurses and physicians agree with the general public that patient risk of infection from HIV-infected HCWs justifies mandatory testing of HCWs, contrary to scientific recommendations (Colombotos et al., 1991).

Clearly, public perception of risk is great while experts continue to estimate a minimal risk of infection from HCWs. Any ethical solution to protecting patients from infection through contact with HIV-infected HCWs must address both perception of risk and expert estimation of risk. These two perspectives place respect for HCW autonomy in conflict with the patient's right to be protected from infected HCWs (El-Mallakh et al., 1992). The nature of the contract between the patient and his or her physicians and nurses requires the promotion of the well-being of patients and the prevention of harm to patients. Fear of infection might prevent some patients from seeking care or from using recommended remedies, such as surgery, if they cannot trust their physicians and nurses to be safe. Still, compulsory testing of all HCWs would be too expensive and too intrusive into privacy for the small margin of safety that might conceivably be added.

The CDC's current recommendations for voluntary testing and minimal restrictions on HCW activity that involves exposure-prone invasive procedures represent a compromise between recognition of differential risk assessment, political expediency, awareness of public fear, and respect for the HCW's autonomy (CDC, 1991; Lo & Steinbrook, 1992). The principle of nonmaleficence supports voluntary HIV testing and restriction of exposure-prone invasive activities to protect patients from harm. An exposure-prone activity,

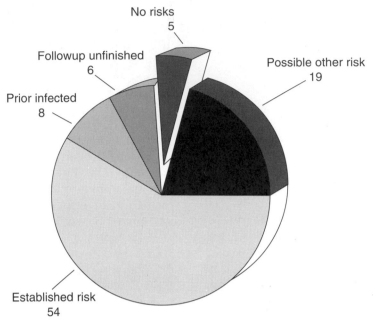

Figure 13–1. Source of infection among 92 HIV positive patients. N = 19,036 patients treated by 57 HIV positive health care workers. (From Centers for Disease Control and Prevention [May 7, 1993] Update: Investigations of persons treated by HIV-infected health-care workers—United States. *Mortality and Morbidity Weekly Report, 42*(17):329–331, 337.)

such as using fingers and a sharp object in a confined or poorly visualized site, presents a risk of percutaneous HCW injury that is likely to bring the HCW's blood in contact with the patient's body cavity, subcutaneous tissues, and/or mucous membranes (Lo & Steinbook, 1992). Other than nurse-midwives, few nurses are likely to engage in exposure-prone invasive activities, and the recommendations of the CDC do not suggest any other restrictions on professional practice. All HCWs who perform invasive procedures are recommended to know their HIV status and to seek counsel from expert panels about clinical activities (U.S. Office of Technology Assessment, 1992). Nurses are less likely than physicians, under current guidelines, to be in a position where their autonomy and right to privacy are in conflict with activities required to protect patients.

Following practices of infection control appropriate to the situation provides protection to the HCW from HIV-infected patients and to the patient from HIV-infected HCWs. Nurses do have a right to privacy, including confidentiality about HIV status. The CDC guidelines about seeking advice from expert panels for HIV-infected nurses and other HCWs who perform invasive procedures weighted HCW autonomy and right to privacy as less compelling than nonmaleficence.

If public pressure continues to propose mandatory testing of HCWs, the consequences could be great. Curtin (1992) cautioned that unnecessarily restrictive practices for HIV-infected HCWs "leads to a 'slippery slope' down which the American people will slide to the lowest levels of bigotry and cruelty." Faced with loss of privacy, loss of access to performing meaningful clinical work, and loss of revenue, HCWs may choose to leave their professions for other work. Recruiting new workers may prove difficult, and new workers require years to develop competency and knowledge that more experienced workers possess. These losses could result in a lower standard of health care—exactly the opposite effect being sought. Table 13–3 provides recommendations to prevent HIV transmission in health care settings.

Other Work-Setting Ethical Issues. Recent rumors suggest that hospitals and health care agencies in the private sector in

Table 13–3. Preventing HIV Transmission in Health Care Settings

NATIONAL COMMISSION ON AIDS RECOMMENDATIONS	CDC RECOMMENDATIONS
Universal precautions	Universal precautions
Improve infection control, including equipment	HCWs who do not perform invasive procedures should not limit clinical activity
Monitoring and education according to OSHA regulations	HCWs who perform exposure-prone procedures should know HIV status
Acknowledge public fears and address them without allowing rational judgment to be overwhelmed	HIV+ HCWs who perform exposure-prone procedures should seek counsel from expert review panel on these activities
Use least restrictive alternatives to reduce or eliminate risk of HIV infection for patients and HCWs	
No mandatory HCW testing for HIV	No mandatory HCW testing for HIV

Adapted from National Commission on AIDS. (1993) *AIDS: An Expanding Tragedy.* The Final Report of the National Commission on AIDS. Washington, D.C.
OSHA, Occupational Safety and Health Administration.

some large urban areas have curtailed the hiring of single male nurses as a method of reducing the possibility of hiring HIV-infected staff. If this rumor is true, it is an unethical and unacceptable discrimination against a group. What are the ethical issues involved, if any, in having HIV-infected nursing staff? Specific problems have included (1) public fear of infection from HIV-infected HCWs in hospitals, clinics, long-term care facilities, or home care agencies that employ infected nurses, causing patients to seek care elsewhere; (2) increased group insurance rates as a result of HIV infected staff, who use their insurance to a much greater extent than other employees; and (3) uneven workload distribution because of HIV-infected nurses who cannot carry a full workload.

These problems have in common an economic concern that is rooted in fear more than in ethical concerns. Staff with HIV/AIDS should receive the same insurance benefits and health care coverage as staff with other chronic, life-threatening illnesses. The Americans with Disabilities Act (1990) protects people from job denial or loss because of their disability, such as HIV infection, but extending hospital privileges to physicians is not included in this act. Health care agencies have a responsibility to educate their patients about the reality of their concerns. Solutions that health care agencies seek in staffing their settings with qualified nurses while attending to their patients' concerns should not create more problems than they solve for any group involved.

San Francisco General Hospital has a large number of HCWs who are HIV infected, and they are assured of job security and the right to carry out clinical practice activities provided they comply with infection control policies (Makulowich, 1992). Barbara Fassbinder (1993) reported that she was reassigned to "paper-shuffling tasks" after she contracted HIV infection on the job, and she proposes that nurses get involved with their own agencies to determine the policies already in place to protect HIV-infected HCWs, or to initiate the needed policies. Table 13–4 identifies workplace principles that many businesses already have initiated to establish fair and standard practices.

ACCESS TO CARE

Access to care involves several important dimensions that blend together into an integrated mosaic: (1) health care facilities and workers must be willing to provide care for people with HIV/AIDS; (2) individuals must have means to pay for their health care, such as medical insurance, independent wealth, or government funds; (3) health care resources

Table 13–4. Workplace Principles

1. Afford people with AIDS or HIV infection the same rights and opportunities as people with other serious illnesses.
2. Set employment policies that, at a minimum, comply with all government regulations.
3. Remember that scientific evidence shows that people with AIDS do not risk infecting co-workers through ordinary workplace contact.
4. Endorse unequivocally—from the highest levels of the company—nondiscriminatory employment policies and educational programs about AIDS.
5. Communicate management support of these policies to workers in simple, clear, and unambiguous terms.
6. Provide employees with sensitive and accurate education about risk reduction in their personal lives.
7. Protect the confidentiality of employee medical information.
8. Prevent work disruption and rejection by co-workers of an employee with AIDS by educating all employees before an incident occurs, and as needed thereafter.
9. Prohibit HIV screening as part of general preemployment or workplace physical examinations.
10. In occupational settings where there may be a risk of exposure to HIV (as in health care, where workers may be exposed to blood), provide specific, ongoing training, as well as the necessary equipment, for appropriate infection control.

Adapted from Citizens Commission on AIDS for New York and Northern New Jersey. (Summer 1991) AIDS Prevention and Education: Reframing the message. *AIDS Education and Prevention, 3*(2), 147–163.

must exist to care for HIV/AIDS patients, in rural or urban areas, locally and abroad; and (4) health care must meet minimal standards of competence and quality. Standards should include delivery of care in a culturally competent manner to the populations being served. Eliason (1993) pointed out that ethical nursing practice requires that the culture and beliefs of the client be considered. Embedded in issues of access to care are individual rights versus the public good, the distribution of society's benefits and burdens and the examination of the consequences, and the outcomes of decisions.

Duty to Provide Care

The following is an excerpt of a letter addressed to the author of a published journal article about AIDS. The letter was from a registered nurse and a writer, and he asserted:

> Yes, I am still a bedside-care nurse, and in keeping with considering myself a true professional, I choose not to care for AIDS patients on a selective basis. If it is an intravenous drug abuser, I'll care for them [sic] without any qualms. You may ask, Why? I blame our own permissive society for it's permissiveness to run amok, insofar as drugs are concerned. These poor igno-

ramus [sic] have "made their bed." out of ignorance, addiction and naivety [sic]. If a homosexual pt. tells me (convincingly) "I know I've sinned and been wrong," I'll take care of him.

The nurse who wrote this letter would be acting contrary to ethical guidelines for professional nursing if he based his refusal to care for persons with HIV/AIDS on his view that homosexuality or drug use is sinful. He also would be subject to legal action. Recently, Attorney General Janet Reno filed civil rights lawsuits against two dental offices because they had refused to treat HIV-infected patients (Ostrow & Cimons, 1993). This legal action was based on the provisions of the Americans with Disabilities Act, which took effect in January 1992 and bars discrimination against individuals with disabilities, including HIV/AIDS. Although unethical and illegal, refusal to care for patients with HIV/AIDS is not uncommon; hence educators and administrators have a responsibility to examine their policies and practices to ensure that students and clinicians have the information they need.

Numerous professional organizations within nursing and other health care disciplines have taken unequivocal stands that their clinicians have a duty to care for HIV/

AIDS patients (ANA, 1988; Council on Ethical and Judicial Affairs, 1988; Halloran et al., 1988). Despite these professional organization guidelines, several surveys reported that many nurses were reluctant to care for HIV/AIDS patients because they feared for their own safety (Kelly et al., 1988; Curry et al., 1990). This reluctance raises ethical questions such as: What justifies the nurse's duty to provide care? And under what circumstances, if any, may a nurse refuse to care for a person with HIV/AIDS?

Nursing is a service profession whose members have a responsibility to use their professional knowledge and skills to benefit society. Most nurses work as employees in health care agencies and form a contract with that agency. This differs from a contract formed directly with patients, which is the traditional model for physicians. For employed nurses, the duty to provide care emerges both from a contract with their employing agency to care for assigned patients and from the accepted tradition that membership in the profession of nursing entails accepting risks involved in caring for patients (Huerta & Oddi, 1992).

Support for this accepted tradition of nurses' acceptance of necessary risk in providing care comes from many sources. Downes (1991) pointed out that the *legal* duty to care is not determined by ethical issues, but ethical standards contribute to the standards of care. She expects health care professionals to provide leadership to other groups and to the public in setting the tone for coping with conflicts between balancing individual rights with public well-being. An ANA position paper (1988) states that the nurse is morally obligated to care for HIV-infected patients if the care presents only the minimal risk, and further suggests that a nurse can exercise a moral option of not caring for the HIV-infected patient only if the nurse's risk exceeds the responsibility to the patient. The ANA position is justified by nursing's responsibility to benefit others and not to cause harm, because the patient could be harmed by being denied care. Additionally, when a nurse refuses to care for a patient, that patient's care becomes assigned to other staff, and this places an undue burden on colleagues. Even though it was feared that requiring nurses to care for HIV/AIDS patients would cause nurses to leave the profession and would impede recruitment efforts, this fear has not been realized.

Means to Pay for Health Care

Americans with HIV infection are drawn from groups who are most likely to be uninsured for health care: young adults, unmarried persons, African Americans, Latinos, and families without a working adult (Short et al., 1989). As HIV/AIDS has become a chronic illness, people live longer and require more medications to prevent and treat their associated opportunistic infections and illnesses. Medications are costly, and some are excluded from insurance coverage. Costs of supplemental therapies, such as nutritional supplements and Chinese herbs, are not covered by private or government payers. Hence the costs of treating HIV disease far outdistance most people's resources to pay. Thus people do not receive the health care that they want and need. The United States continues to struggle to allocate resources for adequate care without a national health plan to guide fair distribution of services.

When money from traditional sources has not been available to help people gain access to the medical care they need, some communities have worked to create resources through political pressure and community action. The gay and lesbian communities united early in the AIDS epidemic to develop resources for people with HIV/AIDS to gain access to medical care and to meet their everyday living needs, such as housing and groceries. Resources included support groups for people to share approaches that they found effective in managing their daily lives and its emotional toll.

Some communities now affected by HIV/AIDS do not have effective resources, nor have they developed strategies to unite to gain needed resources. HIV infection is burrowing more decisively into communities composed of people of color and women—communities where effective medical and social support and everyday living resources and programs are again challenged. Not only do limited income and lack of health insurance coverage impede access to health care among women and people of color, but efforts have been limited in developing culturally competent programs of care or educational programs about the benefits of early treatment and in enrolling women and people of color in clinical trials (Grady, 1991; National Commission on AIDS, 1992). Our society continues to struggle with the question of whether we will regard access to health care as a basic right or a privilege.

The concept of American health care is misleading, because services are offered primarily for illness, rather than health promotion. Current discussions of health care reform seem to favor "universal coverage." This concept endorses the notion that health/illness care is a right. The perspective of health/illness care as a right carries with it a hefty price tag, and the questions of who pays and how to finance the care are pivotal. Health/illness care is a social benefit and, as such, competes with other social benefits, such as education, for public and private dollars.

Healthcare reform, long overdue, will not address all the public policy questions that affect access to health/illness care for those affected by HIV/AIDS. How should money be divided among competing claims for treatment and prevention, and which forms of treatment are most deserving? If treatments are developed that are effective but expensive, how should these treatments be distributed? Is it just that medications and hopefully vaccines will soon be available to Americans but not to others in the world with HIV/AIDS?

Payment for HIV/AIDS care is increasingly challenged as people think of AIDS as a chronic illness and feel less urgency to allocate funds to finance research, treatment, and prevention. As AIDS spreads to communities without cohesion and political power, such as injection drug users and diverse communities of people of color, political pressure may diminish. Many groups are competing for scarce resources instead of creating coalitions to serve their populations and to increase their power. How may programs serve culturally diverse communities competently without also increasing separation?

Adequate Quality of Care

Example. Miguel, a 30-year-old man who usually identifies himself as Mexican American, is half American Indian. When sober, he has a shy grin that masks his characteristic violent reactions when using drugs and drinking. He has applied to detoxification and rehabilitation programs, but nearly all refused to honor his MediCal (Medicaid) coverage. One program accepted MediCal but required that, as a test of motivation, he telephone every day between 9 and 10 AM for a week before they would consider admission. Without an alarm clock, this task proved insurmountable. Now he has been evicted, and because all the shelters are full, he sleeps on a park bench. He has been coughing for a month and has night sweats but has not taken his tuberculosis medicine or other medications for 3 to 4 months. He has not seen his physician for about 6 months. His diagnosis of AIDS was made about 2 years ago, and he is totally discouraged. His caseworker told him, "I can't help you until you stop drugs and drinking," and would not suggest other solutions for health care or housing.

Issues of Quality of Care. Several difficult questions concern quality of care. What is an acceptable quality of care? Is it adequate to diagnose and treat opportunistic illnesses and infections while not offering treatment for the person's substance use problems? Is treatment adequate if we cannot tend to the living context of the sick person to make sure that adequate housing and food are available? Can a person learn how to avoid reinfection if the education is provided in an unfamiliar language or when the person is hungry? Do we blame people for their drug addiction and offer punishment instead of help?

SUICIDE, ASSISTED SUICIDE, AND EUTHANASIA

Example. Donald, who had AIDS, and his lover, Bret, had talked about death but mostly in terms of managing insurance, household belongings, and other property. Donald made out his will and durable power of attorney and told his family that Bret would manage his estate and be his major beneficiary. Donald regretted his limited vision and finally conceded that none of the regimens that he had tried had slowed his rapidly approaching blindness. His diarrhea was worse and his headaches were unrelenting. Donald had tentatively talked with his nurse about reading *Final Exit* (Humphrey, 1992) and wondered whether suicide might be something that he would consider when he became sicker. Without warning, Donald became very confused, had trouble walking without stumbling, and became very forgetful. He wandered outside in the middle of the night and once almost fell into the ravine by the woods adjacent to his house. Soon, though, Donald's energy faded, and he lay in bed fairly motionless unless someone came to help him walk to the bathroom or to sit with him. He rarely spoke, and his words often made no sense. Bret hired an aide for 12 hours a day Monday through Friday, and he and friends shared Donald's care at night and on weekends. Bret's law partners were understanding of his situation and covered for Bret when they could.

Bret spoke with Donald's nurse when she came to see Donald. Once Bret talked with her of how painful it was to see Donald reduced to a shadow of his personhood, for Donald has been such a proud and independent man. Bret wondered about Donald's headaches because he held his head often. Bret wistfully said that he and Donald had never spoken about suicide, and he did not know how Donald felt about it. The nurse struggled with her duty of confidentiality to Donald versus her duty to act as his advocate and spokesperson, because Donald could no longer speak for himself. She told Bret that Donald had begun to explore suicide but that he had not seemed to reach a resolution; indeed, his grasp of the issues involved seemed naive in comparison to the rest of his knowledge about treatments for AIDS. Bret wondered if it was his responsibility as Donald's lover to do for him what he was unable to do for himself. The nurse helped Bret to explore his sense of duty, the practical issues, and his spiritual and existential views about suicide.

Definitions and Ethical Issues. During the past three decades, laws and attitudes about suicide have changed in the United States. Now only a few states have laws against suicide. Changes in the law have allowed a person to seek help after attempting suicide without fear of encountering fines or incarceration. Complex reasons exist for the shift in attitude toward a greater tolerance of suicide and euthanasia. Reasons such as consumerism and technologic advances in maintaining life are factors often cited.

A concise discussion of ethical issues surrounding suicide and euthanasia requires that terms be defined and used consistently. The presence of suicidal thoughts and actions do not imply that a person has any psychiatric disorder. Although suicidal people are often depressed, nurses must recognize that suicide and depression can occur without each other (Saunders & Buckingham, 1988). Suicide is defined as an intentional death that results from injuries or acts by the individual who dies. Assisted suicide is defined as a suicide in which the person kills himself or herself but needs significant help from someone else. Significant help could include providing the gun and ammunition or giving the person access to a lethal dose of medication. "Rational suicide" is a popular but unfortunate term because it incorrectly implies that suicide is either a rational or an irrational act. Rational suicide is defined as a self-inflicted, self-intended death under the following circumstances: (1) unclouded sensorium—that is, without significant depression or mood-altering drugs, (2) capacity to comprehend consequences, and (3) circumstances acceptable to society (Siegel, 1986). Finally, "euthanasia" refers to an action in which one person causes another's death and is usually differentiated into voluntary (killing for the individual's own benefit) and involuntary (killing for society's benefit).

The ethical issues that dominate discussion of these approaches to dying include autonomy, confidentiality, sanctity of life, utility, paternalism, and the "slippery slope." All these terms were defined earlier in this chapter (see Table 13–2) except the concept of the slippery slope. The slippery slope argument, or the wedge argument, refers to the concern that if a limited action is allowed, that action will expand to broader conditions with fewer limitations. Generally, the slippery slope argument has two dimensions: (1) support for one type of action logically implies support for another because the dissimilarities between the actions are too subtle for the underlying principles to differentiate; and (2) social forces might, with time, change the rules from voluntary to involuntary euthanasia.

Ethical Issues. The first issue that must be addressed is differentiating clinical and ethical issues. Quill (1993) argued that transient death wishes among individuals with progressive and incurable illnesses, such as AIDS, are often associated with complex meanings involving untreated physical symptoms, emerging psychosocial problems, spiritual or existential crises, clinical depression, or pain and suffering from various sources. An HIV-infected patient's request to talk about death, suicide, rational suicide or assisted suicide may be a way of exploring control issues, especially after a diagnosis of HIV has been made. A patient's comments about death or suicide need to be met with an open mind by a nurse who is willing to assess the patient's experience and concerns. The nurse should listen to the patient's whole message and avoid responding to a fragment (Quill, 1993; Saunders & Buckingham, 1988).

The nurse who is a strong supporter of patient autonomy and an advocate for easing society's barriers to suicide and euthanasia may miss as many clinical clues as does the nurse from the opposite perspective who believes that suicide violates the sanctity of life and is never defensible. By operating from their own perspectives, both nurses will fail to understand the patient's viewpoint or to assist the patient in clarifying underlying concerns.

A second issue is deciding how the ethical obligations that guide professional actions differ from the ethical duties toward family and friends of a personal nature. In AIDS care, this is even more complex because professional and personal relationships are sometimes mixed. In both situations, it is painful to see individuals lose a meaningful quality of life, but the nurse's roles and resources may differ in personal and professional situations. The California Nurses' Association position paper on suicide (1988) clearly states that nurses do not abandon the care of their suicidal patients; neither can nurses—in their professional role—deliberately act to help patients commit suicide. A nurse who would never think of assisting in the suicide of a patient might have different responses if an aunt or a grandparent requested help in commiting suicide.

Responses to people who are contemplating suicide because of a terminal illness should be thought through carefully. Approaches to considering the issues that have been discussed in the literature provide useful guidelines for practice (Battin, 1991; Saunders & Valente, 1993). Similarly, Jamison (1993) developed a list of questions for the person who is considering assisting another person to die.

Assisting a suicide of a person is a serious act and one that may have traumatic consequences for those who assist. In addition to painful personal responses, the nurse may fear losing professional credentials to practice.

Patients often request confidentiality from the nurse when they discuss their fears and concerns surrounding suicide. The nurse who has promised to keep a patient's suicide plan secret may encounter conflicting obligations that are difficult to resolve. The nurse may wonder whether the patient would benefit from further consultation or treatment, but the nurse would have no way to gain access to that kind of help without breaking a promise and potentially damaging the nurse-patient relationship.

In a society that has demonstrated an increased acceptance of suicide in certain circumstances, many ethical problems remain unresolved. Will increased access to euthanasia or assisted suicide reduce efforts to relieve suffering? Should the same people who are responsible for helping people gain an acceptable quality of life during illness also be responsible for euthanasia and assisted suicide, or should different groups be constituted for this purpose? If voluntary euthanasia is sanctioned to meet the person's request, what conditions might emerge to expand euthanasia to those who don't request death but whose death would benefit society, such as comatose patients or the severely retarded?

Nurses are divided in their beliefs about appropriate responses to suicide and euthanasia. Interviews with 50 oncology nurses found variations in comfort levels in exploring these topics with their patients and divergent views on what is acceptable (Valente et al., 1993). When asked under what circumstances suicide would be considered acceptable, nurses' responses varied: "Patient has to make own decisions about suicide"; "If patient wants to commit suicide, no one can stop him"; and "Nurses should attempt to prevent ALL suicides." One nurse responded that "if he was really serious about suicide, I'd assist the patient."

Nurses seem to have reached no consensus about suicide and euthanasia in U.S. society, nor have they decided on appropriate professional roles. The ethical issues underlying choices about suicide and euthanasia are among the most complex and compelling that we face.

ETHICAL ISSUES AND NURSING RESEARCH

Current Nursing Research

Discussions of patient rights in nursing research have paralleled the general evolution of research in nursing, and yet ethics as a topic of research efforts is very recent (Davis, 1989; Penticuff, 1991). By the mid-1980s, several articles appeared that examined ethics in the context of HIV/AIDS from various perspectives. Studies of ethics and AIDS are now emerging. One of the first is a descriptive, qualitative study of 25 persons with HIV (PWHIV) and five noninfected persons who were significant to the PWHIV (Cameron, 1993). Cameron's sample included women (37%) and people of color (53%). Cameron (1993, p. 8) asked her study participants, "What situation involving AIDS has caused you the most conflict about the right thing to do?" The participants' stories reflect a scope of concerns that expand the more narrowly conceived boundaries of principle-based (normative) ethics, situation ethics, or ethics of car-

ing. All the stories disclosed a struggle to determine the right way to live with AIDS, not classroom discussions of abstract or impersonal situations. These stories capture the reality of the individual's struggle and the immediacy of their consequences. Cameron (1993) reported 10 major categories of ethical concerns that her analysis revealed for these 30 men and women: alcohol and drugs, chronic illness, death, discrimination, finance and business, health care, personhood, relationships, service, and sexuality. Cameron also discussed strategies that she recommends will lead to ethical living, believing that health care professionals themselves grapple with how to live ethical lives and with how to help patients resolve whatever is bothering them.

Other nursing research related to ethics has concentrated on nurses' attitudes about caring for patients with HIV/AIDS (Barrick, 1988; Colombotos et al., 1991; Gignac & Oermann, 1991). These studies have been useful in determining that health care workers continue to be very fearful of providing care to patients with HIV/AIDS and provide useful clues that educators and administrators might take to allay unfounded staff fears and ensure adequate care of patients.

Research Needed in Ethics and HIV/AIDS

So little nursing research has been reported in the literature on ethics and HIV/AIDS that studies can be justified in every aspect of ethics. Nursing especially needs studies that examine the impact of existing and emerging policies and practices on PWHIV. For example, mandatory involuntary testing has been the policy for military recruits and some prisoners, and studies need to compare issues of autonomy, privacy, and utility with people who have been tested in voluntary programs.

Given nurses' continued reluctance to provide care for patients with HIV/AIDS, nursing needs a better understanding of what nurses, in the context of AIDS care, consider moral problems and how they can be resolved. Is the current generation of nurses concerned about a different set of moral issues from those in the past? What are the moral obligations for the nursing profession in this pandemic, and what are the goals and strategies to meet those obligations? How does the moral approach used in resolving moral problems affect the process or outcome for nurses? Does nursing practice differ when the nurse is guided by ethics of caring versus principle-based ethics? What barriers exist to explain the reason that nurses are not using universal precautions or other self-protective measures?

Dumois (1993) expressed concern that HIV-infected babies do not receive the same lifesaving measures (such as forced feeding) as often as do uninfected babies, and this concern is one that warrants full attention. Because testing of infants automatically reveals the mother's HIV status, moving from an autonomous testing program to one in which identities are known poses many potential consequences, and this research should be a high priority.

What are the psychologic and spiritual costs to nurses in AIDS care situations in which their personal ethics conflict with their professional responsibilities? Where do they find support for themselves when they have made tough decisions or been unable to act as they desire? How do administrators and educators provide support for staff and students who are grappling with ethical problems they encounter with their HIV/AIDS patients and their families?

Nursing needs a better understanding of how PWHIV decide that their quality of life is unacceptable and irreparable. Nursing could benefit from learning how nurses assist patients in issues surrounding their quality of life. Which nursing interventions are used when patients broach the topic of suicide or euthanasia, and how do the interventions reflect ethical values? What costs (complicated grief, depression) are incurred by people who do assist their loved ones or their patients with suicide?

Because HIV infection is not distributed evenly across the United States, researchers may have difficulty in gaining access to some subjects, including women or people of color, in their studies. This uneven distribution leads to some individuals' being involved in several studies concurrently, whereas others are never approached to participate in research. Consequently, most of our knowledge about nursing and AIDS may be informed disproportionately by a less diverse core of volunteer study participants than is needed to guide policy or develop nursing intervention. Ethical concerns about participant involvement in nursing research must reach beyond informed consent, autonomous participation, and confidentiality. Nursing should encourage collaboration among researchers that allows comprehensive studies.

AIDS activists have changed the manner of conducting clinical trials research by questioning how long it takes to approve drugs that may mean the difference between life and death for PWHIV. Before these changes, participation in clinical trials was viewed as a burden for patients. This burden was justified because of the public good, and precautions were used to reduce individual risk. Increasingly, HIV-infected individuals regard participation in research as a right and have challenged the practice of excluding women, infants, and people of color as discriminatory, not protective. Research is needed to determine the effects of these changes and to assess current research review processes for adaptation to these changes.

Finally, nurses have been in the forefront of providing direct care to people with AIDS, supporting health promotion efforts of symptom-free patients, and developing prevention strategies. Nurses have provided leadership at national and international conferences but have sometimes seemed invisible. If the nursing profession has ethical obligations to work for better resources for our HIV-infected patients and their families, how can we find our voice to participate in local and international programs and speak of the inequities and injustices that we witness among patients in our clinical practice?

SUMMARY

HIV/AIDS causes nurses to draw on all the traditional principles of ethics and has challenged us to look to new paradigms for guiding our patient care. It also has confronted us as health-care givers with public demands that intrude into our own privacy and personhood. It has caused us to reflect on complex issues of quality of life and death. None of these ethical issues has been studied intensively in any of the health care disciplines. Several suggestions have been identified for nursing research and the ethical issues involved with HIV/AIDS.

REFERENCES

Agich, G.J. (1990). Reassessing autonomy in long-term care. *Hastings Center Report, 12*(6), 12–17.

AIDSline (1992). Women vs. their infants in HIV testing debate. *The Robert Wood Johnson Foundation, 4*(4), 1–4.

Albrizio, M.A., Ozuna, J., Mattheis, R., et al. (1992). A nursing bioethics program. *Clinical Nurse Specialist, 6*(2), 97–103.

American Hospital Association (1985). *Values in conflict: Resolving ethical issues in hospital care.* Report of the Special Committee on Biomedical Ethics. Chicago: American Hospital Association.

American Nurses' Association Committee on Ethics (1985). *Code for nurses with interpretive statements.* Kansas City, MO: American Nurses' Association.

American Nurses' Association Committee on Ethics (1988). Ethics in nursing: Position statements and guidelines. Kansas City, MO: The Association.

Americans with Disabilities Act of 1990 (1990). Public Law No. 101-336, 104 Stat 3 27.

Aroskar, M. (1980). Anatomy of an ethical dilemma. *American Journal of Nursing, 80*(4), 658–663.

Barrick, B. (1988). The willingness of nursing personnel to care for patients with acquired immune deficiency syndrome: A survey study and recommendations. *Journal of Professional Nursing, 4*(5), 366–372.

Battin, M.P. (1991). Rational suicide: How can we respond to a request for help? *Crisis, 12*(2), 73–80.

Beauchamp, T.L., Childress, J.F. (1989). *Principles of biomedical ethics* (3rd ed.). New York: Oxford University Press.

Benner, P., Wrubel, J. (1989). *The primacy of caring: Stress and coping in health and illness.* Menlo Park, CA: Addison-Wesley.

Bishop, A., Scudder, J. (1987). Nursing ethics in an age of controversy. *Advances in Nursing Science, 9*(3), 34–43.

Brown, M.L. (1987). AIDS and ethics: Concerns and consideration. *Oncology Nursing Forum, 14*(1), 69–73.

California Nurses' Association (1988). Nursing and suicide: A position paper. San Francisco, CA: The Association.

Cameron, M.E. (1993). *Living with AIDS: Experiencing ethical problems.* Newbury Park, CA: Sage Publications.

Card, C. (Ed.) (1991). *Feminist ethics.* Lawrence, KA: University of Kansas Press.

Centers for Disease Control and Prevention (July 1991). Recommendations for preventing transmission of human immunodeficiency virus and hepatitis B virus to patients during exposure-prone invasive procedures. *Mortality and Morbidity Weekly Report, 40*(RR-8).

Centers for Disease Control and Prevention (January 1993). Recommendations for HIV testing services for inpatients and outpatients in acute-care hospital settings. *Mortality and Morbidity Weekly Report, 42*(RR-2), 1–6.

Collins, J. (1981). Should doctors tell the truth? In T.A. Mappes & J.S. Zembaty (Eds.), *Biomedical ethics* (pp. 64–67). New York: McGraw-Hill Book Co.

Colombotos, J., Messeri, P., Burgunder, M., et al. (1991). Physicians, nurses and AIDS: Preliminary findings from a national survey, Rockville, MD: Agency for Health Care Policy and Research.

Condon, E.H. (1992). Nursing and the caring metaphor: Gender and political influences on an ethics of care. *Nursing Outlook, 40*(1), 14–19.

Council on Ethical and Judicial Affairs, American Medical Association (1988). *Journal of the Americal Medical Association, 259*(9), 1360–1361.

Curry, C., Johnson, M., Ogden, B. (1990). Willingness of health-professions students to treat patients with AIDS. *Academic Medicine, 65*(7),472–474.

Curtin, L. (1978). A proposed model for critical ethical analysis. *Nursing Forum, XVII*(1), 17–27.

Curtin, L. (1990). The commitment of nursing. In T. Pence & J. Cantrall (Eds.), *Ethics in nursing: An anthology* (pp. 283–286). New York: National League for Nursing.

Curtin, L. (1992). HIV-positive employees. *Nursing Management, 23*(10), 22–25.

Curtin, L., Flaherty, M.J. (1982). *Nursing ethics: Theories and pragmatics.* Bowie, MD: Robert J. Brady Co.

Davis, A.J. (1989). Ethical issues in nursing research. *Western Journal of Nursing Research, 11*(3), 379–381.

Davis, A.J., Aroskar, M.A. (1991). *Ethical dilemmas and nursing practice* (3rd ed.). Norwalk, CT: Appleton & Lange.

Downes, J. (1991). Acquired immunodeficiency syndrome: The nurse's legal duty to serve. *Journal of Professional Nursing, 7*(6), 333–340; *4*(5), 331–336.

Dumois, A.O. (Oct. 19–23, 1993). Social and political strategies for the HIV epidemic. Paper presented at the HIV 6th National AIDS Update Conference, San Francisco, CA.

Eliason, M.J. (1993). Ethics and transcultural nursing care. *Nursing Outlook, 41*(5), 225–228.

El-Mallakh, P.L., Simmons, C., Forman, L., et al. (1992). Mandatory HIV testing of health care workers: A review. *AIDS Patient Care, 6*(4), 164–168.

Fassbinder, B. (Oct. 31–Nov. 3, 1993). My personal story of occupational HIV infection. Panel presentation, Sixth Annual Conference, Association of Nurses in AIDS Care, Century City, CA.

Gadow, S. (1990). A model for ethical decision making. In T. Pence & J. Cantrall (Eds.), *Ethics in nursing: An anthology* (pp. 52–55). New York: National League for Nursing.

Gignac, D., Oermann, M.H. (1991). Willingness of nursing students and faculty to care for patients with AIDS. *American Journal of Infection Control, 19*(4), 191–197.

Gilligan, C. (1982). *In a different voice: Psychological theory and women's development.* Cambridge, MA: Harvard University Press.

Grady, C. (1991). Ethical issues in clinical trials. *Seminars in Oncology Nursing, 7*(4), 228–296.

Halloran, J., Huges, A., Mayer, D.K. (1988). Oncology Nursing Society position paper on HIV-related issues. *Oncology Nursing Forum, 15*(2) 206–210.

Harron, F., Burnside, J., Beauchamp, T. (1983). *Health and human values: A guide to making your own decision.* New Haven: Yale University Press.

Henry, K., Maki, M., Crossle, K. (1988a). Analysis of the use of HIV antibody testing in a Minnesota hospital. *Journal of American Medical Association, 259*(2), 229–232.

Henry, K., Willenbring, K., Crossley, K. (1988b). Human immunodeficiency virus antibody testing. *Journal of American Medical Association, 259*(12), 1819–1822.

Hoagland, S.L. (1991). Some thoughts about "caring." In C. Card (Ed.), *Feminist ethics* (pp. 246–263). Lawrence, KS: University of Kansas Press.

Huerta, S.R., Oddi, L.F. (1992). Refusal to care for patients with human immunodeficiency virus/acquired immunodeficiency syndrome: Issues and responses. *Journal of Professional Nursing, 8*(4), 221–230.

Humphrey, D. (1992). *Final exit.* Eugene, OR: Hemlock Society.

Institute of Medical Ethics Working Party on the Ethical Implications of AIDS (June 1992). AIDS and the ethics of medical care and treatment. *Quarterly Journal of Medicine* (New Series) *83*(302), 419–426.

Jaggar, A.M. (1991). Feminist ethics: Projects, problems, prospects. In C. Card (Ed.), *Feminist ethics.* Lawrence, KS: University of Kansas Press.

Jamison, S. (July 1993). Helping to die: Some practical questions. *Hemlock Quarterly, 7,* 5–7.

Kelly, J.A., St. Lawrence, J.S., Hood, H.V., et al. (1988). Nurses' attitudes towards AIDS. *Journal of Continuing Education in Nursing, 19*(2), 78–83.

Lo, B., Steinbrook, R. (1992). Health care workers infected with the human immunodeficiency virus. *Journal of the American Medical Association, 267*(8), 1100–1105.

Makulowich, G.S. (1992). Retaining the expertise of the HIV-infected health care worker. *AIDS Patient Care, 6*(6), 264–265.

Naccache, H., Fortin, C., Croteau, A., et al. (1993). Universal precautions in a teaching hospital. *AIDS Patient Care, 7*(3), 134–137.

National Commission on AIDS (1992). *The challenge of HIV/AIDS in communities of color.* Washington, DC: The Commission.

National Commission on AIDS (1993). *AIDS: An expanding tragedy. The final report of the National Commission on AIDS.* Washington, DC: The Commission.

Neil, R.M., Watts, R. (Eds.) 1991. *Caring and nursing: Explorations in feminist perspectives.* New York: National League for Nursing.

Noddings, N. (1984). *Caring. A feminine approach to ethics and moral education.* Berkeley: University of California Press.

Ostrow, R.J., Cimons, M. (1993). U.S. alleges bias to AIDS patients by 2 dental offices. (Justice Department files civil rights lawsuits against Castle Dental Center Chain in Houston and dentist Drew B. Morvant in New Orleans. *Los Angeles Times,* V. 112 (Oct. 5, 1993).

Penticuff, J.H. (1991). Conceptual issues in nursing ethics research. *Journal of Medicine and Philosophy, 16*(3), 235–258.

Quill, T.E. (1993). Doctor, I want to die: Will you help me? *Journal of the American Medical Association, 270*(7), 870–877.

Saunders, J.M., Buckingham, S.L. (1988). When the depression turns deadly. *Nursing 88, 18*(7), 60–64.

Saunders, J.M., Valente, S.M. (1993). Nicole: Suicide and terminal illness. *Suicide and Life-Threatening Behavior, 23*(1), 76–82.

Schultz, M., Moore, L. (Oct. 31 to Nov. 3, 1993). Bioethics committee: A subacute model. Paper presented at the Sixth Annual Conference of the Association of Nurses in AIDS Care, Los Angeles, CA.

Shneidman, E.H. (1980). Personal communication.

Short, P., Monheit, A., Beauregard, K. (1989). A profile of uninsured Americans. DHHS publication No. 89–344. National Medical Expenditure Survey Research Findings 1. National Center for Health Services Research and Health Care Technology Assessment. Rockville, MD: U.S. Public Health Service.

Siegel, K. (1986). Psychosocial aspects of rational suicide. *American Journal of Psychotherapy, XL*(3), 405–418.

Stevenson, J.S., Tripp-Reimer, T. (Eds.) (1989). *Knowledge about care and caring: State of the art and future developments.* Kansas City, MO: American Academy of Nursing.

Stoll, J., Mason, P.K. (Oct. 31 to Nov. 3, 1993). Ethics education for nurses in AIDS care. Paper presented at the Sixth Annual Conference of the Association of Nurses in AIDS Care, Los Angeles, CA.

The Hastings Center (1987). *Guidelines on the termination of life-sustaining treatment and the care of the dying.* Bloomington, IN: Indiana University Press.

U.S. Office of Technology Assessment (1992). HIV in the healthcare workplace: A background paper. *AIDS Patient Care, 6*(4), 169–185.

Valente, S.M., Saunders, J.M., McIntyre, L., et al. (Oct. 31 to Nov. 3, 1993). Qualitative analysis of oncology nurses' attitudes toward suicide. Poster session, the Sixth Annual Conference of the Association of Nurses in AIDS Care, Los Angeles, CA.

Walters, L. (1988). Ethical issues in the prevention and treatment of HIV infection and AIDS. *Science, 239*(4840), 597–603.

Watson, J. (1988). *Nursing: Human science and human care: A theory of nursing.* New York: National League for Nursing.

Willy, M., Dhillon, G., Loewen, N., et al. (1990). Adverse exposures and universal precautions practices among a group of highly exposed health practitioners. *Infection Control Hospital Epidemiology, 11*(7), 351–356.

Legal Issues Related to the Care of Persons With HIV 14

Penny S. Brooke

Legal guidelines related to the nursing care of people with HIV and AIDS are derived from information on present regulations, laws, and case precedents. Since the first reported cases of AIDS related illnesses in 1981, the laws affecting HIV issues have been evolving. This chapter discusses the developments to date of regulations, statutory enactments, and case precedents that have evolved and continue to be evolving. The reader is reminded of the fluid nature of the law because the issues surrounding AIDS are far from settled. Our society continues to struggle to balance the conflicting responsibilities and rights of individuals with those of the public, including the rights of HIV-infected persons with those who risk exposure to the virus. To be most informed, nurses themselves must learn of the specific status of the laws in the various jurisdictions in which they practice.

Federal rules, regulations, and statutes are enacted to define the generalized laws of our nation. These topics plus those not yet decided on the federal level may also be discussed in individual state statutes and legal case precedents. Case law from any jurisdiction may be helpful in predicting future developments in other states but may not be binding if the community standards vary too greatly. Juries, judges, and legislatures in the individual states help define the community standards based on the beliefs of the people who make up or elect these decision-making bodies. Some communities are considered conservative, whereas other jurisdictions may be seen as progressive. Much like the ethical dilemmas discussed in Chapter 13, whichever direction a state leans may be considered right or wrong by persons who are affected by these decisions. Whatever the individual states or various legal jurisdictions decide, the legal protections guaranteed by the Constitution of the United States, the case decisions made by the U.S. Supreme Court, and the statutory enactments made by Congress, including the rules and regulations enacted by administrative agencies such as the Occupational Safety and Health Administration (OSHA), must be followed (Covner, 1993). Congress and legislatures delegate their authority to administrative agencies composed of experts in the various health care fields. These delegations of authority empower the administrative agency to enact specific rules and regulations which provide guidelines that the states must follow. Private agencies that do not receive federal funding may have more flexibility when creating their private policies and procedures, but public agencies that receive federal funding are bound by the federal mandates and must comply or lose their financial support.

LEGAL ISSUES AND NURSING

Several legal issues associated with HIV are of concern to nurses. The first of these issues involves the nurse's duty of care and the standards of care owed to patients. Nurses who refuse to care for HIV-infected patients may be reprimanded or fired for insubordination. It is important for the nurse to understand the employer's policies and procedures regarding the nurse's duty of care to HIV-infected patients. A home health care nurse who was in the first trimester of her pregnancy and worried about contracting opportunistic infections common in AIDS patients refused to care for an HIV-infected patient. Her employer had a policy that provided no exceptions for those who refused patient care assignments. The nurse was fired; she consequently charged the employer with discrimination based on gender because of her pregnancy. The court upheld the employer's right to fire the nurse (*Armstrong v Flowers Hospital, Inc.*, 1993). The nurse in *Armstrong* was fired for insubordination, but the legal theory of abandonment also is related. Standards of care direct hospitals to avoid abandoning, or "dumping," patients by sending them to another facility. The patient's legal rights to privacy and to confidentiality of information possessed regarding their health must alert the nurse and other health care providers to the risk of disclosures of this information to persons who fall outside the definition of those who have a need to know this information to provide competent care.

Connected to this legal responsibility to provide care are the issues of the right of the patient to refuse treatment and the questions of the rights of health care providers when they are treating infected individuals. At the core of the patient's right to refuse treatment is the patient's right to consent to treatment. Legal consent includes the concept of a competent patient who has the legal capacity to voluntarily make and to understand the consequences of his or her decisions. Legal concerns regarding mandatory testing of both patients and health care providers will be discussed in this chapter as they relate to professional organization guidelines, the Centers for Disease Control and Prevention (CDC) guidelines, and case precedent. Discussion of the patient's rights and the legal tools to protect these rights, including living wills, special medical directives, and medical powers of attorney, will alert the nurse to understand the legal authority of surrogate decision makers. Finally, employment-related legal issues include workers' compensation, the Americans with Disabilities Act (ADA), and health and disability insurance rights of employees.

FEDERAL DIRECTIONS AND STATE ACTIONS

Transmission of HIV in Health Care Settings

National guidelines regarding blood and body fluid precautions were first issued by the CDC in 1983. By 1985, recommendations for universal precautions were issued (CDC, Nov.

15, 1985). The CDC provided supplementary information in 1986, taking a position against placing practice restrictions and against routine testing of health care providers. Further supplementary recommendations from the CDC, given in 1987, recommended a case-by-case assessment of practice restrictions when a health care worker is seropositive for HIV. Again, in July 1991, the CDC promulgated guidelines emphasizing the importance of the use of universal precautions in infection control and again rejecting mandatory testing of all health care workers; rather, the CDC recommended that health care workers who perform exposure-prone invasive procedures voluntarily submit to testing. The CDC recommended that a review panel be empowered to impose conditions of practice when an AIDS-infected health care worker desires to continue performing exposure-prone invasive procedures and further recommended that physicians advise their patients of the physicians' AIDS status before invasive procedures. Disclosure to former patients was recommended on a case-by-case basis with consideration of the specific risks of exposure and confidentiality obligations (Covner & Wicher, 1993a; Wicher, 1993).

The *American Journal of Nursing* (AJN) "Newscaps" (Staff, *AJN*, 1992c) identified that the CDC guidelines urge infected practitioners to receive written permission from patients as well as clearance from a panel of experts before performing procedures that pose the possibility that their blood will come into contact with a patient's tissue, cavities, or organs. "Newswatch" (Staff, *RN*, May 1993) reported that 27 states had complied with the CDC's directive to develop guidelines to protect patients from HIV-infected health-care workers. The same report described the individual approaches that different states are taking. For example, Minnesota law requires infected workers who know of their condition to notify the health commissioner regarding their HIV status. If the worker's duties pose a risk to patients, the health care worker may be required to appear before the expert review panel. Whereas in New York health care workers are required to use universal precautions and to take periodic courses in infection control. Disclosure of illness is voluntary in

New York. In a survey taken of the Columbia University public health team, it was reported that 63% of registered nurses and 57% of physicians queried were in favor of mandatory AIDS testing of health care workers (Staff, *AJN*, 1991a). Yet, at the July 1991 American Nurses' Association (ANA) House of Delegates meeting, the 600-member delegation rejected mandatory testing and the disclosure of HIV status as unwarranted. The ANA delegates expressed the belief that disclosure will not prevent transmission of the disease (Staff, *AJN*, 1991b).

In December 1991, OSHA issued regulations mandating the use of universal precautions and requiring hospitals and other employers to establish written plans directed toward protecting employees (Covner, 1993). These regulations became effective in March of 1992. The Health Care Finance Administration, U.S. Department of Health and Human Services (DHHS), drafted a rule, to be finalized in August 1993, that would require hospitals to notify patients who have received blood and blood products potentially infected with HIV. The rule would ask the physician to inform the patient of the need for HIV testing and counseling. If the physician was unavailable or declined to comply, the hospital would be required to notify the blood recipient and inform him or her that counseling and testing will be needed. The U.S. Food and Drug Administration also proposed a new rule related to the manufacture of blood and blood products. The new rule discusses the procedures related to protecting persons from donors who subsequently have positive HIV test results, the specific testing used, as well as notification of recipients of infected blood products (*Fresh News*, 1993).

Antidiscrimination: Worker Protection

Discrimination is the disparate treatment of people, whether the discrimination is direct or indirect (*Alexander v. Choate*, 1985). The Civil Rights Act of 1964 underlies the federal law that seeks to protect workers against discrimination. Section 504 of the Vocational Rehabilitation Act of 1973 forbids discrimination against disabled persons. This act applies to federal employees and to employees of com-

panies that receive funding from or are contracting with the federal government. In March 1987 a U.S. Supreme Court case, *School Board of Nassau County, Florida v. Arline,* included the class of persons with infectious diseases as a protected class under the handicap and disability laws.

The Americans with Disabilities Act (ADA) is the most explicit law to date on how employers must treat people with disabilities, including people who are HIV infected or who have AIDS. Although the *Arline* case dealt with the disease of tuberculosis, a majority of states have now set up guidelines prohibiting discrimination against workers who are infected with HIV. Specific jurisdictions may enact rules, regulations, or laws that limit these protections. For example, Tennessee specifically excluded contagious diseases from its definition of handicap. In states where handicap statutes neither include nor exclude AIDS, the courts are left to determine the protections on a case-by-case basis. In the *Arline* case the court ruled that an employee could not be dismissed because of "fear of contagion." The 1990 ADA codified this ruling in stating that if the risk is not significant nor speculative nor remote, the determination should not be based on generalizations, fears, ignorance, or misperceptions (Wicher, 1993). In June 1993 the U.S. Equal Employment Opportunity Commission (EEOC) issued interim enforcement guidance instructions in terms of the employer-provided health insurance plans in relation to the ADA. Title I of the ADA prohibits private employers, state and local governments, employment agencies, and labor unions from discriminating against individuals with disabilities in their employment. Employees with disabilities must be afforded equal access to insurance plans provided to employees without disabilities. Further, an employer cannot make an employment decision based on whether the prospective employee has a relationship with someone who causes concern about the impact on the health plan (Covner & Wicher, 1993b, 1993c; Wicher, 1993).

Although many companies have not issued formal policy statements on how they will respond to employees with AIDS, most employers have not yet denied health care benefits to these employees. This fact appears to be due to the strength of the antidiscrimination laws, including the ADA. The CDC data estimate that most employers, of all sizes, industries, and locations, will be confronted with the reality of the HIV-infected employee. Indirect or subtle discrimination from co-workers who may refuse to work with infected persons may also leave companies open to charges of discrimination if the employer does not oversee and correct the discriminatory work environment. Education of employees has been suggested as a means of avoiding work disruption because of employees' fears of working with an HIV-infected co-worker (Covner & Wicher, 1993b, 1993c). Courts at both the federal and state levels have held in favor of employees who have been fired when their employer learned of their AIDS infection status. However, some courts have allowed self-insured plans more leeway in restricting health benefits for people with AIDS. The scope of the protections afforded by the ADA are most likely to be determined by case precedent in future specific circumstances.

Employees are also protected by the ADA at the time of hiring and when advancements, compensation, or other terms or conditions or privileges of employment are being considered. Only if the employee poses a direct threat to the health and safety of others or if he or she is not qualified for the job may a disabled employee be kept out of a workplace. Under the ADA an employer must provide "reasonable accommodations" for disabled employees, including those with HIV infection or AIDS. Reasonable accommodations may include transferring the employee to another position where the risk of exposure is eliminated or adapting work schedules or the physical environment itself. Persons whose infections are asymptomatic or who have early symptomatic infections may be healthy enough not to need special accommodations. However, under the ADA, these persons have the same rights and protections as others. An employee must disclose his or her need for special accommodations, but the standard of "known or should have known" is applied to an employer who discriminates and later claims not to have been aware of an obvious

disability. State and federal handicap laws protect against this subtle type of discrimination as well (Covner & Wicher, 1993b, 1993c).

The ADA is being more clearly defined as it relates to discrimination based on HIV status through court decisions. A recent 1993 case, *Buckingham v. United States of America,* discusses the reasonable accommodations required when a disability such as AIDS exists. The employer was obligated to transfer the employee to another city where better medical care could be obtained as a reasonable accommodation of the employee's illness (*Buckingham v. USA,* 1993).

Antidiscrimination: Insurance Plans

Section 310 of the Employment Retirement Income Security Act of 1974 prohibits insurance plans from denying or limiting benefits to an employee because of a catastrophic illness that would incur additional costs to the plan. Self-funded plans may have fewer restrictions, fewer employer mandates, and therefore fewer employee protections. Additionally, medical plans may limit payments for certain types of coverage such as mental illness, pharmacy payments, vision needs, and so forth. If an employer can prove that the medical plan was modified for a legitimate business reason, a case can be made for the exclusion of the coverage. Case precedents regarding insurance coverage of AIDS-related illness have developed rapidly. In 1988 a nationwide convenience store chain dropped a controversial "personal lifestyles claims exclusion" from its plan after pressure from civil liberties groups and AIDS activists, and a Georgia manufacturer also dropped its $10,000 lifetime ceiling for AIDS treatment costs for workers and dependents who contracted AIDS voluntarily through sex or drug use (Covner & Wicher, 1993c).

The EEOC issued interim enforcement guidelines in June 1993, reiterating that the ADA does not provide a "safe harbor" for health insurance plans adopted before the July 1990 enactment if it is being charged that the plan is adopted to avoid coverage of a disability. The same guidelines state that if an

Table 14–1. Issues to Consider in the Development of a Comprehensive AIDS Policy

Compliance with state, federal, and local law, including the new ADA

Compliance with labor union contracts or agreements

Issues related to confidentiality and privacy

Prevention of discrimination

First-aid and infection control procedures

Identification of internal and external resources

Benefits options—including long-term disability provisions

Need to find a balance between the needs of the organization, management, co-workers, customers, and individuals

Adapted from Youngberg, B. (1993). *Risk Managers Law Alert,* 2(6), 5–7, Aspen Publishers, Inc.

Table 14–2. Ten Principles for the Workplace

1. People with AIDS/HIV have the same rights and opportunities as others with serious illness.
2. Employment policies must comply with legal obligations.
3. Policies should be based on scientific information.
4. Management should endorse nondiscrimination policies.
5. Support of nondiscrimination should be communicated to all employees.
6. Provide employees with sensitive and accurate information.
7. Protect confidentiality.
8. Educate employees to reduce conflicts between HIV-infected and noninfected employees.
9. Do not require HIV screening for employment.
10. For settings where there may be occupational exposure, provide ongoing evaluation of the risk and education of the employees on how to reduce risk.

Adapted from Youngberg, B. (1993). *Risk Managers Law Alert,* 2(6), 5–7, Aspen Publishers, Inc.

employer claims that a disability-based distinction is not being used to discriminate, the employer must justify this distinction with a detailed explanation of the rationale, including the actuarial conclusions and the factual data that support their decision (U.S. EEOC, 1993). Cases in support of allowing an employer to offer disparate insurance benefits include *Doe v. Colautti* (1979), which upheld Pennsylvania's medical assistance statute to provide disparate benefits for inpatient hospital treatment of mental illness and *Doe v. Devine* (1982), which held that the Blue Cross cutbacks in mental health benefits for federal employees were reasonable and did not discriminate on the basis of disability. The EEOC notice of June 8, 1993, explained that broad distinctions which apply to a multitude of dissimilar conditions and which constrain individuals both with and without disabilities are not distinctions based on disability. Therefore they do not intentionally discriminate on the basis of the disability and do not violate the ADA (U.S. EEOC, 1993).

The employment issues of concern to nurses focus on the desire to prevent transmission of HIV and not to discriminate against patients or health care workers who are HIV infected while also remaining sensitive to the needs of persons with whom they work. Providers must work with their employers to develop supportive policies and programs. Tables 14–1 and 14–2 offer guidelines for development of these policies.

Limits on Protection

Cases dealing with HIV as a handicap protected by law include a 1992 case wherein an HIV-infected pharmacist was supported by a DHHS Review Board decision, which based its ruling on Section 504 of the Vocational Rehabilitation Act of 1973. The DHHS judge ordered the medical center to hire the pharmacist without limiting his duties, or the agency would forfeit all federal reimbursement funding (Staff, *AJN,* 1992b). Employers who receive federal funds are prohibited from discriminating against any otherwise qualified individual on the basis of his or her handicap. The ADA expands protection to employees with disabilities even in the private sector, requiring employers to make reasonable accommodations for HIV-infected employees (Kolasa, 1993; Westchester County Medical Center, 1992).

The 1990 *Leckelt* case involved a plaintiff who was living with a person who died of AIDS. When the hospital infection control department demanded that the employee be tested for HIV antibody, he refused and was fired for failing to comply with hospital policy. The court upheld the termination, relying on CDC guidelines that identify invasive procedures that Leckelt had performed. The fact that the employee refused to be tested was held to prevent the hospital from conducting the necessary inquiry to protect patients, coworkers, and the plaintiff himself. The *Leckelt* court based its finding on the fact that AIDS is fatal and that even a minor risk is unacceptable. This case limits the protection of health-care givers, in comparison with the previous case discussed. In the previous case, the hospital's federal funding was threatened for refusing to hire the HIV-infected pharmacist. Similarly, an HIV-infected intensive care nurse who was reassigned to a "nurse liaison" position was supported by the DHHS. The hospital's federal funding was threatened because the DHHS found that the employee's transfer violated both CDC and handicap guidelines in that intensive care nurses do not practice "exposure prone" procedures under the CDC definitions (Staff, *AJN*, 1992d). However, it is important to note that in the *Leckelt* case the employee was merely suspected of being infected with HIV and yet was fired for refusing to be tested.

Both civil and criminal cases must be brought before the court within a designated time frame called the statute of limitations. Each state and jurisdiction legislate the amount of time allowed to bring cases under various charges. A 2-year statute of limitations is usually the minimum in which a case must be filed or the person's right to bring the case is lost. The New Jersey Supreme Court has held that a discrimination case must be brought within 2 years. In New Jersey the antidiscrimination law did not have its own statute of limitations, and therefore federal and state courts borrow such a statue from other places. The 2-year statute of limitations was found by New Jersey to be appropriate because this shorter time frame would promote more accurate testimony while information was fresh in witnesses' minds (McKenna & Cuneo, 1993; *Montells v. Haynes*, 1993). This case is another example of the many laws and statutes that the nurse must be aware of when evaluating liability issues related to AIDS.

Legislated AIDS Policy

In addition to case law, individual states are taking action to define AIDS policy through legislation. The State of Texas adopted the Human Immunodeficiency Virus Act after a statewide task force recommended that the state develop guidelines covering HIV infection and AIDS specifically related to college campus life (Staff, *Perspective*, 1990).

The New York State Department of Health issued a policy statement and guidelines for health care facilities and HIV-infected medical personnel based on the premise that the limited research available argues against the ready transmission of AIDS by health care workers to their patients and vice versa if universal precautions are followed. Under the New York policy, only when health care workers pose a significant risk of transmitting disease because of their inability to meet basic infection control standards or when they are functionally unable to care for patients is the limiting of their practice justified.

Invasive procedures are defined also by the New York policy guidelines as "those in which there is a significant risk of patient contact with health care workers' blood or body fluids." New York's guidelines encourage workers to voluntarily obtain HIV testing to delay the progression of their disease and the onset of opportunistic infections. New York State law does prohibit involuntary or coerced testing by employers, and nothing in the new guideline encourages employers to require that a health care worker undergo HIV testing (New York State Department of Health Memorandum 89-74, 1989; New York State Department of Health Memorandum 89-67, 1989).

PRIVACY, CONFIDENTIALITY, AND DISCLOSURE

The discussion thus far has focused mainly on the prevention of transmission and on antidiscrimination protections of the ADA. Legal issues of privacy and confidentiality are also contained in the ADA. Issues of privacy and confidentiality involve the element of disclosure. Health care workers in New York are not required to disclose information about their own HIV status to patients. If a facility should choose to disclose that a worker's HIV status is positive in New York, it must obtain a worker's written consent to release his or her identification. Otherwise the facility may choose to provide information to patients but cannot identify the worker (New York State Department of Health Memorandum 89-74, 1989; New York State Department of Health Memorandum 89-67, 1989). The ADA regulations protect the privacy of an HIV-infected person by giving the individual the opportunity to disclose his or her disability. If special accommodations are needed, the employer must disclose only the accommodations that have been identified, without disclosing the specific details of the individual's disability.

Most states require physicians in hospitals to report all cases of contagious diseases, including AIDS, to the CDC, Atlanta, Ga. Some jurisdictions also require the reporting of AIDS and of early symptomatic and asymptomatic HIV disease to the state department of health. Confidentiality provisions contained in these reporting laws prohibit the physician or hospital from releasing medical information to persons other than the patient or the department of health. Many statutes contain exceptions to the rule, however, allowing disclosure of AIDS-related information to persons who have a need to know, such as medical and emergency personnel, spouses, persons with whom the patient has shared needles, or others at risk of acquiring the disease without this knowledge, such as funeral directors. Additionally, courts can order disclosure of AIDS patient records in situations not addressed by state statute. These laws and case precedents are important because they allow the release of confidential information without the patient's consent and perhaps even if the patient is protesting. However, in 1991 the New York State Court of Appeals rejected the Medical Society of New York State's request that AIDS be classified as a sexually transmitted disease, thereby allowing for AIDS test results to be made available to physicians without a medical consent from the patient. The state upheld the privacy protection for AIDS patients (*New York Society of Surgeons v. Axelrod*, 1991).

Disclosure of AIDS-related information has serious implications for persons in our society because of the nature of the disease. The law attempts to balance the individual's rights against the rights of the public. Society has an interest in preventing organ and blood donations by infected individuals, in allowing the government to gain access to AIDS-related information for the conduct of scientific research, and in allowing individual persons such as spouses to know whether their partners are carrying the deadly disease. These conflicting interests have resulted in additional confidentiality legislation on a state-by-state basis, governing the disclosure of AIDS-related information contained in medical records. These statutes not only describe the circumstances under which information may be released but also prohibit disclosure of the identity of persons who have received the results of HIV testing. Both civil and criminal liability can result for unauthorized disclosures.

All 50 states have rules requiring the reporting of AIDS. The rules vary regarding who is required to report the information, such as the physician or the institution, and the details of the information to be reported. Many jurisdictions require specific name, address, age, race, sex, and marital status. Other jurisdictions prohibit any identifying information. It is important for nurses to understand the reporting laws in the jurisdiction in which they practice. The reporting laws make a distinction between cases of clinical AIDS on one hand and positive results on tests for HIV infection and early symptomatic disease on the other.

Several states require only that a person who dies of an AIDS-related illness be reported to the health authorities (Roach & Handler, 1990). In Maryland, laboratories that collect blood, semen, or tissue samples from potential donors must report positive HIV test results, although personal identifying information is not revealed. Similarly, in Iowa, a physician must report a positive HIV test result but may not include personal identifying information. Yet, if AIDS has been diagnosed in a patient, the physician must release the identifying information to the health department.

Several state statutes make clear that the patient waives the physician-patient privilege with regard to reportable information in order to allow the physician to disclose identifying data. Under the Indiana code, the physician is given greater leeway under a permissive reporting law which suggests that the physician may notify the health department if the patient is a serious and present danger to the health of others and is demonstrating noncompliant behavior. No liability exists for the physician if this report is made in good faith. Noncompliant behavior would include the continuation of exposure of others to the HIV virus by engaging in behavior that has been shown to transmit the disease.

Patients have a limited right to gain access to their own medical records and also the right to authorize release of their test results to third parties. As an example, a patient may need to release information to his or her insurance company, employer, or school. It is recommended that a written release, signed by the patient, be included with the medical record before this confidential information is released to any third party.

Most statutes allow information related to AIDS to be released to medical personnel who have a need to know because they are involved in the treatment of the patient. These statutes allow the results of an HIV test to be placed directly in a patient's record. Although confirmation of AIDS or HIV test results found in the patient's record may give additional notice to health care providers, universal precautions must still be taken with all patients. Statutes that authorize the disclosure of positive HIV test results and AIDS diagnoses to health care personnel may give health care workers a false sense of security because the diagnosis may not yet have been made in other patients. These disclosure laws reflect a concern for the safety of health care workers who are placed at risk during the performance of their duties; however, it is important that health care workers protect themselves through recognition of universal precaution procedures.

Many of the laws regarding AIDS disclosure are unclear as to whether they are permissive laws that allow disclosure or mandatory laws requiring disclosure. Additionally, not every health care worker who comes in contact with a patient has a need to know of the patient's HIV status. In California, the results of an HIV test may be recorded in the patient's record and revealed to persons who provide direct patient care and treatment. The California law reflects a concern for the safety of direct-care workers.

Other statutes, such as a Delaware law, restrict disclosure of HIV test information except under certain circumstances and seem to reflect concern for the patient's privacy rather than the safety of the health care worker, because only those persons with a specific need to know may be informed. Illinois has adopted a similar statute under which only those who have a need to know the information may be informed. Hawaii allows the physician to decide who needs this information. Kentucky releases information only to the physician taking care of the patient, whereas Maine allows the HIV test results to be given to those designated by the patient.

Utah's and New York's laws address concern for persons in addition to the patient and the health care worker. Whereas the Utah statute does not create a duty to warn third parties, it authorizes disclosure not only to medical personnel who work with the patient but also family members, sexual partners, and needle partners. Colorado holds all HIV and AIDS reports strictly confidential. None of the exceptions to the Colorado rule refer to medical personnel. In Louisiana, when a patient is transferred to a nursing home, the law requires that the hospital notify the nursing home of a patient's HIV condition. The corresponding duty from a nursing home to a hospital exists in Louisiana. When a body is picked up for disposition in Indiana, the law requires that a conspicuous notice of the deceased person's AIDS or HIV status be attached so that "body fluid precautions" can be observed.

In some states, specific statutes exist to protect emergency personnel, allowing confidential information to be released to protect those who have come in contact with blood or body fluids of an HIV-infected person. Most of these statutes leave to a physician's best medical judgment the determination of whether to disclose the information. A few states impose a duty on the physician to notify emergency personnel who cared for a patient who is later tested and found to have HIV disease. Some confidentiality statutes allow the physician to notify spouses and others at risk for infection of a patient's status. Usually these statutes give permission, but do not impose a duty to provide such notification. Whenever possible, these statutes require the physician to protect the identity of the patient. California has such a law, which further imposes the duty to confer with the patient before such disclosure. South Carolina law states that when a spouse or a known contact is told of a patient's HIV status, the physician is not liable for damages resulting from this disclosure. Although these statutes do not create a duty or responsibility to disclose this information, other states' laws may impose this obligation (Roach & Handler, 1990).

Disclosures without the consent of the patient to a third party may also be statutorily allowed to agencies who have a need to know, such as foster care and adoption agencies and correctional facilities. In Texas, blood banks may be authorized to release the fact that an infectious disease was found in a blood product if the blood was used in a transfusion. The identity of the recipient, however, is kept confidential. Some confidentiality statutes allow disclosure under a court order when a compelling need is shown. The balancing test is used to determine whose rights demand protection—those of the patient, the public, or the persons inquiring as to the status of the

patient's health. Pseudonyms are used in these court-ordered cases to protect the identity of the patient. In a Florida case, *Rasmussen v. South Florida Blood Services* (1987), an automobile accident victim petitioned the court for the names of blood donors from whom he may have received a transfusion. The court denied the request, holding that the public interest, including that of donors, outweighed the plaintiff's need for information. No statute relating to disclosure existed in Florida when this case was decided, and the court relied on its own powers to resolve the conflict. The Florida court relied on federal and state constitutional rights to privacy and on public policy, which encourages persons to be blood donors.

Although most courts agree with the public policy decision of the *Rasmussen* case, a contrary decision was found in the *Tarrant County* case, in which the court ordered the list of donors to be provided to the plaintiff. The *Tarrant* case recognized the *Rasmussen* case but emphasized that limitations would be placed on the plaintiff's use of the list in this case and that the patient's case could not go forward without this list. In the *Tarrant* case the plaintiff was allowed to contact donors only with the court's approval.

The *Tarrant* case, as well as other cases, has reached the additional decision that blood bank donors are not protected under the same physician client privilege that protects other patients. In *Belle Bonfils Memorial Blood Center v. District Court* (1988), the plaintiffs claimed that the blood donor had not been properly screened. The court authorized questions to be asked of the donor with the donor's identity protected. Each plaintiff was allowed to contact the donor through questions directed to a court clerk. Under most confidentiality statutes the burden is placed on the plaintiff to show both a compelling reason that access to donor information is needed, and a lack of alternative sources of information, rather than applying the traditional balancing test of weighing the public interest in encouraging blood donors versus the individual's rights.

In a similar case, *Doe v. American Red Cross* (1989), the plaintiff wished to question a particular donor. A federal court denied this request. The court reasoned that the need to maintain an adequate donor blood supply outweighed the individual plaintiff's need to contact an individual donor. Other cases, such as *Mason v. Regional Medical Center* (1988), have not protected the identity of the donor and have released information to a limited number of persons with a need to know. The case of *Doe v. American Red Cross* further emphasized the fact that voluntary blood donors may be less likely to have contagious diseases than paid blood donors, and yet all donors must be encouraged to provide accurate and honest health history information and not to fear that their identity will be exposed (Roach & Handler, 1990).

LIABILITY FOR EXPOSURE AND RISK

Two civil cases have held that a duty exists to warn a partner of the danger of transmission of a contagious disease. The publicized case in which the plaintiff was given an award against the estate of actor Rock Hudson for concealment of his illness and also a case in which the plaintiff transmitted the herpesvirus to his sexual partner imposed liability for concealing a health threat (Staff, *AIDS Litigation Reporter,* 1989). An obligation of health care providers to disclose their HIV status was found in the case of *Faya v. Almaraz* (1993), in which patients were allowed to proceed with their negligence claim against the surgeon who had performed surgery without disclosing his HIV status, and in the case of *Kerins v. Hartley* (1993), wherein the court held that a claim of battery could be brought against a physician who did not disclose his HIV status as part of his informed consent obligation. Even the fear of contracting AIDS has led to civil suits in which partners have been successful in claiming the reasonableness of their fear and anxiety when they learned of their physician's positive HIV status (*Faya v. Almaraz,* 1993; *Carroll v. Sisters of St. Francis Health Services, 1992; Kerins v. Hartley,* 1993). A patient's visitor who had a needle stick was allowed damages on the basis of the reasonableness of his or her fear of contracting AIDS (*Carroll v. Sisters of St. Francis Health Services,* 1992).

In some states, criminal liability is imposed on HIV carriers who knowlingly engage in activities likely to spread the virus. Florida is one such state. Additionally, Colorado law permits restrictions on reckless, negligent, or criminal behavior that exposes others to HIV infection. Of 20 known individuals in Colorado who persisted in exposing others, 14 have had restrictive measures placed on them by health officers who were allowed by the court to intervene (Woodhouse et al., 1993).

Currently health care providers are not legally obligated to disclose their HIV status. However, as can be seen from the previous discussion, patients are individually filing civil suits against health care providers who fail to disclose. A study reported in 1993 in the *Journal of the American Medical Association* was conducted retrospectively on 2,317 patients of an orthopedic surgeon who followed recommended infection control procedures and was himself infected with HIV (von Reyn, 1993). The authors concluded that the risk of contracting HIV from a surgeon who adheres strictly to safe practices is extremely low (von Reyn, 1993). The *Kerins v. Hartley* case, previously discussed, involved a California surgeon who did not reveal his HIV status and was sued for battery and emotional distress. The plaintiff claimed that she had disclosed her immense fear of contracting AIDS during surgery to her physician, and the court believed that there was an intentional deviation from the consent process. This case is interesting in that the court limited the period in which the plaintiff could claim emotional distress to that period when she received notification that she was not infected and when counseling, more than 18 months after the surgery, was given to reassure the plaintiff of the reliability of the test and the remote possibility of her converting to a positive HIV status (Staff, *American Bar Association Journal,* 1993).

A nurse with positive HIV test results several months after being stuck by a needle during a struggle with a prisoner has received a $5.4 million judgment against the State of New York because the guards who were assigned to the prisoner did not intervene and refused to help control the patient despite the nurse's repeated requests (Staff, *RN* Update,

1992). This suit is under appeal (Staff, *RN Letters*, 1992).

In a well-publicized case, a Florida dentist infected with HIV was claimed to have infected six of his patients during dental procedures. This case prompted researchers to study, for the purpose of documenting the probability of exposure, more than 1,100 patients who had undergone 9,000 procedures by another dentist who was infected with HIV but who followed universal precautions. Infection was documented in five patients, including four patients who evidenced other risk factors for acquiring the HIV virus. The authors concluded that if universal precautions are strictly observed, the risk of transmission is minimal (Dickinson, 1993).

RISK MANAGEMENT FOR HEALTH CARE PROVIDERS

With the growing concern for transmission of the HIV virus to health care providers, insurance companies are moving to market new policies, for both group and individual coverage, to hospital workers who have direct contact with patients. The complicated alternative of filing for workers' compensation when HIV infection is acquired in the workplace is used as a rationale for these insurance policies because it is often difficult to document that the infection was acquired while serving as an employee. State nursing associations are taking an active role in encouraging hospitals to set up funds to protect nurses who become infected at work. The Oregon and Massachusetts nurses' associations have intervened on behalf of nurses in their states. This activity was stimulated by a 1990 case involving an intensive care nurse who had positive test results after a needle stick. The nurse was originally accommodated by being transferred to a clerical job, and then she was placed on workers' compensation at a rate half of her normal salary. Because the nurse was a part-time employee, long-term disability benefits were not available to her (Staff, *AJN*, 1992a).

Other risk management protections for health care workers exist. The OSHA bloodborne pathogens standard mandates that employers enforce universal precautions effective March 1992 (Covner, 1993). This mandate is intended to protect both health care workers and patients (Pugliese, 1992). The Family and Medical Leave Act of 1993 allows employees of companies with more than 50 employees up to 12 weeks of unpaid leave (Youngberg, 1993). The law, however, does not allow release time for caretakers who are friends or companions and therefore may exclude persons who may desire release time to care for HIV-infected friends.

LIVING WILLS, SPECIAL DIRECTIVES, AND MEDICAL POWER OF ATTORNEY

While I was writing this chapter, my close canine friend of 17 years was lying beside me, dying. This personal thought is shared not to be maudlin but perhaps because of a need to memorialize him and to humanize this factual legal content related to the right to make choices during the time of dying. Whereas the guardians of animals are offered choices to relieve the pain of dying, human friends and loved ones have legal guidelines describing the decisions society finds permissible. Death does not come suddenly for many, especially those dying of AIDS. The grieving process is complicated by the choices that must be made within the restrictions set by the law. The choices that our laws presently support for persons dying of AIDS include the legal right to consent to treatment and, accordingly, the legal right to refuse treatment that is not desired. Persons dying of AIDS very often are candidates for life support systems and many extraordinary medical treatments available today. Individuals in our society do not live their lives alike and therefore do not choose to die in the same manner. It is important for the nurse, and also is legally mandated for institutions, to ask the patient whether he or she has a living will or special directive.

The Patient Self-Determination Act, which became effective in 1991, requires all health care agencies to inquire of patients whether they have created a living will or a special directive. Most states have enacted living will statutes that enable a person to request that extraordinary life support be withheld. However, many living will statutes do not afford the protections necessary unless at least two physicians have determined that the patient fits within the definitions of "dying" outlined in the statute. Even patients in a vegetative state may not qualify under many states' living will statutes. It is safer for a patient to create a special medical directive and a special medical power of attorney that identifies a surrogate decision maker who is empowered to express the patient's wishes should the patient become unable to do so. Special medical directives give more details as to what the patient does or does not want performed on his or her person than does a basic living will.

The power of attorney for health care decisions is also an important safeguard because it is a legally recognized delegation of authority to a surrogate decision maker. Some persons who are dying of AIDS may desire to have a friend, partner, or significant other be the surrogate decision maker, rather than a family member as traditionally defined by legal standards. The law recognizes birth families, spouses, and legally created surrogate decision makers as empowered to decide for the patient who is incompetent or no longer capable of understanding the consequences of his or her decisions. If the appropriate legal documentation has not been prepared in advance, the persons most understanding of what the patient would desire may be prohibited from legally speaking for the patient.

SUICIDE AND EUTHANASIA

Our society does not legally sanction suicide or euthanasia. Most states have statutes that specifically direct that suicide is against public policy and illegal. Dr. Jack Kevorkian has brought physician-assisted suicide to the public's attention. Dr. Kevorkian chose the State of Michigan to test his suicide machine because of two cases that had established the legality of assisted suicide (*People v. Roberts, 1920; People v. Campbell, 1983*). He was charged with murder after the first use of his suicide machine, but the charges were dropped by a judge who ruled that the patient had caused her own death and that Michigan had no law against assisting a suicide. In

December 1992, Michigan's governor signed an anti-assisted-suicide bill. This bill temporarily criminalized assisted suicide. The law was written to allow a physician still to prescribe medications to relieve pain and discomfort and not to cause death, even if the patient should take a fatal overdose (Annas, 1993). On Nov. 5, 1993, Dr. Kevorkian was jailed for refusing to post a bond for violating the anti-assisted-suicide bill. The NBC televised news report of this story also stated that Dr. Kevorkian had been involved in 19 previous assisted suicides (NBC Newscast, Nov. 5, 1993).

As of 1992, 19 states had enacted separate statutes that criminalize assisting suicide. An additional eight states include this act under elements of manslaughter, and three states have statutes that make it a felony to cause a person to attempt suicide or to aid a person in attempting it. Nurses must be advised that counseling, encouraging, or intentionally advising suicide is classified as a crime in all 30 of these states. The reader is referred to Chapter 13, which discusses the ethical dilemmas encountered by nurses when a patient is facing a painful, debilitating, slow death. In addition to these 30 states, six states and the Territory of Puerto Rico have separate statutes criminalizing the "causing" of suicide. Seven states include participation in suicide as an element of manslaughter, and four states consider causing suicide to be murder. Tables 14–3 and 14–4 list these states under the categories described above (Logue, 1993; Young, 1993).

LEGAL ISSUES AND NURSING RESEARCH

The research previously discussed in this chapter focused on physicians and dentists with HIV infection and their risk of transmitting the disease to their patients. Nursing research is needed to understand the risk of infection transmission from nurses to patients. An article in *Today's OR Nurse* (Wicher, 1993) reported a conversation in July 1992 with a CDC official who reported that "29 health care workers in the United States have seroconverted to HIV positive due to occupational exposure to the virus. Of these 29,

Table 14–3. States and Territories that Have Statutes Criminalizing "Assisting Suicide"

SEPARATE STATUTE	ELEMENTS OF MANSLAUGHTER	PROMOTING SUICIDE
California	Alaska	Delaware
Florida	Arizona	New York
Kansas	Arkansas	Washington
Maine	Colorado	
Minnesota	Connecticut	
Mississippi	Missouri	
Montana	New York	
Nebraska	Oregon	
New Hampshire		
New Jersey		
New Mexico		
Oklahoma		
Oregon		
Pennsylvania		
Puerto Rico		
South Dakota		
Texas		
Virgin Islands		
Wisconsin		

From Young, H.H. Assisted suicide and physician liability. Published originally in 11 *The Review of Litigation* 623 (1992). Copyright 1992 by The University of Texas Law School Publications, Inc. Reprinted by permission.

Table 14–4. States and Territories that Have Statutes Criminalizing "Causing Suicide"

SEPARATE STATUTES	ELEMENT OF MANSLAUGHTER	ELEMENT OF MURDER
Indiana	Arkansas	Alaska
New Hampshire	Colorado	Connecticut
New Jersey	Connecticut	Delaware
Pennsylvania	Delaware	Maine
Puerto Rico	Hawaii	
Texas	New York	
	Oregon	

From Young, H.H. Assisted suicide and physician liability. Published originally in 11 *The Review of Litigation* 623 (1992). Copyright 1992 by The University of Texas Law School Publications, Inc. Reprinted by permission.

three have AIDS. Eleven are nurses." A nationwide survey, reported in this same article, revealed that more than half of the people surveyed would not wish to be cared for by a health care worker if they knew that the person had AIDS or HIV infection. Of those surveyed, 80% believed that a duty to disclose should be imposed on health care workers (Wicher, 1993).

To date there are only five documented cases of HIV transmission by an infected health care worker to patients. All these cases involve the Florida dentist previously discussed. Although the mode of transmission remains unknown, evidence has indicated that prescribed procedures may not have been used in this dentist's office. Other than this Florida case, 10 years of epidemiologic studies of health care workers who are infected with HIV and who perform invasive procedures have shown no transmission of the disease. Three other studies involving the patients of surgeons with AIDS have shown no evidence of transmission (Wicher, 1993). The CDC reported in May 1992 that continuing investigation of more than 15,000 patients has revealed no further transmission of HIV from health care worker to patient.

The CDC has not recommended mandatory testing. Congress enacted Public Health Service Law 102-141, Section 663, requiring that each state's public health officials certify to the Secretary of the DHHS that CDC guidelines or the equivalent had been instituted by October 28, 1992. Failure to comply will make the state ineligible under Public Health Service Act 42 USC Section 301 to receive federal assistance (Wicher, 1993).

The American Medical Association (AMA) guidelines on employability of HIV-infected physicians state that if a risk of transmission to a patient exists, then disclosure of that risk does not end the physician's responsibility. The AMA not only urges physicians to disclose their status to colleagues in order to gain assistance in assessing the risk to patients but also prompts physicians not to engage in activities if a risk exists. This position is stronger than the standard used by the Supreme Court in *Arline* (*School Board v. Arline*, 1987) and the CDC recommendations. However, mandatory testing for HIV/AIDS is not supported by the AMA. The American Nurses' Association, which also has recognized the seriousness of the implications of the disease on the profession of nursing, is opposed to mandatory testing and has supported policies that encourage the safety of both the health care worker and the patient (Wicher, 1993). The May 1992 policy enacted by New York encourages adherence to universal precautions and allows practitioners to continue to practice without disclosing their status to anyone as long as their abilities are not impaired.

Research related to the transmission of AIDS from nurse to patient has not been documented. Because of the great number of patients and nurses who interact in hospitals, this research is necessary although difficult to conduct. The August 1991 *American Journal of Nursing* reported a study of 1,520 registered nurses and 958 physicians (Staff, *AJN*, 1991a). Ninety-three percent of the registered nurses said that they would wear gloves while performing venipuncture on HIV-infected patients, whereas only 59% would take precautions if the patient's HIV status was unknown. It is also disturbing that two thirds of the registered nurses surveyed reported believing AIDS and hepatitis B to be equally transmissible. The registered nurses in the study were asked to estimate the risk of acquiring HIV if stuck by a needle used on a patient known to be infected with HIV, and only 20% of those surveyed correctly guessed that the risk was less than 1%. Only 33% of the group were willing to care for AIDS patients, but 76% of physicians and 82% of registered nurses said that they would not refuse to treat HIV-infected patients (Staff, *AJN*, 1991a). Although this research is broader than the legal issues discussed, research is recommended in the area of nurse-patient transmission of the disease, and continuing research is recommended on the knowledge base and utilization of universal precautions by nurses. If legislation and case precedents are truly going to reflect the needs of nurses and their patients, nurses must take a proactive position and gather data that can correctly reflect the risk of transmission of disease between the nurse and the patient. The legal questions that have not been totally resolved relate to the necessity or the impropriety of mandatory testing of nurses or their patients. The balancing test between the nurse's rights and the individual

patient's rights continues to be debated. Again, the practice of universal precautions may resolve these legal issues. Evaluation of the threat of harm to the patient and to the nurse could be established through nursing research and will be valuable in assisting legislatures and courts when determinations of whose rights need protection are being made.

It has been argued that nurses do not routinely conduct invasive procedures. Research describing the specific responsibilities of nursing and how they may or may not fall within the invasive procedures category would be helpful. Nursing research that describes how a nurse who is infected with HIV may reasonably be accommodated in his or her employment also would be worthwhile. Questions related to this issue are the reasonableness of the nurse employee's requests, the impact on other employees and patients, and the undue hardship an employer may experience through special accommodations.

Advance practice nurses are establishing relationships with patients similar to those of physicians with patients. Nursing research regarding the issues previously related only to physicians and dentists would be helpful in establishing the advance practice nurse's responsibilities under the law. Advance practice nurses should study the rules and regulations, as well as statutes, both federal and state, that have an impact on their practice. As has been stated, jurisdictions vary widely in their treatment of disclosure, privacy, and confidentiality laws related to AIDS.

SUMMARY

The legal issues of concern to nurses deal with balancing the rights of the individual and society when HIV/AIDS is present. Patients and health care workers are afforded protections against discrimination when they are infected with HIV or have AIDS. The corresponding need to protect the privacy and confidentiality of persons infected with AIDS through strict compliance with disclosure regulations and statutes must be understood by the nurse. Where broadly stated federal and state statutes leave room for definition, courts are filling in the details and determining the rights of persons already infected with AIDS and those who risk infection. Mandatory HIV testing does not exist except in situations where public policy clearly indicates a need to direct persons to receive testing. Health care workers to date have not received mandates that they must be tested.

Patient-assisted suicide is illegal today. Trends in the law develop as society speaks and cases scrutinize the changing needs of our society. The patient's right to refuse treatment and the legal right to give consent to treatment should encourage all people to create a living will and a special medical directive and, if necessary, to identify a surrogate decision maker through a special power of attorney in case they become incompetent or incapable of making these decisions on their own.

Legal research is conducted by studying case developments and looking at the particular similarities and differences between the facts of cases. Where a statute, rule, or regulation does not dictate the behavior of individuals within our society, the courts are given leeway to determine these rights. The balancing test of looking at whose rights—the individual's or society's—demand the protection of the law is used in most AIDS-related cases. The compelling interest of a plaintiff to know and the unreasonableness of denying the plaintiff disclosure of private AIDS-related information have also been utilized in determining whose rights must be protected under case precedent. Public policy is critical to these determinations. Legal research discloses that most cases involving nurses and AIDS today relate to protections needed by the nurse as an employee. Further research is recommended to gather data regarding the risks of transmission of the disease between nurses and patients so that legislators and courts can be educated as additional laws are developed. Individual nurses must take responsibility to inform themselves regarding the laws in the states and jurisdictions in which they practice nursing.

REFERENCES

Alexander v. Choate, 469 U.S. 287 (1985).

Americans With Disabilities Act of 1990. 42 U.S.C. §1210 et. seq. Public Law No. 101–336, 140 Stat 327.

Annas, G.J. (1993). Physician-assisted suicide: Michigan's temporary solution. *New England Journal of Medicine, 328,* 1573–1576.

Armstrong v. Flowers Hospital, Inc., U.S. District Court for the Middle District of Alabama, Southern Division, CV-92-1-101-S, Feb. 9, 1993, cited in "Court dismisses complaint of pregnant nurse who refused to treat AIDS patient." *BNA's Health Law Reporter, 2,* 20.

Belle Bonfils Memorial Blood Center v. District Court, 763 P.2d 1003 (CO 1988).

Buckingham v. United States of America (July 13, 1993). *93 Daily Journal D.A.R.,* 8976.

Carroll v. Sisters of St. Francis Health Services (1992). W.L. 276717 (TN App. Ct., Oct. 12, 1992).

Centers for Disease Control (Nov. 15, 1985). Summary: Recommendations for preventing transmission of infection with human T-lymphotropic virus type III/lymphadenopathy–associated virus in the workplace. *Morbidity and Mortality Weekly Report, 34*(45), 681–695.

Centers for Disease Control (April 11, 1986). Recommendations for preventing transmission of infection with human T-lymphtropic virus type III/lymphadenopathy–associated virus during invasive procedures. *Morbidity and Mortality Weekly Report, 35*(14), 221–223.

Centers for Disease Control (Aug. 21, 1987). Recommendations for prevention of HIV transmission in health-care settings. *Morbidity and Mortality Weekly Report, 36*(2S), 3S–18S.

Centers for Disease Control Guidelines (July 12, 1991). Recommendations for preventing transmission of human immune deficiency virus and hepatitis B virus to patients during exposure-prone invasive procedures. *Morbidity and Mortality Weekly Report, 40*(RR-8), 1–9.

Covner, A.L. (1993, October). Occupational Safety and Health Administration universal precautions. Regulations December 1991, effective March 1992. The American Association of Nurse Attorneys (TAANA) Proceedings, New Orleans, LA.

Covner, A.L., Wicher, C.P. (1993a, October). AIDS: An update on the impact to the health care environment. The American Association of Nurse Attorneys (TAANA) Proceedings, New Orleans, LA.

Covner, A.L., Wicher, C.P. (1993b, October). AIDS: No employer is immune employers ill prepared for AIDS. The American Association of Nurse Attorneys (TAANA) Proceedings, New Orleans, LA.

Covner, A.L., Wicher, C.P. (1993c, October). Disability law to clarify employer's duty. The American Association of Nurse Attorneys (TAANA) Proceedings, New Orleans, LA.

Dickinson, G.M. (1993). Absence of HIV transmission from an infected dentist to his patients. *Journal of the American Medical Association, 269,* 1802–1806.

Doe v. American Red Cross, 125 F.R.D. 646 (D.S.C. 1989).

Doe v. Colautti, 592 F. 2d 704 (3rd Cir. 1979).

Doe v. Devine, 545 F. Supp. 576 (D.D. C. 1982).

Faya v. Almaraz, 620 A. 2d 327 (1993).

Federal Rehabilitation Act of 1973, 29 U.S.C., § 504, 12101 et. seq.

Fresh News—Federal Register Executive Summary for Healthcare (1993). Three Summit Communications, *1*(3).

Kerins v. Hartley, *93 Daily Journal D.A.R.,* 9850 (July 30, 1993).

Key Case Review (1992, August). AIDS and discrimination: What precedent suggests. *Perspective, 7*(8), 1.

Kolasa, E.U. (1993, January). HIV v. A nurse's right to work. *RN, 56*(1), 63–64, 66.

Leckelt v. Hospital District No. 1, 714 F. Supp. 1377, aff'd 909, F2d 820 (5th Cir. 1990).

Logue, K. (1993, October). Medically assisted suicide. The American Association of Nurse Attorneys (TAANA) Proceedings, New Orleans, LA.

Mason v. Regional Medical Center, 121 F.R.D. 300 (W.D. KY 1988).

McKenna & Cuneo (1993, September). New Jersey's Discrimination Law Subject to Two-Year Statute of Limitations. *Labor and Employment Law Bulletin, 93*(9), 18.

Montells v. Haynes, 627 A. 2d 654 (NJ 1993).

NBC Newscast (Nov. 5, 1993). Dr. Jack Kevorkian jailed.

New York Society of Surgeons v. Axelrod (1991). 77 N.Y. 2d 677, 569, N.Y.S. 2d 922.

New York State Department of Health Memorandum: Amendments to Title X (Health) (Aug. 23, 1989). New York City Regional Recommendations Memorandum 89–67.

New York State Department of Health Memorandum 89-74 (Sept. 15, 1989).

New York State Department of Health Policy (1991, January). Guidelines for health care facilities and HIV-infected medical personnel.

People v. Campbell, 335 NW 2d 27 (MI App. 1983).

People v. Roberts, 211 MI, 187, 178 N.W. 690 (1920).

Public Health Service Act, 42 U.S.C. §301 et. seq. (1993).

Pugliese, G. (1992). Universal precautions: Now they're the law. *RN 55*(9), 63, 65–66, 69–70.

Rasmussen v. South Florida Blood Services, 500 So. 2d 533 (FL 1987).

Roach, W.H., Handler, M.S. (1990). Legal review: AIDS patient records—legal issues of access and disclosure. *Topics in Health Record Management, 12*(4), 71–86.

School Board of Nassau County, Florida v. Arline, 480 U.S. 273 (1987).

Staff (April 28, 1989). *AIDS Litigation Reporter;* p. 2576. Edgemont, PA: Andrews Publications.

Staff (1990). Texas passes AIDS legislation. *Perspective, 5*(4), 3.

Staff (1991a, August). Headline news: Majority of RNs favor mandatory testing for AIDS. *American Journal of Nursing, 91*(8), 11.

Staff (1991b, August). News: ANA members say no to mandatory AIDS testing. *American Journal of Nursing, 91*(8), 68–69.

Staff (1992a, May). As demand for HIV insurance grows, insurers move to market new policies. *American Journal of Nursing, 92*(5), 93, 96.

Staff (1992b, July). Headline news: An HIV-infected pharmacist. *American Journal of Nursing, 92*(7), 9.

Staff (1992c, August). Newscaps: States to set AIDS rules for workers. *American Journal of Nursing, 92*(8), 65.

Staff (1992d, December). Headline news: An HIV-infected nurse must be reinstated. *American Journal of Nursing, 92*(12), 9.

Staff (1992, September). Update: A nurse who contracted AIDS wins megasuit. *RN, 92*(9), 14.

Staff (1992, November). Letters: New York shouldn't contest a court's decision for a nurse with AIDS. *RN, 92*(11), 8.

Staff (1993, October). AIDS update. I. *American Bar Association Journal, 79,* 105,

Staff (1993, May). Newswatch: States grapple with guidelines for HIV and workers. *RN, 93*(5), 17.

Tarrant County Hospital District v. Hughes, 734 S.W. 2d 675 (TX Ct. App. 1987).

U.S. Equal Employment Opportunity Commission (June 8, 1993). EEOC issues interim enforcement guidance on the application of the ADA to disability-based provisions of employer-provided health insurance. *EEOC News,* N-915.002.

Vocational Rehabilitation Act of 1973, §504.

von Reyn, C.F. (1993). Absence of HIV transmission from an infected orthopedic surgeon. *Journal of the American Medical Association, 269,* 1807–1811.

Westchester County Medical Center, No. 91-504-2 (Decision No. CR 191 April 20, 1992).

Wicher, C.P. (1993, March/April). AIDS and HIV: The dilemma of the health care worker. *Today's O.R. Nurse, 15*(2), 14–22.

Woodhouse, D.E., Math, J.D., Potterat, J.J., et al. (1993, March/April). Restricting personal behavior: Case studies on legal measures to prevent the spread of HIV. *International Journal STD AIDS, 4*(2), 114–117.

Young, H.H. (1993, October). Assisted suicide and physician litigation. *Review of Litigation, 2,*623–656.

Youngberg, B.J. (1993, October). The employment challenge of AIDS in the workplace meeting. *Risk Managers Law Alert, 2*(6), 5–7.

Culture and Ethnicity

Jacquelyn Haak Flaskerud

Culture and ethnicity have become important concepts in understanding the transmission and prevention of HIV/AIDS because of the disproportionate occurrence of the disease in ethnic communities of color and because AIDS affects so many aspects of life that have cultural meaning: reproduction, birth, death, the roles of women, sexuality, and so forth. The public health service has become aware that standard prevention messages about condom use, mutliple sexual partners, anal-receptive intercourse, and sharing of needles have met cultural roadblocks that increase the complexity of the AIDS education campaign. The nature of HIV/AIDS lends itself to different cultural interpretations and explanations (Nicoll et al., 1993). It is a sexually transmitted disease; it appeared relatively recently without a demonstrable reason; it has a long incubation period, separating infection from death by about 10 years; it is lethal and spreading worldwide; and after only 12 years, scientific knowledge of HIV is growing but frequently changing (Nicoll et al., 1993; Sontag, 1990; Strong, 1990). Therefore AIDS is important, mysterious, and subject to legitimate speculation. It is a strong candidate for alternative lay beliefs and explanations. Frequently these are rooted in existing, workable lay explanations of the cause, transmission, prevention, and treatment of disease. Beliefs and practices acquired through the family and cultural explanations about other illnesses will also be applied to AIDS. Values and practices related to sexuality, the role of women, the importance of children, and so forth will not be changed simply because of the threat of a new and dangerous disease. This is especially so when the lay public perceives the health professional and scientific communities as limited in their knowledge of the disease, frequently changing their explanations and proscriptions, and, in some cases, not to be trusted. The force of a cultural worldview is much more persuasive and pervasive than a scientific explanation not only in ethnic communities of color but in all sociocultural groups.

Health care workers will need to become culturally competent if they are to work credibly and effectively with their various client groups in preventing and treating HIV disease (California Nurses' Association [CNA], 1993). Cultural competence involves a set of congruent behaviors, attitudes, and policies between a health care system, health care professionals, and their clients (Cross et al., 1989). Cultural competence facilitates effective assessments and interventions in cross-cultural situations. A culturally competent system of care (health care agency) acknowledges and incorporates at all structural and management levels the importance of culture; an assessment of cross-cultural relations between workers, workers and clients, and communities; and vigilance in policies, procedures, and methods toward the dynamics resulting from cultural differences (Cross et al., 1989). Culturally competent caregivers acknowledge and actively pursue expansion of cultural knowledge specific to their clients and the communities they serve, and adapt their services to meet culturally unique needs. This adaptation might include a change in focus, method, timing, and emphasis, as well as concrete services and treatments that will be accepted. Before cultural competence can be achieved, a basic understanding of the constructs of culture and ethnicity is needed.

CULTURE AND ETHNICITY

There are as many definitions of culture as there are cultural theorists and conceptual models of culture, including those specific to nursing (Leininger, 1991). The definition of culture given here was chosen because of its universality and its goodness-of-fit with the current situation of HIV disease, particularly as it affects ethnic communities of color in the United States. Theories of cultural ecology or cultural adaptation (Anderson, 1973; Edgerton, 1971) provide a conceptualization of culture and environment that include the major variables identified by the relevant social, behavioral, and medical scientists in the field (see Belgrave & Randolph, 1993; Carrier, 1989; Cochran & Mays, 1993; DeCarpio et al., 1990; Jenkins et al., 1993; Magaña & Carrier, 1991; Marin, 1989; Marin & Marin, 1990; 1992).

Culture is passed on through the family from infancy onward; it is learned, shared, and transmitted in patterned ways. The theory of cultural ecology or cultural adaptation proposes that the culture of a social group arises in response to the environmental resources available to that particular group. The environment includes natural and physical habitat, resources available, and other human groups competing for these same resources. Culture embodies and consists of economic structures, social structures, ideology, and art and artifacts. Economic structures include the economic opportunities, sources of income, and available occupations provided by the particular environment into which one is born. Social structures arise to support the economic structures. Type and function of social structures are influenced by the economic structures and income opportunities. Social structures include family, kin, fictive kin and friend networks, political organizations, social and religious organizations, and so forth. Finally, an ideology arises that endorses, validates, and legitimates the social structures and economy. Ideology consists of values, beliefs, attitudes, behaviors, morals, ideals, ethics, and so forth. Art and artifacts are expressions of ideology, social structures, and economic structures. Members of a particular social group, who share a culture, learn and transmit it in patterned ways, often without being cognitively aware that their worldview differs from that of persons with other cultural backgrounds (Wenger, 1993).

The term "culture" has been used in a more popular sense than the formal definition given here. In that sense it has been used to describe gay culture, teen culture, rock culture, drug culture, and so on. Often the term "subculture" is used in this context (Friedman et al., 1990). From this perspective, culture is taught through the social group rather than the family (Britton et al., 1993; Friedman et al., 1990). It is acquired as a teen or young adult and not from infancy on. It embodies the beliefs and practices of social groups other than the family. Finally, it functions to integrate a person into his or her social group. In some groups—for instance, white gay men—the culture may be well developed, strong, supportive, and sustaining. It may include shared social and community structures and resources; shared political structures; a political agenda; shared discrimination, stigma, and isolation; and shared values, lifestyle, and practices (Grossman, 1991). In other cases—for example, teen culture—it may mark only a passing phase in one's life.

Ethnicity differs from the formal definition of culture given here. Ethnicity is based on a shared sense of peoplehood related to national or regional origin, and sometimes on shared language, religion, and customs. However, despite this difference, Rosenthal (1986) argued persuasively that there is such a phenomenon as ethnic culture. Ethnic culture includes a body of shared cultural meanings that influences beliefs, practices, and relationships with other members of the ethnic group and with the larger society. The term "ethnicity" is chosen here as opposed to race or racial groups because of its better fit with HIV disease. Use of the term "race" would imply a biologic or genetic risk factor for HIV disease in members of a particular racial group; in the case of HIV, this risk factor is not known to exist (Centers for Disease Control and Prevention [CDC], June 25, 1993; Wyatt, 1991). Ethnicity, on the other hand, reflects cultural or learned values, behavioral patterns, social class and other psychosocial factors, and demographic and regional variations (CDC,

June 25, 1993; Wyatt, 1991). Ethnicity is here considered a risk marker rather than a risk factor for HIV disease (CDC, June 25, 1993).

It should be established at the outset that levels of ethnic identification differ within ethnic groups and with individual members of a particular ethnic group (CNA, 1993). Levels of ethnic identification are usually observed in frequency and exclusivity of personal and social contacts, language used and preferred, preferred media, values endorsed and practiced, and preference for foods, dress, and other customs (Keefe & Padilla, 1987; Marin et al., 1987; Marin & Marin, 1990; Wyatt, 1991). For persons with low levels of ethnic identification, ethnicity might be recognized only at holidays or in awareness of surnames.

ETHNICITY AND EPIDEMIOLOGY OF HIV DISEASE

HIV surveillance data are collected for four broad ethnic communities of color in the United States and for an equally broad community of white persons. These groups are categorized as African Americans, Latinos/Hispanics, Asian Americans and Pacific Islanders, American Indian and Alaskan Natives, and European Americans. These broad divisions do not account separately for other groups, such as those from the Middle East or Near East.

African Americans comprise the largest ethnic community of color in the United States, making up 12% of the population. African Americans include those whose ancestors were brought here as slaves in the seventeenth century, as well as recent immigrants from the Caribbean, Africa, and Europe (National Commission on Acquired Immune Deficiency Syndrome [NCA], 1992). Latinos/Hispanics make up 9% of the U.S. population and include Spanish-speaking and -surnamed people from Central and South America, the Caribbean, and Spain. The largest group are Mexican Americans (64%), followed by other Central and South Americans (14%), Puerto Ricans (11%), and Cubans (5%) (NCA, 1992). Asian Americans and Pacific Islanders are the third largest community of color in the United States (3%) and the fastest growing. They

speak more than 100 different languages and are grouped together because of similar regional origins. Asian Americans include Japanese, Chinese, Koreans, Pilipinos, and Southeast Asians. Pacific Islanders include Native Hawaiians and immigrants from Guam, Samoa, and other small island nations having a close relationship with the United States (NCA, 1992). American Indians and Alaskan Natives include more than 500 tribes and villages with government-to-government relationships with the United States. Each has its own language, customs, and history. About half live in urban areas of the United States, one fourth on reserved lands, and one fourth in rural areas (NCA, 1992). For HIV surveillance purposes, European Americans (whites) compose the remainder of the U.S. population, presumably including Australians and New Zealanders and encompassing people from the Middle East (Arab countries) and Near East (e.g., India, Pakistan). As may be seen from each of these broad categorizations, a wide range of ethnic groups, cultures, languages, value systems, beliefs, and practices are included within each category.

The African American community has been affected the most severely by the HIV epidemic. African Americans make up 31% of all AIDS cases (CDC, October 1993). Among African American men, those who risk exposure to HIV are men who have sex with men (MWSM) (42%), injection drug users (IDUs) (36%), and MWSM who are also IDUs (7%). HIV screening of active-duty military and Job Corps applicants found a seroprevalence rate of 5.1/1,000 and 5.3/1,000, respectively, among African Americans (Conway et al., 1993; Kelley et al., 1989). These data represent a spread of HIV disease to youthful populations. African American women make up 53% of all adult women in the United States with AIDS (CDC, October 1993). Injection drug use is the most common means of exposure (52%), followed by heterosexual contact with an IDU (19%), followed by heterosexual contact with an HIV-infected person who is not an IDU (17%). The AIDS rate as a result of sex with a bisexual man is five times higher among black women than among white women (Chu et al., 1992).

Table 15–1. Percentage of Total AIDS Cases in Men (Total N = 293,642) by Ethnicity and Exposure Category, October 1993

EXPOSURE CATEGORY	EUROPEAN AMERICAN (N = 160,923)	AFRICAN AMERICAN (N = 82,174)	HISPANIC/ LATINO (N = 47,351)	ASIAN/PACIFIC ISLANDER (N = 2007)	AMERICAN INDIAN/ ALASKAN NATIVE (N = 614)
Male-male sexual contact (MWSM)	78	42	45	79	63
Injection drug use (IDU)	8	36	38	4	10
MWSM/IDU	7	7	6	3	17
Receipt of blood products*	3	1	1	6	4
Heterosexual contact	1	8	3	1	2
Unidentified risk	3	6	6	8	4

*Includes factor VIII concentrate (hemophilia).

Although the highest seroprevalence rates are concentrated in urban areas, primarily along the East Coast, several studies have documented the spread of HIV to nonurban African American women, principally those living in the U.S. South and East (Conway et al., 1993; Schoenbach et al., 1993; St. Louis et al., 1991; Wasser et al., 1993). In these studies, women were unaware that they were at risk of acquiring infection that was occurring principally through heterosexual exposure. African American children account for 55% of all pediatric AIDS cases in the United States. Of these, 95% acquired HIV infection perinatally from an infected mother and 4% from transfusion with blood products. Contrasting rates of AIDS by ethnic group are provided for men, women, and children in Tables 15–1 to 15–3.

Latinos/Hispanics make up 17% of reported AIDS cases and, together with African Americans, account for 48% of all cases. Among Latino men, 45% were exposed to HIV through male-male sexual contact, 38% through injection drug use, and 6% through male-male sexual contact and injection drug use. Of the total AIDS cases among U.S. adolescents (13 to 19 years of age), 20% are Latino/Hispanic. Latina women account for 20% of the total AIDS cases. For women, exposure is principally through injection drug use (47%) and heterosexual contact with IDUs or bisexual men (41%) (CDC, October 1993; Chu et al., 1992). Pediatric cases of AIDS among Latinos make up 24% of all U.S. pediatric cases. Perinatal transmission accounts for 90% of cases. Mothers were infected principally through heterosexual contact with an IDU (32%) or were themselves IDUs (47%).

Exposure to HIV varies among Latinos according to ethnicity (Diaz et al., 1993a). Among men born in Central and South Amer-

Table 15–2. Percentage of Total AIDS Cases in Women (Total N = 40,702) by Ethnicity and by Exposure Category, October 1993

EXPOSURE CATEGORY	EUROPEAN AMERICAN (N = 10,293)	AFRICAN AMERICAN (N = 21,728)	HISPANIC/ LATINO (N = 8,273)	ASIAN/PACIFIC ISLANDER (N = 230)	AMERICAN INDIAN/ ALASKAN NATIVE (N = 103)
IDU	43	52	47	15	50
Sexual contact (with IDU, MWSM, or other)	35	36	41	45	31
Receipt of blood products	14	3	4	26	8
Unidentified risk	8	9	8	14	11

Table 15–3. Percentage of Total AIDS Cases by Ethnicity in Children (Total N = 4,906) and by Exposure Category, October 1993

EXPOSURE CATEGORY	EUROPEAN AMERICAN (N = 980)	AFRICAN AMERICAN (N = 2,683)	HISPANIC/ LATINO (N = 1,194)	ASIAN/PACIFIC ISLANDER (N = 22)	AMERICAN INDIAN/ ALASKAN NATIVE (N = 14)
Perinatal	68	95	90	45	93
Receipt of blood products	17	3	6	41	—
Hemophilia	14	1	3	14	7
Risk not identified	1	1	1	—	—

ica, Cuba, and Mexico, about 65% of cases were associated with male-male sexual contact and less than 10% with injection drug use. In contrast, among Puerto Rico–born men, 61% were exposed through injection drug use and 22% through male-male sexual contact. A similar pattern was seen in women. Women born in Central and South America, Cuba, and Mexico were exposed through heterosexual contact with an HIV-infected man. According to Chu and colleagues (1992), about 45% of these men were infected through sex with other men. In contrast, women born in Puerto Rico or in the United States but of Puerto Rican ancestry were infected through injection drug use (45%) or sex with an IDU (30%) (Diaz et al., 1993a).

Currently, Asian Americans and Pacific Islanders account for only 0.7% of AIDS cases in the United States, whereas these groups make up 3% of the total population of the United States. For a variety of reasons, there may be underreporting in this group (Lee & Fong, 1990). The distribution of AIDS in these groups resembles the epidemiology of HIV disease in the early years of the epidemic for other ethnic groups. Among men, 79% have been exposed through male-male sexual contact, 4% through injection drug use, and 3% through male-male sexual contact combined with injection drug use. Women have been exposed to HIV through heterosexual contact (45%), receipt of blood products (26%), and injection drug use (15%). Asian American and Pacific Islander children have been exposed through perinatal transmission (45%) and receipt of blood or blood products (55%). The Asian American–Pacific Islander community is considered to be in the early

stages of a growing HIV epidemic in this group in the United States (NCA, 1992). Because of the relative insularity of the ethnic groups composing these communities, once an infectious disease takes hold, it spreads rapidly. If prevention efforts are not instituted, the epidemic in the United States in these groups is expected to resemble that in the African American and Latino communities. Meanwhile, a changing epidemiology is projected worldwide by the year 2000, with the largest proportion of HIV infections occurring in Asian and Pacific Rim countries (Mann et al., 1992).

Currently, fewer than 1% of AIDS cases in the United States have occurred among American Indians and Alaskan Natives. However, there is substantial evidence that AIDS may be undercounted in these groups and misrepresented as white or Latino cases (Conway, 1990; NCA, 1992; Rowell, 1990). AIDS surveillance data show that among Native American men, 63% were exposed through male-male sexual contact, 10% through injection drug use, and 17% through a combination of these exposure routes (CDC, October 1993). Among women, 50% were exposed through injection drug use, 31% through heterosexual contact, and 8% through receipt of blood products. Of pediatric cases, 93% occurred through perinatal transmission. Seroprevalence studies of HIV infection in Native Americans have demonstrated that rates may be much higher than those reflected in AIDS surveillance data (NCA, 1992; Rowell, 1990). In the Military Recruit Study, seropositivity among Native Americans was reported at 4.4/1,000, second only to African Americans (Rowell, 1990). AIDS cases have been reported in every age group for Native Americans and in every Indian Health Service Area (NCA, 1992). From 1989 to 1990, AIDS cases in Native Americans increased by 23%, faster than cases among any other ethnic group: compared with 13% for Latinos, 12% for African Americans, and 2.5% for whites (Metler et al., 1991).

Americans of European origin (whites) account for the remainder of AIDS cases (51%) (CDC, October 1993). European Americans comprise 75.7% of the total population of the United States. White men account for 55% of AIDS cases among men. White men were exposed through male-male sexual contact (78%) and through injection drug use (8%); 7% were exposed through these two categories combined (CDC, October 1993). White women account for about 25% of total AIDS cases among women. White women have been exposed to HIV through injection drug use (43%), heterosexual contact (35%), and receipt of blood products (14%). Of children with AIDS, 20% are European Americans. White children with AIDS were exposed principally through perinatal transmission (68%) and through the receipt of blood products, including factor VIII concentrate (31%). The epidemiology of AIDS makes it clear that the disease is affecting ethnic communities of color disproportionately in the United States.

ENVIRONMENTAL CONSTRAINTS

As noted in the discussion of the conceptualization of culture, a group's economic and social structures and values, beliefs, and practices do not arise in isolation. Instead, they are a response to the environmental resources available and to constraints imposed on the group. So, too, AIDS is not only the result of individual behavior but occurs in an environmental and societal context. For ethnic communities of color, this environmental context includes poverty, urban decay, drug use, racism and discrimination, and often an absence of social, political, and economic structures and of health and human services (Cochran & May, 1993; Friedman et al., 1990; Gallagher, 1992; Jenkins et al., 1993; Singer, 1991).

Ethnic communities of color are affected adversely by differentials in income and employment. On average, people of color have lower income and higher unemployment than whites. The poverty rate in 1991 for African Americans was 32.7%, for Latinos 28.7%, for Asian Americans and Pacific Islanders 13.8%, and for whites 11.3% (Bureau of the Census, 1992). The unemployment rate was 13.7% for African Americans, 11.9% for Latinos, and 6.7% for whites in 1992 (Department of Labor, 1992). Poverty and ill health are often correlated, probably because of decreased access to resources, health education, and health care. Duh (1991) proposed the relationship of poverty and ill health as an explanation for the proportionately high prevalence of HIV disease among people of African descent in both the United States and Africa.

Since World War II, African Americans have become an increasingly urbanized population, moving from rural areas in the South to Northern urban centers experiencing inner-city decay (abandonment by commerce, by social, political, and economic structures, and by health and human services). The same kind of migration from rural to urban areas has occurred in several of the Latino ethnic groups and in Native Americans. The inner-city areas to which people have migrated are characterized by open drug markets, oppressive environmental and social conditions, and few economic opportunities (Singer, 1991). High rates of addiction to injection drugs have been disproportionately associated with inner-city urban life, especially in the Northeast (Courtwright et al., 1989). Significantly, injection drug use has played a major role in spreading HIV not only through the use of shared needles but also through sexual contact and perinatal transmission.

Racism and discrimination have resulted in differentials in the reporting of cases of HIV, in health education, and in health care (McBride, 1991). According to a report of the Institute for Urban Affairs and Research at Howard University, AIDS cases in blacks and Hispanics are counted more stringently than in whites, and blacks and Hispanics are undercounted in the census (McBride, 1991). This results in underreporting of cases in whites rather than overreporting in other groups. Health education is limited in communities of color from several perspectives. There are fewer resources and programs in black and Hispanic middle and secondary schools; a higher dropout rate in these schools results in less education; ethnic people of color entering the health professions are underrepresented; and much of prevention education focuses on a white gay lifestyle (McBride, 1991). Conversely, in the Asian community, HIV infection may be underreported because of the stigma and the masking of illness as cancer or leukemia for fear of deportation (Lee & Fong, 1990). Underreporting also leads to differentials in health education and health care.

Health care is limited in impoverished urban communities. The preexisting health of populations in these communities is poor, increasing the cofactors of transmission. Concurrent sexually transmitted diseases (STDs), pregnancy, and drug use may all undermine immunity and thereby facilitate transmission. The quality of health care may also be lower in poor urban areas because there are fewer health professionals and other resources (McBride, 1991). Significantly, clinical trials of drugs for the treatment of HIV disease have failed to adequately enroll people of color (El-Sadr & Capps, 1992). This failure may be related to the high numbers of IDUs in these communities and the stigma of drug abuse and to issues related to poverty (Brown, 1993). However, as a result, ethnic people of color have not had early access to experimental treatments available through clinical trials. Easterbrook and colleagues (1991) reported ethnic differences in survival time of patients treated with zidovudine. African Americans had decreased survival time because their disease was more advanced when zidovudine therapy was started and because use of prophylaxis therapy for *Pneumocystis carinii* pneumonia was less frequent.

The social, political, and economic resources that the gay white community has been able to mobilize in the fight against HIV are not available in poor communities. The absence of health and human services has resulted in notable disparities in health status between the U.S. population in general and ethnic communities of color. Average life expectancy is lower and the infant and maternal mortality rates are higher in African Americans, Latinos, and Native Americans than the general population. Particular diseases affect each community disproportionately. High rates of other STDs, substance abuse, tuberculosis, and death from cardiovascular disease, stroke, and homicide affect the African American community (CDC, August, 1993; Finelli et al., 1993; Hammett & Biddlecom, 1992; Jenkins et al., 1993; NCA, 1992; Staples, 1991c). Among Latinos, the rates of tuberculosis, gonorrhea, and diabetes are disproportionately high (Flegal et al., 1991; Moran et al., 1990; NCA, 1992). Health problems are exacerbated in this population by alarmingly low levels of health insurance coverage. The health status of Native Americans is affected by high rates of STDs, tuberculosis, diabetes, and alcoholism (Nickens, 1991; Rowell, 1990; Toomey et al., 1989; West, 1993). Among other health problems, Asian Americans and Pacific Islanders are affected by two infectious diseases at much higher rates than the general population: hepatitis B and tuberculosis (NCA, 1992). Poor health status and the various diseases described contribute to the AIDS epidemic by compromising immunity and facilitating transmission of the virus or expression of disease. It is possible also that competing health and social concerns of ethnic communities of color (cancer, heart disease, poverty, violence) dominate people's attention and thereby indirectly contribute to the AIDS epidemic (Elder-Tabrizy et al., 1991; Kalichman et al., 1992; Shayne & Kaplan, 1991). Lack of access to health care means that the opportunistic infections and neoplasms associated with AIDS go untreated and the death rate from AIDS is higher than in those persons with adequate health care and treatment (Easterbrook et al., 1991). With this background in environmental constraints and societal conditions, the knowledge, attitudes, and practices of the various ethnic groups are discussed. These are placed in the context of lay and ethnic culture.

KNOWLEDGE AND BELIEFS

Since 1987 the National Health Interview Survey has included questions about AIDS (Biddlecom & Hardy, 1991; Hardy & Biddlecom, 1991). From this survey it is possible to compare by gender, ethnicity, and age the knowledge, attitudes, beliefs, and behaviors of African Americans, Latinos, and whites. Asian and Native Americans have not been included in this national survey to date. More regional surveys of AIDS knowledge, attitudes, and behaviors have been conducted in all these groups (see Amaro & Gornemann, 1992; Aruffo et al., 1991; DiClemente et al., 1988; Eversley et al., 1993; Flaskerud & Nyamathi, 1988; 1990; Flaskerud & Uman, 1993; Hall et al., 1990; Kalichman et al., 1992; Livingston & Johnson, 1993; Marin & Marin, 1990; St. Lawrence, 1993). In all studies, general knowledge of the virus and the three primary modes of HIV transmission was uniformly high. Greater levels of knowledge were correlated with higher education and level of acculturation; however, the large majority of all respondents were aware of the major exposure categories (Flaskerud & Uman, 1993; Marin & Marin, 1990). Moreover, people of color have expressed an increased willingness to learn more about AIDS (Elder-Tabrizy et al., 1991).

Despite knowledge of transmission and willingness to learn, perception of personal risk often was not related to knowledge or, in other cases, to actual practices (Amaro & Gornemann, 1992; Eversley et al., 1993; Kalichman et al., 1992; St. Louis et al., 1991; Wasser et al., 1993). It is possible that women may be unaware of their risk even though they are aware of the major transmission routes because bisexual behavior is often not acknowledged in ethnic communities of color (Chu et al., 1992; Jenkins et al., 1993). Additionally, perception of risk (multiple sexual partners) did not affect risk behaviors of a sample of women attending a family planning clinic because of a perception of invulnerability to HIV (Eversley et al., 1993). In other cases, perception of risk among women did not affect behavior because of power differentials in the male-female relationship (Amaro & Gornemann, 1992; Fullilove et al., 1990; Jen-

kins, 1993; Livingston & Johnson, 1993; St. Louis et al., 1991).

There is less knowledge of the availability of HIV testing than there is of modes of transmission. Additionally, in several studies fewer respondents were aware of the availability of medications to extend life. The majority of respondents were aware of the efficacy of condoms but, again, fewer than were aware of the modes of transmission (Amaro & Gornemann, 1992; Flaskerud & Uman, 1993; Hardy & Biddlecom, 1991).

Although correct knowledge of HIV transmission was high, many misperceptions about casual transmission have continued. Chief among these are beliefs about transmission via mosquitos, airborne transmission through coughing and sneezing, and transmission through eating food or from dishes handled by someone with HIV (Amaro & Gornemann, 1992; Biddlecom & Hardy, 1991; Flaskerud & Uman, 1993; Marin & Marin, 1990). Beliefs also persist about transmission through other body fluids (sweat, tears, saliva) or through contact with germs, dirty toilet seats or furniture, or water in swimming pools and spas. Additionally, there are beliefs that AIDS is the result of evil forces, "bad" spirits, offense of ancestors, or a punishment from God for individual or collective sins characterized by sexual excess and drug use (Flaskerud & colleagues, 1989; 1991a; 1991b; Kerr, 1993; Lee & Fong, 1990; Nicoll et al., 1993). Many of these beliefs persist because of their congruence and intuitive fit with general conceptualizations of the cause of disease (Flaskerud & colleagues, 1989; 1991a; 1991b; Kerr, 1993; Nicoll et al., 1993). Misperceptions about casual transmission, although they are not dangerous, must be corrected because they lead to unnecessary fear, stigmatization, and isolation of persons who are infected.

More dangerous misperceptions are those concerned with beliefs about how AIDS may be prevented or avoided. Among these are beliefs that AIDS can be prevented by washing after sex or by ejaculating outside the partner and then drinking a lot of water to induce copious urination. Other dangerous misperceptions are that one can use antibiotics prophylactically, that antibiotics (especially penicillin), if taken immediately after intercourse, can prevent or cure AIDS, and that there is a vaccine available to cure AIDS. Furthermore, there are misperceptions about vulnerability. For example, some believe that people who are thin or look sick are more vulnerable to infection or are already infected. Conversely, some believe that people who are fat or well nourished are protected from AIDS and are therefore safer as sexual partners (Amaro & Gornemann, 1992; CDC, August 1993; Flaskerud & colleagues, 1989; 1991a; 1991b; Nicoll et al., 1993). Unlike misperceptions about casual transmission of HIV, these misperceptions represent an increased risk of infection if they are used to justify unsafe behavior.

Finally, there may be a distrust of government and fears born of past and current government practices in ethnic communities of color that may discourage people from following public health service proscriptions for the prevention of HIV transmission. Several beliefs related to genocide exist. In African American communities, one powerful source of the fear of genocide has a basis in past experience with public health professionals and the government—the Tuskegee syphilis study (Guinan, 1993; Thomas & Quinn, 1991). The Tuskegee study by the U.S. Public Health Service of untreated syphilis in black men extended from 1932 to 1972, long beyond the advent of effective treatment. The legacy of that study in the AIDS epidemic has led to legitimate mistrust by African Americans of the public health service and to the belief that AIDS is a form of genocide (Thomas & Quinn, 1991). Current fears of genocide include the belief that HIV was deliberately introduced into the African American community by scientists who were studying the virus (Cochran & Mays, 1993). An alternative belief is that U.S. scientists accidentally introduced the virus but are allowing its spread among African Americans because of racist motives to control population (Guinan, 1993; Nicoll et al., 1993). Fueling these beliefs are reports from South Africa that the AIDS prevention campaign in the black townships has been abandoned. The suspicion is that the intention of this move is to allow the majority black population to be devastated by AIDS within the next 10 years, so that it will pose no political threat (Carswell, 1993). Additionally, in both Africa and the United States the emphasis on the use of condoms to prevent AIDS is viewed as an attempt to reduce pregnancies and births among African Americans and thus control the size of the black population on both continents (Carswell, 1993; Cochran & Mays, 1993; Nicoll et al., 1993). Finally, needle exchange programs are viewed as an attempt to increase the use of injection drugs in the African American community (NCA, 1992). The unchecked rise in AIDS, substance abuse, and violent death in the Bronx, New York City, has been characterized as a program of "planned shrinkage" directed against African American and Latino communities (Wallace, 1990).

Among Latinos and other immigrant populations, there is a distrust of government related to HIV testing programs. These programs are seen as a means of locating undocumented immigrants and deporting them. Alternatively, HIV testing is seen as a means of uncovering infection in documented immigrants and then deporting them because persons with HIV are not eligible to immigrate (Flaskerud, personal communication, 1994b; Gallagher, 1992; NCA, 1992; Romero, 1988). In a study offering free HIV testing and counseling to low income Latina women in Los Angeles, these barriers to testing had to be overcome before participants would enroll (Flaskerud, personal communication, 1994b). The same fears of deportation may affect HIV testing and prevention programs in Asian American communities (Lee & Fong, 1990; NCA, 1992). Compounding this situation is the fact that persons who have HIV disease may not seek treatment because of fear that they will be reported to the Immigration and Naturalization Service.

Several other lay beliefs about prevention and treatment practices may have positive influences on the prevention of HIV transmission and on the expression of disease. These are addressed in depth later in this chapter, in the section on Behaviors and Practices.

ATTITUDES AND VALUES

In addition to knowledge and beliefs, attitudes, moral ideals, and values also influence behaviors and practices. Homophobia and the stigmatization of gay men is a major problem in ethnic communities of color as well as in the society at large (Grossman, 1991). Homophobia results in social and emotional isolation from family and friends, disapproval, prejudice, judgments of shame and immorality, and even violence against persons identified as gay (Carrier, 1976; 1989; Cochran & Mays, 1991; Grossman, 1991; NCA, 1992). Homophobia and the stigmatization of gay men has been reported to be especially intense in ethnic communities of color, causing both the community and gay individuals to practice denial and concealment (Carrier, 1976; 1989; Cochran & Mays, 1991; NCA, 1992; Ostrow et al., 1991). These attitudes have been reported for African Americans, Latinos, Asian Americans and Pacific Islanders, and Native Americans (Lee & Fong, 1990; NCA, 1992). In these communities, homosexuality is generally denied, AIDS is often seen as a gay white disease, and bisexuality is practiced frequently to conceal male-male sexual contact (Bonilla & Porter, 1990; Carrier, 1976; Ceballos-Capitaine et al., 1990; Flaskerud, 1988; Jenkins et al., 1993; NCA, 1992). In contrast, in some Native American communities, homosexuality has a traditional social role for men but not for women; bisexuality is less accepted (CNA, 1993; Rowell, 1990).

Negative attitudes of families toward homosexuality may be one reason for concealment and denial (Ceballos-Capitaine et al., 1990; Grossman, 1991; Ostrow et al, 1991; Turner, et al., 1993). The absence of a viable gay subculture to support and sustain gay men may be another reason for concealment (Carrier, 1989; Cochran & Mays, 1991). Gay subcultures may not develop in communities of color because of severe stigma, hatred, and even violence, and additionally for economic reasons. Living separately from one's family may be a choice available only in affluent communities. Choices of living situations may be limited in ethnic communities of color for both economic and social-attitudinal reasons. Another reason for concealment of homosex-

uality may be related to the primacy of social group identification (Icard, 1985; Morales, 1990). If a man who has sex with men considers his ethnic identity to be primary, he may conceal his sexual identity out of deference to community morals and attitudes. If, on the other hand, his sexual orientation is considered primary, he may join a gay community rather than remain part of an ethnic community (Carrier, 1989; Cochran & Mays, 1991; Grossman, 1991; Icard, 1985). If economic and material resources are not available, he may have no choice but to remain with his family and ethnic community.

Within mainstream society, people of color who are homosexual or bisexual experience prejudice and discrimination based on their ethnic identity and their sexual orientation (Lee & Fong, 1990; Morales, 1990). AIDS creates additional stigma (Grossman, 1991). First, it may reveal or expose persons as those who have engaged in a stigmatizing lifestyle: for instance, male-male sexual contact or injection drug use. Second, the disease itself creates a stigma because of its infectious, or "dirty," nature and its association with death and dying. Both of these circumstances make people want to distance themselves from persons with HIV disease. According to several investigators, AIDS was not considered a problem in ethnic communities of color until 1986 (Jenkins et al., 1993; Morales, 1990; Rowell, 1990). This may still be the belief among Asian Americans (Lee & Fong, 1990; NCA, 1992). Denial of AIDS by leaders in the Asian community and promulgation of this information by the Asian-language media has resulted in a common belief that Asians are immune to AIDS (Lee & Fong, 1990). Reasons for denying the existence of AIDS in communities of color are related to the stigma associated with the disease, with homosexuality, and with drug use. Person(s) with HIV disease (PWHIV) may face tremendous alienation within their own ethnic and cultural communities. The stigma is compounded by the revelation of homosexuality or injection drug use.

Several investigators have discussed differences in stress, coping, and social support among African American, Latino, and white men with HIV disease as a result of this multiple stigma. Ceballos-Capitaine and colleagues (1990) found that HIV-seropositive Hispanic men reported higher levels of stress than whites in their daily interactions with family and friends related to their homosexual lifestyle. This stress was related to trying to conceal a gay identity. Hispanic men also reported more anger than white men. Other investigators have also discussed the stress on Latino MWSM from families who wish to keep homosexuality a secret or who enforce a masculine role expectation (Kaminsky et al., 1990; Morales, 1990). Morales (1990) suggested that the method of coping of these men may include substance abuse. Ostrow and colleagues (1991) found that African American gay men with HIV received less support from their family network than white men received. This situation was extremely stressful for black respondents because family support, as opposed to friend support, is customarily considered more available to blacks than whites.

Attitudes of the family toward homosexuality and AIDS play a large role in determining both who will care for PWHIV and the stresses on the caregiver (Kaminsky et al., 1990). In most ethnic communities of color, the value of the family overrides that of the individual (Cochran & Mays, 1993; Kaminsky et al., 1990; Morales, 1990; NCA, 1992). PWHIV, to protect their family from the disgrace of public exposure, may choose not to seek support from the family (Kaminsky et al., 1990; Morales, 1990; Ostrow et al., 1991). However, support agencies and services for PWHIV in ethnic communities are limited, and the health of the PWHIV is therefore affected. When families do provide care for the PWHIV, they may be overly protective and overly involved in an effort to keep the disease a secret (Andrews et al., 1993; Kaminsky et al., 1990). By not using or not having available support agencies and services, families may become stressed and even overwhelmed by the care of the PWHIV. In communities of color, the caregivers most often are female family members (mothers, sisters) (AIDS Institute, New York, 1991; Carrier, 1989; Mays & Cochran, 1988; Stowe et al., 1993; Worth & Rodriquez, 1987).

Attitudes of various ethnic communities toward homosexuality, drug use, and AIDS may be influenced by organized religion, conceptualizations of male-male sexual contact, and the value placed on civil liberties (Bonilla & Porter, 1990; Friedman et al., 1990). Bonilla and Porter (1990) found that African Americans were least tolerant on a morality dimension of homosexuality, in comparison with Latinos and whites. They attributed this attitude to the strong disapproval of homosexuality expressed by black churches with Southern fundamentalist origins. Latinos have a narrower conceptualization of homosexuality, considering only the receptive partner to be homosexual. This view, combined with a folk-Catholic religious orientation that does not stress dogma, results in less moral judgment. On the other hand, African Americans were most tolerant on a civil liberties dimension for homosexuals, and Latinos were least tolerant. These attitudes were attributed to black identification with civil liberties for all minorities and to the lesser acculturation of Latinos to American values (Bonilla & Porter, 1990). In this same study, African Americans were more tolerant of departures from mainstream norms in many areas of sexuality such as teen pregnancy and single motherhood (Bonilla & Porter, 1990).

Attitudes toward male and female sexuality in general also influence the transmission of HIV. Bowser (1992) noted several sexual values of lower-class and working-class African Americans that are barriers to AIDS prevention. One is the myth of black male sexual superiority that has carried over into the nation's conventional wisdom but is believed also by some African Americans. Placing a value on sexual superiority carries with it a need to demonstrate and affirm this superiority through sexual contacts. According to Jenkins and colleagues (1993), these "machismo behaviors" play a part in the increasing heterosexual transmission of HIV among African Americans. Similar values have been described in Latino and Pilipino cultures (Carrier, 1989; Lee & Fong, 1990; Marin & Marin, 1992; Pavich, 1986; Vasquez-Nuttall et al., 1987). Carrier (1989) reported that Mexican men measure themselves against other men through an emphasis on multiple uncommitted sexual contacts that begin in adolescence. Marin & Marin (1992) found high rates of sexual activity among Hispanic men outside their primary relationship. These investigators related this activity to traditional values that emphasize the need for men to express themselves sexually. Such values may encourage the transmission of HIV.

A second sexual value of African Americans and Latinos that may be a barrier to AIDS prevention is the importance of children in affirming masculinity or femininity and in claiming status as an adult (Bowser, 1992; Mayfield, 1991; Shayne & Kaplan, 1991; Staples, 1991a). Staples (1991a) noted that in U.S. society in general, employment and income are the measure of a man's masculinity and adult status. When these are not available because of ethnic discrimination and prejudice, fathering children becomes the mark of manhood. There are also strong social incentives for women to have children (Castro de Alvarez, 1990; Shayne & Kaplan, 1991). The value placed on having children is one of the reasons for the reluctance to use condoms, which in turn may contribute to the spread of HIV. Another negative attitude toward condoms is their association with prostitution and extramarital relationships in Latin American culture (Marin & Marin, 1992).

Finally, attitudes toward the role of women in society and in sexual relationships cannot be minimized in their effect on the transmission of HIV. The unequal status of women in U.S. society extends to many aspects of HIV disease and may be more pronounced in ethnic communities of color, where power differentials are more apparent. Cultural attitudes toward the role of women that appear to have a direct association with the spread of HIV often involve sexual relationships. Dual standards for men and women extend to cultural attitudes toward virginity, monogamy, expression of sexuality, talking about sexuality, condom use, who may initiate sexual intercourse, and reproduction (Carrier, 1989; Castro de Alvarez, 1990; Chu et al., 1992; Flaskerud, 1988, Flaskerud & Uman, 1993; Marin & Marin, 1992; Mays & Cochran, 1988; Shayne & Kaplan, 1991). Women are expected to be virgins until married, to be monogamous during marriage, to bear children, and not to initiate sexual activities. They are not expected to negotiate condom use or to question their partners' sexual activities. As a consequence, women are frequently unaware of a partner's risk behaviors, such as multiple sexual partners or male-male sexual contact (Chu et al., 1992). In 1989 the AIDS rate from sex with a bisexual man was three and five times higher among Latino and African American women, respectively, than among white women. Additionally, according to investigators studying IDUs, women also are expected to share their needles with their partners, a behavior tied to gender role socialization (Parra et al., 1993; Wayment et al., 1993). Furthermore, addicted women may be more stigmatized than their male counterparts because of society's expectations of nurturant role obligations. Attitudes toward the role of women in gender and sexual relationships places them at increased risk of exposure to HIV. Attitudes that lead to exposure of women to HIV also lead to perinatal transmission.

BEHAVIORS AND PRACTICES

Knowledge, beliefs, cultural attitudes, and values are all related to the behaviors and practices that put people at risk of exposure to HIV. Sexual behaviors and drug use behaviors are either directly or indirectly related to the majority of exposures to HIV for all ethnic groups. Sexual behaviors in association with condom use, reproductive practices, and drug use account for the majority of all adult and pediatric exposures.

Sexual Behaviors

It is important to note that there is a difference between sexual identity and sexual behaviors. A man who has sex with men may label himself as heterosexual, bisexual, or homosexual (Chu et al., 1992; Doll et al., 1992; Magaña & Carrier, 1991). These labels are probably influenced by middle socioeconomic class and white ethnocentric distinctions but may have different interpretations among the

Table 15–4. Ethnicity and Bisexuality

ETHNICITY	BISEXUALITY (%)			
	CHU ET AL.	KRAMER ET AL.	DOLL ET AL.	NY STATE
European American	21	27	33	16
African American	41	47	48	37
Latino/Hispanic	31	—	36	29
Asian/Pacific Islander	29	—	—	24
Native American	28	—	—	56

various ethnic groups. Cultural values, moral ideals, and attitudes influence sexual practices and how sexual behavior is labeled. Jenkins and colleagues (1993) reported that African Americans are taught that homosexuality is not indigenous to the black community—men who are homosexual are pressured also to maintain heterosexual relationships. Men who are bisexual are expected to conceal homosexual contacts. Similar values and consequent practices are ascribed to Asian Americans (Lee & Fong, 1990; NCA, 1992). In the traditional Latino community, a narrower conceptualization of homosexuality has been described by several investigators (Bonilla & Porter, 1990; Carrier, 1989; de la Vega, 1987; Morales, 1990). Only men who practice anal receptive intercourse ("feminine" men) are labeled as homosexual. "Masculine" men, who play the anal insertive role, are not stigmatized as homosexual. In this role, their masculine self-image is not threatened by sexual contact with other men as long as they also have sex with women.

As a result of these cultural values, norms, and labels, African American and Latino MWSM may not self-identify as homosexual (Magaña & Carrier, 1991). A study of HIV-1–seropositive blood donors examined the relationship between sexual identity, ethnicity, and sexual behavior (Doll et al., 1992). All subjects in the study were MWSM. Self-reported sexual identity differed with ethnicity: 54% of white MWSM, 34% of African American MWSM, and 49% of Latino MWSM self-identified as homosexual; 25% of white MWSM, 44% of African American MWSM, and 17% of Latino MWSM self-identified as bisexual; and 21% of white MWSM, 23%

of African American MWSM, and 34% of Latino MWSM self-identified as heterosexual. MWSM who engaged in insertive versus receptive roles did not differ by ethnicity. Those MWSM who self-identified as bisexual and heterosexual perceived their HIV risk as low and cited not being in a risk group as their reason for low-risk perception. Because of such findings, researchers have begun to use categories based on sexual behaviors rather than on sexual self-identification (Chu et al., 1992; Doll et al., 1992).

Several studies suggest that bisexuality might be more common among ethnic men of color than among white men (Bureau of Communicable Disease Control, New York, 1993; Chu et al., 1992; Doll et al., 1992; Kramer et al., 1980; Lee & Fong, 1990). These studies are summarized in Table 15–4. In two of these studies, the same trend in bisexuality was reported in Asian American and Native American men (Bureau of Communicable Disease Control, New York, 1993; Chu et al., 1992).

Bisexuality (the sexuality of men who have sex with men and women) carries with it several risks for HIV infection. The first risk comes from failure to recognize risk because of failure to perceive oneself in a risk group and practice risk-reduction behaviors (Doll et al., 1992; Magaña & Carrier, 1991). Nationally, AIDS incidence continues to increase in MWSM among African Americans and Latinos (Karon & Berkelman, 1991; Peterson et al., 1989; Peterson et al., 1992). A second risk comes from higher rates of injection drug use in the bisexual group than in other sexual groups (Bureau of Communicable Disease Control, New York, 1993; Chu et al., 1992;

Diaz et al., 1993b). Morales (1990) suggested that Latino men who practice bisexual behavior because of cultural proscriptions against homosexuality may abuse drugs because of the stress of concealment and denial. Supporting this assumption, Diaz and colleagues (1993b) found that bisexual men were more often IDUs than were heterosexual men. Bisexuality carries with it also the risk of HIV transmission to women and by extension to children through perinatal transmission (Rogers & Turner, 1991). Chu and colleagues (1992) reported that the AIDS rate from sex with a bisexual man was three times higher among Latino women and five times higher among African American women than among white women. Latin American bisexual men are more likely to be married than are other ethnic bisexual men (Diaz et al., 1993a). It has been suggested that bisexuality may be even higher in ethnic people of color but may not be reported because of the stigma or, in the case of women, because they are unaware of a partner's bisexuality. The relatively high numbers of cases that fall in the "unidentified risk" category in these communities is thought to be related to a failure to report bisexual behavior (Chu et al., 1992; Jenkins et al., 1993; McCray, 1991; Rogers & Turner, 1991) (see Tables 15–1 and 15–2).

Sexual behavior may differ in relation to the level of acculturation, ethnic identification, and social class (CNA, 1993; Carrier & Magaña, 1991; Diaz et al., 1993b; Magaña & Carrier, 1991; Staples, 1991b; van Oss Marin et al., 1993). In one study, married Latino men were more likely to have additional sex partners than were non-Latinos. However, highly acculturated Latino men were less likely to have multiple partners than were less acculturated men. The opposite was true of Latino women (van Oss Marin et al., 1993). Staples (1991b; 1991d) described differences in the number of sexual partners and preferences for monogamy in African American sexual behavior in relation to social class. Furthermore, level of acculturation and sexual socialization were found to be the most important determinants of whether adult men of Mexican origin who have sex with men were influenced by Mexican or Anglo ho-

mosexuality (Carrier & Magaña, 1991; Magaña & Carrier, 1991). Unacculturated and less acculturated MWSM in California preferred a single sexual role (i.e., either anal insertive or receptive but not both) and a focus on anal intercourse, whereas more acculturated men played both roles and engaged in a variety of behaviors, fellatio being most common (Carrier, 1989; Carrier & Magaña, 1991).

Condom use is a practice related to sexual behavior and is promoted by the public health service as a method of reducing the risk of HIV transmission. According to some reports, Latinos and African Americans may not use condoms because of cultural proscriptions against their use except with prostitutes and in extramarital affairs, because of suspicion that condoms are being promoted out of motivation to control the population and because of feelings of invulnerability to HIV or, conversely, fatalistic beliefs about the outcome of diseases such as HIV and cancer (Eversley et al., 1993; Jenkins et al., 1993; Kalichman et al., 1992; Marin & Marin, 1992; Marin, 1989; Peterson et al., 1989; 1992; Sangree, 1993; Schilling et al., 1991; van Oss Marin et al., 1993). Very little is known about condom use among Asian and Native Americans. Early in the HIV epidemic, it was assumed by some Asian leaders and health professionals that AIDS might not occur in the Asian community (Lee & Fong, 1990; NCA, 1992). This assumption may have provided a false sense of security, in addition to any cultural proscriptions against the use of condoms as a risk-reduction practice. Furthermore, the lack of gay and bisexual subcultures in communities of color and the lack of funding for prevention programs with these same populations allow risk behaviors to continue unchecked (Jenkins et al., 1993; Morales, 1990; NCA, 1992).

Among women, other reasons for not using condoms are the personal desire and the cultural mandate to bear children (Castro de Alvarez, 1990; Marin, 1989; Mays & Cochran, 1988; Shayne & Kaplan, 1991). Women may choose to have a child because it makes them feel good about themselves—special, worthwhile, mature, and responsible (Castro de Alvarez, 1990; Mayfield, 1991; Shayne & Kaplan, 1991). They may bear children also because fertility is highly valued in their sociocultural group and/or because they have no choice but to take on a maternal role (CDC, May 28, 1993; Marin, 1989; Mayfield, 1991; Mays & Cochran, 1988; Schilling et al., 1991). Negotiating safer sexual practices with a partner may encounter male resistance anchored in class and culture and may jeopardize a woman's economic survival (Mays & Cochran, 1993; Schilling et al., 1991). These same reasons may extend to women with HIV disease. In addition, for a woman with HIV disease, having a child ensures leaving a legacy of herself after death (Andrews et al., 1993; Shayne & Kaplan, 1991).

Finally, both women and men may not use condoms because they do not perceive a risk of acquiring HIV disease. MWSM who do not identify themselves as homosexual or bisexual may not perceive themselves at risk when prevention messages are couched in these terms (Eliason, 1993). Likewise, women who are unaware of a partner's bisexuality or drug use may not perceive themselves at risk. Finally, for poor people the perceived risk of HIV infection may be low on a list of priorities of more serious life problems, such as employment, child care, and single parenting (Kalichman et al., 1992).

Drug Use Behaviors

Injection drug use and/or being the sexual partner of an IDU is the leading route of exposure to HIV for women of color (CDC, October 1993). The great majority of perinatal exposure of children of color is linked to injection drug use (CDC, October 1993). For men of color, injection drug use is the second most frequent exposure category after male-male sexual contact. Behaviors associated with the use of injection drugs that increase the risk of exposure to HIV are unprotected sexual practices and sharing of injecting equipment. In addition to the reasons cited above for unprotected sexual behavior, the use of crack cocaine and amphetamines has been associated with high-risk sexual practices. High-risk sexual behaviors were related to both crack injection and crack smoking (Booth et

al., 1993; Diaz & Chu, 1993; Klee, 1993; Rivera et al., 1990). Cocaine and amphetamine injectors report a greater interest in sex and a greater frequency of intercourse. They also report exchanging sex for drugs, money, or a place to sleep, and the use of drugs before or during sex (Booth et al., 1993; Crisp et al., 1993; Friedman et al., 1990). The use of opioids and alcohol has recently been differentiated from the use of cocaine and amphetamines in the effects on sexual practices. Some investigators have found that the use of alcohol and opioids does not appear to increase sexual risk practices (Klee, 1993; Temple et al., 1993). Others continue to report an association between high-risk sexual practices and alcohol and opioid use, sometimes in relation to the degree of addiction and the necessity of exchanging sex for drugs (Gossop et al., 1993; Kim et al., 1993). Puerto Rican women in New York City and Puerto Rico who were sexual partners of HIV-infected IDUs were reported to use alcohol, marijuana, and noninjection cocaine frequently (Rivera et al., 1990). Despite knowledge of sexual risk behaviors and perception of their own risk, IDUs were reported often to continue high-risk sexual behaviors (Eversley et al., 1993; Parra et al., 1993).

Behaviors related to cleaning injection equipment, sharing equipment, using needle exchange programs, and using "shooting galleries" to inject have been related to the type of drug used, the degree of dependence on the drug, and the gender, ethnicity, and social relationship of the users. In San Francisco and New York City, cocaine injection has been associated more strongly with HIV seropositivity than has heroin injection (Friedman et al., 1990). Cocaine users inject more frequently, up to four or five times an hour during bingeing. Cocaine binges create anxiety for the drug, resulting in less ability to follow guidelines for bleach decontamination and reduced willingness to delay injection long enough to use bleach. Heroin injectors are typically more able to follow guidelines for using bleach (Friedman et al., 1990). However, severely dependent heroin injectors are more likely than less dependent users to share equipment (Gossop et al., 1993). More dependent users share with dealers because of the urgency of their need for drugs during withdrawal.

Women (more so than men) have been found repeatedly to share injection equipment (Castro de Alvarez, 1990; Klee, 1993; Shayne & Kaplan, 1991; Wayment et al., 1993). Women most commonly share equipment with drug-injecting partners (Parra et al., 1993). This behavior has been related to gender role socialization: the woman's most significant social relationship may be with her injecting partner, who also may be her sexual partner. The status and role of the woman in the relationship require that she be giving and attentive to the needs of a male partner in this situation, just as she is in all other aspects of the female-male relationship (Rivera et al., 1990; Shayne & Kaplan, 1991; Wayment et al., 1993).

Sharing injection equipment is also a means of expressing mutual friendship between persons in the drug-using community (Friedman et al., 1990). Sharing is a behavior that tends to integrate the individual into a social group and makes him or her part of the subculture (Castro de Alvarez, 1990).

Unsafe drug use practices have been related to ethnicity. African Americans are reported to have reduced their risk behaviors (sharing, not cleaning equipment) since AIDS became recognized as a threat, whereas Latinos have not (Friedman et al., 1990). Other investigators have confirmed the behaviors of Latinos in sharing uncleaned equipment and using "shooting galleries" to inject. The majority of Mexican American men and women (81.6%) in a Los Angeles study (N = 100) who injected drugs shared uncleaned needles (Parra et al., 1993). The use of "shooting galleries" has been reported to be more frequent among Puerto Ricans in New York City than among whites and other Latinos (Diaz et al., 1993a; Friedman et al., 1990). It has been speculated that Latinos may be less likely to reduce their risks because of language barriers, sociocultural differences derived from specific histories of an ethnic group, or traditional cultural differences (Diaz et al., 1993a; Friedman et al., 1990). Current place of residence in the United States and a traditional lack of experience with organizational behavior and power have been cited as examples (Diaz et al., 1993b; Rivera et al., 1990). In any case, the social dynamics of ethnicity seems to have an important impact on risk.

Finally, the use of and support for needle exchange programs as a means of reducing HIV risk has created skepticism and received criticism in some parts of the African American community (NCA, 1992). These programs have been viewed by some in the community as encouraging drug use and as part of a racist conspiracy to commit genocide against the black population (Staples, 1991c). It has been argued persuasively that ethnic communities of color need drug rehabilitation programs instead. Other African American leaders have encouraged risk-reduction programs that provide needle exchange, bleach to clean equipment, and information on not sharing equipment, in conjunction with more drug rehabilitation programs made available to African Americans and Latinos (McBride, 1991; Staples, 1991c).

Several other behaviors and practices are related to HIV risk reduction and/or disease progression. One of these is HIV testing practices and the others are health promotion behaviors and practices. All may be related to ethnicity and traditional cultural practices.

HIV Antibody Testing

Several investigators have noted that ethnic communities of color do not participate in voluntary HIV testing programs at the same rate as whites (Berrios et al., 1993; CDC, Oct. 15, 1993; Kalichman et al., 1992; Schwarcz et al., 1993; Shayne & Kaplan, 1991). These data may be influenced by the high rates of gay white men who participate in voluntary testing and parturient women who participate knowingly or unknowingly through the testing of umbilical cord blood and placental tissue. Additionally, Latinos and other immigrants are tested involuntarily as part of an immigration requirement. Various reasons have been given for failure to participate in HIV testing. One is skepticism among people of color about medical research and medical professionals. The stigma associated with AIDS or the behaviors that put persons at risk for HIV may be another reason. An additional reason may be that mandatory testing has been widely viewed as punitive; voluntary testing may engender a similar attitude. Other reasons are related to perception of risk. Many persons are unaware of their risks because of failure to identify culturally with the risk behaviors as they are currently labeled. In the case of women, lack of perception of risk may be related to lack of awareness of a partner's drug use or sexual activity (CDC, Oct. 15, 1993). Finally, some persons may not be tested because of a fatalistic attitude toward HIV disease: "If I am positive there's nothing to be done about it anyway, why make myself worried?" Many of these reasons should carry less weight because HIV testing is thought of differently today than in the past. Today, early testing can result in enrollment in clinical trials, prophylactic treatment, better treatment outcomes, and increased longevity (Brown, 1993; Easterbrook et al., 1991; El-Sadr & Capps, 1992). Efforts to increase voluntary testing among people of color are warranted for these reasons.

Health Promotion Practices and Behavior

Despite attributions of fatalism to some social and cultural groups, studies of low-income Latina, African American, and white women in Los Angeles revealed that all groups were involved in lay disease prevention and treatment practices that were being applied to HIV/AIDS (Flaskerud, 1994a; Flaskerud & Calvillo, 1991a; Flaskerud & Rush, 1989; Flaskerud & Thompson, 1991b). In these studies, AIDS was conceptualized generally as an attack from external forces on the immunity or resistance of the person. This conceptualization is congruent with beliefs in an external locus of control, often attributed to persons of color and lower social class (Jenkins et al., 1993; Marin, 1989) and to the military metaphors used to describe the epidemic in the United States (Sontag, 1990; Wenger, 1993). Regardless the women in

these studies had well-developed prevention and treatment practices that were being used to ward off illness in general and also were being applied to AIDS. These practices involved the use of foods, vitamins, and herbs to keep the body healthy and as remedies for illness. Preventing chills, avoiding extremes in temperature, and keeping the body warm during illness were other common practices. An emphasis on cleanliness to decrease germs in the body, the home, and the environment was practiced by all three groups for both prevention and treatment. Moderate lifestyle behaviors, or a balance in rest and exercise, work and play, and food and fluids, together with a limited use of alcohol and tobacco, were endorsed by all to promote health and to treat illness. All three groups also noted the importance of spirituality, friends, and family in maintaining health and in combating illness. These behaviors and practices were recommended for all illnesses and for AIDS as well. The usefulness and applicability of these practices to AIDS are apparent in their relation to both HIV prevention and progression to disease in PWHIV. The use of traditional healing practices, many of which are preventive in nature, has been reported also among Native Americans to treat and prevent AIDS (Rowell, 1990).

Although not related to AIDS, these practices and behaviors and the beliefs and values they are founded on have been reported by other investigators who have studied the same groups (see Andrews, 1989; Foster, 1981; Freimer et al., 1986; Gonzalez-Swafford & Guttierrez, 1983; Hautman & Harrison, 1982; Helman, 1978; Roberson, 1987; Snow 1983). Similar practices and beliefs have been described for Asians, Middle Easterners, and East Indians (Pliskin, 1992; Ramakrishna & Weiss, 1992; Wei, 1976; Whang, 1981). These beliefs and practices should be viewed as a rich foundation for integrating and implementing HIV prevention and intervention programs. Education, prevention, and treatment within the context of existing ethnocultural beliefs and practices (rather than in the context of biomedical and nursing beliefs) are more likely to succeed because they represent the worldview of the community served.

HIV PREVENTION AND TREATMENT

Numerous investigators, clinicians, and community-based organizations have made similar recommendations for designing and delivering HIV prevention and treatment services in communities of color (Bowser, 1992; De Carpio et al., 1990; Flaskerud & colleagues, 1989; 1991a; 1991b; Kalichman et al., 1993; Kerr, 1993; Marin et al., 1992; Nicoll et al., 1993; Singer, 1991). The majority of these suggestions have come from people of color and from community-based organizations that can be relied on to provide the best direction and guidance for prevention and treatment services. These recommendations are summarized here.

Communities of color have benefited most from programs that have been funded directly to national minority organizations and to community-based organizations (NCA, 1992). However, better targeting of these programs is needed: programs specifically designed for men of color who have sex with other men (50% or more of AIDS cases among men of color occur in this group), for IDUs (about 70% of cases are in people of color), and for women (about 74% of cases are in women of color) (CDC, October 1993; Jenkins et al., 1993; Morales, 1990; NCA, 1992). The unwillingness and inadequacy of traditional leadership organizations and efforts such as churches, tribal councils, and beneficent societies to confront AIDS suggest that funding should go to new organizations and leaders who are more fully involved in HIV/AIDS efforts (Morales, 1990; NCA, 1992). Traditional organizations may provide inadequate leadership because of long-standing cultural and moral proscriptions against homosexuality, drug use, and abortion; the perceived need to remain focused on long-standing social, political, and health problems in the community; and the fear that AIDS will tarnish their image (Castro de Alvarez, 1990; Jenkins et al., 1993; Morales, 1990; NCA, 1992).

A second recommendation is that programs be part and parcel of the target community: that they emerge from the community and be delivered by persons of that same community. These persons include not only professionals, policy makers, and customary leaders but also lay persons indigenous to the community representing homosexuals and bisexuals, IDUs, women, poor persons, and persons of varying levels of education and acculturation. Individuals delivering HIV prevention and treatment services should speak the language(s) of the community and share the cultural values and practices. In some cases they also should share the gender of the group served. Both staff and agencies should be culturally competent. Even staff who share gender, language, and ethnicity with their clients and are indigenous to the community need workshops on homophobia, sexuality, and drug use. Agencies must formulate clear, explicit, and enforceable policies, and agency leaders and managers must enforce these policies. Programs should be communicated by common, familiar, and accepted methods— for example, by the use of oral traditions, storytelling, popular novellas, small discussion groups, role playing and role models (Bowser, 1992; Castro de Alvarez, 1990; Flaskerud & colleagues, 1989; 1991a; 1991b; Finlinson, et al., 1993; Kalichman et al., 1993; Morales, 1990; NCA, 1992; Rowell, 1990; Singer, 1991).

In ethnic communities of color, AIDS occurs within the context of ongoing, serious health problems, as well as social and political problems, including drug abuse, unemployment, violence, teen pregnancies, and STDs. Many community leaders, health professionals, and minority national organizations have recommended that AIDS prevention should be integrated into broad, comprehensive goals of community change and service. This integrated approach is believed to carry with it a greater efficacy in reducing HIV infection than an isolated HIV prevention approach (Castro de Alvarez, 1990; Jenkins et al., 1993; Kalichman et al., 1992; Morales, 1990; NCA, 1992; Rivera et al., 1990; Singer, 1991). In Chapter 2 a case was made for integrating AIDS prevention programs and treatment services into existing community programs and institutions such as the U.S. Public Health Service nutrition program for Women, Infants, and Children (WIC), STD clinics, family planning clinics, drug rehabilitation programs, and the school system. It was argued that these agencies have a history, expertise, and experience and are currently accepted and used by the members of the community.

An alternative argument is given here. These existing programs and institutions may reflect the current negative attitudes toward homosexuality, drug use, and AIDS; they may be perceived by the community as external rather than internal sources of help; and they may be viewed as tired and ineffective in meeting the health and social problems of the community. In such an argument, established programs and institutions would be ineffective in meeting and defeating AIDS at a community level. It could be argued persuasively that new institutions are needed to provide a broad, comprehensive approach to health care, including AIDS treatment. These new institutions would enhance ethnic group identity, solidarity, and political advocacy and activism. They would enlist community members in the development of effective responses to the conditions that contribute to AIDS, drug abuse, teen pregnancies, STDs, tuberculosis, cancer, heart disease, and so forth. These agencies would develop, implement, and enforce social policy strategies that enhance sensitivity to the groups most affected by HIV, eradicate discrimination and prejudice within the community, and build a sense of unity and support throughout the community. Additional benefits of such activities are the therapeutic effect on participants and the community when purpose, direction, and self-determination are fostered, and the degree of power and control over participants' lives that they provide (Hein, 1993; Kalichman et al., 1992; Morales, 1990; NCA, 1992; Singer, 1991).

On the basis of cultural proscriptions, several specialized interventions have attempted to change AIDS knowledge, beliefs, attitudes, and practices among Latino, African American, Southeast Asian, and white (European American) program participants. Other studies have made recommendations for culturally competent interventions based on study findings (Bowser, 1992; DeCarpio et al., 1990; Carrier & Magaña, 1991; Flaskerud & Nyamathi, 1988; 1990; Flaskerud & Rush, 1989; Flaskerud & Uman, 1993; Jemmott & Jem-

mott, 1990; 1991; Jemmott et al., 1992; Jemmott, 1993; Kalichman et al., 1993; Kaminsky et al., 1990; Marin et al., 1990; Nyamathi & Vasquez, 1989; Nyamathi & Lewis, 1991; Rowell, 1990). These studies employed risk-reduction interventions and measured changes in knowledge, beliefs, attitudes, and practices. All studies reported significant changes, and some of the interventions were related to sustained change with time. To measure changes in behavior, almost all studies employed self-report measures. A few measured actual behavior changes: HIV antibody testing, requests for condoms, maintenance of seronegativity. Some innovative approaches utilized the extended family in the intervention, life-enhancement counseling, videotapes, games, counseling, role playing, demonstration–return demonstration, problem solving, coping, oral traditions and storytelling, novellas, photo novellas, comic books, and grounding of the intervention in a personal (ethnic and gender match) and cultural (values related to family and community) context. Some programs targeted to persons with little formal education used messages that were concrete and rooted in temporal reality (rather than general premises), that is, messages related to current environment and life circumstances (Carrier & Magaña, 1991; Lee & Fong, 1990). Acknowledging the environmental constraints on subjects, many studies reimbursed participants with cash, subway tokens, and video game tokens; some provided child care and food. Although all these studies offered specialized AIDS interventions, some of the interventions were offered in such existing community agencies and services as WIC programs, the school system, homeless shelters, STD clinics, and drug rehabilitation programs. Some also utilized an existing social network—the family—in the intervention. Less traditional locations, such as gay bars, migrant labor camps, pornographic book stores, street corners, county jails, and alternative test sites, were also used.

Recommendations drawn from the literature on community-based programs and specialized AIDS interventions pertinent to ethnic communities of color emphasized cultural values, customs and traditions, and social networks. On the basis of these studies and building on existing beliefs and practices, HIV prevention and treatment programs can be based on five goals:

1. Consciously mobilize and enhance cultural beliefs, values, and roles as core elements of the intervention process.
2. Use traditional gender roles and the role of the family in health education and care as a starting point.
3. Enhance beneficial beliefs and practices as they may be related to HIV disease.
4. Clarify misperceptions that may create fear and stigma.
5. Modify detrimental beliefs or negative attitudes and practices within the context of positive ethnocultural and community values (Bowser, 1992; De-Carpio et al., 1990; Flaskerud & colleagues, 1989; 1991a; 1991b; Kalichman et al., 1993; Kerr, 1993; Marin et al., 1992; Nicoll et al., 1993; Singer, 1991).

NURSING RESEARCH IN CULTURE, ETHNICITY, AND AIDS

Summary of Research

Although some studies have included ethnicity as a variable in HIV research, very few nursing investigations have focused on culture: values, beliefs, and attitudes; social structures, roles, and social networks; and economic structures and environmental constraints. These aspects of culture are involved with behavior and provide a framework for culturally competent interventions (see Flaskerud and colleagues, 1988; 1989; 1991a; 1991b, 1993; Jemmott & Jemmott et al., 1992; Jemmott & Jemmott, 1990; 1991; Jemmott, 1992–1996; Nyamathi & colleagues, 1989; 1990; 1991). It should be noted that nurses across the country are beginning to work in this area of research in urban areas where the rates of HIV/AIDS are high and in rural areas where the disease is spreading. This author has personal knowledge of studies by at least 12 nurse researchers in Alaska, California, Texas, Arkansas, Louisiana, Massachusetts,

New York, Puerto Rico, and Nigeria, who are conducting research with ethnic women of color. These studies have involved almost exclusively Latino and African American ethnic groups (one study is with Alaskan Native women). Nursing research is lacking for Asian and Native American ethnic groups relative to AIDS prevention or treatment. However, nursing has a tradition of culturally based research, and some previous studies of health behaviors and practices are particularly applicable to AIDS research on cultural beliefs and practices (see Gonzalez-Swafford & Guttierez, 1983; Hautman & Harrison, 1982; Roberson, 1987).

Issues in Research

Studies of culture and HIV disease are susceptible to a plethora of methodologic pitfalls that result essentially from taking "shortcuts." Some of these pitfalls are summarized here. Chief among them is the use of Anglocentric measures based on an Anglocentric worldview or conceptualization of the values, attitudes, and behaviors related to HIV disease. An obvious example is the use of the Anglocentric labels "homosexual" or "bisexual" in questioning of persons about their sexual preferences and activity. As several investigators (Bonilla & Porter, 1990; Carrier, 1989; Chu et al., 1992; Doll et al., 1992) have pointed out, some MWSM identify themselves as homosexual, others as bisexual, and still others as heterosexual. These labels appear to be related to ethnic culture and community and to societal homophobia and stigma. The difficulties that arise from the bias inherent in these labels results in inaccurate data about how AIDS is being transmitted, uninformed intervention protocols, and a waste of resources on community prevention programs that are addressing the wrong set of behaviors. One devastating result is a total lack of community services for members of some ethnocultural groups with HIV who, as a consequence, are physically sicker and die earlier, psychologically and spiritually bereft. Compounding this situation is the Anglocentric value placed on these labels, which asserts that MWSM should be calling themselves homosexuals, and would if they were just a little better educated.

Another construct that has been applied frequently to research with ethnic people of color is locus of control (Jenkins et al., 1993). The importance of control is apparent in most Western biomedical and psychologic writing about health and illness. *Internal control* is valued by European Americans and considered necessary to a health-promoting and disease-preventing lifestyle. According to the locus-of-control conceptualization, when disease does occur, internally controlled persons are more likely to believe that they have some control over its course and to marshall their personal, social, and spiritual resources to fight it. Most frequently, ethnic people of color, lower-class persons, and older individuals are found to have an *external locus of control.* Theoretically, external control is associated with fatalism; in practice, it is greeted with frustration and labels such as "hard to reach" and "noncompliant" by health professionals and academicians. Persons with an external locus of control believe that illness is the result of external forces and that they have little control over their environment. When they become ill, they are more likely to accept their fate gracefully and not embarrass, shame, or dishonor themselves or their family by anger, complaining, or resistant behavior. Some of the difficulties with using this construct in research occur because of the Anglocentric positive value placed on internal control, the negative attitudes toward external control, and consequent interventions designed to change a person's locus of control if it is external. Furthermore, an uninformed and incorrect assumption that accompanies the findings of an external locus of control is that persons with this orientation are believed not to possess or engage in health promotion, disease prevention, and illness treatment behaviors. As noted in the earlier section on behaviors and practices, many health promotion, disease prevention, and treatment behaviors are practiced by persons who believe that illness is caused by external forces. Given the different worlds and environments in which people live, it is difficult to say whether an internal or external orientation is better or

more realistic when a person is confronted with a life-threatening disease.

There are many other concepts that are equally problematic when they are defined and developed in one ethnocultural group and then applied to other groups (Flaskerud, 1988). Depression is one such concept that has been investigated and clarified cross-culturally, with the result that it is now known that there are different idioms for dysphoria in some groups and no idiom for dysphoria in others. The question that researchers must consider seriously is whether the instruments that they are using are measuring the same attribute from one culture to another. In other words, are the instruments valid?

As noted in the beginning of this chapter, in the section on culture and ethnicity, some theoreticians/investigators have questioned whether commonly used attitude-behavior social science models and theories are applicable to research involving people of color (Cochran & Mays, 1993). These same investigators have noted that the health belief model, the theory of reasoned action, and the self-efficacy theory were developed without a view to cultural, ethnic, and socioeconomic class differences. These theories are based on individualistic as opposed to collectivistic values; they do not account for significant concepts/variables such as environmental constraints and economic and social resources; and they assume mainstream defined motivations, decision-making processes, and personal control. The challenge to HIV nursing research is to capture the worldview and life experiences of a specific ethnocultural group and then to design interventions congruent with these situations and instruments that measure these conceptualizations/variables.

A variety of other methodologic problems exist in cross-cultural research. Several problems involve translation of English-language instruments into other languages. One problem is the assumption that labels or concepts from one language can be directly and literally translated into another language (Flaskerud & Nyamathi, 1988; Lee & Fong, 1990). Compounding this problem is the use in many languages of circumlocutions rather than the use of direct and explicit terms for sexual activity and drug use activity. Another problem is the idiomatic differences within the same language from one ethnic or regional group to another (Hendricson et al., 1989). It is clear that establishing semantic equivalence is necessary but not sufficient to understanding or to valid and reliable responses. Rather, idiomatic equivalence is needed and should be based on ethnicity, social class, age, geographic region, and so forth.

Response formats may create additional problems. The use of Likert scale formats may be culturally biased (Flaskerud, 1988). The use of a true/false or dichotomous response format, although decreasing sensitivity and variability, may be preferable because of its universal practicality and familiarity (Flaskerud, 1988; Kelly et al., 1989). Response sets also may be influenced by cultural traits that encourage or minimize extremes or that encourage acquiescence on verbal measures. Acquiescence or extremes may be the result of cultural politeness, social desirability, the reimbursement offered to the participants in a study, or the shock value of the response on the interviewer (Bowser, 1992; Boyd, 1982; Mays & Jackson, 1991). Additionally, Kauth and colleagues (1991) questioned the reliability of retrospective assessments of behavior. They studied biweekly, 3-month, and 12-month self-reports of sexual behavior and found that the consistency and reliability of the data decreased as the recall period lengthened. Flaskerud (1994b) found that low-income women were highly likely to report *no* sexual activity in the preceding 12 months unless they were reminded of certain markers, such as a holiday, their birthday or anniversary, the birth of a child, or an abortion. Part of this failure to report may have been related to difficulty in recall, but part was also attributed to cultural modesty about sexual behavior even with a husband or monogamous partner.

Other issues in measurement involve the use of validated and standardized measures of HIV knowledge, risk, and practices (Kelly et al., 1989). To plan, implement, evaluate, and refine interventions and risk-reduction programs, one must make a systematic outcome assessment. Currently many instruments are in use, but they often do not have a preexisting established validity or reliability and their psychometric properties are not established in the study in which their use is reported. Consequently, data resulting from their use are not comparable. The National Health Interview Survey has included an AIDS knowledge, behavior, and risk survey since 1988. This questionnaire is available in English and Spanish. The results of the survey are published by the National Center for Health Statistics every 2 years for a national sample of African American, Latino, and white respondents. Data are published in a form that allows comparison of local samples with the national sample (see Flaskerud & Uman, 1993) and that allows analysis of the effects of gender, age, and education on responses. Although the instrument is lengthy, if more investigators were to use it either totally or partially, comparisons and measurement of regional differences and changes with time would be facilitated. Arguments against its use are that it was constructed to measure a universal, vast middle of the U.S. population and not persons who have limited literacy, use idiomatic vocabulary, or come from nonacculturated groups.

Measuring change is another issue in nursing research on culture and HIV disease. The reliability of self-report measures of change has been questioned frequently (see Kalichman et al., 1993; Schilling et al., 1991). The extent to which reported behaviors and attitudes correspond with actual skills and behaviors is a limitation cited by most of the investigators whose research provided a basis for this chapter. In addition, the correspondence between intended behavior and actual behavior in the case of HIV disease has been challenged, especially as it applies to ethnic people of color (Cochran & Mays, 1993). The intention to change and the successful prediction of actual behavior are separated by the influences of poverty, racism, economic and social opportunity, and availability of resources. All these influences have an arbitrary and unpredictable nature.

Another measurement issue related to change is how it is conceptualized. Prochaska and colleagues (1983, 1990) conceptualized change in lifestyle and behaviors as a process that occurs in stages. If this conceptualization is applied to change in HIV risk behaviors, then an assessment must first be made of a person's current stage of change. Then interventions are developed to move him or her to the next stage—from A to B (Kalichman et al., 1993). This approach is considered to have a greater chance of success than attempting to move persons from A to Z with one intervention. The approach allows also for the inclusion of concepts/variables related to culture, ethnicity, social class, economic and social resources, and environmental constraints.

Research Needed

As may be noted from the preceding discussion, much of the research that needs to be done in the area of culture, ethnicity, and HIV nursing involves discovery of the cultural basis of behavior, followed by development of culturally valid constructs, concepts, and theoretical models and then by development of instruments to measure these variables. Another research need is for culturally competent interventions that are ethnically approved, targeted to the stage of change of a particular group or community, and scientifically validated. Finally, research is needed that measures actual change in behavior as opposed to reported change or intended change. Some examples of the research base needed in the area of culture and HIV are provided; however, a much wider range of studies is needed than can be summarized here.

1. Research that discovers and describes:
   - Attitude-behavior models for predicting health-related behavior change that include key constructs to ethnic communities of color: values, social roles and structures, economic resources and environmental constraints, racism, and so forth
   - Cultural models of health promotion, disease prevention, and treatment
   - Cultural models of sexuality that include roles, gender, expression, interpersonal relationships, and power

   - Community-based and societal stigma, discrimination, and homophobia
2. Methodologic research that develops and tests culturally valid instruments to measure concepts/variables of values, attitudes, behaviors, behavior change, and so forth
3. Research that tests the effects of culturally competent interventions:
   - Community-based studies that are designed, implemented, and evaluated by ethnic people of color who are most affected by HIV, such as MWSM, IDUs, and women
   - Community-based behavior change interventions that are longitudinal and attempt to move persons across the stages of change: for example, from fear induction to risk sensitization, to risk contemplation, and finally to risk reduction—with the introduction of the necessary skills and resources at each stage to facilitate change to the next stage
   - Behavior change studies that measure actual behavior change on either a personal or community level as the result of a culturally competent intervention: for example, number of condoms requested, participation in HIV testing and returning for test results, maintaining a seronegative HIV status, a decrease in community STDs, a decrease in teen pregnancies, a decrease in the number of new AIDS cases, and an increase in drug rehabilitation enrollment
   - Studies that employ large-enough numbers of participants to detect effects with a high probability
   - Hypothesis-testing interventional studies in community settings that employ experimental field conditions and comparison groups

SUMMARY

Culture and ethnicity are important concepts in understanding HIV disease because they are apparent in values, attitudes, and behaviors associated with reproduction, sexuality, intimacy, family relationships, death and dying, drug use, stigma, and so forth. The disproportionate effect of HIV on ethnic communities of color is related to ethnocultural differences in values and behaviors but also to poverty, racism, discrimination, and lack of opportunity and resources. An understanding of ethnocultural differences in AIDS knowledge and beliefs, attitudes and values, and practices and behaviors is necessary to effective and culturally competent nursing care. The goal of this chapter is to increase an awareness of culture and the consequent competence of nursing practice and research at individual, agency, and community levels.

Nursing practice and research should be based on an understanding of the cultural foundations of behavior; ethnocultural models of health, illness, prevention, and treatment; and culturally valid models of behavior change. Nurses should involve their ethnic clients of color in the assessment of symptoms and behaviors, in the interpretation of illness, and in the planning and implementation of nursing care and interventions. Nurse researchers and clinicians can continue the tradition they have begun in transcultural nursing to discover cultural beliefs and practices. However, they also must go beyond discovery to implementing cultural mandates for health promotion and care as these relate to HIV disease. The progression of HIV disease in ethnic communities of color makes these activities urgently important.

REFERENCES

AIDS Institute, New York (1991). Cultural factors among Hispanics: Perception and prevention of HIV infection, New York: The Institute.

Amaro, H., Gornemann, I. (1992). HIV/AIDS related knowledge, attitudes, beliefs and behaviors among Hispanics in the Northeast and Puerto Rico: Report of findings and recommendations. Study conducted by the Northeast Hispanic AIDS Consortium, Boston University School of Public Health, Boston, MA.

Anderson, J.N. (1973). Ecological anthropology and anthropological ecology. In J.J. Honigman (Ed.), *Handbook of social and cultural anthropology* (pp. 179–246). Chicago: Rand McNally College Publishing Company.

Andrews, M.M. (1989). Culture and nutrition. In J.S. Boyle & M.M. Andrews (Eds.), *Transcultural concepts in nursing* (pp. 333–355). Glenview, IL: Scott Foresman.

Andrews, S., Williams, A.B., Neil, K. (1993). The mother-child relationship in the HIV-1 positive family. *IMAGE: Journal of Nursing Scholarship, 25*(3), 193–198.

Aruffo, J.F., Coverdale, J.H., Vallbona, C. (1991). AIDS knowledge in low-income and minority populations. *Public Health Reports, 106*(2), 115–119.

Belgrave, F.Z., Randolph, S.M. (1993). Introduction: Psychosocial aspects of AIDS prevention among African Americans. *Journal of Black Psychology, 19*, 103–107.

Berrios, D.C., Hearst, N., Coates, T.J., et al. (1993). HIV antibody testing among those at risk for infection: The National AIDS Behavior Surveys. *Journal of the American Medical Association, 270*(13), 1576–1580.

Biddlecom, A.E., Hardy, A.M. (1991). AIDS knowledge and attitudes of Hispanic Americans: United States, 1990. Provisional data from the National Health Interview Survey. *National Center for Health Statistics Advance Data,* October 17.

Bonilla, L., Porter, J. (1990). A comparison of Latino, Black and non-Hispanic White attitudes towards homosexuality. *Hispanic Journal of Behavioral Sciences, 12*, 437–452.

Booth, R.E., Watters, J.K., Chitwood, D.D. (1993). HIV risk–related sex behaviors among injection drug users, crack smokers and injection drug users who smoke crack. *American Journal of Public Health, 83*(8), 1144–1148.

Bowser, B.P. (1992). Cross-cultural medicine a decade later: African-American culture and AIDS prevention—from barrier to ally. *Western Journal of Medicine, 157*(3), 286–289.

Boyd, C. (1982). The effect of research incentive monies on drug-dependent women. *Journal of Addictions and Health, 3*, 106–117.

Britton, P.J., Zarski, J.J., Hobfoll, S.E., et al. (1993). Psychological distress and the role of significant others in a population of gay/bisexual men in the era of HIV. *AIDS Care, 5*(1), 23–33.

Brown, L.S., Jr. (1993). Enrollment of drug abusers in HIV clinical trials: A public health imperative for communities of color. *Journal of Psychoactive Drugs, 25*(1), 45–52.

Bureau of the Census, U.S. Department of Commerce (1992). Poverty in the United States: 1991. Current Population Reports, Series P-60, No. 181, Washington, DC.

Bureau of Communicable Disease Control, New York State Department of Health (1993, March). *AIDS Surveillance Quarterly Update,* New York.

California Nurses' Association (1993). Cultural issues. *Women at risk: AIDS/HIV Training for Care Providers* (pp. III-1 to III-58). San Francisco, CA: The Association.

Carrier, J.M. (1976). Family attitudes and Mexican male homosexuality. *Urban Life, 5*(3), 359–375.

Carrier, J.M. (1989). Sexual behavior and spread of AIDS in Mexico. *Medical Anthropology, 10*(2-3), 129–142.

Carrier, J.M., Magaña, J.R. (1991). Use of ethnosexual data on men of Mexican origin for HIV/AIDS prevention programs. *Journal of Sex Research, 28*(2), 189–202.

Carswell, W. (1993). HIV in South Africa. *Lancet, 342*(8864), 132.

Castro de Alvarez, V. (1990). AIDS prevention program for Puerto Rican women. *Puerto Rican Health Science Journal, 9*(1), 37–41.

Ceballos-Capitaine, A., Szapocznik, J., Blaney, N.T., et al. (1990). Ethnicity, emotional distress, stress-related disruption, and coping among HIV seropositive gay males. *Hispanic Journal of Behavioral Sciences, 12*, 135–152.

Centers for Disease Control and Prevention (May 28, 1993). Childbearing patterns among selected racial/ethnic minority groups—United States, 1990. *Morbidity and Mortality Weekly Report, 42*(20), 398–403.

Centers for Disease Control and Prevention (June 25, 1993). Use of race and ethnicity in public health surveillance. *Morbidity and Mortality Weekly Report, 42* (RR-10), 11–12.

Centers for Disease Control and Prevention (1993, August). Study of behavior—non-identifying gay men. *HIV/AIDS Prevention, 4*(2), 6–7.

Centers for Disease Control and Prevention (October 15, 1993). Self-reported HIV-antibody testing behaviors—Southern Los Angeles County, 1991–1992. *Morbidity and Mortality Weekly Report, 42*(40), 786–789.

Centers for Disease Control and Prevention (1993, October). *HIV/AIDS Surveillance Report, 5*(3), 1–19, Atlanta, GA: The Centers.

Chu, S.Y., Peterman, T.A., Doll, L.S., et al. (1992). AIDS in bisexual men in the United States: Epidemiology and transmission to women. *American Journal of Public Health, 82*(2), 220–224.

Cochran, S.D., Mays, V.M. (1991). Sociocultural facets of the Black gay male experience. In R. Staples (Ed.), *The black family: Essays and studies* (pp. 289–296). Belmont, CA: Wadsworth Publishing Co.

Cochran, S.D., Mays, V.M. (1993). Applying social psychological models to predicting HIV-related sexual risk behaviors among African Americans. *Journal of Black Psychology, 19*(2), 142–154.

Conway, G. (1990, June). Presentation to Indian Health Service Area Office AIDS Coordinators, San Francisco, CA.

Conway, G.A., Epstein, M.R., Hayman, C.R., et al. (1993). Trends in HIV prevalence among disadvantaged youth. Survey results from a national job training program 1988 through 1992. *Journal of the American Medical Association, 269*(22), 2887–2889.

Courtwright, D., Joseph, H., Des Jarlais, D. (1989). Addicts who survived: An oral history of narcotic use in America 1923–1965. Knoxville, TN: The University of Tennessee Press.

Crisp, B.R., Barber, J.G., Ross, M.W., et al. (1993). Injecting drug users and HIV/AIDS: Risk behaviors and risk perception. *Drug Alcohol Dependency, 33*(1), 73–80.

Cross, T.L., Bazron, B.J., Dennis, K.W., et al. (1989). Towards a culturally competent system of care. Washington, DC: CASSP Technical Assistance Center.

DeCarpio, A.B., Carpio-Cedraro, F.F., Anderson. L. (1990). Hispanic families learning and teaching about AIDS: A participatory approach at the community level. *Hispanic Journal of Behavioral Sciences, 12,* 165–176.

de la Vega, E. (1989). Homosexuality and bisexuality among Latino men. *Focus, 4,* 3.

Department of Labor (1992). News release—The employment situation: September 1992–October 2, 1992. Pub. No. USDLA 92–630.

Diaz, T., Buehler, J.W., Castro, K.G., et al. (1993a). AIDS trends among Hispanics in the United States. *American Journal of Public Health, 83*(4), 504–509.

Diaz, T., Chu, S.Y. (1993). Crack cocaine use and sexual behavior among people with AIDS. *Journal of the American Medical Association, 269*(22), 2845–2846.

Diaz, T., Chu, S.Y., Frederick, P., et al. (1993b). Sociodemographics and HIV risk behaviors of bisexual men with AIDS: Results from a multistate interview project. *AIDS, 7*(9), 1227–1232.

DiClemente, R., Boyer, C., Morales, E. (1988). Minorities and AIDS: Knowledge, attitudes, and misconceptions among Black and Latino adolescents. *American Journal of Public Health, 78*(1), 55–57.

Doll, L.S., Petersen, L.R., White, C.R., et al. (1992). Homosexually and nonhomosexually identified men who have sex with men: A behavioral comparison. *The Journal of Sex Research, 29* 1–14.

Duh, S.M. (1991). *Blacks and AIDS: Causes and origins,* Newbury Park, CA: Sage.

Easterbrook, P.J., Keruly, J.C., Creagh-Kirk, T. (1991). Racial and ethnic differences in outcome in zidovudine-treated patients with advanced HIV disease. *Journal of the American Medical Association, 266*(19), 2713–2718.

Edgerton, R.B. (1971). *The individual in cultural adaptation* (pp. 1–22). Los Angeles, CA: University of California Press.

El-Sadr, W., Capps, L. (1992). The challenge of minority recruitment in clinical trials for AIDS. *Journal of the American Medical Association, 267*(7), 954–957.

Elder-Tabrizy, K.A., Wolitski, R.J., Rhodes, F., et al. (1991). AIDS and competing health concerns of blacks, Hispanics, and whites. *Journal of Community Health, 16*(1), 11–21.

Eliason, M.J. (1993). Ethics and transcultural nursing care. *Nursing Outlook, 41*(5), 225–228.

Eversley, R.B., Newstetter, A., Avins, A., et al. (1993). Sexual risk and perception of risk for HIV infection among multiethnic family-planning clients. *American Journal of Preventive Medicine, 9*(2), 92–95.

Finelli, L., Budd, J., Spitalny, K.C., et al. (1993). Early syphilis: Relationship to sex, drugs, and changes in high-risk behaviors from 1987–1990. *Sexually Transmitted Diseases, 20*(2), 89–95.

Finlinson, A.A., Robles, H.M., Colon, J.B. (1993). Recruiting and retaining out of treatment injecting drug users in the Puerto Rico AIDS Prevention Project. *Human Organizations, 52,* 169–175.

Flaskerud, J.H. (1988). Is the Likert scale format culturally biased? *Nursing Research, 37*(3), 185–186.

Flaskerud, J.H. (1994a). AIDS and traditional food therapies. In R. Watson (Ed.), *Nutrition and AIDS* (pp. 235–247). Ann Arbor, MI: CRC Press.

Flaskerud, J.H. (1994b). Personal communication.

Flaskerud, J.H., Calvillo, E.R. (1991a). Beliefs about AIDS, health, and illness among low-income Latina women. *Research in Nursing and Health, 14*(6), 431–438.

Flaskerud, J.H., Nyamathi, A.M. (1988). An AIDS education program for Vietnamese women. *New York State Journal of Medicine, 88*(12), 632–637.

Flaskerud, J.H., Nyamathi, A.M. (1990). Effects of an AIDS education program on the knowledge, attitudes and practices of low income Black and Latina women. *Journal of Community Health, 15*(6), 343–355.

Flaskerud, J.H., Rush, C.E. (1989). AIDS and traditional health beliefs and practices of black women. *Nursing Research, 38*(4), 210–215.

Flaskerud, J.H., Thompson, J. (1991b). Beliefs about AIDS, health, and illness in low-income White women. *Nursing Research, 40*(5), 266–271.

Flaskerud, J.H., Uman, G. (1993). Directions for AIDS education for Hispanic women based on analyses of survey findings. *Public Health Reports, 108*(3), 298–304.

Flegal, K.M., Ezzati, T.M., Harris, M.I., et al. (1991). Prevalence of diabetes in Mexican Americans, Cubans, and Puerto Ricans from the Hispanic health and nutrition examination survey, 1982–1984. *Diabetes Care, 14*(7), 628–638.

Foster, G.M. (1981). Relationships between Spanish and Spanish-American folk medicine. In G. Henderson & M. Primeaux (Eds.), *Transcultural Health Care* (pp. 115–135). Menlo Park, CA: Addison-Wesley.

Freimer, N., Echenberg, D., Kretchmer, N. (1986). Cultural variation: Nutritional and clinical implications. *The Western Journal of Medicine, 139,* 928–933.

Friedman, S.R., Des Jarlais, D.C., Sterk, C.E. (1990). AIDS and the social relations of intravenous drug users. *The Milbank Quarterly, 68*(suppl 1), 85–110.

Fullilove, R.E., Haynes, K., Gross, S. (1990). Black women and AIDS prevention: A view toward understanding the gender rules. *Journal of Sex Research, 27,* 46–64.

Gallagher, M.A. (1992). Human immunodeficiency virus and immigration status in the United States. *Journal of the Association of Nurses in AIDS Care, 3*(2), 32–35.

Gonzalez-Swafford, M.J., Gutierrez, M.G. (1983). Ethnomedical beliefs and practices of Mexican-Americans. *Nurse Practitioner, 8*(10), 29–30, 32, 34.

Gossop, M., Griffiths, P., Powis, B., et al. (1993). Severity of heroin dependence and HIV risk. II. Sharing injecting equipment. *AIDS Care, 5*(2), 159–168.

Grossman, A.H. (1991). Gay men and HIV/AIDS: Understanding the double stigma. *Journal of the Association of Nurses in AIDS Care, 2*(4), 28–32.

Guinan, M.E. (1993). Black communities' belief in "AIDS as genocide": A barrier to overcome for HIV prevention. *Annals of Epidemiology, 3*(2), 193–195.

Hall, R.L., Wilder, D., Bodenroeder, P., et al. (1990). Assessment of AIDS knowledge, attitudes, behaviors, and risk level of Northwestern American Indians. *American Journal of Public Health, 80*(7), 875–877.

Hammett, A.M., Biddlecom, A.E. (1992). Homicide surveillance—United States 1979–1988. *Morbidity and Mortality Weekly Report, 41*(SS-3), 1–34.

Hardy, A.M., Biddlecom, A.E. (1991). AIDS knowledge and attitudes of Black Americans: United States, 1990. Provisional data from the National Health Interview Survey. *National Center for Health Statistics Advance Data,* October 16.

Hautman, M.A., Harrison, J.K. (1982). Health beliefs and practices in a middle-income Anglo-American neighborhood. *Advances in Nursing Science, 4*(3), 49–64.

Hein, K (1993). "Getting real" about HIV in adolescents. *American Journal of Public Health, 83*(4), 492–494.

Helman, C.G. (1978). "Feed a cold, starve a fever": Folk models of infection in an English suburban community, and their relation to medical treatment. *Culture, Medicine and Psychiatry, 2*(2), 107–137.

Hendricson, W.D., Russell, I.J., Prihoda, T.J., et al. (1989). An approach to developing a valid Spanish language translation of a health-status questionnaire. *Medical Care, 27*(10), 959–966.

Icard, L. (1985). Black gay men and conflicting social identities: Sexual orientation versus racial identity. *Journal of Social Work and Human Sexuality, 4,* 83–93.

Jemmott, J.B., III, Jemmott, L.S., Fong, G.T. (1992). Reductions in HIV risk–associated sexual behaviors among black male adolescents: Effects of an AIDS prevention intervention. *American Journal of Public Health, 82*(3), 372–377.

Jemmott, L.S. (Nov. 12–15, 1993). Perceived approval of sexual partner and HIV risk-associated behavior among Hispanic women: Implications for nursing. Paper presented at the 1993 Scientific Sessions of the American Nurses' Association Council of Nurse Researchers, Washington, DC.

Jemmott, L.S. (April 1992 to March 1996). Research project: AIDS and black women—testing risk behavior interventions. Rutgers, State University of New Jersey, Newark, NJ. (National Institute of Nursing Research grant RO1 NR 03123.)

Jemmott, L.S., Jemmott, J.B., III. (1990). Sexual knowledge, attitudes, and risky sexual behavior among inner-city Black male adolescents. *Journal of Adolescent Research, 5,* 346–365.

Jemmott, L.S., Jemmott, J.B., III. (1991). Applying the theory of reasoned action to AIDS risk behavior: Condom use among Black women. *Nursing Research, 40*(4), 228–234.

Jenkins, B., Lamar, V.L., Thompson-Crumble, J. (1993). AIDS among African Americans: A social epidemic. *Journal of Black Psychology, 19*(2), 108–122.

Kalichman, S.C., Hunter, T.L., Kelly, J.A. (1992). Perceptions of AIDS susceptibility among minority and nonminority women at risk for HIV infection. *Journal of Consulting and Clinical Psychology, 60*(5), 725–732.

Kalichman, S.C., Kelly, J.A., Hunter, T.L., et al. (1993). Culturally tailored HIV-AIDS risk-reduction messages targeted to African-American urban women: Impact on risk sensitization and risk reduction. *Journal of Consulting and Clinical Psychology, 61*(2), 291–295.

Kaminsky, S., Kurtines, W., Hervis, O.O., et al. (1990). Life enhancement counseling with HIV-infected Hispanic gay males. *Hispanic Journal of Behavioral Sciences, 12*(2), 177–195.

Karon, J.M., Berkelman, R.L. (1991). The geographic and ethnic diversity of AIDS incidence trends in homosexual/bisexual men in the United States. *Journal of Acquired Immune Deficiency Syndromes, 4*(12), 1179–1189.

Kauth, M.R., St. Lawrence, J., Kelly, J.A. (1991). Reliability of retrospective assessments of sexual HIV risk behavior: A comparison of biweekly, three-month, and twelve-month self-reports. *AIDS Education and Prevention, 3*(3), 207–214.

Keefe, S., Padilla, A.M. (1987). *Chicano ethnicity.* Albuquerque, NM: University of New Mexico Press.

Kelly, J.A., St. Lawrence, J., Hood, H.V., et al. (1989). An objective test of AIDS risk behavior knowledge: Scale development, validation, and norms. *Journal of Behavioral Therapy and Experimental Psychiatry, 20*(3), 227–234.

Kerr, H.D. (1993). White liver: A cultural disorder resembling AIDS. *Social Science Medicine, 36*(5), 609–614.

Kim, M.V., Marmor, M., Dubin, N., et al. (1993). HIV risk–related sexual behaviors among heterosexuals in New York City: Associations with race, sex and intravenous drug use. *AIDS, 7*(3), 409–414.

Klee, H. (1993). HIV risks for women drug injectors: Heroin and amphetamine users compared. *Addiction, 88*(8), 1055–1062.

Kramer, M.A., Aral, S.O., Curran, J.W. (1980). Self-reported behavior patterns of patients attending a sexually transmitted disease clinic. *American Journal of Public Health, 70*(9), 997–1000.

Lee, D.A., Fong, K. (1990). HIV/AIDS and the Asian and Pacific Islander community. *SEICUS Report, 18*(2), 16–22.

Leininger, M.M. (1991). *Culture care diversity and university: A theory of nursing,* New York: National League for Nursing.

Livingston, I.L., Johnson, T.E.M. (1993). Perceived control, specific at-risk and general fear of AIDS: Intraracial variation among African American college students. *Urban League Review, 15*(1), 53–71.

Magaña, J.R., Carrier, J.M. (1991). Mexican and Mexican American male sexual behavior and spread of AIDS in California. *Journal of Sexual Research, 28*(3), 425–441.

Mann, J., Tarantola, D.J.M., Netter, T. (Eds.) (1992). *AIDS in the world: A global report.* Cambridge, MA: Harvard University Press.

Marin, B.V., Marin, G. (1990). Effects of acculturation on knowledge of AIDS and HIV among Hispanics. *Hispanic Journal of Behavioral Sciences, 12*(2), 110–121.

Marin, B.V., Marin, G. (1992). Predictors of condom accessibility among Hispanics in San Francisco. *American Journal of Public Health, 82*(4), 592–595.

Marin, B.V., Marin, G., Juarez, R.A. (1990). Differences between Hispanics and non-Hispanics in willingness to provide AIDS prevention advice. *Hispanic Journal of Behavioral Sciences, 12*(2), 153–164.

Marin, B.V., Marin, G., Juarez, R.A., et al. (1992). Intervention from family members as a strategy for preventing HIV transmission among intravenous drug users. *Journal of Community Psychology, 20*, 90–97.

Marin, G. (1989). AIDS prevention among Hispanics: Needs, risk behaviors, and cultural values. *Public Health Reports, 104*(5), 411–415.

Marin, G., Sabogal, F., Marin, B., et al. (1987). Development of a short acculturation scale for Hispanics. *Hispanic Journal of Behavioral Sciences, 9*(2), 183–205.

Mayfield, L.P. (1991). Early parenthood among low income adolescent girls. In R. Staples (Ed.), *The Black family* (pp. 227–239). Belmont, CA: Wadsworth Publishing Co.

Mays, V., Cochran, S. (1988). Issues in the perception of AIDS risk and risk reduction activities by Black and Hispanic/Latina women. *American Psychologist, 43*(11), 949–957.

Mays, V.M., Cochran, S.D. (1993). Ethnic and gender differences in beliefs about sex partner questioning to reduce HIV risk. *Journal of Adolescent Research, 8*(1), 77–88.

Mays, V.M., Jackson, J.S. (1991). AIDS survey methodology with black Americans. *Social Science and Medicine, 33*(1), 47–54.

McBride, A.D. (1991). A perspective on AIDS: A catastrophic disease but a symptom of deeper problems in the Black community. In R. Staples (Ed.), *The Black family* (pp. 268–274). Belmont, CA: Wadsworth Publishing Co.

McCray, E. (1991, August). AIDS in the racial and ethnic minority populations. Paper presented at the meeting of the National Medical Association, Las Vegas, NV.

Metler, R., Conway, G., Stehr-Green, J. (1991). AIDS surveillance among American Indians and Alaska Natives. *American Journal of Public Health, 81*(11), 1469–1471.

Morales, E.S. (1990). HIV infection and Hispanic gay and bisexual men. *Hispanic Journal of Behavioral Sciences, 12*(2), 212–222.

Moran, J.S., Janes, H.R., Peterman, T.A., et al. (1990). Increase in condom sales following AIDS education and publicity, United States. *American Journal of Public Health, 80*(5), 607–608.

National Commission on Acquired Immune Deficiency Syndrome (1992, December). The challenge of HIV/AIDS in communities of color. Washington, DC: The Commission.

Nickens, H.W. (1991). The health status of minority populations in the United States. *Western Journal of Medicine, 155*(1), 27–32.

Nicoll, A., Laukamm-Josten, U., Mwizarubi, B., et al. (1993). Lay health beliefs concerning HIV and AIDS: A barrier for control programs. *AIDS Care, 5*(2), 231–241.

Nyamathi, A., Lewis, C. (1991). Coping of African-American women at risk for AIDS. *Women's Health Issues, 1*(2), 53–62.

Nyamathi, A., Shin, D.M. (1990). Designing a culturally sensitive AIDS education program for Black and Hispanic women of childbearing age. *NAACOG's Clinical Issues in Perinatal Women's Health Nursing, 1*(1), 86–93.

Nyamathi, A., Vasquez, R. (1989). The impact of poverty, homelessness and drugs on Hispanic women at risk for HIV infection. *Hispanic Journal of Behavioral Sciences, 11*(4), 299–314.

Ostrow, D.G., Whitaker, R., Frasier, K., et al. (1991). Racial differences in social support and mental health in men with HIV infection: A pilot study. *AIDS Care, 3*(1), 55–62.

Parra, E.O., Shapiro, M.F., Moreno, C.A., et al. (1993). AIDS-related risk behavior, knowledge, and beliefs among women and their Mexican-American sexual partners who used intravenous drugs. *Archives of Family Medicine, 2*(6), 603–610.

Pavich, E.G. (1986). A Chicano perspective on Mexican culture and sexuality. *Journal of Social Work, 4*, 47–65.

Peterson, J.L., Coates, T.J., Catania, J.A. (1992). High-risk sexual behavior and condom use among gay and bisexual African-American men. *American Journal of Public Health, 82*(11), 1490–1494.

Peterson, J.L., Fullilove, R., Catania, J., et al. (1989, June). Close encounters of an unsafe kind: Risky sexual behaviors and predictors among Black gay and bisexual men. Presented at the 5th International AIDS Conference, Montreal, Quebec, Canada.

Pliskin, K.L. (1992). Dysphoria and somatization in Iranian culture. *The Western Journal of Medicine, 157*(3), 295–300.

Prochaska, J.O., DiClemente, C.C. (1983). Stages and processes of self-change of smoking: Toward an integrative model of change. *Journal of Consulting and Clinical Psychology, 51*(3), 390–395.

Prochaska, T., Albrecht, G., Levy, J, et al. (1990). Determinants of self-perceived risk for AIDS. *Journal of Health and Social Behavior, 31*, 384–394.

Ramakrishna, J., Weiss, M.G. (1992). Health, illness, and immigration: East Indians in the United States. *The Western Journal of Medicine, 157*(3), 265–275.

Rivera, R.R., Colon, M.H., Gonzalez, A., et al. (1990). Social relations and empowerment of sexual partners of IV drug users. *Puerto Rican Health Science Journal, 9*(1), 99–104.

Roberson, M.H.B. (1987). Home remedies: A cultural study. *Home Healthcare Nurse, 5*(1), 35–40.

Rogers, S.M., Turner, C.F. (1991). Male-male sexual contact in the U.S.A.: Findings from five sample surveys, 1970–1990. *Journal of Sex Research, 28*(4), 491–519.

Romero, A. (1988). Overcoming HIV seropositivity ineligibility: Legal authority from extreme hardship cases. *Immigration Newsletter, 17*, 1–14.

Rosenthal, C.J. (1986). Family supports in later life: Does ethnicity make a difference? *The Gerontologist, 26*(1), 19–24.

Rowell, R.M. (1990). Native Americans, stereotypes and HIV/AIDS. *SEICUS Report, 18*(2), 9–15.

Sangree, S. (1993). Control of childbearing by HIV-positive women: Some responses to emerging legal policies. *Buffalo Law Review, 41*(2), 309–449.

Schilling, R.F., El-Bassel, N., Schinke, S.P., et al. (1991). Building skills of recovering women drug users to reduce heterosexual AIDS transmission. *Public Health Reports, 106*(3), 297–304.

Schoenbach, V.J., Landis, S.E., Weber, D.J., et al. (1993). HIV seroprevalence in sexually transmitted disease clients in a low-prevalence Southern state: Evidence of sexual transmission. *Annals of Epidemiology, 3*(3), 281–288.

Schwarcz, S.K., Bolan, G.A., Kellogg, T.A., et al. (1993). Comparison of voluntary and blinded human immunodeficiency virus type 1 (HIV-1) seroprevalence surveys in a high prevalence sexually transmitted disease clinical population. *American Journal of Epidemiology, 137*(6), 600–608.

Shayne, V.T., Kaplan, B.J. (1991). Double victims: Poor women and AIDS. *Women and Health, 17,* 21–37.

Singer, M. (1991). Confronting the AIDS epidemic among IV drug users: Does ethnic culture matter? *AIDS Education and Prevention, 3*(3), 258–283.

Snow, L.F. (1983). Traditional health beliefs and practices among lower class Black Americans. *Western Journal of Medicine, 139*(6), 820–828.

Sontag, S. (1990). *AIDS and it's metaphors.* New York: Anchor Books.

St. Lawrence, J.S. (1993). African-American adolescents' knowledge, health-related attitudes, sexual behavior, and contraceptive decisions: Implications for the prevention of adolescent HIV infection. *Journal of Consulting and Clinical Psychology, 61*(1), 104–112.

St. Louis, M.E., Conway, G.A., Hayman, C.R., et al. (1991). Human immunodeficiency virus infection in disadvantaged adolescents: Findings from the U.S. Job Corps. *Journal of the American Medical Association, 266*(17), 2387–2391.

Staples, R. (1991a). Changes in black family structure: The conflict between family ideology and structural conditions. In R. Staples (Ed.), *The Black family* (pp. 28–36). Belmont, CA: Wadsworth Publishing Co.

Staples, R. (1991b). The sexual revolution and the Black middle class. In R. Staples (Ed.), *The Black family* (pp. 88–91). Belmont, CA: Wadsworth Publishing Co.

Staples, R. (1991c). Health issues. In R. Staples (Ed.), *The Black family* (pp. 257–267). Belmont, CA: Wadsworth Publishing Co.

Staples, R. (1991d). The political economy of Black family life. In R. Staples (Ed.), *The Black family* (pp. 248–256). Belmont, CA: Wadsworth Publishing Co.

Stowe, A., Ross, M.W., Wodak, A., et al. (1993). Significant relationships and social supports of injecting drug users and their implications for HIV/AIDS services. *AIDS Care, 5*(1), 23–33.

Strong, P. (1990). Epidemic psychology: A model. *Sociology of Health and Illness, 12,* 249–259.

Temple, M.T., Leigh, B.C., Schafer, J. (1993). Unsafe sexual behavior and alcohol use at the event level: Results of a national survey. *Journal of Acquired Immune Deficiency Syndromes, 6*(4), 393–404.

Thomas, S.B., Quinn, S.C. (1991). The Tuskegee syphilis study, 1932–1972: Implications for HIV education and AIDS risk education programs in the Black community. *American Journal of Public Health, 81*(11), 1498–1505.

Toomey, K.E., Oberschelp, A.G., Greenspan, J.R. (1989). Sexually transmitted diseases and Native Americans: Trends in reported gonorrhea and syphilis morbidity, 1984–1988. *Public Health Reports, 104*(6), 566–572.

Turner, H.A., Hays, R.B., Coates, T.J. (1993). Determinants of social support among gay men: The context of AIDS. *Journal of Health and Social Behavior, 34*(1), 37–53.

van Oss Marin, B., Gomez, C.A., Hearst, N. (1993). Multiple heterosexual partners and condom use among Hispanics and non-Hispanic whites. *Family Planning Perspective, 25*(4), 170–174.

Vasquez-Nuttall, E., Romero-Garcia, I., De Leon, B. (1987). Sex roles and perceptions of femininity and masculinity of Hispanic women. *Psychology of Women Quarterly, 11,* 409–411.

Wallace, R. (1990). Urban decertification, public health and public order: "Planned shrinkage," violent death, substance abuse and AIDS in the Bronx. *Social Science and Medicine, 31*(7), 801–813.

Wasser, S.C., Gwinn, M., Fleming, P. (1993). Urban-non-urban distribution of HIV infection in childbearing women in the United States. *Journal of Acquired Immune Deficiency Syndromes, 6*(9), 1035–1042.

Wayment, H.A., Newcomb, M.D., Hannemann, V.L. (1993). Female and male intravenous drug users not-in-treatment: Are they at differential risk for AIDS? *Sex Roles, 28*(1/2), 111–125.

Wei, L. (1976). Theoretical foundation of Chinese medicine: A modern interpretation. *American Journal of Chinese Medicine , 4*(14), 355–372.

Wenger, A.F.Z. (1993). Cultural meaning of symptoms. *Holistic Nurse Practice, 7*(2), 22–35.

West, E.A. (1993). The cultural bridge model. *Nursing Outlook, 41*(5), 229–232.

Whang, J. (1981). Chinese traditional food therapy. *Journal of the American Dietetic Association, 78*(1), 55–57.

Worth, D., Rodriquez, R. (1987). Latina women and AIDS. *SIECUS Report, 79*(7), 836–922.

Wyatt, G.E. (1991). Examining ethnicity versus race in AIDS related sex research. *Social Science Medicine, 33*(1), 37–45.

Personal Perspectives on Nursing Care

16

*Christine Fegan, Thomas E. Emanuele, Deborah L. Wolen, Kathryn J. Foley,
and Maureen Connolly*

The HIV/AIDS epidemic has been described as two parallel nightmares: first, the HIV disease trajectory and the associated suffering and death, and second, the epidemic of fear and discrimination (Sherer, 1990). The history of the first decade of the epidemic in the United States reflects a story of courage and cowardice, hope and despair, and compassion and hostility, and a struggle between scientific facts and irrational fears (Ungvarski & Ballard, 1993). It also reveals the dedicated work of thousands of nurses who, in the wake of adversity and criticism, took up the challenges of caring for people affected by HIV disease. This chapter reflects the stories of five of those nurses.

CHRISTINE FEGAN, SAN DIEGO, CALIFORNIA

In 1982, I began working with HIV-infected patients in New York City. I had been a nurse since 1978 and had worked on various units in a large teaching hospital. Disillusioned with the lack of diversity and autonomy as a staff nurse, I decided to work as a private duty nurse while I contemplated what I would do next. When I started working as a private duty nurse, our hospital was just beginning to see patients with AIDS. They were very ill, needed close observation, and had a myriad of nursing care requirements. In these early days, very little information was known about HIV disease, and many staff and private duty nurses were too frightened to care for the patients. As more of these patients were admitted to the hospital, I began to care exclusively for AIDS patients. One reason that I became involved with them was that a very close friend

of mine had received a diagnosis of AIDS and had eventually died in 1985.

Because I found my work both intellectually and emotionally challenging, this period was an exciting time for me. I felt a sense of pride in caring for patients for whom few other people would provide care. As a result, I became involved in the Gay Men's Health Crisis (GMHC), and for the first time I became politically and socially active within the community.

Fear of contagion was never a consideration, for some reason. I had a couple of minor needle-stick exposures, which never concerned me until I became pregnant in 1987. It was then, when I went to be tested, that I realized I could have become infected and died of this disease. Fortunately, my test results were negative.

As a private duty nurse, I spent long periods with my patients, sometimes caring for them in the hospital and in their homes as well. Although I had had extensive experience in caring for terminally ill patients, they had usually been much older than I. With AIDS, I had to deal with the fact that most of my patients were close to my age and faced premature death. However, their expressed gratitude for having someone to care for them and listen to their problems kept me motivated. In the early days of the epidemic, patients were often left alone.

In 1986 I moved to California, where I have worked in a variety of settings, including hospice, home care, and primary care. Now, in a clinical research center, I provide care for HIV-infected persons. Although I have often felt emotionally drained and tired, I can't imagine doing any other type of nursing. My experiences in the various populations that I have nursed have been related to my employment roles. In New York City, working as a private duty nurse, I primarily cared for affluent gay white men. In California I have been employed as a staff nurse, caring for a racially and ethnically diverse patient population that is poor and that includes women and their families.

After 11 years, what I consider the rewards of this work are different from those of the earlier years of the epidemic. I have always believed that it has been an extraordinary privilege to be a part of my patients' lives, and my experiences with them have changed my life. To be able to continue providing this care for extended periods, nurses must face issues about themselves that they may not choose to confront otherwise.

The experience of allowing yourself to be fully there for these patients may be painful. Your life is changed because you are exposed to so much suffering and death. If you are too involved, you may become "burned out." Some care providers may stay detached and distant to protect themselves emotionally. It is hard not to be affected emotionally because you see both the best and the worst of people, who are courageous and peaceful at the saddest, most frightening time of their lives. Because they have such emotional highs and lows, it's hard to retain your own equilibrium. As a result, my life has become intensely emotional.

Caring for people with HIV disease has drastically changed my perspective on what is important in life, and material concerns and interests no longer seem as important to me. As a nurse, I develop close relationships very quickly with my patients. Shorty after we meet, we are soon discussing everything from sex to death. This has affected my life in many ways. The intensity of my work and my work relationships has made my life intense. This can make people uncomfortable in a normal setting. I find it difficult to have friends who are not somehow involved in the arena of HIV care. My friends must have an understanding of this aspect of my life because it affects all areas of my life. Many people not involved in this type of work are unable to provide on-going support and understanding. What has changed over the years is my understanding that the rewards I have gained are related to the insights I have had about myself while sharing my patients' experiences. The result, although painful, has been personal growth.

An age-old problem in nursing is that we nurses fail to take care of ourselves. Because this work is so compelling, rewarding, and satisfying to me, I have found it easy to become overly involved with my patients and their families, neglecting my own needs in the process. When I worked in home care and hospice situations, in which I visited people in their homes, I became intimately involved with them and their family dynamics. This over-involvement can make a nurse feel responsible for the outcome of events. It is easy for a nurse to forget that although she can be supportive to her clients with HIV disease, she has no control over individual behavior or outcomes.

Remaining objective and outside this process allows the nurse to be a source of education, strength, and support. Nurses are notorious for believing that we have extraordinary reserves of energy and strength. We don't! Our energy is depleted when we give to others, and if we don't replenish it in some way, we won't have it. When my energy was depleted, I would feel anger, resentment, and depression. My coping skills would be very low, and I would continue to work very hard but accomplish less. I would become impatient with co-workers, friends, and family. Although I would educate my patients and their families about stress reduction, I myself did not have time for it. I would start exercise or self-help programs but would not continue with them for long. Does this sound familiar? Certainly, not only nurses caring for HIV-infected patients fail to care for themselves. After many years, I have finally realized how important it is to take care of myself. I believe that I could not have continued to care for patients with AIDS if I had not developed a self-care program. My regular program of exercise and meditation has decreased my level of stress, increased by energy level, and allowed me to cope more effectively with my work.

Grieving is also very important. You must acknowledge your losses and reflect on what that means to you as a nurse and a person. Whenever a patient with whom you are close dies, you are affected. If these losses are not addressed, the feelings will be exhibited in other, unproductive ways. I think that the nurse who allows herself or himself to feel the pain associated with these losses, and reflects on what death means personally, can more effectively care for dying patients.

Boundary setting and detachment are important strategies that we as nurses must learn to use effectively. Using such strategies doesn't mean that you don't care about your patient and their families or that you can't get close to them. The nurse must realize that the family's and patient's experience of HIV disease is ultimately *their* experience and that, as painful as it may be, *they* need to deal with it. No one, including the nurse, can or should shield them from this process. I believe that my role in my patients' living and dying process is to help with their transition. Sometimes the transition is from being well to being ill and then to being well again, and sometimes it is from life to death. When I first started in this work, I thought that I was supposed to save lives. I would get caught up in the patients' anxiety and struggle with their transitions. How unfair it seemed that these young people had to suffer and die. Later I found out how unhealthy it was for me to adopt the patient's struggle as my own. I have found that I can be more effective and helpful as a care provider if I detach myself from this struggle. Still, I remain involved and feel sadness for the suffering and deaths that I witness. I acknowledge my losses when my patients die, but I also recognize how much I have gained by knowing and caring for them. Facing these issues is a personal process for each of us.

Talking with friends and family who understand may be helpful. Support groups at work or within the community may also be a source of comfort. Personally, I have found that no source of comfort was helpful until I truly looked at what the pain I was feeling meant to me. Slowly I found ways of coping with the losses and continuing to enjoy and be happy in my work.

In the past 13 years, I have learned a great deal, both personally and professionally. Opportunity for this type of growth is not possible with many other professions. Although our time at work takes up so much of our lives, many individuals are unhappy with the work they do. I have loved my work since I started working with HIV-infected patients, and I can provide holistic nursing care in ways not possible in other nursing specialties.

THOMAS E. EMANUELE, DALLAS, TEXAS

I first recall reading about this disease in 1981, on a flight to Vancouver, British Columbia. The newspaper article described some strange cases of a rare cancer found in young male patients. As a young gay man, I was particularly struck by the fact that all the men affected were homosexual. Details in the article were sparse, and I remember being left with many questions. The next year, I started to see more information about gay-related immune deficiency (GRID). It did not affect my practice directly, and at that time I did not know enough or was not reading enough about it to worry.

Then in 1982 something happened. I lived in the Bible Belt in Dallas, Texas, which had a very proactive gay community. Flyers began to be distributed, and the weekly gay newspaper announced that community meetings were being held to discuss this "GRID" thing. These meetings were held to tell us how we might protect ourselves from whatever GRID was. There was no information provided to me as a professional, and at work we had not yet seen or knowingly cared for a patient with GRID. My life-partner and I went to the series of meetings. They were attended by many gay men and a few concerned lesbians. I believe that this was my first inkling that GRID was something big. The leaders were trying to make people aware, and they caught my attention. There still was little to read about professionally. There were no books for nurses, and our journals did not mention it. Reading had always been my method of making myself comfortable when I had a knowledge deficit. Still, in 1983 and 1984, I had not yet cared for a patient with AIDS, so I thought that it couldn't be as bad as they said it was in San Francisco and New York.

Late in 1984 I received an unwelcome surprise. A friend called me to say that another friend of ours, a teacher, "had it!" He was a patient in a major Baptist-affiliated medical center here in Dallas. He asked whether, since I was a nurse, I could go and visit him. Until I got to the hospital, I thought that was a silly reason to visit. I went to the nurses' station to find out what room he was in. They told me that he was infectious and couldn't have any visitors. I told them that I knew what he had, was a nurse and had previously worked there, and I wanted to see him. His family is from West Texas, where there is still a frontier mentality. His mom and dad were there but didn't want anyone to know what he had. Finally, I was able to convince the nurses to let me see him. They made me put on a gown, mask, and gloves before entering the room, although I was not caring for him, just visiting.

The horror and shock of that first experience with AIDS will always be with me. I saw derision, isolation, guilt, and blatant discrimination being displayed toward my friend. I saw how it was being done in the name of God and of the American family. I felt anger and rage, fear and anxiety. As a nurse I could not comprehend the scene I was witnessing.

The fear and anxiety were because of my own lifestyle and my own perception that just being gay was enough to get it. My thoughts led me to believe that we (gay men) were all already infected. Despair did not set in, because, although I am not a religious person, I am a very spiritual person. I define spirituality in terms of the parts of me that make me human: those parts, the sum of which allow me to love, nurture, feel, and be able to have compassion for others.

As a gay man I felt whole because my community offered me support for who I am. Altruistically, I felt as a professional nurse that I wanted to be able to offer my support and expertise, to give something back to my community and family of choice. I did not want

to see any more of my friends go through this experience—not just the disease processes itself but everything else that was happening. This was the feeling that made me want to get involved in HIV care. Soon I began receiving call after call to help someone with AIDS. I had a feeling that I had to mobilize against this thing but did not have a clue about how to do it.

My job at the time was clinic manager for a very high volume outpatient clinic at a large teaching hospital in Dallas. One day I was making rounds in the chest medicine clinic, and I saw that the door to the restroom had been taped shut with a sign of a skull and crossbones on it. I asked another nurse what that was about, and she told me that a patient referred from the allergy clinic had used the toilet and his diagnosis was *Pneumocystis carinii* pneumonia. When the staff heard that he had AIDS, they decompensated. I realized that the time was here, and I had to learn more.

The hospital administration had set up a referral clinic to see patients referred by the allergy clinic and the oncology clinic. At this time the ELISA test (enzyme-linked immunosorbent assay) had just been released. The hospital hired a nurse to counsel the patients. She did this for almost a year. Then I heard that we were going to be doing an open-label study of an antiviral agent called azidothymidine (AZT). I wanted to sign on to learn something about this disease. There were some personnel changes, and I obtained the job of AIDS nurse clinician.

Then my uphill struggle began. It started with what was going to be on my name badge. I told them that it was time for people to be made aware that AIDS was here and to become educated. Although I succeeded in getting the correct title printed on the badge, I was shocked at how fast an elevator would clear when people read the thing! My colleagues were almost as bad at times. I was always having to explain why I was not afraid of getting "it." No one knew what I really felt.

In the 1970s I was taught standard infection control procedures, long before universal precautions were implemented, and was comfortable caring for patients with transmissible diseases, as were most nurses. I had hoped that my example and practice of good infection control technique would enable my associates to dispel their fears and provide the necessary care. I soon learned that my example did not stimulate their desire for professional growth but gave them an excuse not to care for those patients with an AIDS diagnosis. They were glad that they were not having to put themselves "at risk." Does this sound familiar?

In 1979, while I was in college, I saw an article in a nursing journal about therapeutic touch. The article included some Kerlian photographs showing the actual energy radiating from the hands and fingers. The article stimulated my interest, and I wanted to learn more about this phenomenon. From what I read, it was an important nursing intervention that had very postive effects. Little did I know that this article would begin a new journey into healing and wellness promotion for me.

I learned the importance and wonderful effects of therapeutic touch, both personally and professionally. I noted that one of the great deficiencies in the care of "isolation" patients was a lack of touch, sometimes caused by fear of contagion and sometimes by the barriers that we set up as necessary protocols. I discovered that patients yearned to be touched and that gowns and gloves, although necessary, did not have to exclude nurturing touch. The effect of therapeutic touch on patients who had nausea, complained of peripheral neuropathy, or were very anxious was unbelievable. At first I started using therapeutic touch in the clinic examining rooms, with the doors closed. Then, after I saw the effect it had on the patients, I told my nurse manager what I was doing and she supported my efforts by increasing the time I spent on direct patient care. Therapeutic touch allowed me to focus on the patient as an individual and provided time for bonding in our relationship.

My work with people with HIV/AIDS began to clarify an emerging role as a facilitator in the personal journey of others. I realize that different people have different goals for their treatment. As a nurse I was a caretaker both physically and emotionally, and I found it difficult to set boundaries. I had to find a way to care for myself as well as my patients. What I learned was to take responsibility for the assessment and intervention and to evaluate the outcomes without feeling personally responsible for what happened. I realized that both the plan of care and the choices to be made belonged essentially to the patient. I was there to help patients make informed choices and achieve their goals.

I realized early that it is necessary to get involved politically to effect change and bring attention to the severity and depth of the problem, as well as to the rights of the people who were living, or trying to live, with HIV disease. Realizing that I was politically naive, I became involved with activists from the local gay and lesbian organization, the Dallas Gay and Lesbian Alliance (DGLA).

To try to deal with my grief, I got involved in the Quilt Project and learned from the DGLA how to push people's buttons. My life-partner, who has supported me through all this, went with me to the March on Washington in 1987. We saw and felt the power that was ours as a community. This translated into getting involved in Dallas, after returning from the March, in funding and access-to-care issues. At work I became involved with the hospital's ad hoc administrative AIDS task force. On the local community level I became part of the advisory group working with the Dallas City Council in planning the budget for the next 2 years.

This political involvement helped distract me from what was happening inside me. As usual, I was able effectively to suppress my feelings of grief and loss. Eventually I started therapy and learned to stay productively involved within boundaries and that I was not personally responsible for the outcomes of my patients' lives. I had to learn to let go of a sense of control, control that I had no right to assert.

The AIDS epidemic had become a journey for me as well. As a gay man, I noticed that I had terrible feelings of guilt as more patients and friends received the AIDS diagnosis. I felt sad and guilty because they were getting sick and I was still well. I started to feel guilty about not being infected. You must understand that I really did not want to be infected, but I realized that because of my sexual lifestyle and occupation, I didn't understand why I wasn't. This became a problem for me, and I learned to deal with it but at times, when I lose a friend or become especially close to a patient, I find that it comes back to me. This is one phase of grieving that I must allow myself.

We must all allow ourselves to grieve. I found this to be a problem for my colleagues as well. We are experiencing loss at a massive rate, and it is normal to grieve. An important lesson to learn is that it's okay to take time to grieve, it's okay to cry, and it's okay to be yourself. You must love yourself before you can effectively love and care for your patients.

One of the most rewarding experiences for me has been my involvement and networking, both nationally and internationally, with some of the leaders in the nursing profession. Many feel that "nurses eat their young," but I have seen something different in nurses who care for HIV-infected patients. I have found concern and support. I suppose that because none of us knew much about AIDS, we banded together to teach each other in a most collegial manner. The Association of Nurses in AIDS Care (ANAC), in particular, has introduced me to a network of nurses who have, with time, become experts in HIV nursing care. ANAC has also provided me with information and education, and my involvement with ANAC not only has benefited me and my patients, but also has served as a source of support for nurses directly affected by HIV/ AIDS.

In summary, I would have to say that the major benefit I have received from caring for people with HIV infection is that I know I care. I have opened myself to the universe for all the love and learning that it can provide. I have had the blessing of meeting some of the most interesting and caring people, both patients and colleagues, and have been able to experience unconditional love. I would never trade the experiences of the past 9 years, because they have truly helped me to grow in unanticipated and profoundly enriching directions.

DEBORAH L. WOLEN, CHICAGO, ILLINOIS

July 22, 1993, was one of my days off work. I was playing a pretend game with my 5-year-old daughter, Naima, a variation of "house." She was the mom, I was the dad, and the stuffed animals were the children. The phone rang, and it was my friend from work, Margaret, another nurse practitioner at the hospital-based HIV primary care clinic where I work. "I heard that Lee died," she said. "What?" I replied. "Oh, no! What happened?" While the "mom" of the pretend game pulled on my arm, protesting my withdrawal of attention, I listened to the few details that Marge had. I would have to learn more at clinic the next day.

I felt numb. Lee was dead? I did not expect this. Just a few weeks ago he had told me that a diagnosis of lymphoma had been made, but he was not near death. I thought of my last encounter with Lee. He was angry with me when he left my examination room. Did he kill himself? I had failed him. "Mommy!" Naima repeated, "we're still playing this game and the children are waiting for you to take them to dance class—Mommy!" Pulled back to the game, I had to put my thoughts and feelings on hold. I wonder if the "children" (stuffed animals) in the game felt their "dad's" lack of enthusiasm and involvement at dance class. Certainly, Naima seemed to be more demanding and irritable.

Lee, a 37-year-old African American gay man, was a delightful, complex person whom I first met during my orientation to the AIDS services in May 1991. Because I had no experience and no knowledge of HIV disease, I was placed on the AIDS consult service and was expected to learn very fast. I was having great difficulty putting the facts of HIV disease together, which made me feel as incompetent as I had felt in the first few weeks as a new mother.

I was sent to do a consultation on Lee after he had come into the hospital through the emergency department without any prior contact with our hospital or clinic. He had had no prior treatment of his HIV infection, though he had known about it for several years. He had generalized weakness and paralysis of both legs, and hydrocephalus was diagnosed. Although Lee was somewhat lethargic, he spent most of our conversation questioning me about the cause of his illness. I had practically no facts to offer him because I knew so little about HIV. When my daughter was a newborn infant and I did not know what to do for her when she cried, I started singing to her and rocking her, two things I did know how to do. With Lee, I fell back on my nursing skills. I asked him about his life, his interests, and what I could do to make life in the hospital more tolerable while he waited on the neurosurgery schedule. He said he was interested in history and international affairs, so I brought him a few books the next day.

Eventually, Lee had neurosurgery for a shunt placement for hydrocephalus, presumed to have been caused by progressive multifocal leukoencephalopathy. Postoperatively, Lee made rapid progress and I followed him in clinic.

When Lee made his first outpatient visit with me 2 weeks after his hospital discharge, we set a pattern for our future encounters. The shunt placement greatly improved Lee's functioning; he walked well, even skipped, and showed no focal neurologic deficit. He said he felt well, and asked a lot of questions about his illness, his hospitalization, and the cause of his hydrocephalus. Although his memory and cognition seemed greatly improved, I needed to repeat information several times, but by this time, 4 months into this job, I was able to answer some of his questions. Lee seemed to be in a good mood and made sarcastic but funny jokes about the books I had brought to him. Expressing hope for the future, he asked me how long he would live. Although I discussed survival rates with him, I explained that no one can predict how long any individual will live.

I felt happy about Lee's progress. The therapeutic goals of cure and prolonging life are definitely a part of my professional fabric. Most of my previous education and experience had focused on cure and maintaining health. In my current practice the more realistic approach was to improve the quality of the remaining life, because its duration is beyond control (Mount, 1986). However relevant this goal was, I was much less experienced and felt much less comfortable with this approach.

I have been a nurse for 18 years. Initially, I worked as a public health/visiting nurse for 6 years. For the past 10 years, I have been a nurse practitioner in several practice areas at a large public hospital in Chicago, working in emergency services and women's health care. My main interests were health maintenance and patient education.

I became interested in working with people with HIV infection after I met a wonderful nurse practitioner, Jim De La Cerda. He not only helped establish the HIV services at the hospital but also gave lectures about HIV to the nurse practitioner staff in emergency services. Although I did not know him well, I found his integrity and generosity of spirit inspiring and, with time, I felt a stronger desire to work in HIV services. For the past 2½ years, I have been a nurse practitioner providing primary health care in the outpatient clinic to persons living with HIV disease. The patients whom we serve are in various stages of HIV infection and AIDS. Our clinic provides care only to men because other clinics provide services to women and children.

At first, my caseload primarily consisted of new patients who had a recent diagnosis of AIDS and were being treated successfully, or people with asymptomatic HIV infection. After several months I inherited a few patients from a clinician who left the clinic. Some of these patients had advanced, symptomatic disease. As some of the men became more ill, I felt increasingly anxious. Painful memories of childhood losses, unresolved, came into sharp focus. Like a scared child, I wanted to run away. The need to support my patients, and sometimes their families, with their greater losses was a responsibility from which I could not run.

I looked to my basic nursing education for help. I recalled lessons learned from two psychiatric nurses, Sherry Soderberg and Noreen Kessel, on the importance of building a therapeutic relationship between patient and nurse and the relevance of reflective and active listening, to be used during every patient contact. I also recalled lessons I had learned as a student of Jackie Flaskerud. It was her warm, friendly way of being there and her companionship that I wished to incorporate into my practice.

For about a year and a half, my clinic visits with Lee followed the pattern set at the first visit. He asked many questions, and I often had to repeat the answers. In common with many patients, Lee was intensely interested in his CD4$^+$ cell counts. In the hospital, his CD4$^+$ cell count was 180 mm^3, but after 6 months of taking AZT the CD4$^+$ cell count was up to 324 mm^3 and stayed between 200 and 300 mm^3 for another year. Lee also told me about economic and housing problems. He was evicted from his apartment while hospitalized, and all his possessions were missing. Although, by profession, he was a social worker employed in an agency serving mentally retarded adults, he was now without a job and living with his mother, sister, and a nephew. He was reluctant to discuss personal relationships on any level. His primary goal in life at this point was to replace his lost possessions, find an affordable apartment, and regain his independence.

Together, Lee and I mapped out a strategy for him to make a claim against his former landlord for compensation for his lost possessions. He was very pleased when he settled with the landlord before going to trial. He made plans to look for an apartment and to find a part-time social work job to supplement his social security benefits.

As Lee's health status stabilized, he was scheduled for clinic visits every 1 to 2 months, but often he simply came to the clinic as a "walk-in." As frequently as every 2 weeks, he would wait to talk to me after I had seen my scheduled patients. Sometimes he had physical complaints and sometimes a list of questions: "How will I know if I am getting worse?" "Why do I cough in the morning? Is it due to smoking?" "Do you think this heavy winter jacket is good, or should I have a coat?" I interpreted these interactions as his expression of a need for support and reassurance.

Because Lee often expressed sadness and distress over the stigma of AIDS and complained bitterly about his uncertain future and shortened life, I suggested a consultation with our psychologist. Although Lee acknowledged a need for help, he resisted. He asked me about the psychologist's education, philosophy, methods, and length of experience in working with gay men. Each month Lee said: "I am under so much stress, I can't stand it. I should make an appointment with the psychologist." However, he refused to accept the name and telephone number of the psychologist. Each month I searched for more persuasive words that would convince him to seek counseling. First I tried reassuring him that many healthy people consult with mental health professionals, and I did not believe that he was mentally ill. Then I tried to empathize, telling him that although he may never have needed help before, he was now experiencing severe stress. Finally, I tried praising him for having the courage to express his need for help. I even tried making jokes about my own lack of competence to provide the counseling for him. Nothing seemed to work, and I felt anxious and ineffective. Eventually the psychologist made contact with Lee, and he began to attend weekly support groups.

Despite his frequent demands for my attention, I usually felt happy to see Lee. Perhaps the memory of his being so disabled in the hospital made me feel more generous. Also, because I try hard not to become a cog in the bureaucracy, I encourage my patients to seek help from me or others when they feel the need. Most important, I liked Lee. He enjoyed teasing me about being a married feminist: "Isn't that a contradiction?" At each visit he asked: "And how's Mr. Wolen? Oh, I forgot, you're a feminist, you don't use your husband's last name!"

In April 1993 a biopsy was performed for central nervous system lymphoma. Afterward, Lee came to the clinic to see me, and although he had lost three pounds he said he felt well. He was to return for the biopsy results on May 10, so I gave Lee a regular appointment for June 7. I wrote in my note, "Pt. to inform me of biopsy results," and he agreed to do so. Because he came to clinic so often, I thought that he would tell me about any abnormal results. However, he did not return for this appointment, and on June 21, his fortieth birthday, a nurse handed me a note from Lee. It said that after he saw his biopsy results, he had been referred to the oncology clinic and had started radiation therapy for lymphoma localized in the nasopharynx. The note continued: "Today, I started my third week of radiation treatment. I can't stand it anymore. This past weekend I did not eat a single meal . . . I have lost 9 pounds. Needless to say, I am very concerned. HELP."

When he returned to the clinic on June 29, he was visibly upset and complained vehemently about his weight loss, being unable to eat, and proclaimed his disdain for liquid supplements. He told me, "I want real food to eat!" He appeared despondent, and although he denied any suicidal intent, he said that he felt that the last 2 years of clinic visits had been useless. "You told me that I would live 7 years!" I felt anxious and concerned. I suggested that his inability to eat was an emotional reaction and that he needed to take the supplements, tasteless or not. Lee became enraged: "I can see that you don't understand at all!" As he stormed out of my examination room, I invited him back anytime and hoped that our relationship could continue but feared it would not.

Afterward, I wrote a letter to Lee, sending him some housing information he wanted and telling him that I was thinking about him and hoped to hear from him soon. Then, on July 22, I got the phone call from Marge about Lee's death. I felt confused and anxious. I spoke to Lee's sister, Linda, who said that after the family did not hear from him for a while, they called the building manager. The manager had found Lee on his apartment floor on July 12, dead, with his face covered with dried blood. According to the coroner's office, he had been dead since July 9. Linda spoke of the funeral and said, "Lee would have liked it." Linda was crying, and I kept repeating, "I'm sorry, I'm sorry."

My first reactions to Lee's death was shock and disbelief. My thoughts seesawed from thinking that there had been a mistake and Lee wasn't dead, to sadness over having missed the funeral. Why hadn't Lee told me

about the biopsy results sooner? He had come in so often with little problems, but it seemed that when he had a serious problem, he stayed away. Perhaps he thought that I was incapable of helping him in certain situations. I wondered whether he had suffered great pain and how he had felt—and had he killed himself? Awful images passed through my mind of Lee lying on the floor, alone, hemorrhaging. Then someone said that I had four patients waiting. Numbly, I walked to the clinic waiting area to call the first patient of the day.

Later, I received a letter from Dana, another of Lee's sisters. She had found the letter that I wrote to Lee and wanted to know more about his illness. One evening, as the sun set, I called her from my office. Why, why, Dana begged me, why had Lee not told her of his lymphoma? Why did he shut her out of his life, always treating her as the inadequate little sister? "Why," she asked, "am I so angry with him?" Because I thought that more facts might help her, I encouraged Dana to obtain the autopsy report and to let me know of the results. More facts might help me, too.

So far, I have heard nothing and I don't want to bother the family. Most days, especially on Fridays, I expect to see Lee coming around the corner, a big gym bag slung over his shoulder. "Ms. Wolen, I'd like to have a word with you, please!" Sometimes I nearly look for him. I feel very lonely and empty without Lee. I have lost a person who was important to me, for whom I cared.

Bowlby (1980) described four stages of bereavement: numbing, yearning and searching, disorganization and despair, and finally reorganization. The initial stage of numbing often results in a stunned state, where the individual goes on with life robotically and may experience panic attacks. Yearning and searching, which can last for several years, is characterized by dissonant feelings that acknowledge the loved one's death while simultaneously disbelieving it, similar to my expecting, and perhaps hoping, to see Lee every Friday. Letting go of my attachment to Lee is difficult for me, partly because it is perpetuated by my continuing to work in the clinic where Lee shared his experience with me. Disorganization and despair are necessary before old patterns of thinking about the deceased person can be discarded and the process of reorganization completed.

As I write this, I am still searching. Loss and grief are predominant characteristics of my work as a nurse practitioner caring for people living with HIV disease. After 18 years of nursing, maintaining professional boundaries is second nature to me, and yet I still become attached to my patients. I miss Lee and all my other patients who have died.

"Intimate attachments to other human beings are the hub around which a person's life revolves, not only when he is an infant or toddler or a schoolchild but throughout his adolescence and his years of maturity as well, and on into old age. From these intimate attachments, a person draws his strength and enjoyment of life and, through what he contributes, he gives strength and enjoyment to others" (Bowlby, 1980, p. 442).

KATHRYN J. FOLEY, BOSTON, MASSACHUSETTS

Yesterday I spent the afternoon digging a yew bush out of my front yard. It was a fairly small bush, only about 3 feet tall, but it took me 2 hours to dig it up because the roots were buried deep into the ground. Even more remarkably, they spread out in a complex and intricate web that varied from thick roots 1 inch in diameter to lacy, delicate rootlets. As I struggled to pull the bush out of the ground, it almost seemd as though it did not want to come out.

At the time I was removing the bush, a patient of mine was being buried about 12 miles away. He was a 41-year-old Haitian immigrant who had battled AIDS for at least 10 years. Last summer, he was critically ill with pneumonia and we were sure that he would die. Instead, he got better and went back to work. Last week he dropped dead at home for no apparent reason. For him, it was probably a quick and painless death, but for those of us left behind, it was extremely difficult. He and many of my patients are like that common yew bush. They are often unnoticed and, when faced with death, cling tenaciously to the earth.

I have been a public health nurse since 1985 and worked previously as a staff nurse and a nurse practitioner in women's health. I became interested in public health nursing because I wanted to work with patients who had significant health problems and limited access to health care. I was also attracted to the opportunity to work independently, and to be "out there," seeing patients in their own homes and building relationships with them in their own communities.

My first position was as a nurse epidemiologist for a city- and state-supported sexually transmitted disease clinic in Boston. It was 1985, when awareness of AIDS was increasing among the public and health care professionals, and I began attending seminars. At the same time, I became involved in a nurse-run AIDS committee that eventually became an official committee of the Massachusetts State Nurses' Association.

After 3 years, budget cuts eliminated my position, and I went to work for the state department of public health as coordinator of partner notification for the AIDS program. Although I enjoyed the work and was able to contribute to policy-making decisions, I missed direct patient contact. I eventually took a position with the city health department in tuberculosis (TB) control, where I currently work. This position offers me independent practice and direct patient contact, primarily with people living with the dual diagnosis of HIV and TB. My nursing goal is to motivate patients to continue their TB medications to treat the disease and prevent its spread. This is simply stated but has become an incredibly challenging and life-changing job for me.

Given the demographics of people with TB and HIV, most of my patients are poor and are from racial and ethnic minority groups. Although some of my patients are homeless, mentally ill, or both, most are disenfranchised. The two most common HIV risk exposures of my patients are injecting drug use and birth in a country where heterosexual transmission predominates. In my caseload, the country of origin for many of my patients is Haiti.

When a case of TB in an HIV-infected

patient is reported to the health department, that patient is assigned to me. My relationships with my patients are usually long term, lasting for at least 1 year. Some patients receive the news that their HIV test result is positive at the same time they learn that they have TB. Consequently, taking care of their TB is often low on their priority list. They may not be used to taking care of their health at all. They are busy worrying about where they are going to live, whether they are going to eat, when they are going to die, and who (if anyone) they are going to tell about being infected with HIV.

It now becomes necessary for the patients to take TB medicine. It is difficult for anyone, including health care providers, to take ampicillin for a week, for example; taking the complicated and sometimes unpleasant drugs for TB is extremely difficult. My strategy for helping patients follow this regimen rests on the building of a trusting and caring nurse-patient relationship. I act as an advocate and a link to a confusing, intimidating health care system for patients previously unable or unwilling to negotiate this system for themselves. I cannot facilitate treatment of their TB disease without helping them address their need for HIV care as well. Because some patients will not obtain any primary care for their HIV illness, out of either fear or denial, I often become the only health care provider working with them. I have no medical backup for HIV related problems, so I must be alert to symptoms that could signal the advancement of HIV disease and then try to convince the patients to seek care. It is scary for me at times. For these patients with HIV and TB, their only link to health care is through the TB program.

Our TB program has many ways to encourage and support compliance with the plan of care. I am convinced that the key to success in this program is the case management system, in which each patient is assigned to a public health nurse–case manager who has special expertise in dealing with the subgroup to which the patient belongs. For many of my patients, having their own public health nurse is the first attempt of the "health care system" to provide care for them.

A major function of my job is to make home visits throughout the course of treatment. A home visit is a very powerful statement to a patient and is an enhancing strategy in building our relationship. Besides giving me the opportunity to assess living conditions, food availability, support systems, family constellations, and so forth, the home visit tells patients that I care about them and that their TB disease is serious. The importance of building nurse-patient rapport and gaining the patient's trust cannot be overestimated in enhancing the patient's ability and motivation to take the prescribed TB medicine. Feeling that someone cares, and believes that she or he is worth an investment of time and effort, can motivate a person to care about himself or herself. The emphasis that I place on relationship building has had a very profound effect on me as well.

I frequently find myself in the position of being a witness to intense and courageous struggle in the face of much adversity. For example, the Haitian patient to whom I referred earlier had great hopes of having his two daughters come to the United States to live with him. He lived alone and had saved most of his meager earnings for many years. He had just purchased a house when active TB was diagnosed. From that time on, he had various health problems that affected his ability to work. Foreclosure on his mortgage was always imminent. He continued to work as much as possible, and he never stopped planning for his daughters' eventual immigration. Despite his many physical discomforts, he never complained. At one clinic visit he arrived febrile and short of breath but in a perfectly ironed shirt. His pride, dignity, stoicism, and perserverance throughout years of suffering were an inspiration to me.

Other Haitian patients have experienced heartless discrimination from landlords because of both TB and HIV disease. One of my patients came home from the hospital to find his belongings on the sidewalk. He remained homeless for weeks afterward. He stayed on his TB medication by coming to the clinic each day to pick them up. When he moved into housing that had recently been renovated for AIDS patients, it was like a miracle.

Some Haitian patients, out of shame or fear, tell no one else in their lives about their HIV status. I am often the only other person who knows. There is great isolation and sadness in these situations. In Creole, there is a saying: *"Derrier mon, kay mon."* Literally it means, "After the mountain, there is the mountain." This saying speaks to the Haitian sense of history and struggle. I have seen it reflected in my Haitian patients' personal lives and have tried to apply it to my own life.

In addition to HIV and TB, many of my patients suffer from the complications of substance abuse. I have taken care of patients in all phases of addictive disease and have witnessed the incredible struggle of their daily lives as well. Many of these patients have difficulty in following treatment plans.

One of the responsibilities of my role is to process papers for an involuntary admission to the locked TB treatment unit (TTU). In my state, as in most, there are public health laws that allow hospitalization against the patient's will if he or she is "unable or unwilling" to comply with TB treatment. The patient is admitted to the TTU, which is located in one of our state hospitals. This decision is made by the public health nurse and involves many ethical and emotional issues for both the nurse and the patient.

A young Hispanic woman in my caseload received a diagnosis of TB after she already knew that she had HIV infection. She had not been involved in any health care until TB was diagnosed after an admission to the hospital. When we met, she was very candid about her lifestyle of drug use and prostitution on the street. Together we worked out several strategies to help her achieve compliance with her TB treatment. Because of her ongoing drug use and her inability to follow through with any of these plans, I had to use the law to hospitalize her to protect her health and the health of those around her. Her activities continued to expose other people to HIV or TB or both. Nevertheless, taking away someone's civil liberties is a serious responsibility. I never undertake this lightly or without consultation with other public health nurses, the program manager, and two physicians.

When I first visited my patient after she had been admitted to the TTU, I was greeted with extreme hostility and verbal abuse, including profane descriptions of me and my character and threats to my physical safety. I felt terrible, and yet my role as public health nurse mandated that I maintain a relationship with her. I continued to visit her regularly on my weekly rounds to the unit, but she refused to talk to me. As she was being detoxified, eating three meals a day, and receiving excellent medical care for both her HIV disease and her TB, she started to gain weight and feel better. Finally she began to talk to me again. We formulated a new plan, which included a signed contract between us, for directly observed therapy in the TB clinic.

Soon after the young woman was discharged from the TTU, she was found to have Stevens-Johnson syndrome, a potentially fatal allergic, dermatologic, and systemic reaction to antibiotics. She was in the medical intensive care unit for many days and in the hospital for many additional weeks. I visited her regularly. When she was discharged, she stopped taking her TB medication again. After a couple of months on the street, she was arrested and ordered by the court to undergo inpatient drug treatment. She was very debilitated, so I intervened and had her admitted to the TTU again, where she could be detoxified, attend Narcotic Anonymous (NA) meetings, and receive medical care for both her TB and her HIV infection. She remained there for a month and was discharged after we devised yet another follow-up plan.

Currently this patient is stable and in recovery, living with her mother, and attending NA meetings regularly. She comes into the TB clinic for directly observed therapy. She often tells me that getting TB was the best thing that ever happened to her, and that I saved her life. She feels a real sense of accomplishment, and I share in that feeling. She is living with HIV, TB, and drug addiction. She survived a life-threatening illness and has continued to make plans for her future.

Working with patients who are chemically addicted is challenging, frustrating, and deeply rewarding at the same time. One patient, for example, has engendered in me love, anger, fear, frustration, and pride. I have witnessed strength, despair, and the incredible tenacity of the human will to live despite incredible odds.

These experiences with patients have greatly affected me. I remember learning in nursing school that professionals do not become "emotionally involved" with patients. I know that that piece of professional myth has no merit. It is impossible not to become emotionally involved, and we would not be human if we did not. In my position, I spend a lot of time with patients in their own environment and get to know their families. I see them through many kinds of crises, while constantly trying to keep my focus on persuading them to complete a full course of TB treatment. When a patient dies, I feel a sense of personal loss. When a patient completes a course of TB treatment, I share her sense of accomplishment. For some patients, the TB treatment is one of the few things they have ever completed. After I have worked with individuals for a year or longer, it is a great feeling to see them reach this milestone.

Working with people with TB and HIV disease has caused me to explore my own feelings about life and death. I have reevaluated what in life is most important to me, I take life much less for granted, and I am grateful for what I have that I value. I also have seen death and therefore have found an appreciation for my own mortality. I have learned how to take care of myself and my own relationships so that I have the stength to do this work. It has also confirmed my belief that people have a lot more in common than separating them, regardless of ethnic and cultural backgrounds, economic status, or personal lifestyle.

The rewards of this job have far outweighed the drawbacks. The feelings of shared accomplishment and the privilege of getting to know patients so well helps me deal with the frustration and loss. Like most nurses who work with AIDS patients, I find that no day is like any other, and I am continually challenged both personally and professionally. The skills that I have acquired in working closely with my patients will be with me throughout my nursing career. The memories that I have of them and what I have witnessed have become a part of the web of my own root system, which holds me to the earth like the yew bush.

MAUREEN CONNOLLY, STATEN ISLAND, NEW YORK

Most of my time at work now involves the administration of programs that provide services or advocacy for people with HIV disease. Although I don't recall ever making a deliberate choice to work in AIDS care, I believe that the spread of this epidemic has forced all health care providers in New York City to deal with it in some way. I cannot think of any type of health care worker in New York City who is not involved with people who are living with this disease. It is too pervasive and too widespread here for any nurse not to have heard of, known of, cared for, or loved an HIV-affected person. Some health care professionals have risen to the occasion, and others have left the field. Regardless of who stays and who leaves, the epidemic remains and is not going away. After reviewing the ever-increasing statistics, a colleague sarcastically stated to me that we are all assured of jobs into the twenty-first century, caring for people living with HIV disease. Unfortunately, his words are true.

From 1979 to 1986, I worked in a New York City emergency department. During the early 1980s, young men with multiple gastrointestinal complaints such as vomiting, diarrhea, food intolerance, weight loss, and severe wasting would come into the emergency department. The staff would evaluate and admit them to the hospital, and we would soon forget them and move on to the next case. However, one day a young man arrived who was severely jaundiced, hypotensive, and actively bleeding. He was accompanied by another young man whom I would later learn was his lover. My recollections of this case are twofold: first, I remember my total bewilderment over what could possibly have caused such illness in a young man in a short time; second, I remember the fright and horror on the faces of these young men as we made a futile effort to save the patient's life. Later I spoke with the physician about possible causes, but he had no answers. Today I know that this experience was most likely my first one of caring for someone dying of complications of HIV infection.

As the years passed, the knowledge grew that something bad was happening and people were dying. Transmission of an organism through blood was discussed, and universal precautions were developed, together with an overwhelming fear of the unknown. In providing care during this time, we not only treated people with this disease but unfortunately we unknowingly transmitted it through contaminated blood products. I believe that my highest risk of acquiring and transmitting this virus occurred during this time. A large number of patients with hemophilia utilized our emergency department to receive factor-replacement blood products. I shudder to think how casually we treated this procedure and how we exposed ourselves directly to the factor when it dripped on our hands during reconstitution. Then we administered this product, ultimately providing a mechanism of transmission. We never considered that our practices could be unsafe, nor did the individual who practiced unprotected sex or who shared needles. Today we all must live with the consequences of our actions, both the known and the unknown.

By 1987, I had become exhausted with emergency nursing and took a staff nurse position in an infusion program in a certified home health agency in Staten Island, New York. I enjoyed the autonomy and the ability to provide direct service in the community setting. For the first time in my career, I felt that the patients and their families understood the role of nursing.

From 1987 to 1989, my role progressed from staff nurse to program director. My promotions were a demonstration of leadership abilities, available resources, and good luck. It is through my home care experience that I have learned about caring for people with AIDS. However, it is not only the disease, but the consequences of this disease for individuals and their caregivers, that present nurses with the greatest challenge and the deepest despair.

Our numbers of AIDS patients have grown, and the demographics of patients admitted with a diagnosis of AIDS in our agency have followed national trends. Our client populations have changed from gay men to injection drug users and the significant others of these individuals. There has been an increase in women, many with small children in single-parent households with little outside support. We have provided services for patients from the ages of 7 months to 75 years, and including all races, ethnicities, and socio-economic levels and involving all communities on Staten Island.

By 1993, Staten Island had a case rate for AIDS of 333 cases per 100,000 adults (Staten Island AIDS Task Force, 1993). This rate is lower than that of the other boroughs but significantly higher than rates in many other cities in the United States. Staten Island is the smallest of the five boroughs that make up the City of New York, with a population of close to 300,000 people. It is separated from the rest of the city by busy harbors. People commute to the other boroughs on ferries and over bridges. People live in Staten Island because of its rural nature and because of their perception of safety and separateness from the rest of the city. This sense of protection and isolation is the way that many communities in Staten Island feel about AIDS and has impeded awareness and sensitivity toward this issue.

During the years of providing home care services for people living with AIDS and their families, I have seen the extraordinary strength and fortitude of patients and their caregivers. Many are faced with overwhelming crises. Both the patients and the families are forced to deal with premature death, multiple losses, lifestyle changes, estranged family relationships, lack of support, isolation, fear of disclosure, and the need to provide direct care to the infected person (Brown & Powell-Cope, 1993).

I have seen two common scenarios in working with patients and their caregivers. In the first scenario, the infected person has been either physically or emotionally estranged from their family, often because of lifestyle choices outside the family norm. The infected individual returns to the family home when he or she is no longer able to live alone. In the second scenario, individuals have found themselves infected years after they have stopped the high-risk behavior. Many have moved on to develop careers and families. This diagnosis forces them and their loved ones to face their mortality and forever changes the course of their lives.

Brown and Powell-Cope (1991) interviewed individuals and their families who were coping with this diagnosis and developed their theory of AIDS family caregiving. They identified the basic social-psychologic problem as uncertainty. The transition through this uncertainty is divided into subcategories of managing and being managed by the disease, living with loss and dying, renegotiating relationships, going public, and containing the spread of HIV. The individual and the family or other caregiver's response will be guided by personal beliefs, cultural and religious beliefs, and the nature of the family's organization and adaptation skills (Walker, 1991).

The home care staff is challenged with helping patients and families deal not only with the uncertainty of the disease process but also with other problems in an attempt to help resolve these conflicts and come to closure. Home care nurses play a vital role in this process.

Home care nurses coordinate services; develop interdisciplinary teams of nurses, social workers, nutritionists, psychologic and bereavement counselors, physicians, and other supportive services as indicated; promote communication among these teams; and act as the advocate for the patient and the caregiver. The epidemic of AIDS has called out for the art of caring, which is the underlying basis of nursing.

When staff members are overwhelmed with the continued loss of patients, we stress the important role that the staff members have played in providing support to the patients and their families and the benefit in making those last days bearable. The staff members gather support from each other, using humor and recognizing the value of tears and their positive influence on the patients' last days, in addition to witnessing supreme acts of strength, grace, forgiveness, and un-

conditional love. I believe that we stay in this field of practice for those reasons.

I have been tremendously saddened by the isolation in which people with HIV disease and their families live their lives. They hide their diagnosis, seek treatment in other boroughs, and avoid seeking needed services for fear of disclosure and possible incrimination. Unfortunately, these fears are not unfounded—13 years into this epidemic, the consequences of disclosure are still a major problem. We have seen patients lose their housing when their diagnosis is discovered, pharmacies refuse to fill prescriptions, and medical staffs of institutions gossiping over patients' diagnosis.

This sense of isolation was demonstrated very clearly to me recently. One of the patients in our program of long-term therapy had another family member who had been ill for a number of years. That individual received his care in another borough and his intravenous therapy from another company. As I continued to visit this home, I could see that this individual was failing and that the family had limited support from the other infusion company. When I offered the services of our agency, I was given an excuse regarding their reason for remaining with the other company. Although I accepted the response, I recognized that the individual's needs were not being met. One day, I received a call from the case manager of the insurance company, who stated that she had the permission to relay some information to me. She said that the individual about whom I had been concerned had AIDS and the family needed additional services. She said that the family could not reveal this diagnosis to anyone. Services were provided, and the individual died a short time later. Many members of this individual's family did not know his cause of death.

I was extremely angry with myself for not identifying the family's fear of the stigma associated with the diagnosis of AIDS. As a professional, I should have been able to identify what was going on in this home and to give the family an opportunity to communicate their needs. Despite the trust and familiarity I had with this family, the family members could not share this information until the very end. The fear of disclosure had placed an additional stress on them and deprived them of services that could have been of benefit.

This incident impressed on me how nursing research could assist nursing practice in this area. Was the need of this family to remain in complete isolation more important than their need to seek services? Would the disclosure of the illness better affect the grieving process? Is the grieving process prolonged when people keep the disease a secret? Are the possible recriminations after disclosure as severe as people perceive them to be?

I still interact with this family, and on the surface, all appears well. However, no one discusses the deceased. Even though the family members have moved on, I am unsure at what cost.

During the past 2 years, there has been an improvement in the sensitivity of people living with AIDS and their families in this community. The increase in numbers has forced awareness of the disease into communities perceived to be immune. Providers of services to people living with AIDS have participated in committees that have focused on education, advocacy, case management, and policy development. Finally, individuals living with AIDS have begun to go public. They have joined organizations that offer support and have integrated into the provider meetings. Some speak publicly of how they contracted their disease and how they live and deal with it. They speak eloquently of the struggle that they have endured and how they wish to help improve awareness of and sensitivity toward this disease. They have offered support and guidance to people in similar situations. This has done a great deal to alleviate the public's fear of the unknown and has brought a human face and personal experience to this disease.

I have found great satisfaction in this work. I have been extremeley proud of my staff members as they have immersed themselves in the problems related to this disease in an effort to improve situations for patients and their families. The patients and their caregivers have been appreciative of the work that has been done for them. Although we cannot create miracles or provide cures, we can provide a support system of caring, understanding, and empathy.

Dane and Miller (1992) stated that "AIDS is a harsh teacher imposing on us a painful tutorial in grief and mourning that has returned death to the vocabulary of everyday life. An abiding legacy of the AIDS epidemic will be the effects on the survivors" (p. 5). The support and help that we offer to the families, the caregivers, and each other will determine whether any of us will survive this epidemic.

SUMMARY

It is interesting to note that none of the nurses contributing to this chapter collaborated with each other while writing about their experiences. In fact, to our knowledge [the editors], none of the authors know each other. However, certain common themes have appeared, including issues related to the degree of emotional involvement that develops between nurses and their patients, setting boundaries, learning to take better care of ourselves, suffering loss, and grieving. Equally interesting are the coping strategies that they have learned because of their experiences, and the fact that they truly enjoy the work that they do. We thank Chris, Tom, Debbie, Kathy, and Maureen for sharing their lives with us and applaud all nurses who continue to improve the lives of people living with HIV disease.

REFERENCES

Bowlby, J. (1980). *Attachment and loss* (vol. 3). New York: Basic Books.
Brown, M., Powell-Cope, G. (1991). AIDS family caregiving: Transition through uncertainty. *Nursing Research, 40,* 338–344.
Brown, M., Powell-Cope, G. (1993). Themes of loss and dying in caring for a family member with AIDS. *Research in Nursing and Health, 16,* 179–191.
Dane, B., Miller, S. (1992). *AIDS: Intervening with hidden grievers.* Westport, CT: Auburn House.
Mount, B.M. (1986). Dealing with our losses. *Journal of Clinical Oncology, 4*(7), 1127–1134.
Sherer, R. (1990). AIDS policy in the 1990s. *Journal of the American Medical Association, 263*(14), 1972–1974.

Staten Island AIDS Task Force (1993, September). *Understanding the HIV/AIDS statistics.* Staten Island, NY: The Task Force.

Ungvarski, P.J., Ballard, K.M. (1993). Nurses, consumers, activists, and the politics of AIDS. In D.J. Mason, S.W. Talbott, & J.K. Leavitt (Eds.), *Policy and politics for nurses: Action and change in the workplace, government, organizations and community* (2nd ed.) (pp. 677–697). Philadelphia: W.B. Saunders.

Walker, G. (1991). *In the midst of winter.* New York: W.W. Norton & Company.

NURSING RESOURCE

Association of Nurses in AIDS Care, 704 Stony Hill Road, Suite 106, Yardley, PA 19067; telephone: (215) 321–2371.

Quick Reference Guide for Clinicians

Number 7

Managing Early HIV Infection

Clinical Practice Guideline

Early HIV Infection

- Disclosure of HIV Status

- Evaluation and Medical Management in Adults

- Caring for Adolescents

- Evaluation and Medical Management in Infants and Children

- Case Management of Persons Living with HIV

- Algorithms

U.S. Department of Health and Human Services
Public Health Service
Agency for Health Care Policy and Research

Attention clinicians:

The *Clinical Practice Guideline* on which this *Quick Reference Guide for Clinicians* is based was developed by an interdisciplinary, private-sector panel comprising health care professionals and consumer representatives. Panel members were:

Wafaa El-Sadr, MD, MPH
   (Co-Chair)

James M. Oleske, MD, MPH
   (Co-Chair)

Bruce D. Agins, MD

Kay Bauman, MD, MPH

Carol Brosgart, MD

Gina M. Brown, MD

Jaime V. Geaga, PA-C

Deborah Greenspan, DDS

Karen Hein, MD, BMS

William L. Holzemer, RN, PhD

Rudolph E. Jackson, MD

Michael K. Lindsay, MD, MPH

Harvey J. Makadon, MD

Martha W. Moon, MSN

Claire A. Rappoport, MS

Walter W. Shervington, MD

Lawrence C. Shulman, MSW

Constance B. Wofsy, MD, MA

For a description of the guideline development process and information about the sponsoring agency (Agency for Health Care Policy and Research), see the *Clinical Practice Guideline, Evaluation and Management of Early HIV Infection* (AHCPR Publication No. 94-0572). To receive another copy of the *Clinical Practice Guideline,* this Quick *Reference Guide* for Clinicians (AHCPR Publication No. 94-0573), or the *Consumer Guides, HIV and Your Child* (AHCPR Publication No. 94-0576) and *Understanding HIV* (AHCPR Publication No. 94-0574), call toll free: (800) 342-AIDS or write to:

AHCPR HIV Guideline
CDC National Clearinghouse
Post Office Box 6003
Rockville, MD 20849-6003.

Note: This *Quick Reference Guide for Clinicians* contains excerpts from the *Clinical Practice Guideline,* but users should not rely on these excerpts alone. Clinicians should refer to the complete *Clinical Practice Guideline* for more detailed analysis and discussion of the available research, critical evaluation of the assumptions and knowledge of the field, health care decision-making, and references.

Managing Early HIV Infection

Purpose and Scope

According to the World Health Organization, 30 to 40 million men, women, and children around the world will be infected with the human immunodeficiency virus (HIV) by the year 2000. By the turn of the century, acquired immuno-deficiency syndrome (AIDS) will be the third most common cause of death in the United States. The increasing presence of HIV in every community necessitates that primary care providers become involved in and knowledgeable about caring for patients with HIV. The growing population of individuals living with HIV and their families also need guidance in seeking and accessing appropriate care.

This *Quick Reference Guide* presents highlights from the *Clinical Practice Guideline on Evaluation and Management of Early HIV Infection.* The *Guideline* focuses on the early stages of HIV infection because early recognition of HIV is becoming more common, and medical intervention in the early stages of HIV infection may be most effective in delaying life-threatening symptoms. In addition, and perhaps most important to primary care providers, early intervention and education often increase patient involvement in treatment, improve access to services, and slow the spread of the disease.

This *Quick Reference Guide* and the *Guideline* were developed both for primary care providers and those who receive care. In the early years of the epidemic, the most severe complications of HIV infection received the most attention. The focus has since evolved to emphasize outpatient care, health maintenance, prevention of hospitalization, and integration of the patient and loved ones into a system that provides supportive services. Thus, primary care providers must be prepared to diagnose HIV infection, disclose test results, and evaluate and manage early HIV infection.

Because the subject of early HIV care is so broad and complex, the *Guideline* is limited to selected elements of adult and pediatric care that are particularly significant for practitioners: disclosure of HIV status, monitoring of CD4 lymphocyte counts; prevention of *Pneumocystis carinii* pneumonia (PCP) and tuberculosis; initiation of antiretroviral therapy; treatment of syphilis; eye and oral care; performance of Papanicolaou (Pap) smears; diagnosis of HIV infection in infants and children; monitoring of CD4 lymphocyte counts and initiation of antiretroviral therapy in infants and children; preventive therapy for PCP and assessment of neurologic problems in HIV-infected children;

pregnancy counseling; and development of a comprehensive case management system for the patient that covers both social services and health care. Algorithms, found at the back of this *Quick Reference Guide*, show the sequence of events related to evaluating and managing early HIV infections in adults, adolescents, infants, and children.

Because advances in the management of HIV infection are occurring át a rapid pace, providers should seek frequent updates.

Published data were used to the greatest extent possible to formulate the recommendations in the *Guideline*. In the *Guideline* and this *Quick Reference Guide*, each recommendation is rated and labeled according to the degree to which it is data-based:

- **Supported by evidence (SPE):** Evidence from at least one well-designed, published, randomized controlled trial in the population for which the recommendation is made; or from at least one well-designed, published population-based study.

- **Suggested by evidence (SGE):** Consistent results from other study designs or studies in populations other than that for which the recommendation is made.

- **Expert opinion (EO):** Expert clinical experience described in the literature or consensus of panel members.

Disclosing HIV Status

Initial disclosure of HIV test results to the patient sets the foundation for the patient's acceptance, knowledge base, and attitudes about his or her condition. This in turn may dramatically affect patients' quality of life and their ability to care for themselves. The manner in which the test results are communicated to the patient is, therefore, extremely important.

Provider Disclosure to Patient, Parent, or Guardian

- Before disclosing the results of HIV testing to a patient or the parent or guardian of a child who has been tested, assess the degree to which that person is prepared to receive the results. Consider the person's social, demographic, cultural, and psychological characteristics, which may be important factors in his or her ability to cope with the test results. (SGE)

- Disclosure and accompanying counseling should take place face-to-face. Discuss the natural history of HIV infection, the potential effects of HIV infection on physical and mental health, prevention of further HIV transmission, the role of health maintenance, and the availability of treatments. For adolescents, encourage the presence of a supportive adult. (SGE)

- Disclosure counseling provides an opportunity both to provide immediate interventions and to involve the patient in medical, mental health, social, and family-support networks. Immediate interventions should include assessing the patient for the potential for violence to himself/ herself or others; ensuring that the patient receives a thorough evaluation, staging, and initial care; informing the patient of available services; scheduling the next appointment; addressing prevention of further HIV transmission; assessing the availability of a key support person (e.g., lover, partner, significant other, roommate, child, friend, parents, spouse, spiritual support person) and other care providers; and providing information on local and national sources of support. (EO)

■ The provider should make referrals for any needed services that cannot be obtained on site. (EO)

Provider Disclosure to Agencies

■ Providers should know their State's HIV reporting requirements and educate patients about them (see page 4 for a State-by-State listing of HIV reporting requirements). (EO)

■ Providers should ensure that patients are aware of the extent and limits of confidentiality of HIV test results. (EO)

Patient Disclosure to Other Individuals and Agencies

Primary care providers should help their patients appreciate why disclosure of their HIV infection may be useful in some situations and detrimental in others. In some States, disclosure of HIV infection enables a patient to become eligible for entitlement benefits.

Disclosure to significant others may result in increased social support; it may also prompt a significant other to consider whether to seek HIV testing. Conversely, disclosure may result in housing discrimination, loss of employment or of child custody, reduction or cessation of health benefits, or rejection by a potential employer or a significant other.

■ Through counseling and referrals as needed, the provider should explain and help the patient to understand the advantages and disadvantages of disclosing HIV status to others, including the potential for discrimination against persons with HIV infection. (EO)

■ The patient should be strongly encouraged to disclose his or her HIV status to significant others, particularly sexual and needle-sharing partners. At the same time, providers must be aware of the potential for domestic violence when one or both partners has HIV infection. (SGE)

Parent or Guardian Disclosure to Infected Children and Other Family Members

■ The provider should assist parents and guardians in making decisions regarding disclosure of HIV infection to an infected child or adolescent and other family members. This assistance should consist of educating parents and guardians, and working with them to ensure that needed support services are in place during the process of disclosure. (EO)

Reporting requirements for human immunodeficiency virus (HIV) infection

By name	Anonymous	Not Required
Alabama	Georgia	Alaska
Arizona	Iowa	California
Arkansas	Kansas	Connecticut
Colorado	Kentucky	Delaware
Idaho	Maine	Florida
Illinois	Montana	Hawaii
Indiana	New Hampshire	Louisiana
Michigan	Oregon	Maryland[2]
Minnesota	Rhode Island	Massachusetts
Mississippi	Texas	Nebraska
Missouri		New Mexico
Nevada		New York
New Jersey[1]		Pennsylvania
North Carolina		Vermont
North Dakota		Washington[2]
Ohio		District of Columbia
Oklahoma		
South Carolina		
South Dakota		
Tennessee[1]		
Utah		
Virginia		
West Virginia		
Wisconsin		
Wyoming		

[1] Implementation date, January, 1992.

[2] Requires reports of symptomatic HIV infection by name.

Note: Current as of March 1, 1993. All States require reporting of acquired immunodeficiency syndrome (AIDS) cases by name at the State/local level.

Evaluation and Management of HIV-Infected Adults

Early identification of HIV infection allows the provider to conduct a thorough medical and psychological assessment to define the immediate and long-term needs of the patient. A detailed medical history is a crucial first step in treatment and should include a review of the HIV test result, previous infections, and sexual and substance use history.

A comprehensive physical examination, including assessments of eye and oral health, neurologic status, skin and lymph nodes, and HIV-associated signs and symptoms, accompanied by open discussion of the patient's concerns and fears, allows the provider to define the stage of HIV infection, determine the best treatment, and lay the foundation for an effective partnership with the patient.

Algorithm 1 presents an overview of the selected elements of early HIV care covered in the Guideline and this Quick Reference Guide. Tables 1, 2, and 3 (see pages 21-24) list the drugs discussed here and in the Guideline, as well as dosages and adverse effects.

Monitoring CD4 Lymphocytes and Initiating Antiretroviral Therapy and PCP Prophylaxis

The assessment of immune status is a key element of the patient's initial evaluation. Measuring the number of CD4 lymphocytes is the primary test for monitoring immune function. It establishes the stage of HIV infection, the prognosis of disease, and helps to determine the appropriateness of initiating antiretroviral therapy [1] and prophylaxis for PCP and other opportunistic infections.

Steps for carrying out this evaluation are presented in Algorithm 2. CD4 testing and specific treatments for pregnant women are shown in Algorithm 3. Other recommendations are listed here:

■ The immune status of an HIV-infected individual should be assessed at the time of his or her initial medical evaluation. A CD4 lymphocyte count should be the primary test for monitoring immune function. (EO)

■ The number of CD4 cells should be measured once every 6 months when the CD4 count is greater than 600 cells/µl and at least every 3 months when the CD4 count is between 200 cells/µl and 600 cells/µl. More frequent measurements may be desirable if there is evidence of rapid decline in cell count of if the patient's symptoms become more severe. (EO)

■ Ongoing measurement of CD4 cells below 200 cells/µl at least every 3 months may be necessary to track the effects of antiretroviral therapy and to

---

[1] Information included in this guide may not represent FDA approval or approved labeling for the particular products or indications in question. Specifically, the terms "safe" and "effective" may be not synonymous with the FDA-defined legal standards for product approval.

determine the appropriate time for initiation of new preventive and therapeutic interventions. (EO)

■ Antiretroviral therapy with zidovudine (the major antiretroviral therapy, formerly known as AZT, now ZDV) should be discussed with all HIV-infected individuals whose CD4 counts are less than 500 cells/μl. (SGE)

■ Those patients who do not tolerate ZDV or have clinical progression of HIV infection on this treatment, should be offered therapy with didanosine (ddI) or dideoxycitidine (ddC). (SPE)

■ Those patients who are tolerating ZDV may remain on ZDV; consider switching to ddI after a period of time, as some evidence suggests a benefit from this change. (EO)

■ PCP prophylaxis should be initiated if any of the following conditions is met: (1) the CD4 count is less than 200 cells/μl (SPE); (2) there has been a prior episode of PCP (SPE); or, (3) oral candidiasis or constitutional symptoms such as unexplained fevers are present (SGE).

■ Oral trimethoprim-sulfamethoxazole (TMP-SMX) is the preferred agent for PCP prophylaxis. (SPE)

■ Other effective prophylactic agents include aerosolized pentamidine, oral dapsone, and a combination of oral dapsone and pyrimethamine. Consider their advantages and disadvantages in determining whether to use them. (SPE)

■ In HIV-infected pregnant women, CD4 counts should be determined at the time of presentation for prenatal care. CD4 counts should be determined at delivery for those women who have received no prenatal care. (EO)

■ If the count is 600 cells/μl or above, it need not be repeated during pregnancy, unless indicated by clinical symptoms. If the count is 200 cells/μl or less, it need not be repeated during pregnancy, according to current data. If the count is between 200 cells/μl and 600 cells/μl, it should be repeated each trimester. (SGE)

■ Discuss antiretroviral therapy with ZDV with HIV-infected pregnant women whose CD4 lymphocyte counts are less than 500 cells/μl. (SGE)

■ Providers should inform HIV-infected pregnant women of the benefits of early ZDV therapy and the potential for risks to the mother and fetus. (SGE)

■ HIV-infected pregnant women should receive PCP prophylaxis according to the same guidelines used for other adults. (SGE)

Testing and Preventive Therapy for Tuberculosis Infection

The reemergence of tuberculosis (TB) as a major public health concern is especially important for HIV-infected individuals because the immunosuppression caused by the virus permits *Mycobacterium tuberculosis* infection to progress at an accelerated pace, and they are more likely to develop active TB. TB merits special consideration in the treatment of HIV-infected patients because it is readily communicable to others, management is different for HIV-infected patients than for non-HIV-infected patients, and, unlike many other opportunistic infections, it is preventable and may be curable if treated promptly.

Screening

■ The medical history for all HIV-infected individuals should include the following steps (see Algorithm 4): (a) assessment of previous TB infection or disease, past treatment or preventive therapy, and history of exposure to *M. tuberculosis;* (b) assessment of the risk for *M. tuberculosis* infection, including predisposing social conditions (e.g., household contacts, country of origin, homelessness, history of incarceration, residence in a congregate living situation); and (c) suggestive symptoms (e.g., cough, hemoptysis, fever, night sweats, weight loss). During the physical examination, the provider should seek indications of active disease (e.g., abnormal pulmonary signs, documented weight loss). (SGE)

■ The medical history for all HIV-infected individuals should also include an assessment of health and social conditions that may affect an individual's ability to complete a course of therapy, specifically, repeated failure to keep medical appointments, alcoholism, mental illness, and substance use. (SGE)

■ All HIV-infected individuals, including those who have received BCG vaccination, should be screened, using purified protein derivative (PPD) for infection with *M. tuberculosis* during their initial evaluation. (SGE)

■ All HIV-infected individuals should be screened for anergy using two control antigens in addition to PPD during their initial evaluation. (SGE)

■ All HIV-infected individuals who are PPD-positive or anergic should receive a chest x-ray and clinical evaluation, and those who have symptoms suggestive of TB should receive a chest x-ray, regardless of their PPD or anergy status. (SGE)

■ PPD and anergy testing should be repeated annually in persons who are neither PPD-positive nor anergic on initial evaluation. Persons who reside in areas where TB prevalence is high should be tested every 6 months. (SGE)

■ All PPD-negative or anergic HIV-infected individuals who have recently been exposed to persons with suspected or confirmed TB should be immediately tested with PPD and anergy antigens. Repeat testing should be performed in 3 months. (SGE)

■ PPD testing should be performed by the Mantoux method, using an intradermal injection of 0.1 ml 5 TU PPD (intermediate strength). (SGE)

■ Reactions should be assessed by a trained observer between 48 and 72 hours after injection. Reactions of 5 mm or greater induration should be considered positive in persons with HIV infection, regardless of prior BCG vaccination. (SGE)

■ Two of the following three antigens can be used for anergy testing: candida, mumps, or tetanus toxoid. Any degree of induration observed in response to intradermal injection of these antigens constitutes a positive reaction and indicates that the individual is not anergic. (SGE)

■ Chest x-rays should be obtained to exclude the presence of active pulmonary TB in all HIV-infected individuals who are PPD-positive, anergic, or have symptoms suggestive of TB. (SGE)

■ If the chest x-ray reveals any abnormality, multiple sputum smears and cultures should be performed. (SGE)

■ If a sputum smear is positive, the patient should be started on anti-TB therapy immediately, pending culture results. Acid-fast bacillus (AFB) isolation should be initiated promptly if the patient is coughing. If the sputum smears are negative and if there is no other etiology for the abnormal chest x-ray, bronchoscopy should be performed and empiric anti-TB therapy should be initiated, pending the results of the mycobacterial culture. AFB isolation should be maintained until the diagnosis is confirmed by smear or culture. (SGE)

■ In many of these clinical situations, diagnostic evaluation and management will need to be individualized. Consultation with an infectious disease or pulmonary specialist may be necessary. (SGE)

Preventive Therapy

■ Preventive therapy for TB should proceed according to the following protocol: (1) isoniazid (INH) preventive therapy should be initiated and continued for 12 months in all HIV-infected individuals who have a positive PPD test but do not have active disease, regardless of their age; (2) preventive therapy should be strongly considered for anergic patients who are known contacts of patients with TB and for anergic patients belonging to groups in which the prevalence of TB infection is 10 percent or higher. Such individuals include injection drug users, prisoners, homeless persons, persons living in congregate housing, migrant laborers, and persons born in countries where rates of TB are high. (SGE)

■ Clinicians should consider factors specific to their geographic areas, including the incidence and prevalence of TB infection, when considering the decision to start preventive therapy. (SGE)

■ In persons with HIV who are exposed to drug-resistant strains of *M. tuberculosis,* an alternative preventive therapy should be considered. Consultation should be sought with a pulmonary or infectious disease specialist. (SGE)

■ The presence of AFB on sputum smear should prompt immediate empiric anti-TB therapy tailored to community drug-susceptibility patterns, pending final determination of drug susceptibility testing. (SGE)

Pregnant Women

■ The evaluation and management of *M. tuberculosis* infection in pregnant women should be performed as described in the recommendations above. Preventive INH therapy is not contraindicated in pregnant women and should be initiated according to these recommendations. (SGE)

■ In asymptomatic women, chest x-ray should be performed only after the first trimester, and a lead apron shield should be used. In women with symptoms that suggest TB, x-rays should be performed irrespective of stage of pregnancy. A lead apron shield should be used. (SGE)

Improving Adherence to Regimens of Preventive Therapy for TB

The failure of patients to complete treatment of their *M. tuberculosis* infection is a common and serious concern because these patients are at increased risk that the infection will progress to the disease, tuberculosis. Additionally, these individuals may infect others and may develop drug-resistant strains of *M. tuberculosis.* Specific recommendations include:

■ TB prophylaxis and treatment regimens should be closely monitored by health care providers to ensure completion of the entire course of therapy. (SGE)

■ Providers should educate their patients about the importance of completing the full course of anti-TB therapy, and should recommend the simplest appropriate regimen. (EO)

■ Case management and directly observed therapy should be used when needed to ensure successful completion of therapy. (EO)

Testing and Treatment for Syphilis

The incidence of HIV infection and syphilis have both increased dramatically in the last 10 years, and co-infection is not uncommon. It is crucial to know whether both are present because HIV infection may alter the natural history, laboratory diagnosis, and patient's response to syphilis therapy.

Sexually experienced adolescents have a high rate of sexually transmitted diseases (STDs). A sexual history, screening pelvic or genital examination, and laboratory assessment are indicated for all adolescents who have had sexual intercourse, including those who are asymptomatic.

Recommendations for the assessment and treatment of syphilis in HIV-infected patients are summarized in Algorithm 5. Specific recommendations include:

Screening and Diagnosis

■ All HIV-infected and sexually experienced adults and adolescents should be evaluated for syphilis. (SGE)

■ Initial serologic screening for current or past syphilis should be performed with nontreponemal tests (i.e., the rapid plasma reagin [RPR] or the Venereal Disease Laboratories [VDRL] test). (SGE)

■ All reactive nontreponemal tests should be followed by a specific treponemal test (i.e., the micro-hemagglutination assay for *Treponema pallidum* [MHA-TP] or the fluorescent treponemal antibody absorption [FTA-ABS] test). (SGE)

■ In patients with clinical findings suggestive of syphilis who have nonreactive nontreponemal tests, the serum should be diluted to overcome the possibility that the high antibody levels have produced a prozone phenomenon. (SGE)

■ In patients with primary syphilis, both nontreponemal and treponemal serologic tests may be nonreactive. If primary syphilis is suspected, dark-field microscopy and direct fluorescent antibody staining for *T. pallidum* (DFA-TP) from a scraping of suspected lesions should be performed. (SGE)

■ If a dark-field examination cannot be done and primary syphilis is suspected, empiric treatment should be instituted. (SGE)

■ Evaluation of the cerebrospinal fluid (CSF) for evidence of neurosyphilis may be prudent for all HIV-infected individuals with positive treponemal serologies. (SGE)

■ HIV-infected pregnant women should be screened for syphilis with a nontreponemal test (RPR or VDRL) at entry into prenatal care, during the third trimester, at delivery, and at any time when they have been exposed to or present with symptoms or signs of an STD. (SGE)

Management

■ CSF evaluation should be discussed with and encouraged in all HIV-infected individuals with primary syphilis. It should be recommended to all HIV-infected patients with secondary syphilis, latent syphilis, or infection of unknown duration. (EO)

■ If neurosyphilis is excluded, primary, secondary, early latent, and late latent syphilis, as well as infection of unknown duration, should be treated with three weekly doses of intramuscular benzathine penicillin, 2.4 million units. (SGE)

- HIV-infected individuals with abnormal CSF findings (presence of cells, increased protein, or positive VDRL test results) should be treated with a regimen effective against neurosyphilis: intravenous (IV) aqueous penicillin, 2 to 4 million units every 4 hours for 10 to 14 days. (SGE)

- Treatment for presumptive neurosyphilis should be encouraged when the CSF cannot be evaluated. (EO)

- Patients with syphilis and a reported reaction to penicillin should be referred to an allergist or infectious disease specialist. (EO)

- All HIV-infected individuals should have a nontreponemal serologic test for syphilis performed at least annually. In addition, serologic tests should be performed after exposure to or diagnosis of any STD. (EO)

- In HIV-infected individuals who have been diagnosed with and treated for syphilis, followup nontreponemal serologies should be performed at 1, 2, 3, 6, 9, and 12 months post-treatment and annually thereafter. The same test should be used each time, because titers are not comparable between different nontreponemal tests. (EO)

- HIV-infected individuals diagnosed with syphilis should be evaluated for other STDs and substance use and should be managed accordingly. The diagnosis of syphilis or other STDs in HIV-infected individuals should alert the provider to counsel the patient on the importance of safe-sex practices. (EO).

- Treatment and followup of syphilis are the same for pregnant women as for nonpregnant adults. To reliably prevent congenital syphilis, penicillin therapy must be completed at least 4 weeks prior to delivery. All infants born to women with syphilis should be assessed for congenital syphilis and managed as appropriate. (SPE)

Oral Examinations

HIV-infected patients experience several unique oral conditions, including frequent oral lesions and in some patients, unusually rapid and destructive periodontal disease. As a result, special attention should be paid to their routine and specialized oral care. Oral lesions, in particular, are important because they may provide the only early indication of HIV infection, and they are key in classifying the stage of HIV disease. Recommendations for oral care include the following:

- Discuss with patients the importance of oral care, including descriptions of common HIV-related oral lesions and associated symptoms.

- Perform an oral examination during every physical examination (EO); all oral mucosal surfaces should be carefully examined. (SGE)

- Recommend that patients have twice-yearly dental examinations; if oral lesions or other problems appear, dental followup should be more frequent. (SGE)

- Primary care providers and dentists should be trained to identify and treat oral lesions associated with HIV infection. (EO)

Eye Examinations

While there are a number of ocular complications associated with HIV disease, they generally occur at a late stage of the disease. Cytomegalovirus retinitis (CMV retinitis) is the most common opportunistic infection associated with visual loss in HIV infection. Providers should take the following steps regarding eye care:

- Take a careful history of any visual disturbances and perform an eye examination, including funduscopy, during the patient's routine visits. Educate the patient about CMV retinitis and visual disturbances (e.g., blurring or vision loss) and the importance of monitoring visual symptoms to maximize early identification. (EO)

- Recommend to patients that they be examined by a qualified eye doctor according to the following schedule: every 3 to 5 years at ages 20 to 39; every 2 to 4 years at ages 40 to 64; every 1 to 2 years at ages 65 and over. More frequent examinations will be necessary if problems develop. (EO)

- Refer patients with any visual symptoms suggestive of CMV to an ophthalmologist for confirmation of diagnosis. (SGE)

Pap Smears

With the increasing impact of the HIV epidemic on women, the evaluation of HIV-associated gynecologic conditions and the provision of appropriate gynecologic care for women with HIV infection have become important areas of concern for the primary care provider.

Evidence shows a higher prevalence of Pap smear, vaginal, and cervical abnormalities among HIV-infected women compared with uninfected women. In addition, cervical abnormalities are likely to be more severe and may progress more rapidly in women with HIV infection. Regular gynecologic examinations, including a Pap smear, are therefore an integral component of primary care for these patients. Recommendations on Pap smears for women with early HIV infection are outlined in Algorithm 6 and in the chart that follows.

- A Pap smear should be done as part of the initial gynecologic examination in all women with HIV infection. For pregnant women, Pap smears should be performed at entry into prenatal care. Women who have not received prenatal care should have a Pap smear before being discharged from the hospital following delivery. (SGE)

- Pap smears should be repeated twice in the first year; annually when the initial Pap smear is normal; every 6 months when there is a history of human papilloma virus (HPV) infection, previous Pap smear showing squamous intraepithelial lesion (SIL), or symptomatic HIV

Suggested classification of squamous epithelial cell cytologic changes

---

1. Atypical squamous cells of undetermined significance (specify recommended followup and/or type of further investigation).

2. Squamous intraepithelial lesions (SILs) [comment on presence or absence of cellular changes consistent with human papilloma virus (HPV) infection]:

   ◼ Low-grade SIL, encompassing:
   Cellular changes consistent with HPV infection
   Mild dysplasia/CIN 1

   ◼ High-grade SIL, encompassing:
   Moderate dysplasia/CIN 2
   Severe dysplasia/CIN 3
   Carcinoma in situ/CIN 3

3. Squamous carcinoma.

---

[1] Summarized from abstract presented at the Workshop on Terminology and Classification of Vaginal Cytology, National Cancer Institute, December 1988.

---

infection; after treatment of the underlying cause of an inflammation; or if no endocervical cells are seen. (SGE)

◼ All women, including those who are pregnant, should be referred to a trained clinician for colposcopy when: the Pap smear indicates atypical cells of undetermined significance; the Pap smear demonstrates either low- or high-grade SILs or carcinoma; there is a history of untreated SIL. (SGE)

Pregnancy Counseling

Counseling HIV-infected women with regard to reproductive issues and options should be a part of primary care practice. The counseling must focus on the health outcomes that might be expected as a result of any choice, for the mother as well as for the infant. These outcomes include the possible effects of pregnancy on the mother's health and the progression of her HIV infection; the issues pregnancy raises with regard to enrollment in clinical trials and access to new agents; the effect of HIV infection on birth outcome; the risk of HIV transmission from mother to infant; the prognosis of HIV infection in infants; and issues related to the care of children who have lost their parents.

Pregnancy counseling remains challenging because evidence shows that a woman's decision to become pregnant or to continue or terminate a pregnancy is not related in a straightforward way to the woman's HIV status and possible HIV-related outcomes. Specific recommendations include:

■ Conduct contraceptive, precon-
ceptional, and prenatal counseling for HIV-infected patients in a
nondirective manner, with the
focus on the woman. Listen more
than talk. (SGE)

■ Assess the psychological state of
the patient and provide the most
recent information in language
she will understand, on possible
effects of HIV infection and
pregnancy on each other, on her
current health status, transmission rates to the fetus and to
sexual partners, and the need for
contingency plans for future care
of children. (SGE)

■ Include maternal characteristics
such as age, attitudes and beliefs,
general health status, and pregnancy history in contraception
and pregnancy counseling for
HIV-infected patients. (SGE)

■ Inform the patient that at present
there is no direct evidence of a
deleterious effect of pregnancy
and childbirth on the course of
early HIV infection and no consistent evidence of adverse birth
outcomes in infants of women
with early HIV infection. (SGE)

■ Explain that breast-feeding is
not recommended for HIV-
infected mothers in the United
States because of the risk of
transmission. (SGE)

■ Inform pregnant patients that
the risk of perinatal HIV transmission ranges from 13 to 39
percent. (SPE)

■ During counseling, discuss the
long-term implications of pregnancy decisions on the family
and encourage the patient to
discuss these issues with significant others. (EO)

■ Respect the woman's decision
regarding conception and continuation or termination of pregnancy. (EO)

Caring for Adolescents with Early HIV Infection

HIV infection is spreading rapidly in
the adolescent population. There are
approximately 30,000 HIV-infected
adolescents in the United States
today.[2] Since 1988, AIDS has been
the sixth leading cause of death
among young persons 15 to 24 years
of age in the United States. Caring
for adolescents with early HIV infection presents a unique set of issues:
differences in the epidemiology of

HIV infection among youth; variable
laws and practices regarding consent
and confidentiality for minors under
the age of 18; special barriers to
receiving HIV care; lack of availability of age-specific clinical services;
special features of the progression of
HIV infection during adolescence;
limited standards for routine
management of HIV infected youth;
difficulties in assuring adolescents'
participation in research, including
clinical trials; and lack of dissemination of effective models for engaging
and retaining youth in HIV care and
prevention efforts.

[2] Adolescents are defined as those from 13
to 21 years of age; children are those from
2 to 12 years of age; infants are those from
birth to 2 years of age; and newborns are
those from birth to 30 days old.

To adequately care for HIV-infected youth, primary care providers must address the barriers that prevent adolescents from accessing care, including payment, consent, and confidentiality. Providers also must be able to offer the appropriate range of laboratory tests, including Pap smears and STD screening tests.

Issues related to the care of adolescents are discussed in this section. In addition, more specific recommendations for adolescent HIV care are integrated throughout this Quick Reference Guide. Recommended drugs and dosages specific to adolescents are detailed in Tables 1, 2, and 3 (pages 21-24).

Age-specific counseling at the time of HIV testing is the first step in appropriate early care for HIV-infected adolescents. For all adolescents, support at the time of test result notification in the form of a supportive adult (parent, guardian, or other) is preferable.

Clinical assessment and care are different for adolescents than for young children or adults. History-taking, physical examination, and laboratory assessment of HIV-infected adolescents should be conducted and interpreted within the context of age-specific issues. An appropriate history should include details about sexual and drug use practices, including age of initiation, same and opposite sex experiences, sexual identity, and use of condoms or other barrier methods. Psychosocial assessment should include details of living situation, peer group associations, and school and work activities, as well as an assessment of cognitive development and psychiatric history (with attention to suicidal ideation).

The physical examination and staging of HIV infection should take into account the marked changes in body size and composition and organ function that occur during puberty. When assessing development during adolescence, use of the Sexual Maturity Rating Scale of Tanner and Whitehouse[3] is a more reliable indicator of pubertal development than is chronologic age.

Progression of HIV infection in adolescents may differ from adults. For example, HIV wasting is defined by weight loss in adults, but during puberty—when height and weight should be increasing dramatically—wasting should be characterized as a failure to gain weight. Because adolescents have the highest rates of STDs of any age group, a screening pelvic or genital examination and laboratory assessment are indicated even for asymptomatic adolescents who have had sexual intercourse.

Antiretroviral treatment should begin with pediatric dose schedules for adolescents who are Tanner stage I or II; adult dose schedules should be used for adolescents who are Tanner stage IV or V. Tanner stage III youths should be monitored particularly closely, as this is the time of most rapid growth. Pubertal changes in body composition and organ function may affect drug distribution and metabolism, thereby necessitating changes in drug dose and interval of administration.

---

[3] Tanner JM. Growth at adolescence: with a general consideration of the effects of hereditary and environmental factors upon growth and maturation from birth to maturity. 2nd ed. Oxford: Blackwell Scientific Publications; 1962.

Evaluation and Management of HIV-Infected Infants and Children

Currently, there are an estimated 15,000 to 20,000 HIV-infected infants and children in the United States. Since the screening of blood products began in 1985, perinatal HIV transmission has accounted for 85 percent of all AIDS cases in children under age 13.

Primary care providers can do much to care for these patients, including identifying at-risk infants and HIV-infected children; performing routine counseling and diagnostic tests for HIV infection; monitoring clinical and immunologic status; providing general pediatric care, including immunizations; and linking families to case management and additional counseling.

Diagnosis of HIV Infection in Infants and Children

Because the interval between infection, development of AIDS, and mortality is compressed in infants and children, the need for early diagnosis of HIV infection is crucial. Diagnostic testing of infants and children of HIV-infected mothers should be incorporated into the schedule of routine pediatric care and immunizations.

Evidence of infants born to HIV-infected mothers shows that most have clinical or immunologic abnormalities by 6 months of age. The first chart on page 17 presents the tests and timetables for determining HIV status in infants. The common clinical manifestations and HIV-associated conditions in infants and children are listed in a second chart on page 17. Because of its complexity, laboratory diagnosis of HIV-infected newborns and infants and evaluation of HIV-related central nervous system (CNS) symptoms should be done in consultation with a pediatric HIV specialist. Specific recommendations include:

- All infants born to HIV-infected mothers should be monitored to determine HIV status. (SPE)

- In the HIV-exposed infant under 18 months of age, virus culture or polymerase chain reaction (PCR) are the preferred methods for diagnosis of HIV infection. If these tests are not available, P24 antigen assays should be used. (SPE)

- One or more of these HIV-specific tests should be done as soon as possible after the infant has reached 1 month of age. If negative, testing should be repeated between 3 and 6 months of age. (SPE)

- Infants with negative diagnostic tests at 6 months of age should have an HIV antibody test (enzyme-linked immunosorbent assay, ELISA) performed at 15 and 18 months of age to document HIV infection status. (SPE)

- In the child over 18 months of age, testing for antibody to HIV using the standard ELISA test with an approved confirmatory test is sufficient for diagnosis of HIV. (SPE)

Diagnosis of infection in HIV-exposed infants

Age	Test	If test is positive	If test is negative
1 month	HIV culture or PCR[1]	Repeat test to confirm diagnosis of infection	Repeat test at age 3 to 6 months
3 to 6 months	HIV culture or PCR[1]	Repeat test to confirm diagnosis of infection	Test with ELISA at age 15 months
15 months	ELISA	Repeat test at age 18 months	Repeat test at age 18 months
18 months or older	ELISA	Child is infected[2]	Child is not infected[3]

[1]If HIV culture and PCR are unavailable, p24 antigen testing may be used after 1 month of age.

[2]Serologic diagnosis of HIV infection requires two sets of confirmed HIV serologic assays (ELISA/Western blot) performed at least 1 month apart after 15 months of age.

[3]Confirmation of seronegativity requires two sets of negative ELISAs after 15 months of age in a child with normal clinical and immunoglobulin evaluation.

Note: This chart presents recommendations only for the items reviewed by the HIV panel.

HIV-associated conditions in pediatric HIV infection

Failure to thrive

Generalized lymphadenopathy

Hepatomegaly

Splenomegaly

Persistent oral candidiasis

Parotitis

Recurrent or chronic diarrhea

Encephalopathy

Lymphoid interstitial pneumonitis (LIP)

Hepatitis

Cardiomyopathy

Nephropathy

Recurrent bacterial infections

Opportunistic infections (recurrent viral infections [herpes simplex, herpes zoster], fungal, parasitic)

Malignancies (lymphoma)

Monitoring CD4 Lymphocytes and Initiating PCP Prophylaxis and Antiretroviral Therapy

HIV infection has more adverse effects on the developing immune systems of infants and children than it does on the mature immune systems of older individuals, thus the onset of clinical symptoms and the progression of disease are more rapid in this group. It is, therefore, crucial to use a marker for immune status in younger patients so that preventive therapies can be instituted while they still can be effective. Algorithm 7 summarizes pertinent recommendations, and Tables 1, 2, and 3 list the common antiretroviral, PCP, and TB drugs used for younger age groups, and their dosages and adverse effects. Specific recommendations include:

- CD4 counts and percentages should be obtained in all infants born to HIV-seropositive mothers at 1, 3, and 6 months of age, and then at 3-month intervals until the HIV status of the child is known. (EO)

- Thereafter, CD4 counts and percentages should be monitored at 3- to 6-month intervals in children proven to be HIV-infected. (EO)

- PCP prophylaxis should be initiated if the CD4 cell count falls below age-adjusted normal values, if the percentage of CD4 cells is 20 percent or lower, or after the patient has had an episode of PCP, regardless of CD4 count. (SGE)

- Emerging data suggest that PCP prophylaxis should be initiated in at-risk and infected infants 1 month to 1 year of age, regardless of CD4 count or percentage. The drug of choice for prophylaxis is trimethoprim-sulfamethoxazole, or TMP-SMX. (SGE)

- Antiretroviral therapy should be initiated for (a) all infants and children with symptomatic HIV infection (SGE); (b) any HIV-infected infant or child whose CD4 count falls below the following age-adjusted thresholds: less than 1,750 cells/μl for infants birth to 12 months; less than 1000 cells/μl for infants 12 to 24 months; less than 750 cells/μl for children between 2 and 6 years of age; and less than 500 cells/μl for children over 6 years of age; and (c) any HIV-infected infant less than 1 year of age with a CD4 percentage of 30 or less; any child between 1 and 2 years with a CD4 percentage of 25 or less; and children of all other ages through adolescence with a CD4 percentage of 20 or less (EO).

Neurologic Testing

HIV infection in infants and children results in a wide spectrum and a high incidence of neurologic disease. In children with perinatal HIV infection, clinical signs of neurologic dysfunction may appear as early as 2 months and as late as 5 years of age. This neurologic dysfunction is caused either directly or indirectly by a primary HIV infection of the brain and is most commonly manifested in impaired brain growth; motor dysfunction; attention and memory difficulties; loss or plateau of previously acquired milestones; and cognitive impairment.

Algorithm 8 outlines the steps in evaluating neurologic status of infants and children with early HIV infection. Specific recommendations include:

■ A neurologic examination, including an age-related developmental assessment, should be performed on all HIV-exposed infants and HIV-infected infants and children at the initial assessment. A neurologic examination should be performed at each clinical visit, and an age-related developmental assessment should be done every 3 months for the first 24 months of life and every 6 months thereafter. (EO)

■ Baseline computerized tomographic (CT) scan or magnetic resonance imaging (MRI) is recommended at the time of diagnosis of HIV infection in infants and children. If CNS symptoms subsequently occur, neuroimaging studies should be repeated and cerebrospinal fluid obtained for analysis. (EO)

■ Serial CT or MRI scans are not indicated for the routine evaluation of HIV-infected infants and children who do not have CNS symptoms. (EO)

■ After exclusion of other diagnoses, infants and children who have primary HIV CNS disease should be treated with antiretroviral therapy and referred to a pediatric neurologist, if available, or a specialist in HIV care. (SGE)

■ Support and rehabilitation services, such as nutritional supplementation; physical, occupational, or speech therapies; and early intervention programs should be part of the comprehensive management of these patients. (EO)

Case Management for Persons Living with HIV

Case management for persons with HIV infection is a mechanism to facilitate provision of comprehensive health and mental health care and social support services. One of its objectives is to empower patients, family members, and significant others. It includes identifying those who need services, assessing their specific needs, developing a written care plan, implementing and monitoring the plan, reassessing and updating the plan as necessary, and terminating the plan when appropriate.

In the early stages of HIV infection, case management centers around the provision of social services, such as housing and financial assistance. As the infection progresses, the focus shifts to a greater emphasis on the provision of medical services.

Case management services can be delivered in a number of different settings, such as physician offices, community health clinics or hospitals, rehabilitation facilities, or within community-based organizations. Specific recommendations are:

■ All primary care providers should be knowledgeable about the uses of case management and should develop referral mechanisms to case-management services in their community (see listing of national and State resources on pages 35 and 36 of this guide). Methods for accomplishing this include providing continuing education and training; contracting with a local or regional case-management system; or employing a case manager in the primary care setting. (EO)

■ Case-management services should include intake; assessment of patient needs; development, implementation, and monitoring of a case-management plan; and periodic assessments. (EO)

■ Case-management services should be comprehensive and formalized in a written care plan that sets forth which services are required, who will provide them, and within what time frame. The patient or his or her parent or guardian should be able to select the specific services required at a given time. (EO)

■ Case-management programs should be directed by individuals knowledgeable about the clinical nature of HIV infection and issues affecting service delivery. (EO)

■ Minimum qualifications for a case manager include a working knowledge of the disease and/or illnesses of their patients, as reported in medical and nursing assessments; knowledge of and contact with services in immediate and neighboring communities as well as with health care, social services, and public entitlement programs; resourcefulness and creativity in accessing required services; the ability to interact effectively with clients and multiple providers in all settings; and the ability to maintain a spirit of hope and to empathize with patients and their loved ones. (EO)

Conclusion

As the number of HIV-infected persons increases throughout this decade, the need for well-informed health care providers also increases. The changing geographic distribution of the disease, with HIV infection no longer concentrated in only a handful of cities but spread across the country, places increasing demands on delivery sites and providers formerly unaffected by the epidemic. Providers will need to acquire new information and skills, and public and private policymakers will need to develop new systems to meet these challenges.

This Quick Reference Guide and the Guideline from which it is drawn present recommendations for early identification and management of HIV infection in infants, children, adolescents, and adults. Early care for HIV-infected individuals can have a major effect on their quality of life and, with appropriate patient education, help stem the spread of the disease.

Table 1. Drug[1] dosage and adverse effects; Antiretroviral therapy[2]

Medication	Dosage Adult/Tanner stage IV and V adolescents[3]	Dosage Infants/children/ Tanner stage I and II adolescents[3]	Adverse effects[4]
Zidovudine (ZDV) formerly azidothymidine (AZT) Retrovir® Formulation: 100 mg capsules Pediatric syrup 50 mg/5 ml	100 mg/dose administered orally every 4 hours or 5 doses given 7 days/week	180 mg/m[2] dose administered orally every 6 hours given 7 days/week	Granulocytopenia Anemia Nausea Headache Confusion Myositis Anorexia Hepatitis Seizures Nail discoloration
Didanosine (ddI) (dideoxyinosine) Videx® Formulation: 25, 50, 100, 150 mg tablets Pediatric powder for oral solution 10 mg/ml	Patients under 45 kg: 100 mg/dose orally given every 12 hours 7 days/week Patients over 45 kg: 200 mg/dose administered orally every 12 hours given 7 days/week (Tablet should be chewed and taken on an empty stomach)	200 mg/m[2]/day administered orally every 12 hours given 7 days per week	Pancreatitis, potentially fatal Peripheral neuropathy Peripheral retinal atrophy (in children only) Nausea Diarrhea Confusion Seizures
Zalcitabine (ddC) (dideoxycitidine) Formulation: 0.375 mg tablets 0.750 mg tablets Pediatric 0.1 mg/ml syrup	Patients under 45 kg: 0.375 mg/dose administered orally every 8 hours given 7 days/week Patients over 45 kg: 0.750 mg dose administered orally every 8 hours given 7 days/week	0.005-0.01 mg/kg/ dose administered orally every 8 hours given 7 days/week	Aphthous ulcers Esophageal ulcers Peripheral neuropathy Stomatitis Cutaneous eruptions Thrombocytopenia Pancreatitis

[1] Contains only drugs discussed or recommended in the *Clinical Practice Guideline for Evaluation and Management of Early HIV Infection.* Not all drugs or combinations of drugs used in the care of HIV-infected individuals are included.

[2] Dosage schedules and recommendations for use are based on review of literature or expert consensus and may not have approval of the Food and Drug Administration (FDA) for indications noted. Information included in this guideline may not represent FDA approval or FDA-approved labeling for the particular products or indications in question. Specifically, the terms "safe" and "effective" may not be synonymous with the FDA-defined legal standard for product approval.

[3] For adolescents who are Tanner stage I or II, pediatric dose schedules should be followed. Adult doses should be used for adolescents who are Tanner stage IV or V. Tanner stage III adolescents should have dose individualized, recognizing that this is the stage of most rapid growth.

[4] For a complete list of adverse reactions to these drugs, consult the *Physicians' Desk Reference* (Medical Economics Data, Montvale, NJ, 1993) or the drug's package insert.

Table 2. Drug dosage[1] and adverse effects; *Pneumocystis carinii* pneumonia prophylaxis[2]

Medication	Dosage Adult/Tanner stage IV and V adolescent [3]
Trimethoprim-Sulfamethoxazole (TMP-SMX) Bactrim® Septra® Formulations: Single-strength tablet: 80 mg TMP 400 mg SMX Double-strength tablet: 160 mg TMP 800 mg SMX Pediatric suspension: (per 5 ml) 40 mg TMP 200 mg SMX	Most commonly used regimens: one double-strength tablet taken orally three times per week on alternate days or daily 7 days per week
Pentamidine Isethionate NebuPent® 300 mg The vial must be dissolved in 6 ml sterile water and used with Respirguard® nebulizer	Aerosolized pentamidine (AP) (NebuPent®) is given as single 300 mg (one vial) dose every 4 weeks. Nebulized dose given over 30-45 min at a flow rate of 5-9 liters/min from a 40-50 lb per square inch air or oxygen source Alternative: if a Fisons ultrasonic nebulizer is used, dose of pentamidine is 60 mg given every 2 weeks after a loading dose of five treatments given over 2 weeks
Dapsone Formulation: 25 and 100 mg tablets	50-100 mg total daily oral dose divided into two doses or administered as a single daily dose given 2-7 times per week daily dose given 7 days per week

[1] Contains only drugs discussed or recommended in the *Clinical Practice Guideline for Evaluation and Management of Early HIV Infection.* Not all drugs or combinations of drugs used in the care of HIV-infected individuals are included.

[2] Dosage schedules and recommendations for use are based on review of literature or expert consensus and may not have approval of the Food and Drug Administration (FDA) for indications noted. Information included in this guideline may not represent FDA approval or FDA-approved labeling for the particular products or indications in question. Specifically, the terms "safe" and "effective" may not be synonymous with the FDA-defined legal standard for product approval.

Dosage Infants/children/ Tanner stage I and II adolescents [3]	Adverse effects [4]
150 mg/m^2 TMP 750 mg/m^2 SMX Total oral daily dose given 3 times/week Can be divided into two doses or administered as a single daily dose and given on 3 consecutive or 3 alternate days per week This same oral daily dose divided into 2 doses can be given 7 days per week	Drug allergy: Skin rash Steven-Johnson syndrome Fever Arthralgia Toxic epidermal necrolysis Hematologic: Anemia Neutropenia Thrombocytopenia Gastrointestinal: Elevation of serum transaminase Nausea Vomiting Anorexia Fulminant hepatic necrosis (rare)
Children over 5 yr can receive same inhalation dose as adults	Pulmonary: Bronchospasm with cough Pneumothorax Other: Extrapulmonary *P. carinii* infection Increased risk of environmental transmission of *M. tuberculosis*
1 mg/kg administered orally as a single daily dose given 7 days per week	Hematologic: Agranulocytosis Aplastic anemia Hemolytic anemia in G6PD deficiency Methemoglobinemia Cutaneous reactions: Bullous and exfoliative dermatitis Erythema nodosum Erythema multiforme Peripheral neuropathy Gastrointestinal: Nausea Vomiting

[3] For adolescents who are Tanner stage I or II, pediatric dose schedules should be followed. Adult doses should be used for adolescents who are Tanner stage IV or V. Tanner stage III adolescents should have dose individualized, recognizing that this is the stage of most rapid growth.

[4] For a complete list of adverse reactions to these drugs, consult the *Physicians' Desk Reference* (Medical Economics Data, Montvale, NJ, 1993) or the drug's package insert.

Table 3. Drug[1] dosage and adverse effects; Preventive therapy (chemoprophylaxis) for *Mycobacterium tuberculosis*[2]

Medication	Dosage: Adult/Tanner stage IV and V adolescents[3]	Dosage: Infants/children/ Tanner stage I and II adolescents[3]	Adverse effects[4]
Isoniazid INHR Nydrazid® Formulation: 50 mg, 100 mg, 300 mg tablets 1 gram vial Syrup 50 mg/5 ml	300 mg administered orally as a single daily dose given 7 days/wk for 12 mo or 900 mg administered orally as a single daily dose given 2 days/week for 12 mo	10-15 mg/kg/day (max 300 mg/day) administered orally as a single daily dose given 7 days/wk for 12 mo	Gastrointestinal: Hepatotoxicity (rare in children) Nausea, vomiting, anorexia Neurologic: Peripheral neuropathy Neuritis, fatigue Weakness Hematologic: Agranulocytosis Hemolytic and aplastic anemia Thrombocytopenia Eosinophilia Drug Allergy: Skin rash Fever Lymphadenopathy and vasculitis (SLE-like syndrome)

[1] Contains only drugs discussed or recommended in the *Clinical Practice Guideline for Evaluation and Management of Early HIV Infection.* Not all drugs or combinations of drugs used in the care of HIV-infected individuals are included.

[2] Dosage schedules and recommendations for use are based on review of literature or expert consensus and may not have approval of the Food and Drug Administration (FDA) for indications noted. Information included in this guideline may not represent FDA approval or FDA-approved labeling for the particular products or indications in question. Specifically, the terms "safe" and "effective" may not be synonymous with the FDA-defined legal standard for product approval.

[3] For adolescents who are Tanner stage I or II, pediatric dose schedules should be followed. Adult doses should be used for adolescents who are Tanner stage IV or V. Tanner stage III adolescents should have dose individualized, recognizing that this is the stage of most rapid growth.

[4] For a complete list of adverse reactions to these drugs, consult the *Physicians' Desk Reference* (Medical Economics Data, Montvale, NJ, 1993) or the drug's package insert.

Algorithms

Algorithm 1. Selected Elements of the Initial and Ongoing Evaluation of Adults with Early HIV Infection

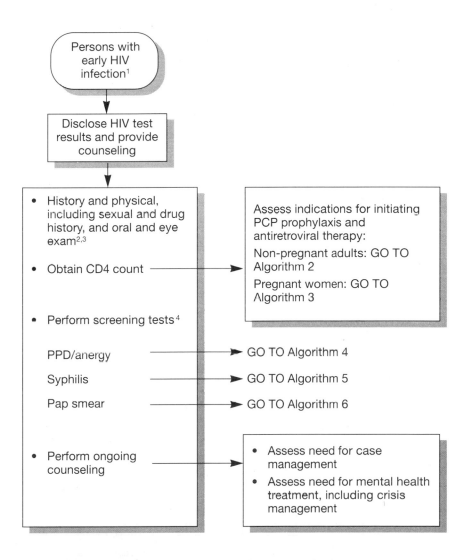

[1] Provider should review and evaluate the adequacy of HIV diagnostic tests.

[2] Appropriate immunizations should be provided (this topic was not reviewed by the HIV panel).

[3] Schedule followup appropriate for patient's condition.

[4] Many other screening tests were not reviewed by this panel, including toxoplasmosis, hepatitis serology, and routine laboratory tests.

Note: The algorithm presents recommendations only for the items reviewed by the HIV Panel.

Algorithm 2. Evaluation for Initiation of Antiretroviral Therapy and PCP Prophylaxis; Men and Nonpregnant Women with Early HIV Infection

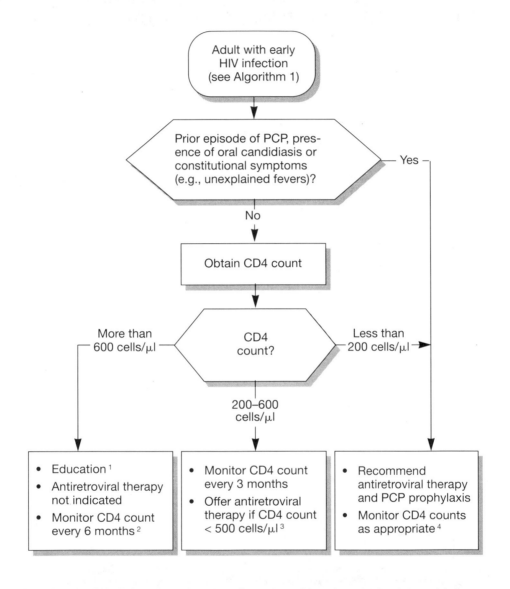

[1] Education should include a discussion of enrollment into relevant investigational drug trials for asymptomatic persons.

[2] If CD4 count has shown great variability or is rapidly declining, repeat the CD4 within 3 months.

[3] If patient develops symptoms, recommend antiretroviral therapy.

[4] If CD4 count < 200 cells/μl, continued monitoring of CD4 counts may be needed to determine eligibility for clinical trials, and prophylaxis for opportunistic infections other than PCP and to guide antiretroviral therapy.

Note: The algorithm presents recommendations only for the items reviewed by the HIV panel.

Algorithm 3. Evaluation for Initiation of Antiretroviral Therapy and PCP Prophylaxis; Pregnant Women with Early HIV Infection

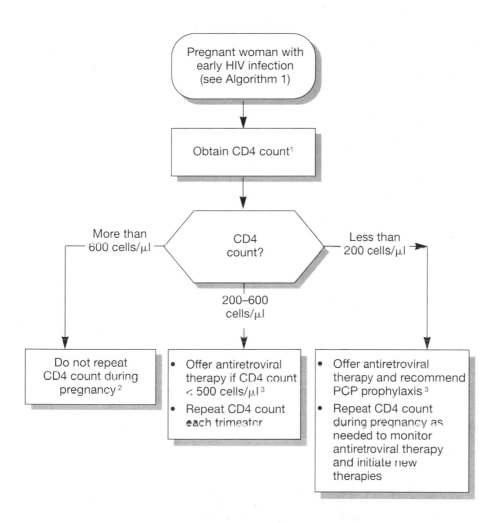

[1] CD4 count should be obtained on presentation for prenatal care; women who have received no prenatal care should have CD4 counts taken at delivery.

[2] Unless indicated by the presence of clinical symptoms.

[3] The possible benefits and risks of antiretroviral therapy to both mother and fetus should be discussed fully with the patient.

Note: The algorithm presents recommendations only for the items reviewed by the HIV panel.

Algorithm 4. Evaluation for *Mycobacterium tuberculosis* Infection in Adults and Adolescents with Early HIV Infection

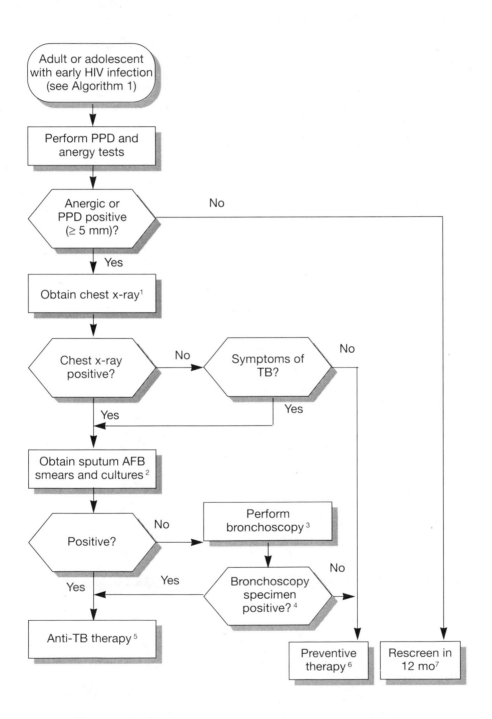

[1]Chest x-ray can be performed, using a lead apron shield, after the first trimester in pregnant women asymptomatic for TB or at any stage of pregnancy in women symptomatic for TB.

[2]At least three sputum smears and cultures should be obtained.

[3]If there is no other etiology for the abnormal chest x-ray.

[4]Both AFB smears and cultures should be obtained at bronchoscopy.

[5]Anti-TB therapy should be guided by local susceptibility patterns and modified appropriately when isolated susceptibilities become available.

[6]Preventive therapy is indicated for PPD-positive patients and should be strongly considered for anergic patients who are known contacts of patients with TB and for anergic patients belonging to groups in which the prevalence of TB is at least 10 percent (e.g., injection drug users, prisoners, homeless persons, persons in congregate housing, migrant laborers, and persons born in foreign countries with high rates of TB).

[7]Individuals who reside in settings where TB prevalence is high should be retested in 6 months; individuals who are exposed acutely to others with suspected or confirmed TB should be retested in 3 months; anergic individuals need not be retested, except in special circumstances.

Note: The algorithm presents recommendations only for the items reviewed by the HIV panel.

Algorithm 5. Evaluation for Syphilis in Adults and Sexually Active Adolescents with Early HIV Infection

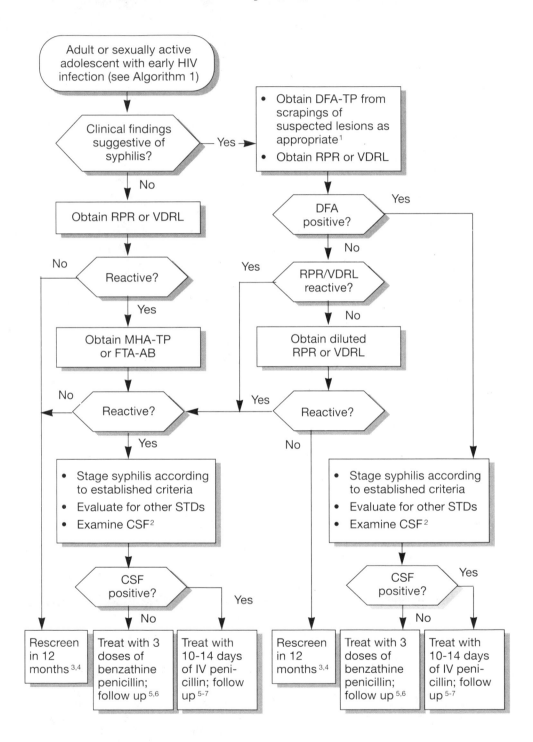

[1] If dark-field exam cannot be performed and primary syphilis is suspected, empiric treatment should be instituted.

[2] Treatment for neurosyphilis recommended if the CSF cannot be evaluated (See *Guideline for Evaluation and Management of Early HIV Infection* for recommended followup).

[3] Or after exposure to or diagnosis of any sexually transmitted disease.

[4] Pregnant women should be screened for syphilis at entry to prenatal care, during the third trimester, or at delivery.

[5] See *Guideline for Evaluation and Management of Early HIV Infection* for recommended followup

[6] For issues specific to pregnant women, see *Guideline for Evaluation and Management of Early HIV Infection* for recommended followup.

[7] Alternative treatments include 10 days of IM procaine penicillin or 10-14 days of 1-2 g of IM ceftriaxome.

Note: The algorithm presents recommendations only for the items reviewed by the HIV panel.

Algorithm 6. Pap Smears in Women with Early HIV Infection

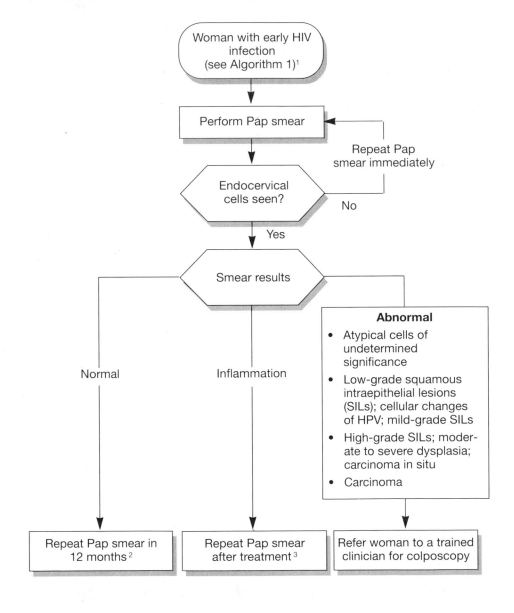

Woman with early HIV infection (see Algorithm 1)[1]

Perform Pap smear

Repeat Pap smear immediately

Endocervical cells seen?

No

Yes

Smear results

Abnormal

- Atypical cells of undetermined significance
- Low-grade squamous intraepithelial lesions (SILs); cellular changes of HPV; mild-grade SILs
- High-grade SILs; moderate to severe dysplasia; carcinoma in situ
- Carcinoma

Normal

Inflammation

Repeat Pap smear in 12 months[2]

Repeat Pap smear after treatment[3]

Refer woman to a trained clinician for colposcopy

[1] Pap smears should be performed at entry to prenatal care for pregnant women and prior to discharge for women who present for delivery without prenatal care.

[2] HIV-infected women with a history of human papilloma virus (HPV) or with previous Pap smears showing SILs should have their Pap smears repeated every 6 months.

[3] Treatment should be guided by diagnosis of the cause of inflammation.

Note: The algorithm presents recommendations only for the items reviewed by the HIV panel.

Algorithm 7: Evaluation for Initiation of Antiretroviral Therapy and PCP Prophylaxis; Infants and Children with Early HIV Infection

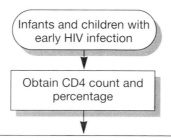

Infants and children with early HIV infection

↓

Obtain CD4 count and percentage

↓

- Initiate antiretroviral therapy as indicated by either CD4 count (Table A) or CD4 percentage (Table B)
- Initiate PCP prophylaxis as indicated by either CD4 count (Figure A) or CD4 percentage (Figure B)[1]
- Infants and children receiving neither antiretroviral therapy nor PCP prophylaxis should have their CD4 counts and percentages monitored[2]

Figure A

Age	CD4 count (cells/ml) 200 300 500 750 1000 1500 1750
<12 mo[1]	
12–24 mo[2]	
2–6 yr[2]	
≥ 6 yr[2]	

■ Initiate PCP prophylaxis
■ Initiate antiretroviral therapy

Figure B

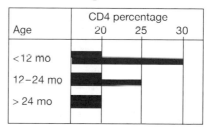

Age	CD4 percentage 20 25 30
<12 mo	
12–24 mo	
> 24 mo	

■ Initiate PCP prophylaxis
■ Initiate antiretroviral therapy

Source: Figure A adapted from Centers for Disease Control and Prevention, 1991.

[1] Patients with prior episode of PCP should receive PCP prophylaxis regardless of CD4 count and percentage.

[2] Obtain CD4 count and percentage at 1 month of age, 3 months of age, and then at 3-month intervals through 24 months of age; thereafter obtain CD4 count and percentage every 6 months, unless values reach an age-related threshold where testing should be repeated monthly.

Note: The algorithm presents recommendations only for the items reviewed by the HIV panel.

Algorithm 8. Neurologic Evaluation of Infants and Children with Early HIV Infection

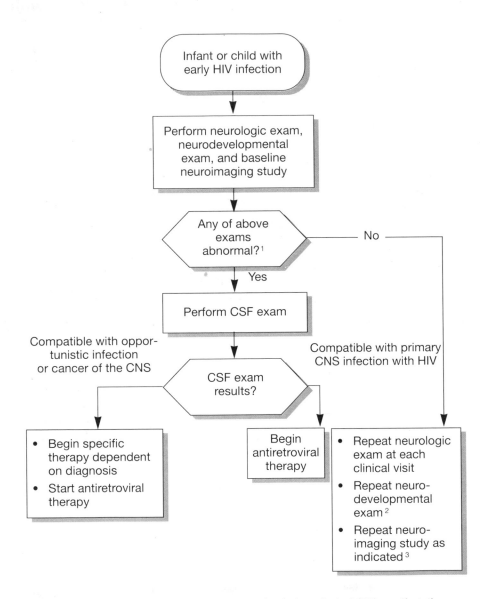

[1] Abnormal exam is defined as focal pathology, obstructive lesion, atypical CNS manifestations, or evidence of progressive neurologic disease (see *Guideline for Evaluation and Management of Early HIV Infection*).

[2] Neurodevelopmental exams should be performed at 3-month intervals up to 24 months of age, then every 6 months thereafter.

[3] Neuroimaging studies should be performed if CNS symptoms occur; such studies should be performed in conjunction with CSF analysis.

Note: The algorithm presents recommendations only for the items reviewed by the HIV panel.

Sources of HIV information

General information:

English: 800-342-AIDS (2437)
Spanish: 800-344-7432
TDD Service for the Deaf: 800-243-7889

General information for health care providers:

HIV Telephone Consultation
Service: 800-933-3413

State hotlines:

For information about HIV-specific resources and counseling and testing services, call your State AIDS hotline:

Alabama 800-228-0469
Alaska 800-478-2437
Arizona 800 548 4695
Arkansas 501-661-2133
California (No.) 800-367-2437
California (So.) 800-922-2437
Colorado 800-252-2437
Connecticut 800-342-2437
Delaware 800-422-0429
District of
Columbia 202-332-2437
Florida 800-352-2437
Georgia 800 551 2728
Hawaii 800-922-1313
Idaho 208-345-2277
Illinois 800-243-2437
Indiana 800-848-2437
Iowa 800-445-2437
Kansas 800-232-0040
Kentucky 800-654-2437

Louisiana 800-922-4379
Maine 800-851-2437
Maryland 800-638-6252
Massachusetts 800-235-2331
Michigan 800-827-2437
Minnesota 800-248-2437
Mississippi 800-537-0851
Missouri 800-533-2437
Montana 800-233-6668
Nebraska 800-782-2437
Nevada 800-842-2437
New Hampshire 800-324-2437
New Jersey 800-624-2377
New Mexico 800-545-2437
New York 800-541-2437
North Carolina 800-733-7301
North Dakota 800-472-2180
Ohio 800-332-2437
Oklahoma 800-535-2437
Oregon 800-777-2437
Pennsylvania 800-662-6080
Puerto Rico 800-765-1010
Rhode Island 800-726-3010
South Carolina 800-322-2437
South Dakota 800-592-1861
Tennessee 800-525-2437
Texas 800-299-2437
Utah 800-366-2437
Vermont 800-882-2437
Virginia 800-533-4148
Virgin Islands 809-773-2437
Washington 800-272-2437
West Virginia 800-642-8244
Wisconsin 800-334-2437
Wyoming 800-327-3577

For HIV/AIDS treatment information, call:

The American Foundation
for AIDS Research
800-39AMFAR (392-6327)

AIDS Treatment Data Network
212-268-4196

AIDS Treatment News
800-TREAT 1-2 (873-2812)

For information about AIDS/HIV clinical trials conducted by National Institutes of Health and Food and Drug Administration-approved efficacy trials, call:

AIDS Clinical Trials Information
Service (ACTIS)
800-TRIALS-A (874-2572)

To locate a physician, call your local or State Medical Society

For more information about HIV infection, call:

Drug Abuse Hotline
800-662-HELP (4357)

Pediatric and Pregnancy AIDS
Hotline
212-430-3333

National Hemophilia Foundation
212-219-8180

Hemophilia and AIDS/HIV
Network for Dissemination
of Information (HANDI)
800-42-HANDI (424-2634)

National Pediatric HIV
Resource Center
800-362-0071

National Association of People
with AIDS
202-898-0414

Teens Teaching AIDS Prevention
Program (TTAPP)
National Hotline:
800-234-TEEN (8336)

Note: This is not an all-inclusive list. For other sources of information, contact your State HIV hotline listed on page 35.

Abstract

This *Quick Reference Guide for Clinicians* contains highlights from the *Clinical Practice Guideline on Evaluation and Management of Early HIV Infection*, which was developed by a private-sector panel of health care providers and consumers. Selected aspects of evaluating and managing patients, both adults and children, who are in the early stages of human immunodeficiency virus infection are presented. Topics covered include disclosure of HIV status, monitoring of CD4 lymphocyte counts, prevention of *Pneumocystis carinii* pneumonia and infection with *Mycobacterium tuberculosis*, initiation of antiretroviral therapy, treatment of syphilis, eye and oral care, performance of Papanicolaou smears, diagnosis of HIV infection in infants and children, preventive therapy for PCP and assessment of neurologic problems in HIV-infected children, pregnancy counseling, and development of a comprehensive case management system. Algorithms are included that show the sequence of events related to evaluating and managing early HIV infection in adults and children, as well as drug dosing tables for antiretroviral, PCP, and *M. tuberculosis* therapies.

El-Sadr W, Oleske JM, Agins BD et al. *Managing Early HIV Infection: Quick Reference Guide for Clinicians.* AHCPR Publication No. 94-0573. Rockville, MD: Agency for Health Care Policy and Research, Public Health Service, U.S. Department of Health and Human Services, January 1994.

Appendix II
Integrating HIV/AIDS Content Into Baccalaureate Nursing Curricula

The three-stage model of HIV/AIDS curriculum development proposed by Duffy (1993) may be used in conjunction with this textbook at any of the three stages. Faculty choosing a curriculum stage should consider the epidemiology of AIDS in their region, their program's philosophy, the availability of nurses with expertise in HIV content, the availability of HIV clinical sites and community resources, and the developmental phase of their program related to HIV content. Any stage may be chosen for the introduction of HIV content into the curriculum. This stage may be an appropriate permanent stage, depending on the factors listed above, or it may be the first step in developing the curriculum through the succeeding stages. Suggestions for use of this textbook and for teaching and learning strategies are included for each stage of the model.

STAGE I. THE GUEST SPEAKER

Characteristics of Stage I

- Introductory
- Content delivered by expert guest(s)
- A one-shot lecture, program, or workshop for each nursing student class

Content of Stage I	Relevant Chapters in This Textbook

Social context of HIV	Chapter 1. Overview of HIV Disease and Nursing
	    History of HIV
	    Nurses' knowledge and attitudes
	Chapter 13. Ethical Issues Related to the Care of Persons with HIV
	Chapter 15. Cultural Issues Related to the Care of Persons with HIV

Epidemiology	Chapter 1. Overview of HIV Disease and Nursing Sociodemographic distribution
Prevention	Chapter 2. Health Promotion and Disease Prevention

Universal precautions	Chapter 10. Infection Control
Clinical course of HIV	Chapter 4. Clinical Manifestations of AIDS in Adults
	Chapter 5. Nursing Management of the Adult
Personal experience of HIV	Chapter 11. Psychosocial Aspects of Nursing Care
	Chapter 16. Personal Perspectives on Nursing Care
Roles in HIV nursing	Chapter 1. Overview of HIV Disease and Nursing
	History of HIV
	Chapter 2. Health Promotion and Disease Prevention
	Chapter 11. Psychosocial Aspects of Nursing Care
	Nurses' roles
	Behavior change
	Complexity of care

Examples of Learning Activities—Stage I

- Reading assignments (noted above)
- Lecture/discussion with visual media
- Small-group discussions with hospital infection control nurses
- Panel of nurses working with person(s) with HIV disease (PWHIV)
- Panel of clergy, ethicist, attorney

STAGE II.   MAINSTREAMING HIV CONTENT

Characteristics of Stage II

- Builds on Stage I content and guest expertise
- Inclusion of lectures on HIV in appropriate places in the traditional curriculum
- Involvement of guest faculty in lectures, curriculum development (teaching objectives, philosophy of program, regional epidemiology)
- Forming of liaisons with community agencies serving PWHIV

Content of Stage II	Course(s)	Relevant Chapter(s) in This Textbook
	Integrate the content of items 1 to 4 into the following courses:	
1. Evaluation of people with asymptomatic HIV	Medical Nursing	Chapter 4: Clinical Manifestations of AIDS in Adults
	Surgical Nursing	Chapter 5: Nursing Management of the Adult
2. Treatment of people with asymptomatic HIV	Gerontologic Nursing	
	Psychiatric Nursing	Chapter 11: Psychosocial Aspects of Nursing Care

3. Evaluation of people with symptomatic HIV	Maternity Nursing	Chapter 8: Nursing Care of Women
	Pediatric Nursing	Chapter 6: Nursing Care of the Child
4. Treatment of people with symptomatic HIV		
	Integrate the content of items 5 and 6 into the following courses:	
5. Human sexuality	Human Sexuality	Chapter 2: Health Promotion and Disease Prevention
		Chapter 5: Nursing Management of the Adult
6. Taking a sexual history	Physical Assessment	Chapter 7: Nursing Care of the Adolescent
		Chapter 8: Nursing Care of Women
7. Infection control procedures	Introduction to the Art and Science of Nursing	Chapter 10: Infection Control
8. Substance abuse	Psychiatric Nursing	Chapter 9: Nursing Care of Chemically Dependent Clients
9. Substance abuse treatment		
10. The immune system	Human Physiology	Chapter 3: Pathophysiology of HIV-1: Clinical Course and Treatment
11. Epidemiology and history of HIV	Community Health Nursing	Chapter 1: Overview of HIV Disease and Nursing
12. Prevention		Chapter 2: Health Promotion and Disease Prevention
13. Community care		Chapter 12: Community-based and Long-term Care
14. Legal and ethical issues	Professional Issues in Nursing	Chapter 13: Ethical Issues Related to the Care of Persons with HIV
		Chapter 14: Legal Issues Related to the Care of Persons with HIV

Examples of Learning Activities—Stage II

- Reading assignments (noted above)
- Expert nurse guest-faculty lectures
- Videotapes on specific topics
- Skills laboratory
- Psychosocial and physical assessment laboratory
- Demonstration and return demonstration
- Role playing

- Visits to community agencies
- Panel of PWHIV
- Panel of substance abusers
- Panel of clergy, ethicist, attorney

STAGE III.   INTEGRATION

Characteristics of Stage III

- Builds on Stage II content and mainstreaming of HIV content into the traditional curricula
- Involvement of core faculty in teaching HIV content in the curriculum
- Identification and teaching of new content based on the challenges of HIV care
- Clinical placement and experience of students with PWHIV

Content of Stage II	Course(s)	Relevant Chapters in This Textbook
All content related to Stage II continues, taught by core faculty accompanied by student clinical experience with PWHIV. Additional new content and courses are listed here.		
	Integrate items 1 to 4 into the following courses:	
1. Sexual history taking and counseling	Psychiatric Nursing	Chapter 2: Health Promotion and Disease Prevention
	Physical, Psychosocial, and Neuropsychiatric Assessment	Chapter 5: Nursing Management of the Adult
2. Substance abuse history taking and counseling		Chapter 9: Nursing Care of Chemically Dependent Clients
3. Neuropsychiatric assessment and care		Chapter 11: Psychosocial Aspects of Nursing Care
4. Pregnancy counseling	Maternity Nursing	Chapter 8: Nursing Care of Women
5. Comorbidity and HIV disease Tuberculosis Syphilis	Medical Nursing Community Health Nursing	Chapter 2: Health Promotion and Disease Prevention Chapter 4: Clinical Manifestations of AIDS in Adults
6. Organic mental disorders	Psychiatric Nursing	Chapter 11: Psychosocial Aspects of Nursing Care
7. Long-term survival	Chronic Care Nursing	Chapter 12: Community-based and Long-term Care
8. Culture, ethnicity, and HIV disease	Cultural Responses to Illness	Chapter 15: Cultural Issues Related to the Care of Persons with HIV
9. Case management	Nursing Management	Chapter 12: Community-based and Long-term Care

Examples of Learning Activities—Stage III

- All activities listed for Stage II
- Clinical practice with PWHIV
- Case management skills and practice
- Discharge planning and referrals
- Involvement in support groups of nurses caring for PWHIV

REFERENCE

Duffy, P.R. (1993). A model for the integration of HIV/AIDS content into baccalaureate nursing curricula. *Journal of Nursing Education, 32*(8), 347–351.

Appendix III
Drugs Used to Treat HIV Infection and AIDS-related Conditions (*Under investigation)

GENERIC NAME (TRADE NAME)	ROUTE OF ADMINISTRATION	INDICATIONS	SIDE/ADVERSE EFFECTS
ACYCLOVIR (Zovirax)	PO IV Topical	Herpes simplex virus infection Herpes zoster infection Varicella infection	Parenteral: skin rash, hives, hematuria, lightheadedness, headache, diaphoresis, confusion, tremors, abdominal pain, difficulty in breathing, decreased frequency of urination, nausea, vomiting, unusual thirst, extreme fatigue Oral: changes in menstrual period, skin rash, diarrhea, dizziness, headache, joint pain, nausea, vomiting, acne, anorexia, somnolence Topical: mild pain, burning, itching, skin rash
ADENINE ARABINOSIDE (Vidarabine) (Vira–A)	IV Ophthalmic	Herpes simplex virus infection Herpes zoster infection Progressive multifocal leukoencephalopathy Varicella infection	Anorexia, nausea, vomiting, diarrhea, tremors, dizziness, confusion, hallucinations, ataxia, psychosis, leukopenia, thrombocytopenia, elevated SGOT and bilirubin levels, anemia
ALBENDAZOLE (Eskazole) (Zentel)	PO	Microsporidiosis Cryptosporidiosis	Stomach upset, headache, dizziness, rash, fever, elevated liver function tests, alopecia
*ALL TRANS RETINOIC ACID	PO	Kaposi's sarcoma	None yet reported
AMIKACIN (Amikin)	IV IM	*Mycobacterium avium* complex infection	Increase or decrease in frequency of urination or amount of urine, increased thirst, loss of appetite, nausea, vomiting, muscle twitching, numbness, any loss of hearing, ringing or buzzing, clumsiness, dizziness, unsteadiness, difficulty in breathing

Continued on following page

GENERIC NAME (TRADE NAME)	ROUTE OF ADMINISTRATION	INDICATIONS	SIDE/ADVERSE EFFECTS
AMITRIPTYLINE (Elavil)	PO	Peripheral neuropathy Depression	Drowsiness, dizziness, excitation, tremors, weakness, confusion, headache, nervousness, orthostatic hypotension, tachycardia, hypertension, blurred vision, tinnitus, mydriasis, dry mouth, constipation, nausea, vomiting, anorexia, paralytic ileus, urine retention, rash, urticaria, sweating
AMPHOTERICIN B (Fungizone)	IV	Candidiasis Coccidioidomycosis Cryptococcosis Histoplasmosis	Fever, chills, hypokalemia (irregular heartbeat, muscle cramps or pain, extreme fatigue), pain at site of infusion, anemia, blurred or double vision, renal failure (increased or decreased urination), paresthesias, impaired hearing, tinnitus, seizures, shortness of breath, skin rash or itching, agranulocytosis or leukopenia, thrombocytopenia
*AMPHOTERICIN B COLLOIDAL DISPERSION	IV	Cryptococcosis	*See* Amphotericin B
*ANTI–B4–BLOCKED RICIN	IV	Lymphoma	Allergic reactions, weight gain, can affect liver
AMPICILLIN (Omnipen) (Omnipen–N) (Polycillin) (Polycillin–N) (Principen) (Totacillin) (Totacillin–N)	PO IM IV	Salmonellosis	Anaphylaxis, serum sickness, neutropenia, platelet count dysfunction, skin rash, fever, hives, itching, pseudomembranous colitis, seizures, diarrhea, nausea, vomiting, thrush, abdominal pain or cramps
*ATEVIRDINE MESYLATE	PO	HIV infection	Rash, fever, palpitations
ATOVAQUONE (Mepron) (formerly 566C80)	PO	*Pneumocystis carinii* pneumonia	Rash, nausea, diarrhea, headache, vomiting, fever, insomnia, asthenia, pruritus, thrush, abdominal pain, constipation, dizziness, anemia, neutropenia, elevated liver enzymes

GENERIC NAME (TRADE NAME)	ROUTE OF ADMINISTRATION	INDICATIONS	SIDE/ADVERSE EFFECTS
AZITHROMYCIN (Zithromax)	PO	Cryptosporidiosis *Mycobacterium avium* complex infection Toxoplasmosis	Diarrhea, nausea, vomiting, abdominal pain, palpitations, chest pain, dyspepsia, flatulence, melena, cholestatic jaundice, *Monilia* infection, vaginitis, nephritis, dizziness, ototoxicity, vertigo, somnolence, fatigue, rash, photophobia, angioedema
*BACI	PO	Cryptosporidiosis	None yet reported
BLEOMYCIN (Blenoxane)	IV	Kaposi's sarcoma Non–Hodgkin's lymphoma Cervical cancer	Cough, shortness of breath, pneumonitis, fever, chills, stomatitis, confusion, syncope, diaphoresis, changes in skin color and texture, rashes, swelling of fingers, nausea, vomiting and anorexia, weight loss, hair loss
*BROVAVIR	PO	Herpes simplex virus infection Varicella-zoster virus infection	None yet reported
*CD4, RECOMBINANT SOLUBLE	IV IM	HIV infection	Local reactions at injection site, fever
CEFTRIAXONE (Rocephin)	IM IV	Neurosyphilis	Bleeding, bruising, abdominal cramps/pain, diarrhea, melena, fever, bronchospasm, hypotension, Stevens–Johnson syndrome, decreased urine output, skin rash, joint pain, itching, redness, swelling, seizures, thrombophlebitis, pseudolithiasis
CHLORAMPHENICOL (Anocol) (Chloromycetin)	PO IM IV	Salmonellosis	Blood dyscrasias, abdominal distention, blue–gray skin color, low body temperature, difficulty in breathing, coma, cardiovascular collapse, skin rash, fever, confusion, delerium, headache, loss of vision, paresthesias, extremity weakness, diarrhea, nausea, vomiting, pale skin, sore throat, bleeding

Continued on following page

GENERIC NAME (TRADE NAME)	ROUTE OF ADMINISTRATION	INDICATIONS	SIDE/ADVERSE EFFECTS
CHLORHEXIDINE GLUCONATE Oral Rinse (Peridex)	Oral Rinse	Prophylaxis for thrush	Change in taste, increased tartar, staining of teeth, fillings, and dentures, mouth irritation
CIMETIDINE (Tagamet)	PO	HIV infection	Diarrhea, headache
CIPROFLOXACIN (Cipro)	PO	*Mycobacterium avium* complex infection	Restlessness, tremors, seizures, crystalluria, blood in urine, dysuria, low back pain, skin rash, itching, redness, swelling of face or neck, joint pains, stiffness, visual disturbances, photosensitivity, dizziness, headache, abdominal pain, diarrhea, nausea, vomiting, insomnia, unpleasant taste in mouth
CISPLATIN (Platinol) (Platinol–AQ)	IV	Cervical cancer	Leukopenia, thrombocytopenia, anemia, nephrotoxicity, ototoxicity
CLARITHROMYCIN (Biaxin)	PO	*Mycobacterium avium* complex infection	Nausea, vomiting, headache, rash, hearing loss, hepatotoxicity, abnormal taste, diarrhea, stomach pain or discomfort
CLINDAMYCIN (Cleocin)	PO IM IV	Toxoplasmosis Pneumocystosis	Pseudomembranous colitis, skin rash, neutropenia, thrombocytopenia, abdominal pain, nausea and vomiting, diarrhea, fungal growth
CLOFAZIMINE (Lamprene)	PO	*Mycobacterium avium* complex infection	Colicky or burning abdominal or stomach pain, nausea, vomiting, pink or red to brownish black discoloration of skin (two suicides have been reported as a result of mental depression secondary to skin discoloration), visual changes, gastrointestinal bleeding, hepatitis or jaundice, dry rough scaly skin, anorexia, dizziness, drowsiness, dryness, burning, itching, or irritation of eyes, skin rash, photosensitivity
CLOTRIMAZOLE (Mycelex Troches)	PO	Candidiasis (oropharyngeal)	Abdominal or stomach cramping or pain, diarrhea, nausea or vomiting

GENERIC NAME (TRADE NAME)	ROUTE OF ADMINISTRATION	INDICATIONS	SIDE/ADVERSE EFFECTS
*CMV IMMUNE GLOBULIN	IV	Cytomegalovirus	Flushing, chills, muscle cramps, back pain, fever, nausea and vomiting, wheezing
COLONY–STIMULATING FACTORS (Leukine) Neupogen)	IV SC	Neutropenia	Hypersensitivity reactions (urticaria, angioedema, bronchoconstriction, anaphylaxis), fever, chills, rigors, bone pain, arthralgias, adult respiratory distress syndrome, rash, pericarditis, local erythema at site of injection, hypoxia
CYCLOPHOSPHAMIDE (Cytoxan) (Neosar)	PO IM IV	Non–Hodgkin's lymphoma	Missing menstrual cycles, darkening of skin and fingernails, loss of appetite, nausea, vomiting, diarrhea, stomach pain, flushing and redness of face, headache, increased sweating, swollen lips, skin rash, hives, loss of hair
CYCLOSERINE (Seromycin)	PO	*Mycobacterium avium* complex infection *Mycobacterium tuberculosis*	Anxiety, confusion, dizziness, drowsiness, increased irritability, increased restlessness, mental depression, muscle twitching or trembling, nervousness, nightmares, other mood or mental changes, speech problems, skin rash, numbness, tingling, burning pain or weakness in the hands or feet, headache, seizures
CYTARABINE (Ara–C) (Cytosine arabinoside) (Cytosar–U)	PO IM IV	Non–Hodgkin's lymphoma Progressive multifocal leukoencephalopathy	Fever, chills, cough, hoarseness, lower back or side pain, difficult urination, diarrhea, sores in mouth or on lips, unusual bleeding or bruising, numbness or tingling in fingers, toes or face, unusual tiredness, swelling of feet or lower legs, pain at injection site, skin rash, reddened eyes, chest pain, shortness of breath, itching of skin, headache

Continued on following page

GENERIC NAME (TRADE NAME)	ROUTE OF ADMINISTRATION	INDICATIONS	SIDE/ADVERSE EFFECTS
DAPSONE (Avlosulfon) (DDS)	PO	Pneumocystosis	Hemolytic anemia, Stevens–Johnson syndrome, agranulocytosis (fever and sore throat), hepatic damage, methoglobinemia (bluish fingernails, lips, or skin, fatigue, dyspnea), mood changes, peripheral neuritis
DEXTROAMPHETAMINE (Dexedrine)	PO	HIV dementia	Restlessness, tremor, hyperactivity, insomnia, dizziness, headache, chills, dysphoria, tachycardia, palpitations, hypertension, hypotension, nausea, vomiting, cramps, dry mouth, diarrhea, constipation, metallic taste, anorexia, weight loss, urticaria, impotence, altered libido
*DICLAZURIL	PO	Cryptosporidiosis	Nausea, vomiting, fever, flu–like symptoms
DIDANOSINE (ddl) (Videx)	PO	HIV infection	Diarrhea, abdominal pain, pancreatitis, peripheral neuropathy, seizures, headaches, abnormal bone marrow function, abnormal liver function, electrolyte abnormalities, cardiac arrythmias, allergic reactions
DOXORUBICIN HYDROCHLORIDE (Adriamycin)	IV	Kaposi's sarcoma Non–Hodgkin's lymphoma	Leukopenia or infection (fever, chills, sore throat), stomatitis, esophagitis, flank, stomach, or joint pain, pain at infusion site, peripheral edema, fast or irregular heartbeat, shortness of breath, gastrointestinal bleeding, thrombocytopenia (unusual bleeding or bruising), changes in skin color, diarrhea, nausea, vomiting, skin rash or itching, hair loss, reddish color to urine

GENERIC NAME (TRADE NAME)	ROUTE OF ADMINISTRATION	INDICATIONS	SIDE/ADVERSE EFFECTS
DRONABINOL (Marinol)	PO	HIV wasting	Irritability, insomnia, restlessness, hot flashes, sweating, rhinnorhea, loose stools, hiccups, anorexia, tachycardia, mood changes, confusion, personality changes, hallucinations, depression, nervousness, anxiety, dry mouth, vision changes, hypotension
EPOETIN ALFA, RECOMBINANT (Epogen) (Eprex) (Procrit)	IV SC	Anemia associated with HIV infection or zidovudine therapy	Chest pain, edema, tachycardia, headache, hypertension, polycythemia, seizures, shortness of breath, skin rash, arthralgias, asthenia, diarrhea, nausea, fatigue, flu–like syndrome after each dose NOTE: Should be temporarily discontinued if the hematocrit reaches or exceeds 36%
ETHAMBUTOL (Myambutol)	PO	*Mycobacterium avium* complex infection *Mycobacterium tuberculosis*	Acute gout, chills, pain and swelling of joints, skin rash, fever, arthralgias, numbness, tingling, burning pain, weakness of hands or feet, blurred vision, eye pain, red–green color blindness, any loss of vision, abdominal pain, anorexia, nausea, vomiting, headache, mental confusion
ETHIONAMIDE (Trecator–SC)	PO	*Mycobacterium avium* complex infection *Mycobacterium tuberculosis*	Yellow skin and eyes, tingling, burning, or pain in hands or feet, mental depression, clumsiness or unsteadiness, confusion, mood or mental changes, changes in menstrual periods, coldness, decreased sexual ability, dry puffy skin, weight gain, hyperglycemia, blurred vision or loss of vision, skin rash

Continued on following page

GENERIC NAME (TRADE NAME)	ROUTE OF ADMINISTRATION	INDICATIONS	SIDE/ADVERSE EFFECTS
ETOPOSIDE (VePesid)	IV	Kaposi's sarcoma Non–Hodgkin's lymphoma	Leukopenia, thrombocytopenia, stomatitis, ataxia, paresthesias, tachycardia, shortness of breath or wheezing, pain at site of injection, nausea, vomiting and loss of appetite, diarrhea, fatigue, loss of hair
FLUCONAZOLE (Diflucan)	PO IV	Candidiasis Cryptococcosis	Abnormal liver function, Stevens–Johnson syndrome, nausea, headache, skin rash, vomiting, abdominal pain, diarrhea
FLUCYTOSINE (Ancobon) (5–Fluorocytosine) (5FC)	PO	Candidiasis Cryptococcosis	Anemia, yellow eyes or skin, skin rash, redness, itching, sore throat, fever, unusual bleeding or bruising, confusion, sensitivity to sunlight, abdominal pain, diarrhea, loss of appetite, nausea, vomiting, dizziness, lightheadedness, drowsiness, headache
FOSCARNET SODIUM (Foscavir)	IV	Cytomegalovirus infection Herpes simplex virus infection HIV infection	Increased thirst, headaches, nausea, anorexia, flank pain, muscle twitching, elevated creatinine, mild proteinuria, renal failure, decrease in calcium, hyperphosphatemia, fatigue, irritability, tremors, seizures, genital ulcers
GANCICLOVIR (Cytovene) (formerly known as DHPG)	PO IV Intravitreal implants	Cytomegalovirus infection	Granulocytopenia, thrombocytopenia, anemia, mood changes, tremors, nervousness, fever, skin rash, abnormal liver function, phlebitis, abdominal pain, loss of appetite, nausea, vomiting
*GENTAMICIN LIPOSOME INJECTION	IV	*Mycobacterium avium* complex infection	Urinary frequency, increased thirst, anorexia, nausea, vomiting, muscle twitching, paresthesias, seizures, impaired hearing, itching, skin rash, impaired vision

GENERIC NAME (TRADE NAME)	ROUTE OF ADMINISTRATION	INDICATIONS	SIDE/ADVERSE EFFECTS
*gp 120 vaccines *gp 160 vaccines	IM	Preventive, therapeutic, and perinatal vaccines	Malaise, myalgia, headache, fever, tenderness and induration at injection site
*HUMAN GROWTH HORMONE (Humatrope) (Protropin)	SC	Immunomodulation	Sodium and water retention, edema, carpal tunnel syndrome, increased intracranial pressure
*HYPERICIN	IV	HIV infection	Elevated liver function tests, photosensitivity, paresthesias
INTERFERON ALFA RECOMBINANT (Intron–A) (Roferon–A) (Kemron) (Alferon)	IM SC PO	HIV infection Kaposi's sarcoma	Parenteral: flu–like syndrome (fever, myalgias, and malaise), leukopenia, elevation in liver enzymes, weight loss, hair loss, fatigue, proteinuria, reversible congestive cardiomyopathy (weight gain and signs of right- or left-sided congestive heart failure) Oral: no side effects have been reported with low dose oral interferon alfa
*INTERLEUKIN–2 RECOMBINANT	IV	HIV infection	Fluid retention, hypotension, fever, chills, elevated creatinine, elevated BUN, oliguria, anuria, azotemia, fatigue, weight gain, tachycardia, nausea, vomiting, transient changes in liver function studies, headache, light headedness, dizziness, mental changes, pulmonary symptoms, anemia, leukocytosis, skin rash, mylagia, arthralgia
ISONIAZID (INH) (Isotamine) (Laniazid) (Nydrazid) (Tubizid)	PO IM	*Mycobacterium avium* complex infection *Mycobacterium tuberculosis*	Loss of appetite, nausea, vomiting, diarrhea, unusual tiredness or weakness, dark urine, yellow eyes and skin, clumsiness or unsteadiness, numbness, tingling, burning or pain in hands or feet, fever, sore throat, unusual bleeding or bruising, skin rash, pain at injection site, arthralgia, seizures, depression, psychosis, blurred vision with or without eye pain

Continued on following page

GENERIC NAME (TRADE NAME)	ROUTE OF ADMINISTRATION	INDICATIONS	SIDE/ADVERSE EFFECTS
ITRACONAZOLE (Sporanox)	PO	Maintenance therapy for: Cryptococcosis Histoplasmosis	Nausea, vomiting, headaches, fatigue, abdominal cramps, rash, loss of potassium, edema, diarrhea, anorexia, fever, headache, dizziness, pruritus, hypotension, hypokalemia, elevated liver enzymes, impotence
KANAMYCIN SULFATE (Kantrex)	IV IM PO	Drug–resistant TB	*See* Amikacin
KETOCONAZOLE (Nizoral)	PO	Candidiasis	Hepatitis, nausea, vomiting, diarrhea, dizziness, drowsiness, gynecomastia, headache, skin rash, itching, impotence, insomnia, photophobia
*LAMIVUDINE	PO	HIV infection	Neutropenia, rash, insomnia, fever, headache, fatigue, diarrhea, vasculitis, photophobia, paresthesias
*LETRAZURIL	PO	Cryptosporidiosis	Nausea, vomiting, rash
LIPOSYN III–2%	IV	HIV wasting	Fever, chills, sore throat, dyspnea, hives, anemia, chest pain, cyanosis, diarrhea, flushing, dizziness, nausea, vomiting, thrombocytopenia, jaundice
LEUCOVORIN (Citrovorum) (Folinic Acid) (Wellcovorin)	PO IM IV	Prophylaxis and treatment of toxic effects related to: Methotrexate Pyrimethamine Trimethoprim	Skin rash, hives, itching, wheezing
MEGESTROL ACETATE (Megace)	PO	HIV wasting	Alteration of menstrual pattern with unpredictable bleeding, pain in chest, visual disturbances, headache, insomnia, pain in abdomen, groin, calf, or leg, loss of coordination, slurred speech, weakness or numbness in extremities, yellow eyes and skin, depression, skin rashes, peripheral edema, brown spots in skin, acne, increased body hair, increased breast tenderness, loss of scalp hair

GENERIC NAME (TRADE NAME)	ROUTE OF ADMINISTRATION	INDICATIONS	SIDE/ADVERSE EFFECTS
METHOTREXATE (Folex) (Folex PFS) (Mexate) (Mexate–AQ)	PO IM IV	Non–Hodgkin's lymphoma	Gastrointestinal ulceration or bleeding, enteritis, intestinal perforation, leukopenia, bacterial infections, septicemia, thrombocytopenia, stomatitis, renal failure, azotemia, hyperuricemia, nephropathy, cutaneous vasculitis, hepatotoxicity, pulmonary fibrosis, pneumonitis, central nervous system toxicity, anorexia, nausea, vomiting, acne, boils, skin rash
METHYLPHENIDATE PMS-methylphenidate (Ritalin)	PO	HIV dementia	Tachycardia, hypertension, chest pain, tremors, allergic reactions, anemia, blurred vision, convulsions, leukopenia, agitation, confusion, anorexia, nervousness, insomnia, headache, nausea, vomiting, stomach pain
MEXILETINE (Mexitil)	PO	HIV peripheral neuropathy	Chest pain, rapid or irregular heart beats (PVCs), shortness of breath, leukopenia, thrombocytopenia, dizziness, lightheadedness, tremors, ataxia, heartburn, nausea, vomiting, confusion, impaired vision, headache, diarrhea, constipation, tinnitus, rash, insomnia, slurred speech
MICONAZOLE (Micatin) (Monistat Derm) (Monistat IV)	PO IM IV Topical	Candidiasis Coccidioidomycosis Cryptococcosis	Fever, chills, skin rash, itching, redness, swelling at injection site, unusual tiredness, weakness, unusual bleeding or bruising, anorexia, diarrhea, nausea, vomiting
MITOMYCIN (Mutamycin)	IV	Cervical cancer	Leukopenia, thrombocytopenia, pneumopathy, nephrotoxicity, stomatitis
*NEVIRAPINE	PO	HIV infection	Rash, thrombocytopenia, fever
NIMODIPINE (Nimotop)	PO	HIV dementia	Decreased blood pressure

Continued on following page

GENERIC NAME (TRADE NAME)	ROUTE OF ADMINISTRATION	INDICATIONS	SIDE/ADVERSE EFFECTS

NYSTATIN
  (Mycostatin)
  (Nilstat)
  (Nystex)
	PO	Candidiasis (oropha-
		ryngeal)
			Diarrhea, nausea, vomiting,
			stomach pain

OCTREOTIDE (Sandostatin)	SC	HIV–related diar- rhea	Hyperglycemia, hypoglyce- mia, abdominal pain, diarrhea, nausea, vomit- ing, pain at injection site, headache, fatigue, dizzi- ness, lightheadedness, edema, flushing of face, hepatic dysfunction
*OXANDROLONE	PO	HIV wasting	Anabolic steroid side effects, masculinizing effects in women (facial hair growth, deepened voice), feminizing effects in men (breast development), edema, jaundice, hepatic carcinoma, nausea, vom- iting

PAROMOMYCIN SULFATE
  (Humatin)
  (Aminosidine)
	PO	Cryptosporidiosis	Nausea, vomiting, diarrhea,
			renal damage

PENTAMIDINE ISETHIONATE
  (Nebupent, inhalation)
  (Pentam parenteral)
	IM
	IV
	Inhalation
		Pneumocystosis	Parenteral: blood dyscrasias,
			rapid and irregular pulse,
			diabetes mellitus, skin
			rash, hyperglycemia, hy-
			poglycemia, hypotension,
			pain or tenderness at site
			of injection, redness or
			flushing of the face, me-
			tallic taste in mouth
			Inhalation: chest pain,
			congestion, coughing,
			dyspnea, pharyngitis,
			wheezing, skin rash, me-
			tallic taste in mouth,
			pneumothorax

*PEPTIDE T	SC Intranasal	Immunomodulation HIV dementia Neuropathy	None reported yet
*PMEA	IV	HIV infection	None reported yet

PREDNISONE
  (Deltasone)
  (Meticorten)
  (Orasone)
  (Prednicen–M)
  (Sterapred)
	PO	HIV myopathy
		Pneumocystis carinii
		pneumonia (as
		adjunctive ther-
		apy)
			Allergic reaction, rectal irri-
			tation, bleeding, impaired
			vision, diabetes mellitus,
			psychic disturbances, skin
			problems, muscle cramp-
			ing, delayed wound heal-
			ing, infection

GENERIC NAME (TRADE NAME)	ROUTE OF ADMINISTRATION	INDICATIONS	SIDE/ADVERSE EFFECTS
PYRAZINAMIDE (PZA)	PO	*Mycobacterium tuberculosis*	Joint pain, loss of appetite, unusual tiredness or weakness, yellow eyes and skin, swelling of joints, itching rash, nausea
PYRIMETHAMINE (Daraprim)	PO	Pneumocystosis Toxoplasmosis	Folic acid deficiency (loss of taste, glossitis, diarrhea, sore throat, dysphagia, ulcerative stomatitis), fever, bleeding, bruising, fatigue, skin rash, trembling, unsteadiness or clumsiness, seizures, anorexia, vomiting
RIFABUTIN (Ansamycin)	PO	*Mycobacterium avium* complex infection (for prophylaxis and treatment of disease)	Increase in both liver enzymes and creatinine, rash, fever, leukopenia, gastrointestinal distress, hemolysis, arthralgias
RIFAMPIN (Rifadin) (Rifadin IV) (Rimactane)	PO IV	*Mycobacterium avium* complex infection *Mycobacterium tuberculosis*	Chills, difficult breathing, dizziness, fever, headache, muscle and bone pain, shivering, rash, itching, skin redness, sore throat, yellow eyes and skin, unusual bleeding or bruising, loss of appetite, nausea, vomiting, unusual tiredness or weakness, bloody or cloudy urine, stomach cramps, diarrhea, sore mouth or tongue, discoloration of urine, feces, sputum, sweat, or tears
*SP303T	Topical	Herpes simplex virus infection	None yet reported
*SPIRAMYCIN	PO IV	Cryptosporidiosis	Parenteral: paresthesias, irritation at injection site, dysesthesia, giddiness, pain, stiffness, burning sensation, hot flashes Oral: nausea, vomiting, diarrhea, fatigue, indigestion, sweating, heaviness in the chest, cool sensation in mouth or pharynx
STAVUDINE (Zerit) (formerly known as d4T)	PO	HIV infection	Peripheral neuropathy, hepatotoxicity, anemia, headache, nausea

Continued on following page

GENERIC NAME (TRADE NAME)	ROUTE OF ADMINISTRATION	INDICATIONS	SIDE/ADVERSE EFFECTS
SULFADOXINE and PYRIMETH-AMINE (Fansidar)	PO	Pneumocystosis	Stevens–Johnson syndrome, toxic epidermal necroly-sis, fulminant hepatic ne-crosis, agranulocytosis, aplastic anemia, photo-sensitivity, bleeding or bruising, folic acid defi-ciency (loss of taste, glos-sitis, diarrhea, sore throat, dysphagia, ulcer-ative stomatitis), skin rash, fatigue, aching in joints or muscles, hema-turia, dysuria, goiter, tremors, seizures, head-ache, dizziness, nausea, vomiting
SULFAMETHOXAZOLE and TRI-METHOPRIM (Bactrim) (Bethaprim) (Cheragan W/TMP) (Cotrim) (Septra) (Sulfamethoprim) (Sulfaprim) (Sulfatrim) (Sulfoxaprim) (Triazole) (Uroplus)	PO IV	Isosporiasis Pneumocystosis Salmonellosis Toxoplasmosis	Skin rash, itching, Stevens–Johnson syndrome (my-lagia, arthralgia, redness, blistering, peeling or loosening of the skin, ex-treme fatigue), dyspha-gia, fever, leukopenia (sore throat), thrombocy-topenia (unusual bleed-ing or bruising), hepatitis (dark urine, pale stools, yellow skin and sclerae), crystalluria, hematuria, diarrhea, dizziness, head-ache, anorexia, nausea, vomiting
SULFAMETHOXAOLE (Gantanol)	PO	Toxoplasmosis	Fever, itching, skin rash, hepatitis, photosensitivity, blood dyscrasias, diffi-culty in swallowing, red-ness, blistering, peeling of skin, hematuria, crys-talluria, thyroid dysfunc-tion, dizziness, headache, anorexia, nausea, vomit-ing, diarrhea
SULFISOXAZOLE (Gantrisin)	PO	Toxoplasmosis	Fever, itching, skin rash, hepatitis, photosensitivity, blood dyscrasias, diffi-culty in swallowing, red-ness, blistering, peeling of skin, hematuria, crys-talluria, thyroid dysfunc-tion, dizziness, headache, anorexia, nausea, vomit-ing, diarrhea

GENERIC NAME (TRADE NAME)	ROUTE OF ADMINISTRATION	INDICATIONS	SIDE/ADVERSE EFFECTS
TAXOL (Paclitaxel) (Taxol A)	IV	Kaposi's sarcoma	Neutropenia, thrombocytopenia, headache, fatigue, peripheral neuropathy, bradycardia, nausea, vomiting, diarrhea, mucositis, hair loss, arthralgia, fever, taste alterations, urticaria, rashes
TESTOSTERONE	PO IM	Depression Muscle wasting	In females: menstrual irregularities, deepened voice, excessive hair growth In males: bladder irritability, breast soreness, frequent or continuing erections Both sexes: edema, dizziness, headaches, fatigue, flushing or redness of skin, bleeding, nausea, vomiting, yellowing of eyes and skin, itching, diarrhea, redness or pain at injection site
*THALIDOMIDE	PO	Immunomodulation	Sedation, severe congenital abnormalities in developing fetuses, neurotoxicity
*THYMIC HUMORAL FACTOR	IM	Immunomodulation	Pain on injection, redness, swelling, fatigue, mental fogginess
*THYMOPENTIN	SC	Immunomodulation	Respiratory congestion, pain at injection site, headache, sleep disorders, fatigue, gastrointestinal side effects, pruritus, elevated liver enzymes
*TNP–470	IV	Kaposi's sarcoma	Anorexia, anemia, thrombocytopenia, neutropenia, seizures, ataxia, hemorrhages in lung, brain, and retina, abnormal liver function
TRIMETHOPRIM (Proloprim) (Trimpex)	PO	Salmonellosis	Blood dyscrasias (bleeding), headache, methemoglobinemia, skin rash, itching, alteration in taste, sore mouth or tongue, anorexia, diarrhea, nausea, vomiting, abdominal pain, cramping

Continued on following page

GENERIC NAME (TRADE NAME)	ROUTE OF ADMINISTRATION	INDICATIONS	SIDE/ADVERSE EFFECTS
TRIMETREXATE GLUCURO-NATE (Neutrexim)	IV	Pneumocystosis	Decrease in neutrophil and platelet counts, nausea, vomiting, diarrhea, reversible liver function abnormalities, skin rash, fever, mucositis, abdominal pain, kidney damage
VINBLASTINE (Velban) (Velsar)	IV	Kaposi's sarcoma	Fever, chills, cough, hoarseness, lower back pain, side pain, painful or difficult urination, pain or redness at site of injection, sores in mouth and on lips, rectal bleeding, dizziness, difficulty in walking, double vision, drooping eyelids, headache, jaw pain, mental depression, numbness or tingling in fingers and toes, pain in fingers or toes, pain in testicles, weakness, nausea, vomiting, loss of hair
VINCRISTINE (Oncovin) (Vincasar PES) (Vincrex)	IV	Kaposi's sarcoma Non–Hodgkin's lymphoma Cervical cancer	Constipation, stomach cramps, bed-wetting, decrease or increase in urination, dizziness, lightheadedness, dysuria, lack of sweating, joint pain, lower back or flank pain, visual changes, ataxia, drooping eyelids, headache, jaw pain, numbness or tingling in fingers or toes, pain in testicles, weakness, hyponatremia, leukopenia, thrombocytopenia, stomatitis Syndrome of inappropriate antidiuretic hormone (SIADH) evidenced by agitation, confusion, dizziness, hallucinations, anorexia, mental depression, seizures, insomnia, loss of consciousness
*WOBENZYM	PO	Immunomodulation	

GENERIC NAME (TRADE NAME)	ROUTE OF ADMINISTRATION	INDICATIONS	SIDE/ADVERSE EFFECTS
ZALCITABINE (HIVID) (ddC)	PO	HIV infection	Pancreatitis, peripheral neuropathy, oral aphthous ulcers, fever, rash, stomatitis
ZIDOVUDINE (Retrovir) (formerly known as AZT)	PO IV	HIV infection	Anemia, leukopenia, neutropenia, platelet count changes (either increased or decreased), anorexia, asthenia, diarrhea, dizziness, fever, headache, nausea, insomnia, malaise, myalgia, pain in abdomen, rash, somnolence, taste alteration

Sources: American Foundation for AIDS Research (1993). Opportunistic infections and related disorders. *AIDS/HIV Treatment Directory, 4*(4), 1–108; United States Pharmacopeial Convention, Inc. (1994). USPDI (Vol. I) (14th ed.). Rockville, MD: The Convention.

Appendix IV
Health Teaching for the Client With HIV Disease

TOPIC	ENCOURAGE	DISCOURAGE	RATIONALE
Stress	A proactive response style to HIV disease	Passive attitude and/or self-destructive behaviors	Stress may negatively affect the immune response and favor progression of HIV-related disease (Evans et al., 1991; Flescher et al., 1992; Hassan & Douglas, 1990).
	Identifying stressor categories (Pivar & Temoshok, 1990): 1. HIV diagnostic testing 2. Severe symptom or illness episodes 3. Treatment issues 4. Complications with family, work, school (or finances) 5. Physical and psychologic limitations or losses 6. Concerns about future		
	Psychoeducational support groups to reduce stress and improve coping (Moulton et al., 1990; Perry et al., 1991)		
	Individual strategies to reduce stress such as: 1. Exercise 2. Meditation 3. Use of visualization 4. Relaxation techniques 5. Use of therapeutic touch		
	Seeking factual information related to HIV disease from knowledgeable health care professionals	Relying on friends, gossip in the media for the "latest" information	
Exercise	A daily schedule of exercise activities	Continuing or adapting a sedentary lifestyle	Exercise may be physiologically, immunologically, and psychologically beneficial to HIV-infected persons and may favorably influence the course of HIV disease (LaPerriene et al., 1990; 1991; MacArthur et al., 1992; Rigsby et al., 1992; Schlenzig et al., 1992).
Sexual practices	Safer sexual practices (see Chapter 2)	Unsafe sex	Latex condom use reduces the risk of gonorrhea, herpes simplex virus, genital ulcers, and pelvic inflammatory disease and provides a barrier to HIV, hepatitis B virus, and *Chlamydia trachomatis* (Centers for Disease Control and Prevention [CDC], 1993).
	Proper use of male condoms, including: 1. Using a latex condom only 2. Using a new condom with each sexual act and/or partner	Improper use of a male condom, including: 1. Using natural-membrane condoms 2. Reusing condom or using same condom for insertive sex when having sex with multiple partners at the same time	

TOPIC	ENCOURAGE	DISCOURAGE	RATIONALE
Sexual practices —cont'd	3. Carefully handling the condom	3. Damaging condom with fingernail, teeth, or other sharp objects	
	4. Putting on the condom before genital contact with partner and when penis is erect	4. Using condom only for vaginal or anal penetration or attempting to apply condom to a flaccid penis	
	5. Ensuring that no air is trapped in tip of condom	5. Leaving air bubble at tip of condom	
	6. Ensuring adequate lubrication during vaginal or anal intercourse	6. Engaging in "dry" intercourse	
	7. Using only water-based lubricants (e.g., K-Y jelly, glycerine) with latex condom	7. Using oil-based lubricants (e.g., petroleum jelly, shortening, mineral oil, massage oils, body lotions, or cooking oil), which can weaken latex	
	8. Holding the condom firmly against base of penis during withdrawal and withdrawing penis while still erect	8. Allowing slippage or spillage when withdrawing	
	9. Storing of condoms in cool, dry place, away from direct sunlight	9. Using damaged condoms, as evidenced by brittleness, stockiness, or discoloration	
	10. Checking expiration date	10. Using outdated condoms	
	Proper use of the female condom; second choice to male latex condom (see Chapter 8)	Improper use of the female condom	The female condom has limited information available on its effectiveness in preventing sexually transmitted diseases, and has a relatively high pregnancy rate (26%) (Food and Drug Administration, 1993).
	Use of nonoxynol-9 (a nonionic surfactant spermicide); no studies have shown that the use of nonoxynol-9, used with a condom, increases the protection provided by use of a latex condom alone (CDC, 1993)		
	Use of barrier protection for fellatio and cunnilingus (condoms and dental dams)	Performing fellatio or cunnilingus without a barrier	
	Using latex gloves for digital insertive manipulative practices	Inserting finger(s) into vagina or rectum without a barrier	
Procreation	Providing unbiased information regarding HIV disease so that client can make informed reproductive decisions, including (Berman, 1993; Smeltzer & Whipple, 1991):	Negating the fact that the client does have reproductive options	Through counseling the client may achieve sufficient knowledge to make informed choices about procreation (Berman, 1993).

Continued on following page

TOPIC	ENCOURAGE	DISCOURAGE	RATIONALE
Procreation— cont'd	1. Illness may occur in the mother during pregnancy, and choices regarding treatment will have to be made that may be toxic to the fetus. 2. The HIV status of the child may not be known until approximately 15 months after birth. 3. Either the child or the mother, or both, may become ill and die. Additional considerations 1. Possible illness and death of the father 2. Finances 3. Support systems 4. Guardianship and adoption Choices including 1. Contraception 2. Abortion		Maternal antibodies are found in a child's blood for 12 to 15 months after birth. A new test to identify infected newborn infants accurately by 3 months of age is available, but not yet in widespread use (Miles et al., 1993).
Nutrition	Increased intake of protein (fish, chicken, meat, eggs, milk, cheese, dried beans, nuts, and tofu)	Diets that are inadequate in protein intake	Nutritional counseling and support can improve the nutritional status of people (Beach, 1992; Bradley-Springer, 1991; Kotler, 1992).
	Increased intake of carbohydrates as a source of calories (bread, cereals, rice, macaroni, noodles, potatoes, dried beans, plantain, fruits, cakes, cookies, and candy)	Diets that are calorically sparse	High nutrient intake is associated with higher $CD4^+$ T-cell counts and can reduce the rate of AIDS development (Abrams et al., 1993).
	Increased intake of fat (butter, margarine, oils, mayonnaise, salad dressing, cheese, sour cream, whole milk, sausages, salami, bacon, bologna, and other cold, high-fat meats, and cold cuts)		
	Increased vitamin and mineral intake by taking a multivitamin daily and eating the above-mentioned foods as well as fruits and vegetables	Inadequate intake of vitamins and minerals	
	Increased intake of water and juices on a daily basis		
	Participation in meal programs for people with HIV disease as an opportunity to learn more about nutrition as well as socialize		
	Building on the client's current dietary patterns	Introduction of an entirely new menu or standardized menus that may be irrelevant to the client	

TOPIC	ENCOURAGE	DISCOURAGE	RATIONALE
Food safety	Prevention of food-borne diseases (CDC, 1989a; Life Sciences Research Office, 1990) by: 1. Eating and drinking pasteurized dairy products (only) 2. Cooking meats, fish, and poultry to "well done" 3. Considering all animal-derived foods as contaminated, and: a. Washing hands immediately after handling b. Using meat thermometer to ensure thorough cooking c. Cooking to achieve internal temperatures of 165° F for poultry and stuffed meats; 150° F for pork, and at least 140° F for other foods (Nadakavukaren, 1990) d. Using separate cutting boards for raw and cooked foods 4. For microwave cooking, following directions carefully, especially standing time, which allows heat to fully penetrate food 5. When barbecuing, precooking meat first (especially chicken) 6. Washing utensils used for meats before reuse or before use on other foods 7. Wearing disposable gloves if there are cuts or abrasions on hands 8. Washing all fruits and vegetables thoroughly before eating 9. When food shopping: a. Placing raw meat or poultry into plastic bags to prevent juices from leaking onto other foods b. Reading expiration or "sell by" dates and pasteurized labels c. Refrigerating perishables as soon as possible	The nine factors most often implicated in bacterial food poisoning (Nadakavukaren, 1990, p. 219) 1. Eating of raw protein foods, such as uncooked eggs, rare meat, and sushi 2. Failure to refrigerate foods properly 3. Preparing food a day or more before it is to be served 4. Failure to cook foods thoroughly 5. Poor personal hygiene when handling food 6. Improper "hot" holding (keeping foods in heating trays at temperatures under 140° F) 7. Inadequate reheating of cooked foods 8. Failure to avoid moldy or spoiled foods 9. Use of foods after labeled expiration date	Infectious complications can be prevented by avoiding ingestion of contaminated food (Filice & Pomeroy, 1991).

Continued on following page

TOPIC	ENCOURAGE	DISCOURAGE	RATIONALE
Water safety	At home, use of boiled water for drinking or boiling of unsafe water for 10 minutes to sterilize it (CDC, 1990) When away from home, drinking bottled or canned carbonated water or soft drinks	Adding ice cubes to drinks	Infectious complications can be prevented by avoiding ingestion of contaminated water (Filice & Pomeroy, 1991). Water-borne diseases continue to occur from relatively sophisticated community water systems (CDC, 1991; Gold, 1993).
	After using swimming pools, hot tubs or whirlpools, showering well and using an antimicrobial soap	Swallowing water during recreational activities	Water-borne diseases can occur as a result of surface contact with or swallowing contaminated water (CDC, 1991).
Skin care	Keeping skin moist and intact (Hardy, 1992) Showering daily for at least 10 minutes Maintaining water temperature of 90° to 105° F Using a superfatted soap Patting skin dry and, while damp, applying an emollient cream	Tub baths Using drying, perfumed soap Using creams and lotions that have a high alcohol content and are drying	Secondary skin infections or transfer of infections from one part of the body to another can be prevented and the effects of xerosis (dry skin) and ichthyosis (rough, thick, scaly skin), the most common dermatoses seen in HIV infection minimized. (Duvic, 1991).
Hair care	Washing hair infrequently Using mild soap Using conditioner Covering head while in bed Combing hair	Washing hair daily Using drying, perfumed shampoo Brushing hair	Hair loss related to telogen effluvium (decrease in number of hair follicles), caused by severe stress, recurrent infections, and high fevers can be minimized (Cockerell, 1991).
Mouth care	Using a soft toothbrush Using nonabrasive toothpaste (or baking soda) Brushing surface of teeth only Using Toothettes for mucosal surface cleaning Performing mouth care t.i.d.	Using firm or hard toothbrush Using abrasive toothpaste Brushing mucosal surfaces Performing mouth care only q.d. or b.i.d.	The incidence and/or severity of secondary oral infections, especially thrush, can be reduced.
Hand washing	Washing frequently after activities of daily living Using soap in a pump dispenser Rinsing well Applying emollient cream to protect the skin Wearing rubber or latex gloves when cleaning Demonstrating hand washing	Using hot water Using bar soap Teaching hand washing without demonstrating correct method	Secondary infections related to poor hand-washing practices can be prevented.
Environmental cleaning and safety	Using household bleach (5.25% sodium hypochlorite) diluted; ¼ cup of bleach per gallon of tap water (CDC, 1989b)	Using expensive ineffective (for disinfection) household detergents	Secondary infections related to unclean environment and contamination of environment with HIV can be prevented.

TOPIC	ENCOURAGE	DISCOURAGE	RATIONALE
Environmental cleaning and safety—cont'd	Discarding solution daily and remixing when necessary Cleaning up blood or body fluids with this solution Using household bleach for laundry soiled with blood or body fluids	Using cleaning solutions beyond 24 hours after mixing	
	Using securely fastened plastic bags to discard disposable items contaminated with blood or body fluids	Discarding soiled disposable items without using secured bags	
	Placing used needles and sharps in puncture-resistant containers such as detergent containers or coffee cans (United States Environmental Protection Agency, 1990) Cleaning or changing air conditioner filters frequently	Throwing used needles and sharps directly into household garbage	
Pet care	Having pet care performed by someone other than person with HIV disease When necessary, wearing gloves and washing hands when finished Always washing hands, face, etc., after having direct contact with body secretions or excretions from pets or when scratched Keeping domestic pets, especially cats, indoors	Handling pet excreta or cleaning litter boxes, bird cages, or aquariums	Certain infectious complications that are zoonotic can be prevented (Filice & Pomeroy, 1991).
	Feeding only commercially prepared canned or dry pet food and meats that are cooked thoroughly	Feeding raw meat or poultry to domestic animals	
Alcohol drinking	Abstinence or modification	Regular consumption of alcohol	Although Kaslow and colleagues (1989) found no effect on the progression of HIV disease, Bagasara and associates (1993) found that alcohol intake did increase HIV replication.
Smoking	Reduction in smoking Avoidance of smoking Or starting a smoking cessation program	Continued smoking Returning to smoking as a means of coping with stress	Smoking may negatively influence the course of HIV disease and increase the propensity for development of pulmonary opportunistic infections, oral mucosal lesions, and periodontal disease (Buskin et al., 1992; Clarke et al., 1993; Forthal et al., 1992; Neiman et al., 1993; Royce & Winkelstein, 1990; Swango et al., 1991).

Continued on following page

TOPIC	ENCOURAGE	DISCOURAGE	RATIONALE
Intravenous drug use	Cessation of drug use and referral for treatment Not sharing drug paraphernalia with others Disinfecting drug paraphernalia before sharing equipment (if client persists in sharing) Open dialogue regarding continued drug use Referral to needle exchange program (if locally available)	Sharing of contaminated drug paraphernalia Client and health care professional avoiding discussion of drug use	Prevent transmission of blood-borne disease. Cessation of intravenous drug use may result in slowing of HIV disease progression (Weber et al., 1990).
Travel	Travel planning	Travel to middle, central, and south central United States, including the Ohio and Mississippi river basins, as well as the Caribbean and South America (to avoid histoplasmosis); travel to Arizona, California, Nevada, New Mexico, Utah, and western Texas, as well as Mexico and Central and South America (to avoid coccidiomycosis)	Prevent opportunistic infections (Jewett & Hecht, 1993).
	Nutrition safety 1. Cooking all meat, fish, poultry, and eggs well done and served hot 2. Eating only fresh fruits and vegetables that can be peeled 3. Drinking only bottled water or canned carbonated water or soft drinks 4. Purchasing food in restaurants or hotels Planning for special needs 1. Requesting in advance a room with a refrigerator (for medication storage), a request honored by most hotels 2. Requesting a wheelchair in advance for movement into and out of airports, as well as for transfers between connecting flights. Consulting with a health care provider before traveling to discuss the possible need for chemoprophylaxis for traveler's diarrhea	1. Eating undercooked or raw meat, fish, poultry, or eggs 2. Eating prepared fruits and vegetables that are not cooked (e.g. salads) 3. Adding ice cubes to drinks (even to alcoholic drinks) 4. Buying food from street vendors 1. Waiting until checking in to request the special need 2. Waiting until arriving at an airport to request wheelchair transport	Prevent gastrointestinal infection (DuPont & Erickson, 1993).

TOPIC	ENCOURAGE	DISCOURAGE	RATIONALE
Health care follow-up	Establishing a pattern for health care follow-up (e.g., physician, nurse practitioner, visiting nurse, clinic)	Changing patterns of health care follow-up	Patients with CD4$^+$ T-cell counts greater than 500 cells/mm^3 can be reassured that they are at the same risk for developing any pathologic condition as HIV-negative person and can handle most minor symptomatic problems without professional consultation. Patients with declining CD4$^+$ counts less than 500 cells/mm^3 should be taught signs and symptoms that may indicate serious disease (Hecht & Soloway, 1993).
	Establishing a relationship with health care professional knowledgeable about HIV disease	Seeking health care from professionals with knowledge deficits of HIV disease	
	Watching for signs and symptoms indicating secondary complications of HIV disease including but not limited to:	Ignoring warning signs	
	1. Skin lesions, rashes, itching, lumps, or bruising		
	2. Lesions or exudate in mouth		
	3. Persistent fever, night sweats		
	4. Extreme fatigue even when getting plenty of rest		
	5. Weight loss		
	6. Changes in digestion, difficulty in swallowing, and diarrhea		
	7. Shortness of breath, persistent coughing		
	8. Headache, visual changes, numbness in arms and legs, forgetfulness, dizziness, seizures		
	9. Unusual bleeding (e.g., bleeding gums)		
Additional considerations	Receiving TB testing and influenza vaccination annually		
	Using own personal care items (e.g., razors, toothbrushes, makeup)	Sharing personal care items	
	Refraining from donating blood or organs	Donating blood or making plans to donate body organs	
	Informing health care professionals responsible for primary care that the client has HIV disease	Withholding information about HIV disease from health care professionals responsible for coordinating care	Preventing transmissions and withholding information on current HIV diagnosis could result in a delay in diagnosing and treating problems related to HIV disease.
	Planning financially	Waiting until a crisis occurs to access entitlements	

REFERENCES

Abrams, B., Duncan, D., Hertz-Picaotto, I. (1993). A prospective study of dietary intake and acquired immune deficiency syndrome in HIV seropositive homosexual men. *Journal of Acquired Immune Deficiency Syndrome, 6*(8), 949–958.

Bagasra, O., Kajdacsy-Balla, A., Lischner, H.W., et al. (1993). Alcohol intake increases human immunodeficiency virus type I replication in human peripheral blood mononuclear cells. *Journal of Infectious Diseases, 167*(4), 789–797.

Beach, R.S. (1992). Nutrition and people with HIV/AIDS: A summary for data presented at the VIII International Conference on AIDS. *Nutrition and HIV/AIDS, 1*(1), 107–108.

Berman, N. (1993). Family and reproductive issues: Reproductive counseling. *AIDS Clinical Care, 5*(6), 45–47.

Bradley-Springer, L. (1991). Nutrition and support in HIV infection: A multilevel analysis. *Image: Journal of Nursing Scholarship, 23*(3), 155–159.

Buskin, S.E., Hopkins, S.G., Farizo, K.M. (1992). Heavy smoking increases the risk of *Pneumocystis carinii* pneumonia (PCP). *International Conference on AIDS* (abstract No. WeC1030). *8*(1), We50.

Centers for Disease Control (1989a). *Eating defensively: Food safety advice for persons with AIDS.* (videorecording). Atlanta: CDC.

Centers for Disease Control (1989b). Guidelines for prevention of transmission of human immunodeficiency virus and hepatitis B virus to health care and public safety workers. *Morbidity and Mortality Weekly Report, 38*(S-6), 1–37.

Centers for Disease Control (1990). *Health information for international travel.* (HHS Pub. No. CDC 90-8280). Washington, DC: U.S. Government Printing Office.

Centers for Disease Control (1991). Waterborne-disease outbreaks. *Morbidity and Mortality Weekly Report, 40* (SS-3), 1–13.

Centers for Disease Control and Prevention (1993). Update: Barrier protection against HIV infection and other sexually transmitted diseases. *Morbidity and Mortality Weekly Report, 42*(30), 589–591, 597.

Clarke, J.R., Taylor, I.K., Fleming, J. (1993). The epidemiology of HIV-1 infection in the lung in AIDS patients. *AIDS, 7*(4), 555–560.

Cockerell, C.J. (1991). Noninfectious inflammatory skin diseases in HIV-infected individuals. *Dermatologic Clinics, 9*(3), 531–541.

DuPont, H.L., Ericsson, C.D. (1993). Prevention and treatment of traveler's diarrhea. *The New England Journal of Medicine, 328*(25), 1821–1827.

Duvic, M. (1991). Papulosquamous disorders associated with human immunodeficiency virus infection. *Dermatologic Clinics, 9*(3), 523–530.

Evans, D.L., Lesserman, J., Perkins, D.O., et al. (1991). Stress related reduction of natural killer cells in HIV. *International Conference on AIDS.* (abstract No. TH.B. 91). *7*(2), 79.

Filice, G.A., Pomeroy, C. (1991). Preventing secondary infections among HIV-positive persons. *Public Health Report, 106*(5), 503–517.

Flescher, M., Watkins, L.R., Lockwood, L.L., et al. (1992). Specific changes in lymphocyte subpopulations: A potential mechanism for stress-induced immunomudulation. *Journal of Neuroimmunology, 41*(2), 131–142.

Food and Drug Administration (1993). Female condom approval. *FDA Medical Bulletin, 23*(2), 4.

Forthal, D., Gordon, R., Larsen, R. (1992). Cigarette smoking increases the risk of developing cryptococcal meningitis. *International Conference on AIDS.* (abstract No. PoB 3172). *8*(2), B115.

Gold, D. (1993). Treatment briefs: Risky drinking water. *Treatment Issues: The Gay Men's Health Crisis Newsletter of Experimental AIDS Therapies, 7*(7), 6.

Hardy, M.A. (1992). Dry skin care. In G.M. Bulechek & J.A. McCloskey (Eds.), *Nursing interventions: Essential nursing treatments* (2nd ed.) (pp. 34–47). Philadelphia: W.B. Saunders.

Hassan, N.F., Douglas, S.D. (1990). Stress-related neuroimmunomodulation of monocyte-macrophage functions in HIV-1 infection. *Clinical Immunology and Immunopathology, 54*(2), 220–227.

Hecht, F.M., Soloway, B. (1993). Identifying patients at risk for HIV infection. In D.J. Cotton & G.H. Friedland (Eds.), *HIV infection: A primary care approach* (rev. ed.) (p. 307). Waltham, MA: Massachusetts Medical Society.

Jewett, J.F., Hecht, F.M. (1993). Preventive health care for adults with HIV infection. *Journal of the American Medical Association, 269*(9), 1144–1153.

Kaslow, R.A., Blackwelder, W.C., Ostrow, D.G., et al. (1989). No evidence for a role of alcohol or other psychoactive drugs accelerating immunodeficiency in HIV-1 positive individuals. A report from the Multicenter AIDS Cohort Study. *Journal of the American Medical Association, 261*(23), 3424–3429.

Kotler, D.P. (1992). Nutritional effects and support in the patient with acquired immunodeficiency syndrome. *Journal of Nutrition, 122*(Suppl. 3), 723–727.

LaPerriere, A.R., Antoni, M.H., Schniederman, N., et al. (1990). Exercise intervention attenuates emotional distress and natural killer cell decrements following notification of positive serologic status for HIV-1. *Biofeedback and Self Regulation, 15*(3), 229–242.

LaPerriere, A.R., Fletcher, M.A., Antoni, M.I., et al. (1991). Aerobic exercise training in an AIDS risk group. *International Journal of Sports Medicine, 12*(Suppl. 1), 553–557.

Life Sciences Research Office, Federation of American Societies for Experimental Biology (1990, November). *Nutrition and HIV infection* (FDA No. 223-88-2124). Washington, DC: Center for Food Safety and Applied Nutrition, Food and Drug Administration, Department of Health and Human Services.

MacArthur, R.D., Levine, S.D., Birk, T.J., et al. (1992). Cardiopulmonary, immunologic and psychologic responses to exercise training in individuals seropositive for HIV. *International Conference on AIDS.* (abstract No. PuB 7327). *8*(3), 103.

Miles, S.A., Balden, E., Megpantay, L., et al., (1993). Rapid serologic testing with immune-complex–dissociated HIV p24 antigen for early detection of HIV infection in neonates. *New England Journal of Medicine, 328*(5), 297–302.

Moulton, J.M., Gurbuz, G., Sweet, D., et al. (1990). Outcome evaluation of eight-week educational support groups: Validating the model using control group comparisons. *International Conference on AIDS.* (abstract No. S.B. 400). *6*(3), 186.

Nadakavukaren, A. (1990). *Man and environment: A health perspective* (3rd ed.). Prospect Heights, IL: Waveland Press.

Nieman, R., Fleming, J., Coker, R.J., et al. (1993). The effect of cigarette on the development of AIDS in HIV-1 seropositive individuals. *AIDS, 7*(5), 705–710.

Perry, S., Fishman, B., Jacobsberg, L., et al. (1991). Effectiveness of psychoeducational interventions in reducing emotional distress after human immunodeficiency virus antibody testing. *Archives of General Psychiatry, 48*(2), 143–147.

Pivar, I., Temoshok, L. (1990). Coping strategies and response styles in homosexual symptomatic seropositive men. *International Conference on AIDS.* (abstract No. S.B. 382). *6*(3), 181.

Rigsby, L.W., Dishman, R.K., Jackson, A.W., et al. (1992). Effects of exercise training on men seropositive for the human immunodeficiency virus-1. *Medicine and Science in Sports and Exercise, 24*(1), 6–12.

Royce, R.A., Winkelstein, W. (1990). HIV infection, cigarette smoking and CD4+ T-lymphocyte counts: Preliminary results from the San Francisco men's health study. *AIDS, 4*(4), 327–333.

Schlenzig, C., Jaeger, H., Wehrenberg, M., et al. (1992). Physical exercise favorably influences the course of illness in patients with HIV and AIDS. *International Conference on AIDS.* (abstract No. PoB 3401). *8*(2), B153.

Smeltzer, S.C., Whipple, B. (1991). Women and HIV infection. *Image: Journal of Nursing Scholarship, 23*(4), 249–256.

Swango, P.A., Kleinman, P.V., Konzelman, J.L. (1991). HIV and periodontal health. A study of military personnel with HIV. *Journal of the American Dental Association, 122*(8), 49–54.

United States Environmental Protection Agency (1990, January). *Disposal Types for Home Health Care.* (EPA/530-SW-90-014A). Washington, DC: United States Environmental Protection Agency.

Weber, R., Ledergerber, B., Opravil, M., et al. (1990). Progression of HIV infection in misusers of injected drugs who stop injecting or follow a program of maintenance treatment with methadone. *British Medical Journal, 301*(6765), 1362–1365.

Appendix V

Case Management: Initial Database for Client Assessment

I. Demographics
   A. Personal data: name, age, date of birth, sex, race ethnicity, marital status
   B. Address, telephone number(s)
   C. Social security number
   D. Occupation/profession
   E. Country of origin
   F. Immigration status if not a citizen
   G. Language(s) spoken (note primary/preferred language)
   H. Risk behavior/factor for acquiring HIV infection
II. Support Person(s)
   A. Person living with client (note relationship)
   B. Person designated by the client to act on the client's behalf in an emergency (telephone number[s])
   C. Person who is willing to participate in the plan of care and to provide care when necessary
      1. Is the person available 24 hours a day, 7 days a week?
      2. If not, who can be designated as an alternative-care partner?
   D. Family members
      1. Who are the persons aware of the client's diagnosis?
      2. Where do they live (nearby or in another city, state, or country)?
      3. Are they in agreement with the client's chosen care partner/significant other?
   E. Community-based AIDS services
      1. Is the client, at present, receiving services from AIDS organizations?
      2. Types of services
III. Functional Status
   A. Physical impairments
      1. Sensory—speech, sight, hearing, or areas of anesthesia and/or paresthesias
      2. Motor—dominant arm and hand dysfunction; hemiparesis, paraparesis, or tetraparesis; hemiplegia, paraplegia, quadriplegia
      3. Functional limitations caused by neurologic, cardiovascular, or respiratory disease
      4. Bladder and bowel control—continent, occasionally incontinent, or always incontinent
   B. Mental impairments
      1. Cognitive impairment—disoriented, short-term memory impairment, impaired judgment, calculation problems
      2. Communication—can the client make needs known, and can the client direct others?
      3. Emotional status—anxious, agitated, angry, abusive, depressed, or danger to others
      4. Does the client wander when left unattended?
      5. Any sleep disorder?
      6. Does the client need safety monitoring (e.g., because of smoking)?
   C. Activities of daily living
      1. Personal care—bathing, grooming, dressing, toileting, ambulation, feeding (independent or needs assistance)
      2. Chore services—cleaning, laundry, shopping, meal preparation, reheating prepared meals (independent or needs assistance)
IV. Clinical Needs of the Client
   A. Medical diagnoses—include all, noting whether chronic or resolved

B. Medications
1. Allergies—allergy and type of reaction
2. Current drug therapy—names, dosages, routes, and frequency
3. Client's ability to self-medicate— needs reminding, help with preparation, needs supervision or requires preparation and administration by another person
4. Can the client be taught to self-medicate?
5. What arrangements need to be made for medication administration?

C. Clinical trials
1. Type
2. Location of trial
3. Frequency of visits
4. Special information on trial

D. Nutrition
1. Method—oral, enteral, or parenteral
2. Is the client independent or in need of assistance?

E. Rehabilitation therapy
1. Does the client require occupational, physical, and/or speech therapy?
2. What are the goals—functional, restoration, or maintenance?
3. What is the frequency of therapy sessions?

F. Treatments
1. Does the client require special treatments, including decubitus care; turning, positioning, and exercising because of confinement to bed; incontinence care; ostomy care (type); catheter care (type); tube irrigation; oxygen therapy; inhalation therapy (including pentamidine aerosol); suctioning; infusion therapy?
2. Has frequency of special treatments been noted?
3. Who is available to perform treatments, and has this person been taught how to perform the procedures?

G. Equipment needed for care
1. Assist devices—cane, crutches, walker, wheelchair, hospital bed with trapeze bar, side rails, commode, bedpan, urinal, bath bar, bath seat, handheld shower, Hoyer lift, etc.
2. Disposable supplies—incontinence pads, diapers, dressing supplies, etc.
3. Infusion and/or tube feeding supplies
4. Respiratory equipment

H. Medical follow-up
1. Frequency of physician visits required
2. Laboratory abnormalities that should be monitored—actual and/or potential and frequency

I. Addictions treatment
1. Does the client wish:
   a. To seek addictions treatment?
   b. Needle exchange program (if available)?
   c. To continue to use drugs (specify type and route)?
2. Is the client, if needed, enrolled in an addiction treatment program?
3. Specify type of treatment program and frequency of contact visits.

V. Family Data
A. Has the client's sexual partner been tested for HIV? What were the test results?
B. Is the sexual partner in need of health care?
C. If the client is pregnant:
   1. How many months?
   2. Is she receiving prenatal care? Where?
   3. Does she want abortion information?
D. If the client is a parent:
   1. Is the client living with sexual partner?
   2. Or is he or she a single parent?
   3. What are the children's names, ages, and HIV status?

4. What are the health care problems of the children?

VI. Legal Data
  A. Has the client legally:
    1. Provided for durable power of attorney?
    2. Appointed a health care proxy?
    3. Drawn up:
       a. A living will?
       b. A will for the estate?
    4. Provided for guardianship of children?
  B. Does the client wish to complete any of these tasks?

VII. Social Data
  A. Living arrangements
    1. Housing
       a. Owns own home
       b. Rents an apartment in the home of another
       c. Rents a room (shares facilities) in the home of another
       d. Rents home
       e. Rents apartment
       f. Rents hotel room
       g. Lives in shelter for homeless persons
       h. Lives in special housing— supportive housing for persons with AIDS
       i. Lives in senior citizen housing
    2. Facilities
       a. Wheelchair accessible, both inside and outside
       b. Utilities—heat, hot water, electricity, air conditioner, sink, tub, shower, telephone
       c. Toilet—own or shared
       d. Cooking facilities—stove, hot plate, toaster oven, microwave, refrigerator
       e. Elevator or walk-up—can or cannot be managed by the client
       f. Laundry—appliances in the home, in the building, or nearby
  B. Community assessment
    1. Safety—neighborhood where in-home services can be provided if needed
    2. Available services—grocery shopping, pharmacy, etc.
    3. Transportation
       a. Does the client own a car and is he or she able to drive?
       b. Is public transportation available near client's home, and can client negotiate public transportation?
  C. Spiritual needs
    1. What are the client's spiritual (religious) preferences?
    2. Does the client participate in religious services? With what frequency?
    3. How important is religion to the client?

VIII. Financial Picture
  A. Is the client able to continue employment?
    1. How many hours per week?
    2. Benefits?
  B. Monthly income versus monthly expenditures
  C. Savings and financial assets
  D. Health care payments—including insurance and payments for service care or drugs not covered
  E. Eligibility for entitlements:
    1. Medicaid
    2. Medicare
    3. Special programs for financial aid to persons with AIDS

IX. Current Services Received by Client
  A. List all agencies and individuals providing service to the client.
  B. Identify contact persons and telephone numbers to facilitate case planning and management.

Appendix VI
Deciding to Enter an AIDS/HIV Drug Trial

1. About the trial
    a. What is the name of this trial? What kind of trial is it? Phase I? Phase II? Phase III? Double-blind design? Open label? Placebo?
    b. What type of drug is being tested? Antiretroviral? Immunomodulator? Antineoplastic? Treatment or prophylaxis for a specific opportunistic infection or illness?
    c. How often must the drug be taken? How will the drug be given in this trial? Orally? Intravenously? Other?
    d. If the participant is a child, will this affect how often the drug is taken? Will any physical restraints be used (for instance, in the case of intravenous drugs)? How long will the drug's effectiveness be monitored in children?
    e. Must the drug be taken in the hospital or at a test site, or can I take the drug at home?
    f. Do I need to be in the hospital to be in this trial? For how long?
    g. How often must I visit the test site? What will happen on these visits? How long will each visit take?
    h. Is the trial being conducted at any other locations? Is there a location easier for me to get to? Is there a site that may meet my particular needs (for instance, Spanish-speaking counselors, or child care)?
    i. What if I have to miss a visit or forget to take the drug?
    j. When can I start in the trial? How long will the trial last?
    k. Do I have to do any special activities while I am at home? Do I have to write down these activities?

2. About the drug
    a. What other drugs are being used today for my problems? How does the trial drug compare in safety and success? What is the evidence that this substance can be helpful in treating my problem?
    b. Has this drug been used before? For what conditions? What were the results? Were there any risks with taking the drug?
    c. What are the immediate side effects of this drug? What are the long-term effects of my using this drug? Are any of the above effects permanent?
    d. If I have any side effects, how will I be helped to deal with them? Whom can I call?
    e. How will taking the drug affect my day-to-day activities? Are there things I cannot do during the trial? Will I be able to continue working? Exercising? Having sex?
    f. Is this drug available outside this trial? If so, where and how could I get it?

3. Financial concerns
    a. Do I need to have my own doctor to get into this trial? If I cannot afford my own doctor, will the trial provide one?
    b. Do I need health insurance to be in the trial?
    c. Do I have to pay for laboratory tests or any other costs?
    d. If I experience side effects requiring emergency treatment, which hospital can I go to and who pays for the treatment?
    e. Will I be given any money for participating in the trial?
    f. Will I be given carfare for traveling to and from any visits?
    g. If I am caring for a child, is child care available?

From AIDS Treatment Resources (1990). Deciding to enter an AIDS/HIV drug trial (6th ed.). New York: AIDS Treatment Resources, Inc.

4. Laboratory tests
   a. What tests will be given before I start? Will I be given the results of these tests?
   b. What tests will be given during the trial? How often? Will I be given the results of these tests?
   c. How often will the researchers tell me how I am doing while I am in the trial?
5. Medical history
   a. What do the researchers need to know about my medical condition to see how the drug may affect my health?
   b. If I am a person with a medical problem, including hemophilia, how will the drug affect my specific condition?
6. Foods, special diets, and other considerations
   a. If the drug is a pill or capsule, should I take it on an empty stomach? With food? Which foods?
   b. Are there any special foods that I need to eat while in this trial? If I am already on a special diet, may I continue? Can I take vitamins?
   c. Are there any foods or other substances that I shouldn't have while taking this drug? Can I drink alcoholic beverages? Can I take any over-the-counter (non-prescription) drugs? Aspirin? Nonaspirin pain killers (such as Tylenol or other forms of acetaminophen)? Cold tablets? Cough syrup?
   d. Can I use prescription drugs while I am in this trial? Can I use other experimental drugs? Can I take drugs against HIV? Can I take immunomodulators? Can I take prophylaxis or treatment for opportunistic infections, cancers, or any other illnesses I may get?
   e. What type of contraceptives can I use? Are oral contraceptives permitted? Will my use of contraceptives be monitored? Are pregnant women allowed in the trial?
7. Informed consent
   a. Is this trial confidential? Will anyone outside the trial know about my health condition without my permission?
   b. How will information about me be coded to protect my privacy?
   c. Do the consent papers that I am signing describe all the risks and benefits of my participating in the trial?
   d. What written information will be given about the trial and the drug?
   e. How often will the institutional review board (IRB) review the trial for any changes?
   f. How will I be informed of those changes? If this trial changes significantly, or if I'm put into another trial, will I receive an updated informed consent form to sign?
8. Leaving the trial/end of the trial
   a. If my condition gets worse while I am on the drug, will I be taken out of the trial? If I am in a placebo group, can I get the drug if my condition gets worse during the trial?
   b. If I develop health problems as a result of being in the trial, will treatment be available to me even if I leave the trial before it is over?
   c. If the trial was successful, can I take the drug once the trial is over? Will the sponsors of the drug supply it to me free until it is marketed and available to the public? If the drug worked for me, can I continue to take the drug even if the trial was declared a failure? How is the success of this trial defined by the protocol?
   d. How will decisions about stopping the trial be made? How is failure defined in the protocol?
   e. Will my health continue to be checked after I stop taking the drug? For how long and under what conditions? Will this be done even if I decide to leave the trial before it is over? Even if the entire trial is stopped early by the researchers?
   f. Will there be long-term follow-up on how I am doing? Will this be done even if I leave the trial before it is over? Even if the entire trial is stopped early by the researchers?
   g. How can I find out the results of the trial?
   h. Will I be able to participate in future trials of this drug? Will I receive the results of future trials using this drug?

Index

Note: Page numbers in *italics* refer to illustrations; page numbers followed by t refer to tables.